Emergency Medicine
Second Edition

The National Medical Series for Independent Study

Emergency Medicine

2nd EDITION

Editors

Scott H. Plantz, M.D., FAAEM
Associate Professor
Department of Emergency Medicine
Chicago Medical School
Mount Sinai Medical Center
Chicago, Illinois

E. John Wipfler, III, M.D., FACEP
Associate Professor
Department of Emergency Medicine
Medical Director Disaster Medical Services
University of Illinois College of Medicine
OSF Saint Francis Medical Center
Peoria, Illinois

⊞ Lippincott Williams & Wilkins
a Wolters Kluwer business
Philadelphia · Baltimore · New York · London
Buenos Aires · Hong Kong · Sydney · Tokyo

Acquisitions Editor: Donna M. Balado
Managing Editor: Kathleen H. Scogna
Marketing Manager: Emilie Linkins
Production Editor: Julie Montalbano
Designer: Terry Mallon
Compositor: Circle Graphics, Inc.
Printer: Data Reproductions Corporation

351 West Camden Street
Baltimore, MD 21201

530 Walnut Street
Philadelphia, PA 19106

Printed in the United States of America

First Edition, 1998

Library of Congress Cataloging-in-Publication Data

Emergency medicine / editors, Scott H. Plantz, Jonathan N. Adler, E.
 John Wipfler, III. — 2nd ed.
   p. ; cm. — (The national medical series for independent study)
 Includes index.
 ISBN-13: 978-0-7817-8884-7
  1. Emergency medicine—Outlines, syllabi, etc. 2. Emergency medi-
cine—Examinations, questions, etc. I. Plantz, Scott H. II. Adler,
Jonathan. III. Wipfler, E. John. IV. Series.
  [DNLM: 1. Emergency Medicine—Examination Questions.
 2. Emergency Medicine—Outlines. 3. Emergencies—Examination
Questions. 4. Emergencies—Outlines. 5. Emergency Medical Ser-
vices—Examination Questions. 6. Emergency Medical Services
—Outlines. WB 18.2 N738 2007]
RC86.7.E5793 2007
616.02'5—dc22
                                                                      2006019402

To purchase additional copies of this book, call our customer service department at **(800) 638-3030** or fax orders to **(301) 223-2320**. International customers should call **(301) 223-2300**.

Visit Lippincott Williams & Wilkins on the Internet: *http://www.LWW.com*. Lippincott Williams & Wilkins customer service representatives are available from 8:30 am to 6:00 pm, EST.

07 08 09 10
2 3 4 5 6 7 8 9 10

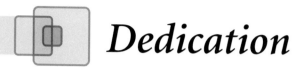

Dedication

We would like to dedicate this book to our parents, Alan H. and Pauline G. Plantz, and Jack and Shirley Wipfler, for their love, support, and guidance.

Dr. Plantz would also like to dedicate this book to the emergency department attendings at Christ Hospital and Medical Center and Butterworth Hospital, who provided the clinical foundation on which we build: Lance Kreplick, M.D.; Barb McCreary, M.D.; Bernard Feldman, M.D.; Stewart Reingold, M.D.; Robert Harwood, M.D.; Joseph Wood, M.D.; Peter Fried, M.D.; Denise Fligner, M.D.; Barb Shufeldt, M.D.; Herbert Wigder, M.D.; Steve Anneken, M.D.; Larry Cohen, M.D.; Sue Nezda, M.D.; Mike Lambert, M.D.; Denise Bielefeld, M.D.; Sheila Bonaguro, M.D.; Harvey DeMaagd, M.D.; Sue N. VandenBerg, M.D.; George Drew, M.D.; Henry Hammersmith, M.D.; Gwen Hoffman, M.D.; Steven Holt, M.D.; Jeff Jones, M.D.; Jon Krohmer, M.D.; Robert LaFleur, M.D.; Maureen Prendergast, M.D.; Ralph Rogers, M.D.; Dale McNinch, D.O.; Daryl Wisdom, M.D.; Bruce W. Nugent, M.D.; and Robert Heacox, M.D.

Dr. Wipfler would also like to dedicate this book to his wife, Diane K. Wipfler, and to his friends and colleagues at OSF Saint Francis Medical Center and the 3rd Order of Saint Francis Sisters, who pursue a most worthy mission in this world. Special thanks also to his lifetime mentor, Dr. Hugh E. Stephenson, who has provided inspiration and encouragement to pursue excellence.

Preface

Emergency medicine is one of the most comprehensive and difficult specialties; ready knowledge of all aspects of medical training is essential. The typical 1- to 2-month student rotation in emergency medicine is often challenging because students are expected to quickly acquire a knowledge base and procedural skills to face an ever-changing array of patient problems.

In keeping with the purpose of the National Medical Series, this textbook has been written to provide residents, medical students, physician assistants, and nurse practitioners with a basic introduction to the core content of emergency medicine in a format that can be quickly assimilated for practical use in the evaluation and treatment of patients in the emergency department. The narrative outline allows the concise presentation of large amounts of material. Clinical features, differential diagnoses, patient evaluation, therapy, and patient disposition are discussed for most disorders. Each chapter is followed by study questions that mimic those found in the U.S. Medical Licensing Examination (USMLE), accompanied by complete explanations. A comprehensive examination, also with complete answers and explanations, is available online to allow for additional self-testing.

The authors hope that you will find the book practical and the subject matter exciting.

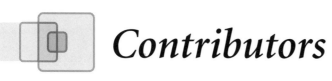

Contributors

Jonathan N. Adler, M.D., M.S., FAAEM
Assistant in Emergency Medicine
Massachusetts General Hospital
Instructor of Medicine
Harvard Medical School
Boston, Massachusetts

Kathleen M. Beaver, M.D.
Assistant Professor of Emergency Medicine
Medical College of Pennsylvania Hahnemann
    School of Medicine
Allegheny University of the Health Sciences
Philadelphia, Pennsylvania

Rodney Berger, M.D., FAADEP
Assistant Professor
Department of Emergency Medicine
Mount Sinai Medical Center
Chicago, Illinois

Jon A. Buras, M.D., Ph.D.
Emergency Medicine Resident
Harvard-Affiliated Emergency Medicine
    Residency
Brigham and Women's Hospital
Boston, Massachusetts

Leslie S. Carroll, M.D.
American Board of Emergency Medicine
American Board of Medical Toxicology
Mount Sinai Hospital
Chicago, Illinois

Katherine C. Clark, M.D.
Department of Emergency Medicine
Hennepin County Medical Center
Minneapolis, Minnesota

David C. Cone, M.D.
Chief, Division of Emergency Medical Services
Assistant Professor of Emergency Medicine
Medical College of Pennsylvania Hahnemann
    School of Medicine
Allegheny University of the Health Sciences
Philadelphia, Pennsylvania

C. James Corrall, M.D., M.P.H.
Clinical Associate Professor of Pediatrics
Clinical Assistant Professor of Emergency
    Medicine AP Surgery
Clinical Assistant Professor of Pharmacology
University of Indiana
Peoria, Indiana

Judith A. Dattaro, M.D.
Attending, Emergency Department
The New York Hospital
Instructor, Department of Surgery
Cornell University Medical College
New York, New York

Anthony J. Dean, M.D., FAAEM
Assistant Professor of Emergency Medicine
Medical College of Pennsylvania Hahnemann
    School of Medicine
Allegheny University of the Health Sciences
Associate Medical Director, Emergency
    Department, Misericordia Hospital
Philadelphia, Pennsylvania

Susan E. Farrell, M.D., FAAEM
Assistant Professor
Department of Emergency Medicine
Division of Toxicology
Medical College of Pennsylvania Hahnemann
    School of Medicine
Allegheny University of the Health Sciences
Philadelphia, Pennsylvania

William Gossman, M.D.
Project Medical Director
Mount Sinai Hospital
Clinical Instructor of Emergency Medicine
Finch University/The Chicago Medical School
Chicago, Illinois

B. Zane Horowitz, M.D.
Associate Professor, Emergency Medicine and
    Clinical Toxicology
University of California, Davis
Sacramento, California

Donna J. Kinser, M.D.
Associate Professor of Emergency Medicine
Associate Director, Division of Emergency
  Medicine
University of California, Davis
Sacramento, California

David C. Lee, M.D.
North Shore University Hospital
Manhasset, New York
Assistant Professor
Medical College of Pennsylvania Hahnemann
  School of Medicine
Allegheny University Hospital of the Health
  Sciences
Philadelphia, Pennsylvania

Nicholas Lorenzo, M.D., DABPN
Editor-in-Chief
eMedicine, Neurology
Private Practice
Omaha, Nebraska

Eric C. Miller, M.D., FAAEM
Emergency Physician
Yakima Memorial Hospital
Yakima, Washington

Edward J. Mlinek, Jr., M.D.
Associate Professor
Section of Emergency Medicine
Department of Surgery
University of Nebraska Medical Center
Omaha, Nebraska

R. Konane Mookini, M.D., J.D., FCLM
Medical Board of California
Sacramento, California

David L. Morgan, M.D., FACEP
Assistant Professor
University of Texas Southwestern Medical School
Parkland Memorial Hospital
Dallas, Texas

Edward A. Panacek, M.D.
Associate Professor and Residency Director
Division of Emergency Medicine
University of California, Davis
Sacramento, California

Amarjit Singh, M.D.
Associate Professor of Emergency Medicine
Mount Sinai Hospital
Finch University/The Chicago Medical School
Chicago, Illinois

Peter E. Sokolove, M.D.
Assistant Professor
Division of Emergency Medicine
University of California, Davis
Sacramento, California

Dana A. Stearns, M.D., FACEP
Instructor in Medicine
Harvard Medical School
Attending Physician
Department of Emergency Medicine
Massachusetts General Hospital
Boston, Massachusetts

Jack Stump, M.D., FAAEM
Rogue Valley Medical Center
Medford, Oregon

Joan Surdukowski, M.D.
Assistant Professor of Emergency Medicine
Chicago School of Medicine
Attending Physician, Emergency Medicine
  Department
Mount Sinai Medical Center
Chicago, Illinois

Stephen Thomas, M.D.
Instructor
Harvard Medical School
Department of Emergency Medicine
Massachusetts General Hospital
Boston, Massachusetts

Richard C. Urgo, M.D.
Attending Physician
Emergency Medicine
Northwest Community Hospital
Arlington Heights, Illinois

Thomas Widell, M.D., FACEP
Program Director, Emergency Medicine
    Residency
University of Chicago
Mount Sinai Medical Center
Assistant Clinical Professor
The Chicago Medical School
Chicago, Illinois

David E. Williams, M.D.
Assistant Professor
Department of Emergency Medicine
Mount Sinai Medical Center
Chicago, Illinois

Leslie S. Zun, M.D., MBA, FACEP, FAAEM
Associate Professor of Emergency Medicine
Chicago Medical School
Chairman, Department of Emergency Medicine
Mount Sinai Hospital Medical Center
Chicago, Illinois

Contents

PART I

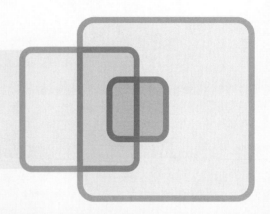

Acute Resuscitation

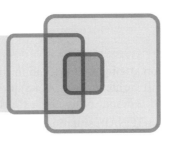

chapter 1

Resuscitation

JON A. BURAS · JONATHAN N. ADLER

I DISCUSSION

A Definitions

1. **Cardiopulmonary arrest** is defined as the sudden cessation of cardiac and respiratory function.

2. **Resuscitation** is the revival of a patient from potential or apparent death. Clinically, death is defined by the loss of heartbeat, respirations, and cerebral function. The limiting factor in resuscitation is the ability to perfuse the brain and myocardium with oxygened blood.

3. **ABCs.** Successful resuscitation must restore ventilatory and circulatory function while maintaining cerebral viability. The overall hierarchy of management during resuscitation is directed toward restoring or preventing loss of the physiologic systems most immediately responsible for supporting cerebral function. Preventing anoxic brain damage and death requires function of **airway patency, breathing,** and **circulation.**

   a. **Airway.** A patent airway is necessary for gas exchange.

   b. **Breathing.** Airway patency alone does not ensure adequate ventilation. Breathing (ventilation) allows oxygenation of the blood and elimination of carbon dioxide.

      (1) **Normal ventilatory control** is mediated by the:

         (a) **Central** and **peripheral chemoreceptors,** which detect changes in the pH and arterial oxygen tension (PO_2), respectively.

         (b) **Respiratory control center** (brain stem–integrating and motor neurons)

         (c) **Respiration effectors**

            (i) **Neuromuscular** (spinal cord, nerves, muscles)

            (ii) **Ventilatory** (chest wall, pleura, airways, lung parenchyma)

      (2) **Hypoventilation** may occur if any aspect of normal ventilatory control is disrupted. The chemoreceptors, brain stem, and effector neurons are sensitive to prolonged hypoxia and acidosis. The spinal column, chest wall, and lung parenchyma may all be affected by ischemia, acidosis, or traumatic injury.

   c. **Circulation.** Circulatory function is necessary to distribute oxygen to, and remove carbon dioxide from, distal end organs. Circulatory failure typically represents either inadequate blood volume or inadequate pump function.

B Prognosis The general outcome of cardiac arrest is poor. Factors influencing outcome include the time between arrest and the institution of therapy, the type of cardiac arrest, and the underlying cause. Irreversible hypoxic brain damage is noted after 4 minutes of cardiac arrest.

1. **Predictors of outcome.** Studies of comatose survivors of cardiac arrest suggest that a definitive prognosis of poor outcome can be made on the basis of the neurologic examination 72 hours after the hypoxic–ischemic event. The lack of motor response to pain is the best predictor of poor outcome at 72 hours.

2. **Termination of resuscitation attempts.** Resuscitation attempts may be terminated following adequate trial of advanced cardiac life support (ACLS) protocols if no reversible causes of arrest are identified and arrest persists despite resuscitative efforts.

3. **Do not attempt resuscitation (DNAR) situations.** Cardiopulmonary resuscitation (CPR) and ACLS protocols should be withheld under the following circumstances:
   a. A valid DNAR order has been established prior to arrest.
   b. Successful resuscitation is deemed impossible given the patient's underlying medical condition.

II   APPROACH TO THE PATIENT

A **Primary survey** of the patient includes a **rapid (10-second) assessment of the ABCs.**

1. **Airway** and **breathing** are assessed by visualizing spontaneous respirations while hearing or feeling expired air from the patient's airway. Head-tilt and chin-lift procedures may be performed for patients without risk of cervical spine injury. If spontaneous respirations are not present, ventilation should be assisted by mouth-to-mask or bag-valve-mask breathing.

2. **Circulation** is assessed by palpating either a carotid or femoral pulse. If no pulse is palpable, chest compressions should be performed to promote blood flow until a defibrillator is available. Cardiac rhythm should be assessed immediately with the defibrillator paddles to identify ventricular fibrillation or another rhythm responsive to cardioversion. **Early defibrillation [direct current (DC) cardioversion] is the most important intervention for successful resuscitation during known ventricular fibrillation cardiac arrest and should take precedent over intravenous line placement and intubation. In a witnessed arrest, the initial therapy should be immediate application of an automatic external defibrillator.**

B **Secondary survey** of the patient is directed toward **more definitive management of the ABCs** and **investigating the underlying cause.**

1. **Airway management.** The decision to perform **endotracheal intubation** or use **other airway adjuncts** to maintain and protect the airway must be made.

2. **Breathing management** entails the **administration of oxygen** and **assessment of the need for ventilatory support** with positive pressure. **Arterial blood gas (ABG) determinations** should be considered to guide ventilatory management.

3. **Circulatory management**
   a. **Intravenous access** should be obtained for the delivery of fluids and medications required for resuscitation. Standard intravenous access for resuscitation is two 14- to 16-gauge peripheral intravenous catheters. Central venous access may be obtained.
   b. **Electrocardiographic monitoring** should be instituted, and the cardiac rhythm identified and treated using ACLS guidelines. The underlying cause of the arrest should be identified and treated if possible.

4. **Other interventions**
   a. **Laboratory studies,** including creatine kinase levels, electrolytes, and serum and urine toxin screens, should be considered.
   b. **Bladder catheterization** with a Foley catheter should be considered to assist in fluid management.
   c. **Nasogastric tube placement** should be considered for patients who are being mechanically ventilated (to decrease aspiration risk). Nasogastric tube placement should also be considered for patients suspected of drug overdose (to allow administration of decontamination agents).

C **Reassessment**   The patient should be reassessed frequently using both the primary and secondary surveys until the patient has been stabilized.

III AIRWAY

A **Assessment** The most important part of airway management is assessing immediate airway patency as well as determining future risk of airway compromise. Tasks to protect the airway, such as endotracheal intubation, are often easier to perform than making a decision about future airway risk.

1. **Airway patency**
   a. The airway should be assessed for patency first by **looking, listening,** and **feeling for air exchange.** The patient without spontaneous respirations requires an attempt at ventilation to assess airway patency.
   b. The most common cause of airway obstruction is prolapse of the tongue into the posterior oropharynx, causing obstruction of airflow. Physical examination may also reveal foreign bodies or facial, mandibular, or tracheal–laryngeal fractures that may result in airway obstruction.

2. **Airway protection**
   a. Testing the **gag reflex** is one way to assess airway protection. This method predominantly assesses the sensory afferent component of cranial nerves IX and X.
   b. A superior alternative is to assess the posterior oropharynx for pooled secretions and, time permitting, to observe the patient for the **ability to swallow.** Swallowing is the natural means of protecting the airway and clearing secretions; a patient with pooled oral secretions requires definitive airway management. Intact swallowing requires coordinated function of the sensory and motor components of cranial nerves V_2, V_3, IX, and X.

B **Interventions**

1. **General guidelines**
   a. **Protection of the cervical spine.** All trauma victims should be placed in a **protective cervical spine collar** (this step is often performed in the prehospital setting). However, intubation is best performed with the collar off and experienced hands maintaining spinal immobilization.
   b. **Prevention of aspiration.** Vomiting and aspiration are common events associated with resuscitation. Immediate suctioning of the lower pharynx and oropharynx with a Yankauer device is mandatory for proper airway management. A vomiting patient should be rolled to the left lateral decubitus position and the entire spine properly protected so that the airway can be cleared.

2. **Simple maneuvers and airway adjunct devices**
   a. **Head tilt/chin lift.** This maneuver is performed by simultaneously lifting the chin forward while applying pressure to the forehead and is contraindicated if neck trauma is suspected.
   b. **Jaw thrust.** Applying pressure behind the angles of the mandible to thrust the entire mandible forward simultaneously lifts the tongue and epiglottis forward. The jaw-thrust maneuver is the preferred method for patients with possible cervical spine injury.
   c. **Oropharyngeal airway (OPA).** An OPA is a curved, hollow plastic device that is placed over the top of the tongue. Its curved shape allows the distal portion of the device to fit behind the base of the tongue, lifting it forward and preventing obstruction.
      (1) **Indications** for use are an obstructed airway in an obtunded individual. Conscious patients will not tolerate an OPA.
      (2) **Sizing.** The device is sized by comparing its length to the distance between the corner of the mouth and the angle of the mandible externally.
   d. **Nasopharyngeal airway (NPA, nasal trumpet).** An NPA is a soft rubber tube, 15–20 cm long, which is lubricated and passed through an open nasal passage so that the distal tip lies behind the tongue.
      (1) **Indications.** Conscious and semiconscious patients can tolerate an NPA. The trumpet is indicated when oral trauma precludes OPA usage or when an OPA may not be tolerated by a semiconscious or conscious patient requiring limited airway management.

      (2) Complications include nasal trauma (sustained during placement) and laryngospasm and vomiting in a conscious patient with a sensitive oropharynx.

    e. Laryngeal mask airway (LMA). The LMA is a new device composed of a mask with an inflatable rim attached to a 15- to 20-cm long tube. The mask fits over the larynx the same way a face mask fits over the nose and mouth. The tube communicates with the mask and allows for direct ventilation of the larynx or trachea.

      (1) Indications. The LMA is very easy to place, even in the neutral position, and is indicated when the airway cannot be secured by endotracheal intubation in an unconscious patient. However, this device does not protect the airway from aspiration and should be replaced as soon as possible with an endotracheal tube.

      (2) Although the LMA is used frequently in the operating room, there is limited experience with this adjunct in the emergency department (ED).

  3. Intubation provides a more secure airway than simple interventions and is the treatment of choice for any patient who is unable to safely maintain a patent airway or who cannot sustain adequate ventilation.

    a. Orotracheal intubation. Guidelines for orotracheal intubation are given in Table 1–1.

    b. Nasotracheal intubation is easiest if the patient is awake and spontaneously breathing. Use of a tube with directional tip control (e.g., a "ringed" or Endotrol tube) may also facilitate the procedure. Guidelines for nasotracheal intubation are given in Table 1–2.

    c. Rapid sequence induction (RSI) is directed at preparing the patient for intubation; it is a series of steps to maximize success and minimize complications. RSI incorporates paralysis of

---

TABLE 1–1 Guidelines for Performing Orotracheal Intubation

1. **Determine tube size.** Usual endotracheal tube sizes are 7.0–9.0 mm for women and 7.5–10.0 mm for men. In children, the diameter of the tube is calculated by adding 16 to the patient's age and dividing by 4.
2. **Assemble all equipment** (e.g., suction device, supplemental oxygen, bag-valve-mask device, endotracheal tubes, cricothyroidotomy or needle-jet equipment, carbon dioxide indicator, laryngoscope, pulse oximeter).
3. **Prepare medications** in the event that sedation or paralysis (or both) is necessary. Medications necessary for rapid sequence induction (RSI) should also be assembled.*
4. **Position the patient's head** in the "sniffing" position (i.e., with the head flexed at the neck and extended). If necessary, elevate the patient's head with a small pillow or towel. Maintain cervical immobilization when spinal instability is of concern (e.g., in trauma victims).
5. **Preoxygenate the patient** by allowing him or her to breathe 100% oxygen. Avoid unnecessary gastric filling by minimizing assisted bag-valve-mask ventilation. Ideally, the patient should be oxygenated to an oxygen saturation of 100%.
6. **Position the laryngoscope** handle with the left hand, inserting the laryngoscope along the right side of the mouth to the base of the tongue and pushing the tongue to the left. If using a curved blade, advance the laryngoscope to the vallecula (superior to epiglottis) and lift anteriorly. If using a straight blade, place the laryngoscope beneath the epiglottis and lift anteriorly.
7. **Intubate the patient,** stopping just after the cuff disappears behind the vocal cords. If the intubation attempt is unsuccessful after 30 seconds, stop and resume bag-valve-mask ventilation before reattempting intubation.
8. **Inflate the cuff** with a syringe and attach the tube to an Ambu bag or ventilator.
9. **Confirm the placement of the tube** by checking for equal bilateral breath sounds and the absence of gastric air. Carbon dioxide monitoring, a syringe test, or a chest radiograph may also be useful for checking tube location. If any question remains regarding the placement of the endotracheal tube, repeat laryngoscopy with the tube in place to be sure it is endotracheal.
10. **Secure the tube** with tape and note the centimeter mark at the mouth. Suction the patient's oropharynx and trachea.

---

*If sedation or paralysis is employed, the patient is at risk for vomiting and aspiration; therefore, application of pressure to the cricoid cartilage (the Sellick maneuver) should be performed as soon as the patient loses the ability to protect the airway.

TABLE 1–2 Guidelines for Nasotracheal Intubation

1. **Determine tube size.** Common tube sizes are 6.0–7.0 mm for women and 7.0–8.0 mm for men.
2. **Administer medications**
   a. Spray the nasal passage with a **vasoconstrictor spray** such as cocaine 4% (4 mL) or phenylephrine 0.25% (2 mL), unless contraindicated.
   b. Apply a **topical anesthetic** (e.g., viscous lidocaine 2% or a topical spray).
   c. If **sedation** is required, administer fentanyl (1 µg/kg) or midazolam (0.05–0.1 mg/kg) and titrate to effect.
3. **Position the patient.** Nasotracheal intubation may be performed with the patient sitting up.
4. **Intubate the patient.** Place the tube in the nasal passage and guide it into the nasopharynx. Monitor progress by listening for air movement and observing fogging of the tube. As the tube enters the oropharynx, gradually guide the tube downward. If using a tube with a directional tip control, pull on the ring at this time to direct the tube anteriorly. If the sounds stop, withdraw the tube approximately 1–2 cm until breath sounds can be heard again. Reposition the tube, extending the patient's head if necessary. If difficulty is encountered, perform laryngoscopy or use Magill forceps. Successful intubation occurs when the tube passes through the cords; the patient may cough and breath sounds will reach maximum intensity if the tube is correctly positioned.
5. **Confirm the placement of the tube** by checking for equal bilateral breath sounds and the absence of gastric air. Carbon dioxide monitoring, a syringe test, or a chest radiograph may also be useful for checking tube location. If any question remains regarding the placement of the endotracheal tube, repeat laryngoscopy with the tube in place to be sure it is endotracheal.

a patient, ideally in association with sedatives. Sedative agents are not nearly as effective as paralytic agents in decreasing muscle tone, and they are not able to facilitate intubation to the degree provided by paralytics.

(1) **Overview**
   (a) **Indications and contraindications**
      (i) **Relative indications** for RSI include the inability to cooperate with intubation while awake, combative behavior, a depressed level of consciousness, active seizure activity, clenched oral musculature, a postictal state, severe trauma, and risk of complications resulting from intubation in the setting of head injury, stroke, or aortic dissection [e.g., increased intracranial pressure (ICP) or increased systolic blood pressure].
      (ii) **Relative contraindications** include airway distortion (which could interfere with the ability to intubate once the patient is paralyzed) and the presence of viable alternatives to RSI.
   (b) **Goals.** The goals of RSI are to:
      (i) Preoxygenate the patient
      (ii) Avoid positive-pressure ventilation
      (iii) Induce unawareness
      (iv) Prevent complications, including aspiration
      (v) Atraumatically intubate the patient
   (c) **Guidelines** for performing RSI are summarized in Table 1–3.
(2) **Pharmacologic adjuncts**
   (a) **Atropine** (0.01 mg/kg) prevents muscarinic bradycardia, which can be associated with the administration of succinylcholine (especially in children). Atropine should be strongly considered for children younger than 6 years who require RSI.
   (b) **Lidocaine** (1.5 mg/kg administered intravenously approximately 3 minutes before intubation) may blunt the increases in ICP, systolic blood pressure, and pulse that are usually associated with intubation, and it may have other direct benefits in patients with injured brain tissue. Although the efficacy of lidocaine administration is controversial,

---

TABLE 1–3   Guidelines for Performing Rapid Sequence Induction (RSI)

1. Decide whether to use a depolarizing or nondepolarizing agent.
2. Decide whether a priming dose of a nondepolarizing agent is indicated.
3. Assemble and check all equipment, including a pulse oximeter, a cricothyroidotomy tray, a Yankauer suction, laryngoscope blades, and a carbon dioxide detector. Be sure to include equipment necessary for an alternative plan if the intubation attempt is unsuccessful (e.g., cricothyroidotomy, bag-valve-mask ventilation, transtracheal needle-jet insufflation).
4. Reassure the patient and describe the procedure.
5. Preoxygenate the patient with 100% oxygen. Avoid unnecessary gastric filling by avoiding unnecessary respiratory assistance.
6. Premedicate the patient to block increases in intracranial pressure (ICP) and blood pressure as indicated by the patient's condition. Consider lidocaine for patients in whom increased ICP and blood pressure are a concern and fentanyl for patients in whom increased blood pressure is a concern.
7. Administer a priming dose of the nondepolarizing agent if the decision is made to prime.
8. Sedate the patient using the agent of choice.
9. Paralyze the patient using the agent of choice.
10. Intubate the patient.
11. Confirm placement of the tube by checking for equal bilateral breath sounds and the absence of gastric air. Carbon dioxide monitoring, a syringe test, or a chest radiograph may be useful for checking tube location. If any question remains regarding placement of the endotracheal tube, repeat laryngoscopy with the tube in place to be sure it is endotracheal.
12. Continue sedation, analgesia, and paralysis as appropriate for the patient's condition.

---

overall, the administration of lidocaine may be helpful and is unlikely to be harmful, and lidocaine is readily available and inexpensive.

(3) **Induction of unawareness. Sedative–induction agents** are used to decrease consciousness during intubation. Properties of these agents are summarized in Tables 1–4 and 1–5.

(a) **Thiopental**

(i) **Effects.** Thiopental lowers the ICP by reducing cerebral blood flow. Rapid redistribution of thiopental out of the brain results in a short duration of action and can cause light anesthesia. Thiopental, a myocardial depressant, decreases systolic and mean arterial pressure.

(ii) **Adverse effects** may include airway hyperactivity and laryngospasm following mechanical stimulation of the airway during instrumentation. Hypotension may also occur.

(iii) **Contraindications.** Thiopental is contraindicated in patients who are not hemodynamically stable.

(b) **Methohexital** lowers the ICP and has the same adverse effects as thiopental.

(c) **Fentanyl** is not commonly used as a sole inducing agent.

(i) **Effects.** Fentanyl appears to blunt increases in blood pressure and pulse associated with intubation and thus may be useful for patients in whom such increases could be catastrophic.

(ii) **Adverse effects.** Fentanyl can cause bradycardia and hypotension secondary to parasympathetic stimulation and blunting of catecholinergic activity.

(d) **Midazolam** has minimal cardiovascular effects and may blunt the increase in ICP associated with intubation. Additionally, it is a drug familiar to most emergency physicians.

(e) **Etomidate.** The primary advantage of etomidate is that it has minimal cardiovascular effects (as compared with thiopental) and it can play a role for induction of select trauma victims. It has a rapid onset and short duration of action.

TABLE 1–4   Sedative–Induction Agents

Agent	Class	Onset	Duration	Induction Dose
Thiopental	Barbiturate	30–60 seconds	5–10 minutes	3.0–5.0 mg/kg intravenous push in adults and children (approximately 300 mg), may be titrated
Methohexital	Barbiturate	30–60 seconds	5–10 minutes	5–12 mL of 1% solution at 1 mL/5 sec (1–2 mg/kg)
Fentanyl	Opiate	2–4 minutes	45 minutes	3–5 µg/kg (approximately 200–300 µg) for adults; 2–3 µg for children 2–11 years
Midazolam	Benzodiazepine	1–5 minutes	30 minutes	0.1 mg/kg (approximately 5 mg) for adults; 0.05–0.1 mg/kg for children*
Etomidate	Benzodiazepine derivative (imidazole)	30–60 seconds	4–6 minutes	0.3 mg/kg (approximately 20 mg); not recommended for children younger than 10 years
Propofol	Diisopropylphenol	30 seconds	5–10 minutes	1.5–3.0 mg/kg (approximately 140 mg)
Ketamine	Arylcyclohexylamine	1 minute	10–20 minutes	1–2 mg/kg

*Midazolam may also be administered rectally, intranasally, or orally. Lower doses can be used to assist in sedation.

(i) **Adverse effects.** Etomidate can suppress cortisol production, even with a single dose.
(ii) **Contraindications.** Etomidate is currently contraindicated in children younger than 10 years and in pregnant or lactating women.
(f) **Propofol** lowers the ICP and causes as much or greater hypotension when compared with thiopental. In addition, it has a rapid onset of action as well as rapid resolution of sedation.
(g) **Ketamine**
(i) **Effects.** Chemically, ketamine is related to phencyclidine (PCP) and causes a dissociative, cataleptic state. Ketamine also has analgesic properties. Ketamine relaxes bronchial smooth muscle and causes little respiratory depression. These characteristics make ketamine a particularly appropriate induction agent for patients with isolated respiratory failure, especially asthmatics.

TABLE 1–5   Hemodynamic and Intracranial Effects of Sedative–Induction Agents

Agent	Effect on MAP	Effect on Pulse	Effect on ICP
Thiopental	↓	↑	↓↓
Methohexital	↓	↑↑	↓↓
Fentanyl	No effect or ↓	No effect or ↓	No effect
Midazolam	No effect or ↓	↓↑	↓
Etomidate	No effect	No effect	↓↓
Propofol	↓↓	↓	↓
Ketamine	↑↑	↑↑	↑

ICP = intracranial pressure; MAP = mean arterial pressure; ↑ = increase, ↓ = decrease.

(ii) Adverse effects. Dreams or hallucinations occur in 30%–50% of adults and 5%–10% of prepubescent children. These may be recalled as being dysphoric. Benzodiazepine medications are often given to minimize this side effect. Ketamine increases skeletal muscle tone and is associated with nonpurposeful movements. It increases the mean arterial pressure (MAP), the pulse rate, and the ICP.

(iii) Contraindications. Ketamine is contraindicated for patients with elevated ICP and for patients in whom an increase in the MAP could be harmful.

(4) Neuromuscular blockade is used to relax musculature to facilitate intubation. Neuromuscular transmission is mediated by acetylcholine (ACh), which is created from acetyl coenzyme A (acetyl CoA) and choline. ACh is stored in synaptic vesicles in axon terminals and, after it is released, is hydrolyzed by acetylcholinesterase in the synaptic cleft or by pseudocholinesterase in the plasma. An action potential in the terminal motor nerve causes the release of ACh, which diffuses across the synaptic cleft, binds to postsynaptic end-plate receptors, and depolarizes the end-plate membrane, producing an action potential.

(a) Depolarizing blockade is achieved with **succinylcholine,** which binds to end-plate ACh sites and causes depolarization in the same manner as ACh. Succinylcholine results in a brief period of repetitive muscle contractions manifested by fasciculations, followed by block of neuromuscular transmission.

(i) Dose. Succinylcholine is given intravenously (1.5 mg/kg for adults and children older than 10–12 years); 100 mg is the average adult dose. Dosing is increased to 2.0 mg/kg for children younger than 10–12 years of age.

(ii) Onset and duration of action. Succinylcholine is the fastest acting paralytic agent—satisfactory relaxation occurs within 30–60 seconds. Succinylcholine is hydrolyzed rapidly by pseudocholinesterase and as a result has the shortest duration of action of the paralytic agents (3–5 minutes, occasionally as long as 10 minutes).

(iii) Adverse effects. Succinylcholine has been associated with **increased intragastric and intraocular pressures.** It is unclear whether succinylcholine alone causes increased ICP. Succinylcholine has also been associated with **malignant hyperthermia** and **arrhythmias** (especially bradycardia in children). Succinylcholine is associated with **risk for prolonged paralysis in patients with abnormal pseudocholinesterase levels** (e.g., some pregnant women, patients with severe hepatic dysfunction, patients with renal failure, and patients with bronchogenic carcinoma).

(iv) Contraindications. Succinylcholine is contraindicated in patients with penetrating ocular trauma or glaucoma, in patients with unstable fractures (which may be worsened by fasciculations), in patients with neuromuscular diseases, and in burn patients more than 24 hours after injury.

(b) Nondepolarizing blockade is achieved via competitive inhibition of postsynaptic ACh sites. In general, nondepolarizing agents cause more prolonged paralysis than can be achieved with succinylcholine (Table 1–6).

(i) D-Tubocurarine (dTc) is the prototypical nondepolarizing agent. The incidence of bronchospasm, bradycardia, and myocardial depression limits the utility of dTc in the ED.

(ii) Vecuronium lacks any histamine-releasing or ganglion-blocking activity. Advantages include no fasciculations and no increase in ICP, intragastric pressure, or intraocular pressure. Vecuronium has a long duration of action; therefore, it must be used with caution because if the attempt at intubation fails, the patient will require prolonged ventilatory support using bag-valve-mask ventilation until another attempt can be made.

TABLE 1–6   Neuromuscular Blocking (Paralytic) Agents

Agent	Onset	Duration	Induction Dose
Depolarizing Agents			
Succinylcholine	30–60 seconds	3–5 minutes; occasionally as long as 10 minutes	1.5 mg/kg for adults and children older than 10–12 years (approximately 100 mg for adults); 2.0 mg/kg for children younger than 10–12 years
Nondepolarizing Agents			
D-Tubocurarine (dTc)	1–5 minutes	40–60 minutes; longer in infants	0.03 mg/kg for children younger than 1 week; 0.06 mg/kg for children older than 6 weeks
Vecuronium	2–3 minutes	20–40 minutes	0.1 mg/kg (approximately 7 mg for adults)
Pancuronium	2–3 minutes	40–80 minutes	0.1 mg/kg (approximately 7 mg for adults)
Rocuronium	1.5 minutes	30 minutes	0.6 mg/kg

        (iii) **Pancuronium** can slightly increase the pulse and blood pressure, although the increase is not usually clinically significant.

        (iv) **Rocuronium** is a newer nondepolarizing agent that has been created in an attempt to achieve the rapid onset and short duration of action of succinylcholine. Rocuronium has the fastest onset of the nondepolarizing agents (see Table 1–6).

    (c) **"Priming"** is a technique that consists of the administration of a less-than-paralytic dose of a nondepolarizing agent (e.g., vecuronium, 0.01 mg/kg) to bind postsynaptic ACh receptor sites prior to the administration of a second dose of a paralytic agent. Evidence supporting use of priming for various purposes is controversial. Priming will block succinylcholine-induced fasciculations and their sequelae and likely decreases the onset time and duration of action when followed by an appropriate dose of a nondepolarizing agent. However, there is little evidence that priming affects the ICP or provides significant benefit when succinylcholine is used for paralysis.

  4. **Techniques for managing the difficult airway**

    a. **Cricothyrotomy.** A longitudinal skin incision is made over the cricothyroid membrane and extended through the membrane. The hole is dilated and maintained with a dilator, or a hook and tracheostomy tube are inserted into the trachea.

    b. **Transtracheal jet insufflation.** Needle cricothyrotomy is performed by inserting a large-caliber (12- to 14-gauge) plastic cannula into the trachea, again through the cricothyroid membrane. The cannula is attached to a high-pressure oxygen source; oxygen is delivered with manually controlled intermittent insufflation.

    c. **Fiberoptic intubation.** Fiberoptic laryngoscopy precedes intubation and the endotracheal tube is advanced over fiberoptic cable into the trachea.

    d. **Lighted stylet intubation.** A stylet with a bright light source at the tip is used in a darkened room to help identify the trachea. An endotracheal tube is advanced over the stylet into the airway.

    e. **Video-assisted laryngoscopy.** A modified laryngoscope is used to improve visualization of the oropharynx and pass the endotracheal tube into the trachea.

    f. **Retrograde wire intubation.** A needle and subsequently a long wire are passed from the cricothyroid membrane up the pharynx and out the nose or mouth, which is then used to guide the endotracheal tube into position.

IV BREATHING (VENTILATION)

A Assessment Spontaneous ventilation requires function of the nervous system, lungs, chest wall, and diaphragm. Each component should be examined and evaluated rapidly.

1. **Physical examination.** This aspect of assessing the patient's ability to ventilate can be combined with the initial assessment of airway patency.
   a. **Observation.** The physician should observe and palpate the chest wall, searching for spontaneous respirations and evidence of crepitus or trauma. It is also necessary to feel and listen for oral air exchange (it may be difficult to hear in the setting of a noisy ED).
      (1) Patients may present with **agonal gasps** at varied rates.
      (2) In the nonarrest patient, **tachypnea** is an indication that additional airway management is necessary.
   b. **Auscultation** of the chest for breath sounds provides clues to possible causes of respiratory arrest or distress, including pneumothorax, congestive heart failure (CHF), pulmonary edema, or pleural effusions.
2. **Monitoring.** Although its usefulness may be limited by low peripheral circulation, **pulse oximetry** monitoring should be instituted for all resuscitation patients. In pulse oximetry, oxygen saturation is estimated based on spectrophotometric analysis of light absorption by oxyhemoglobin and deoxyhemoglobin using red and infrared light. Oxygen saturations of 100%, 90%, 60%, and 50% correlate with arterial oxygen tensions of 90 mm Hg, 60 mm Hg, 30 mm Hg, and 27 mm Hg, respectively.
3. **Diagnostics.** A portable chest radiograph may aid in diagnosis of pneumothorax, CHF, or pericardial tamponade. However, acute intervention based on clinical grounds should always supersede radiologic investigation.

B Interventions

1. **Administration of supplemental oxygen** is mandatory for all resuscitation patients. Initially, oxygen should be provided at a concentration as close to 100% as possible (oxygen toxicity from 100% concentrations requires an average of 6 continuous hours of exposure). Concentrations may be decreased once the patient has been stabilized. Oxygen may be delivered by the following methods:
   a. **Nasal cannula.** A nasal cannula delivers oxygen at concentrations of 25%–45% at a flow rate of 1–6 L/min and may be useful for **conscious patients with chronic obstructive pulmonary disease (COPD) in a nonarrest setting,** where the respiratory drive depends on oxygen sensors alone. This device is not optimal for resuscitation due to the low concentration of oxygen delivered and the fact that delivery of oxygen requires spontaneous respirations and the actual inspired oxygen concentration depends on the respiration depth.
   b. **Simple (standard) face mask.** This is a plastic mask with side holes that allow inhalation and exhalation of room air and supplemental oxygen. An oxygen flow rate of greater than 5 L/min is necessary to fill the mask reservoir; the recommended flow rate is 8–10 L/min for delivery of oxygen at a concentration of 40%–60%. The limitations of a simple face mask in an arrest setting are the same as those of the nasal cannula.
   c. **Venturi mask.** A Venturi mask is similar to a simple face mask, but the Venturi mask is modified to allow more precise delivery of oxygen. The Venturi mask is appropriate for **conscious COPD patients in whom tight control of the oxygen concentration is required.** The limitations of the Venturi mask in an arrest setting are the same as those of the nasal cannula and the simple face mask.
   d. **Nonrebreather mask.** A one-way exhalation valve prevents mixing of room air and expired air with the reservoir bag of 100% oxygen. In order to be effective, the patient must have spon-

taneous respirations, the mask must fit tightly, and the reservoir bag must be completely filled (necessitating an oxygen flow rate of 10–15 L/min). A nonrebreather mask is the **first-line method for the delivery of oxygen at concentrations approaching 100% in a patient with spontaneous respirations.**

2. **Assisted ventilation** should be guided by the patient's serum pH and arterial oxygen and carbon dioxide levels. Pulse oximetry monitoring should be in place and ABG determinations to assess acid–base status and guide prolonged mechanical ventilation may be considered. The recommended tidal volume for resuscitation is 10–15 mL/kg.

   a. **Rescue breathing.** Direct mouth-to-mouth, mouth-to-mask breathing is still advocated by the American Heart Association (AHA).

      (1) Concern from bystander rescuers about infection transmission may limit the use of rescue breathing; however, the estimated rate of infectious disease transmission is very low.

      (2) Exhaled gas contains 16.6%–17.1% oxygen and 3.5%–4.1% carbon dioxide.

   b. **Bag-valve-mask ventilation ("bagging the patient")** allows manually controlled delivery of tidal volumes and is the standard of ventilation for **apneic, nonintubated patients.** Bag-valve-mask ventilation can allow the operator to estimate lung compliance through the amount of force required to ventilate the patient.

      (1) **Components** include a clear mask with an air-cushion rim to provide a tight face seal; a true nonrebreathing valve; a no-pressure release valve; and an attached bag and reservoir that may accept oxygen flow at a rate of 12–15 L/min for a delivered oxygen concentration of almost 100%.

      (2) **Disadvantages**

         (a) Personnel inexperienced in the use of the bag-valve-mask may find it difficult to maintain the mask seal while coordinating bag ventilation, and often two operators are required for optimal usage. (Alternatively, the bag apparatus can be attached to an endotracheal tube for manual ventilation.)

         (b) Large tidal volumes may inadvertently cause gastric distention, increasing the risk of aspiration and limiting the effective tidal volume. Large tidal volumes also increase the risk of pneumothorax.

   c. **Endotracheal intubation** is the optimal means of ventilating the **unconscious patient** or the **patient with severe respiratory compromise.** Endotracheal intubation allows for the delivery of 100% oxygen directly to the trachea and for direct monitoring of expired carbon dioxide, which may be helpful in optimizing chest compressions during CPR [see V B 1 a (3) (c)]. In addition, endotracheal intubation affords some increase in protection against aspiration.

   d. **Mechanical positive-pressure ventilation** allows maximal control of the tidal volume and airway pressures, decreasing the risk of barotrauma, and is the optimal method of ventilating unconscious patients. However, this method of ventilation may be difficult to initiate during the immediate resuscitation phase.

C **Failure to oxygenate or ventilate** may occur for multiple reasons.

   1. **Mechanical failure.** The ventilatory circuit should be systematically evaluated.

      a. Check for monitor malfunction/accuracy.

      b. Ensure that all interventional equipment is properly positioned. (Is the endotracheal tube in the esophagus? Is the mask seal tight?)

      c. Ensure that the oxygen supply is adequate.

   2. **Organic source.** Development of tension pneumothorax or the existence of preexisting conditions [e.g., pleural effusions, acquired respiratory distress syndrome (ARDS), pulmonary edema, CHF] can all lead to inadequate oxygenation or ventilation. Any specific cause that can be identified should be treated appropriately (e.g., chest tube thoracostomy, furosemide, thoracocentesis).

V CIRCULATION

A Assessment

1. **Physical examination**
   a. The physical examination may provide clues to the cause of arrest (e.g., shock, pericardial tamponade, dysrhythmia, tension pneumothorax, etc.).
   b. The pulses, neck veins, skin color, and quality of the heart sounds should be rapidly assessed. Pulses may correlate roughly with the systolic blood pressure: a palpable radial pulse = a systolic blood pressure greater than 80 mm Hg, a palpable femoral pulse = a systolic blood pressure greater than 70 mm Hg, and a palpable carotid pulse = a systolic blood pressure greater than 60 mm Hg.

2. **Monitoring**
   a. **Quick look.** A quick look with **defibrillator paddles** to identify convertible dysrhythmias (e.g., ventricular tachycardia, ventricular fibrillation) is the most important step in treating cardiac arrest.
   b. **Continuous three-lead electrocardiographic monitoring** to assess variable rhythms and **noninvasive blood pressure monitoring** (updated every 2 minutes) should also be instituted, regardless of the cause of arrest.

3. **Diagnostics**
   a. A **12-lead electrocardiogram (ECG)** and a **stat potassium level** should be considered for patients with non–DC-convertible rhythms (as identified during the quick look).
   b. **Immediate bedside ultrasound** may be useful in diagnosing pericardial tamponade–induced pulseless electrical activity (PEA).

B Interventions

1. **Maintaining cerebral and cardiac perfusion**
   a. **Noninvasive (closed chest) compression.** Standard closed chest compressions provide only 25%–30% of normal cardiac output. Successful cardiopulmonary–cerebral resuscitation is dependent on the **return of spontaneous circulation (ROSC).** ROSC is directly related to the ability to supply myocardial blood flow [i.e., the **coronary perfusion pressure (CPP)**]. The CPP is the gradient across the coronary vasculature and is equal to the difference between the aortic diastolic pressure and the right atrial pressure. During CPR, the maximal CPP occurs between chest compressions. Standard CPR provides a CPP of only 1–8 mm Hg, and the estimated CPP required for ROSC is 15–30 mm Hg. Epinephrine, which increases systemic vascular resistance and the aortic diastolic pressure, thereby increasing the CPP, is a useful adjunct in CPR.
      (1) **Standard technique.** Closed chest compressions are performed by placing the heel of one hand two finger breadths above the xiphoid on the sternum, with the other hand covering the first. Force is transmitted downward with the elbows locked so that the patient's chest is compressed (1.5–2 inches for adults; 1–1.5 inches for children) at a rate of 80–100 compressions per minute. Proper technique requires a firm backboard. The individual performing compressions should also be comfortably positioned above the patient, with the aid of a footstool if necessary, to minimize rescuer fatigue.
      (2) **Mechanism of action.** The mechanism of action of closed chest compressions is unknown. The two leading theories are:
         (a) **Cardiac pump theory.** This theory suggests that the heart is squeezed between the sternum and spine, leading to the forward flow of blood. Backflow is prevented by the cardiac valves and the heart passively fills between compressions. Criticisms of this theory are that the arteriovenous pressure gradient may be equalized during arrest and the mitral or semilunar valves may be incompetent.

(b) **Thoracic pump theory.** This theory suggests that the intrathoracic veins collapse with chest compression and blood is forced forward through the aorta. Backflow of blood in the venous circulation is prevented by valves located in the large veins at the thoracic inlet. Between compressions, the central venous circulation fills and the cycle is repeated.

(3) **Monitoring the effectiveness of chest compressions** is not currently the accepted standard, despite the fact that compressions are often not optimally applied during resuscitation. Monitoring techniques include the following:

    (a) **Invasive blood pressure monitoring** allows direct calculation of the CPP.

    (b) **Assessment of central venous oxygen saturation** may be predictive of the ROSC: a central venous oxygen saturation of 72% is associated with 100% ROSC, whereas a central venous oxygen saturation of 30% is associated with 0% ROSC.

    (c) **Capnometry.** Measurement of the end-tidal carbon dioxide concentration correlates directly with cardiac output when the minute ventilation is constant. The monitoring device is attached to the endotracheal tube or ventilator system. Calorimetric capnometry may provide an inexpensive and readily available means of gauging CPR effectiveness.

(4) **Complications** are mostly the result of inappropriately placed or excessive force.

    (a) **Rib fractures** (30%)

    (b) **Sternal fractures** (20%)

    (c) **Pneumothorax, cardiac contusion, pericardial hemorrhage, cardiac laceration, gastroesophageal tears,** and **liver or splenic lacerations**

(5) **Modifications to the standard closed chest compression technique**

    (a) **Interposed abdominal counterpulsation** involves alternating standard chest compressions with abdominal compressions and is thought to improve the CPP and cerebral blood flow by increasing the intrathoracic pressure and aortic pressure. An additional trained rescuer must be present. Early investigation suggests improvement in outcome when performed on patients experiencing in-hospital arrest.

    (b) **Circumferential chest compression** involves the use of a pneumatic vest, which inflates to compress the chest circumferentially. Circumferential chest compression generates greater fluctuations in intrathoracic pressure and increases intrathoracic airway collapse, resulting in air-trapping. Air-trapping increases the intrathoracic pressure by increasing the intrathoracic volume, potentiating the external compressive force. Use of a pneumatic vest has been shown in early studies to increase short-term survival in humans, but disadvantages include cost and availability.

    (c) **Active compression–decompression.** Active decompression of the chest during the relaxation phase of chest compression is provided through a hand-held suction cup device. Active compression–decompression CPR is thought to increase the net negative intrathoracic pressure during the relaxation/decompression phase (following the thoracic pump model). A possible advantage is the simultaneous ventilation of the patient provided through chest wall compression–decompression.

    (d) **High-impulse CPR.** Standard chest compressions are performed at a faster rate (e.g., 120–150 compressions/min). Although it has been found that cardiac output increases linearly with the compression rate, operator fatigue and an increased risk of rib fractures are disadvantages of this approach.

b. **Open chest compression.** Open massage provides up to 55% of the baseline cardiac output, as compared with the 25%–30% output generated by closed chest compression.

(1) **Standard technique.** Open chest compression is performed after thoracotomy by positioning the heart between both hands, with the palms at the base. Massage is conducted by compressing the heart from the palms at the apex toward the fingertips at the base. Defibrillation may be carried out with internal paddles at 0.5 joule/kg.

(2) Indications
  (a) Cardiac arrest in the setting of penetrating chest trauma
  (b) Following blunt trauma, when signs of life are present in the prehospital setting but absent in the ED
  (c) In patients with chest deformities that preclude effective closed chest compressions
  (d) In some patients with pulmonary embolism, hypothermia, pericardial tamponade, or abdominal hemorrhage

c. Cardiopulmonary bypass. Extracorporeal support has been described as successful in several reports. Access is obtained via the femoral artery and vein. Disadvantages include the need for a skilled operator and for special equipment.

d. Investigational techniques
  (1) Selective aortic arch perfusion involves the placement of an intra-aortic balloon at the level of the descending aorta to isolate the cerebral and myocardial circulations. This technique may increase perfusion pressures and allow the instillation of pharmacologic agents to improve cardiac function and enhance cerebral protection.
  (2) Selective aortic perfusion and oxygenation (SAPO) entails the use of an intra-aortic balloon in conjunction with oxygenated bovine polymerized hemoglobin solution and has been successful in animal models. Advantages include direct access to the cardiac and cerebral circulations and the possible feasibility of using this technique in the prehospital setting. The main disadvantage is the need for invasive catheterization of the femoral artery.

2. Restoring rhythm. Defibrillation (countershock) is the passing of energy through the chest in an attempt to produce momentary asystole, allowing the natural pacemaker and electrical conduction tracts of the heart to reestablish normal function. Success of defibrillation in restoring rhythm is inversely proportional to the time between arrest and countershock. **Early defibrillation is the only intervention consistently proven to improve outcome in cardiac arrest.** Energy may be passed through the chest by mechanical or electrical means.

a. Mechanical defibrillation. Precordial thump is performed by raising the fist 8–10 inches above the chest and delivering a firm blow to the center of the sternum. This method provides 0.5–1 joule of energy.
  (1) Disadvantages. Precordial thump may cause degeneration of ventricular tachycardia to ventricular fibrillation, asystole, or PEA.
  (2) Indications. Precordial thump is indicated only in patients with cardiac arrest resulting from witnessed ventricular fibrillation. DC countershock should not be delayed.
  (3) Contraindications. Precordial thump is contraindicated in infants and children.

b. Electrical defibrillation. Automatic external defibrillators (AEDs) are portable devices that monitor the cardiac rhythm and automatically deliver DC countershock of 0–360 joules if ventricular fibrillation is detected. [The appropriate energy for countershock varies according to the underlying rhythm (see VI A).] Some AED devices read the rhythm but require an operator to initiate countershock delivery. The goal of the AED is to provide early defibrillation without expert training.
  (1) Synchronized versus unsynchronized countershock
    (a) In the **synchronized mode,** the defibrillator delivers the countershock within milliseconds of the ECG R wave to prevent administration of the shock during the absolute refractory period of the ECG cycle.
    (b) In the **unsynchronized mode,** the defibrillator delivers countershock on demand, irrespective of the point in the ECG cycle. The unsynchronized mode should be used initially for patients with ventricular fibrillation or pulseless ventricular tachycardia. It may also be used for patients with unstable ventricular tachycardia with a pulse if an undue delay in synchronization occurs.

    (2) Considerations

        (a) Transthoracic resistance, which is increased by the skin and air-filled lungs, limits the effective current. Successive rapid shocks, firm pressure of the electrodes (e.g., 25 pounds) on the chest wall, the use of conduction gel, increased paddle size, and end expiration can decrease transthoracic resistance.

        (b) Implantable cardioverter-defibrillator (ICD) systems (see Chapter 2 V B) are typically implanted in survivors of non-myocardial infarction (MI)–related ventricular fibrillation or ventricular tachycardia arrest, or in patients with recurrent ventricular tachycardia that is not responsive to pharmacotherapy. When externally defibrillating a patient with an ICD or other pacemaker, the paddles should be positioned 5 inches away from the device to prevent damage to the implanted device.

    (3) Pharmacologic adjuncts to defibrillation. In patients with ventricular fibrillation, the administration of epinephrine, lidocaine, amiodarone, procainamide, or magnesium sulfate may be indicated. Antiarrhythmics have not been proven to improve survival from cardiac arrest; however, they may raise the fibrillation threshold and prevent recurrent fibrillation following successful countershock.

        (a) Lidocaine is the first-line antiarrhythmic for patients with ventricular fibrillation, because most emergency medical system (EMS) personnel and emergency physicians are familiar with its use.

        (b) Magnesium sulfate (2–4 g administered as an intravenous bolus) dilates coronary vascular beds and increases the effective refractory period in the atrioventricular (AV) node. Magnesium sulfate has been proven useful in arresting polymorphic ventricular tachycardia and may also be useful in terminating ventricular fibrillation arrest.

3. Electrical pacing is used to maintain cardiac rhythm when contractions initiated by the natural pacemaker are inadequate to maintain sufficient blood pressure.

  a. Indications. Electrical pacing is indicated for patients with:

    (1) Refractory tachycardia

    (2) Polymorphic ventricular tachycardia (torsades de pointes)

    (3) Bradycardias with unstable presentation (i.e., a systolic blood pressure of less than 80 mm Hg, a change in mental status, MI, or pulmonary edema):

        (a) Complete heart block

        (b) Symptomatic second-degree heart block

        (c) Symptomatic sick sinus syndrome

        (d) Drug-induced bradycardias (e.g., from β blockers, calcium channel blockers, digoxin, procainamide)

        (e) Permanent pacemaker failure

        (f) Idioventricular rhythms

        (g) Symptomatic atrial fibrillation with slow ventricular response

        (h) Refractory bradycardia during hypovolemic shock that does not respond to volume restoration attempts

        (i) Right bundle branch block with left anterior or posterior fascicular block

        (j) Bradysystolic arrest (electrical pacing is only effective within 20 minutes of arrest in this situation)

  b. Pacer settings depend on the clinical setting. In general, output should be set at the maximum and decreased after control of rhythm is achieved. The target rate should be 80–100 beats/min. The mode should be asynchronous in the setting of emergency pacing for arrest.

  c. Methods

    (1) Transcutaneous pacing is the fastest and least invasive technique; pacing leads are applied directly to the anterior and posterior chest wall.

      (a) The ability to capture is related to the energy of pacing and transthoracic resistance. Higher energy may be required in obese, barrel-chested individuals, and in the setting of a large pericardial effusion.

      (b) Defibrillation paddles should be placed a minimum of 2–3 cm from the pacing leads to prevent arcing.

    (2) **Transvenous pacing** requires the placement of temporary pacing wires through a central vein so the catheter tip lies against the apex of the right ventricle. Transvenous pacing may be instituted after successful transcutaneous pacing.

4. **Establishing intravenous access.** Intravenous access is required for the administration of drugs and fluids during resuscitation.* The type of intravenous catheter and the placement site vary according to the resuscitation situation. The standard recommendation for intravenous access is two 14- to 16-gauge catheters inserted peripherally in the upper extremity.

    a. **Complications** of all types of intravenous access include hematoma formation, cellulitis, thrombosis, phlebitis, sepsis, pulmonary thromboembolism, catheter-fragment embolism, and air embolism.

    b. **Flow rate.** The flow rate is directly proportional to the radius of the catheter raised to the fourth power and inversely proportional to the catheter length. Therefore, flow rate is limited by the catheter diameter and length, not the size of the vein cannulated. The fastest flow rate has been observed in large-bore (9 French), short-length (5½-inch) introducer catheters, which may be placed at any central access point (Table 1–7).

    c. **Circulation time.** The circulation time of drugs is increased in patients with cardiac/circulatory arrest.

      (1) Drugs administered centrally generally achieve the fastest onset of action.

      (2) Drugs administered via upper extremity peripheral intravenous sites require 1–2 minutes to reach the central circulation. Medications administered by a peripheral intravenous push and followed immediately with a 20-mL bolus of intravenous fluid and elevation of the extremity arrive at the heart as quickly as those given centrally.

      (3) Use of a femoral or lower extremity vein for drug administration during cardiac arrest is not recommended due to prolonged circulation time and altered blood flow with chest compressions. A long femoral vein catheter extending above the diaphragm is acceptable for central administration of drugs during arrest.

    d. **Access site.** From a practical standpoint, site selection is limited by the success of line placement, the potential for interference with other resuscitative measures (e.g., chest compressions, intubation), and preexisting injuries (e.g., cervical trauma).

      (1) **Peripheral sites**

        (a) The **basilica** or **median veins** in the antecubital fossa are the first choices for intravenous access, because these sites are associated with ease of cannulation, lack of interference with chest compressions, acceptable circulation time of infused drugs, and minimal complications. Access may be more difficult to obtain in hypovolemic patients, intravenous drug abusers, and morbidly obese individuals.

        (b) The **external jugular vein** is a peripheral vein that may be easily cannulated and provides rapid access to the central circulation. Disadvantages include difficult placement in hypovolemic patients, interference with airway management measures, easy dislodgement, and variable function with head movement (e.g., turning of the head may cause the catheter to kink).

---

*In emergency resuscitation circumstances when intravenous access is not available, lidocaine, atropine, naloxone, and epinephrine may be administered endotracheally via the endotracheal tube. The doses should be increased 2- to 2.5-fold over the intravenous dosage. Medications should be diluted to a final volume of 10 mL of normal saline to ensure distal delivery to the absorption site.

TABLE 1–7 Flow Rates Through Standard Resuscitation Catheters

Catheter Type	Location	Tap Water Flow Rates by Gravity (mL/min)
USCI 9-French introducer, 5½"	Central	247
USCI 8-French introducer, 5½"	Central	243
Deseret Angiocath (gauge 16, 5½")	Central	91
Deseret subclavian jugular catheter (gauge 16, 12")	Central	54
Deseret Angiocath (gauge 14, 2")	Peripheral	173
Deseret Angiocath (gauge 16, 2")	Peripheral	108

Modified with permission from Mateer JR, et al. Rapid fluid resuscitation with central venous catheters. *Ann Emerg Med* 1983;12:149–152.

(2) **Central sites.** Central venous catheterization is indicated if peripheral access attempts fail, if central pressure monitoring or pulmonary artery catheterization is required, or if administration of hypertonic or irritating fluids (pressor agents) is required.

(a) The **right internal jugular vein** is preferred over the left because it is directly aligned with the right atrium, the dome of the diaphragm and pleura are lower on the right side, and there is no thoracic duct on the right side. Intravenous access is usually obtained using the Seldinger (catheter over a guidewire) technique (Table 1–8).

TABLE 1–8 Guidelines for Right Internal Jugular Vein Catheterization (Middle Approach)

1. Prepare a percutaneous central venous access kit.
2. Position the patient in the Trendelenburg position (10°–15°), with the head turned to the left if possible.
3. Identify landmarks. The insertion site is the cephalad apex of the triangle formed by the two heads of the sternocleidomastoid muscle and the clavicle. Use ultrasound to identify and guide placement, if necessary.
4. Sterilely prepare and drape the area.
5. In conscious patients, infiltrate the skin overlying the area of puncture with 1% lidocaine.
6. With the finder needle attached to a 5-mL syringe, puncture the skin at a 45° angle at the apex of the triangle and advance the needle toward the ipsilateral nipple while gently drawing back on the syringe plunger.
7. Entry into the internal jugular vein is marked by the return of nonpulsatile venous blood into the syringe. Typically, the internal jugular vein should be entered no more than 5 cm from the skin surface. Return of pulsatile arterial blood indicates puncture of the carotid artery. If this occurs, remove the needle and apply direct pressure for 5–10 minutes.
8. Following successful cannulation of the internal jugular vein, advance the larger needle along the tract of, or right over, the finder needle. Some operators skip the step of using the finder needle.
9. Holding the needle firmly in place, remove the syringe and insert the guidewire through the needle. Note that whenever the needle hub is open to air, there is a threat of air embolism. **Always cover the open hub to prevent air entry.** The wire should advance smoothly. Do not let go of the guidewire.
10. While controlling one end of the wire, remove the needle. Puncture the skin at the site of wire entry with a scalpel. Some kits have the catheter over a dilator; some require a separate step of advancing a dilator over the wire before advancing the catheter over the wire. Remove the wire.
11. Attach a syringe to the line and demonstrate easy draw of blood. Flush the line with heparin solution or initiate fluid flow through the line and suture in place.
12. Obtain a portable chest radiograph to rule out pneumothorax and confirm line placement.

      (i) **Advantages.** The internal jugular vein is preferred for central venous access because it is associated with a rapid circulation time, easier access during chest compressions, easy compression in the event of a hematoma, and decreased risk of pneumothorax (as compared with a subclavian approach).

      (ii) **Disadvantages** of internal jugular vein catheterization include interference with airway management and increased rate of carotid artery puncture (2%–10%), pneumothorax, and hemothorax.

   (b) The **subclavian vein** is easily cannulated and allows for rapid central administration of drugs. Left subclavian vein catheterization is the preferred route for placement of transcutaneous pacing wires. The infraclavicular approach to obtaining intravenous access via the subclavian vein is summarized in Table 1–9.

      (i) **Advantages.** Subclavian vein catheterization is associated with a low infection rate and is more comfortable for long-term access.

      (ii) **Disadvantages** are the increased risk of pneumothorax (1%–2%), subclavian artery puncture (1%), and interference with chest compressions.

   (c) The **femoral vein** is considered a central access point and is easily cannulated (the success rate is 90%). Guidelines for femoral vein catheterization are given in Table 1–10.

      (i) **Advantages.** Catheterization of the femoral vein does not interfere with airway management or chest compressions and there is no risk of pneumothorax.

      (ii) **Disadvantages** include the highest rate of infection of all central lines, increased risk of thrombosis (10%) and femoral artery puncture (5%), and prolonged circulation time in arrest situation if the catheter does not reach above the diaphragm.

TABLE 1–9   Guidelines for Subclavian Vein Catheterization (Infraclavicular Approach)

1. Prepare a percutaneous central venous access kit. Attach the needle to a syringe.
2. Position the patient in the Trendelenburg position if possible.
3. Identify landmarks. The insertion site is 1 cm inferior to the clavicle at approximately the distal third of the clavicle length. This point is also identified as the superior inflection point of the clavicle, and is just lateral to the insertion of the sternocleidomastoid muscle on the clavicle.
4. Sterilely prepare and drape the area.
5. Infiltrate the skin at the insertion point with 1% lidocaine. Direct the needle down to the clavicle and infiltrate the periosteum with 1% lidocaine.
6. Insert and advance the needle parallel to the skin along a horizontal line between the shoulders toward the sternal notch. Apply gentle back pressure on the syringe plunger while advancing the needle. The needle should just skirt the clavicle (on the underside) while being advanced toward the sternal notch.
7. Entry into the subclavian vein is marked by the return of nonpulsatile venous blood. Sudden aspiration of air is a marker of entry into the pleural space and indicates induction of a pneumothorax. In the event of pneumothorax, remove the needle, obtain a stat chest radiograph, and prepare to perform tube thoracostomy.
8. Following successful cannulation of the subclavian vein, advance the needle several millimeters so that the tip is in the lumen of the vein.
9. Holding the needle firmly in place, remove the syringe and insert the guidewire through the needle. Note that whenever the needle hub is open to air, there is a threat of air embolism. **Always cover the open hub to prevent air entry.** The wire should advance smoothly. Do not let go of the guidewire.
10. While controlling one end of the wire, remove the needle. Puncture the skin with a scalpel at the site of wire entry. Some kits have the catheter over a dilator; some require a separate step of advancing a dilator over the wire before advancing the catheter over the wire. Remove the wire.
11. Attach a syringe to the line and demonstrate easy draw of blood. Flush the line with heparin solution or initiate fluid flow through the line and suture in place.
12. Obtain a portable chest radiograph to rule out pneumothorax and confirm line placement.

TABLE 1–10   Guidelines for Femoral Vein Catheterization

1. Prepare a percutaneous central access kit. The catheter may be the large introducer type (e.g., an 8.5-gauge French catheter) for rapid volume administration, or a 16- to 20-cm 16-gauge catheter.
2. Identify landmarks. If the femoral artery is palpable just below the inguinal ligament, then the femoral vein lies 1–2 cm medial to the palpable pulse. If no palpable pulse is present, then the insertion point is blind. Imagine a line between the superior iliac crest and the pubic tubercle. Divide the line into three intervals. The femoral artery lies at the junction of the medial and middle intervals. The femoral vein lies 1–2 cm medial to this junction. Remember the NAVEL mnemonic (nerve, artery, vein, empty space, lymphatics) to help visualize the anatomy.
3. Sterilely prepare and drape the groin.
4. Guard the femoral artery pulse with one hand and insert the needle attached to a 5-mL syringe 1–2 cm medially with the other hand. Advance the needle cephalad at a 30° angle to the skin.
5. Entry into the femoral vein is marked by the return of nonpulsatile venous blood. If pulsatile arterial flow is noted, withdraw the needle and compress the site for 5–10 minutes.
6. Following successful cannulation of the femoral vein, advance the larger needle along the tract of, or right over, the finder needle. Some operators skip this step if using the small finder needle.
7. Holding the needle firmly in place, remove the syringe and insert the guidewire through the needle. Note that whenever the needle hub is open to air, there is a threat of air embolism. **Always cover the open hub to prevent air entry.** The wire should advance smoothly. Do not let go of the guidewire.
8. While controlling one end of the wire, remove the needle. Puncture the skin at the site of wire entry with a scalpel. Some kits have the catheter over a dilator; some require a separate step of advancing a dilator over the wire before advancing the catheter over the wire. Remove the wire.
9. Attach a syringe to the line and demonstrate easy draw of blood. Flush the line with heparin solution or initiate fluid flow through the line and suture in place.

VI   SPECIFIC RESUSCITATION SITUATIONS

A **Dysrhythmias**   The AHA prepared the first **ACLS guidelines** in 1974 to provide an organized algorithmic approach to victims of cardiac arrest based on presenting cardiac rhythm. In addition, **all patients with arrest caused by a dysrhythmia should receive standard resuscitation measures** (i.e., **ABCs, establishment of intravenous access, administration of supplemental oxygen,** and **monitoring**).

1. **Ventricular fibrillation** may be the most common arrest rhythm and occurs commonly in the setting of CAD. Ventricular fibrillation has the best outcome of all arrest rhythms because of its responsiveness to DC countershock; the survival rate associated with ventricular fibrillation arrest is estimated at 15%.
   a. **Clinical evaluation**
      (1) **Patient history.** Ventricular fibrillation is often seen in the setting of CAD accompanied by angina, with or without MI.
      (2) **Physical examination.** There is no palpable pulse.
   b. **Differential diagnoses** include asystole and a motion artifact from the ECG leads.
   c. **Therapy.** The ACLS algorithm for ventricular fibrillation is shown in Figure 1–1.
      (1) **Immediate defibrillation,** beginning at 200 joules and increasing to 360 joules as needed, and **chest compressions** are indicated.
      (2) **Epinephrine** (1 mg every 3–5 minutes) should be administered, followed by **countershock** within 30–60 seconds. Escalating or high-dose epinephrine should be considered.
      (3) **Second-line agents,** such as **amiodarone 300** (300 mg, repeat doses 150 mg), **magnesium sulfate** (1–4 g intravenously), and **procainamide** (30 mg/min to a maximum dose of 17 mg/kg), should be considered for patients with refractory ventricular fibrillation.

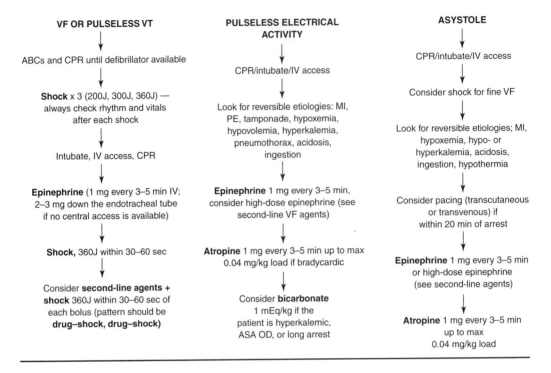

| VF OR PULSELESS VT | PULSELESS ELECTRICAL ACTIVITY | ASYSTOLE |

VF OR PULSELESS VT

↓

ABCs and CPR until defibrillator available

↓

Shock x 3 (200J, 300J, 360J) — always check rhythm and vitals after each shock

↓

Intubate, IV access, CPR

↓

Epinephrine (1 mg every 3–5 min IV; 2–3 mg down the endotracheal tube if no central access is available)

↓

Shock, 360J within 30–60 sec

↓

Consider **second-line agents + shock** 360J within 30–60 sec of each bolus (pattern should be **drug–shock, drug–shock**)

PULSELESS ELECTRICAL ACTIVITY

↓

CPR/intubate/IV access

↓

Look for reversible etiologies: MI, PE, tamponade, hypoxemia, hypovolemia, hyperkalemia, pneumothorax, acidosis, ingestion

↓

Epinephrine 1 mg every 3–5 min, consider high-dose epinephrine (see second-line VF agents)

↓

Atropine 1 mg every 3–5 min up to max 0.04 mg/kg load if bradycardic

↓

Consider **bicarbonate** 1 mEq/kg if the patient is hyperkalemic, ASA OD, or long arrest

ASYSTOLE

↓

CPR/intubate/IV access

↓

Consider shock for fine VF

↓

Look for reversible etiologies; MI, hypoxemia, hypo- or hyperkalemia, acidosis, ingestion, hypothermia

↓

Consider pacing (transcutaneous or transvenous) if within 20 min of arrest

↓

Epinephrine 1 mg every 3–5 min or high-dose epinephrine (see second-line agents)

↓

Atropine 1 mg every 3–5 min up to max 0.04 mg/kg load

Second-line agents

Amiodarone: 300 mg IV, repeat doses 150 mg

Lidocaine: 1.5 mg/kg (avg dose 100 mg) IVB, repeat in 3–5 min to max 3 mg/kg load

Magnesium sulfate: 1–2 g IV, especially consider if patient is in torsades de pointes, known hypomagnesemia, or refractory VF

Procainamide: infuse 30 mg/min to max 17 mg/kg load (avg dose 1–1.2 g)

Bicarbonate: 1 mEq/kb, consider for nephrine hyperkalemic patients, TCA OD, ? long arrest

Epinephrine: 1 mg 3–5 min apart

FIGURE 1–1 Advanced cardiac life support (ACLS) algorithms for the treatment of pulseless dysrhythmias. *ABCs* = airway, breathing, circulation; *ASA* = acetylsalicylic acid; *CPR* = cardiopulmonary resuscitation; *IV* = intravenous; *MI* = myocardial infarction; *OD* = overdose; *PE* = pulmonary embolism; *TCA* = tricyclic antidepressant; *VF* = ventricular fibrillation; *VT* = ventricular tachycardia. Reprinted with permission from the *Massachusetts General Hospital Medical Housestaff Manual 1996–1997.*

2. **PEA** is electrical activity that does not result in significant contraction of the heart muscle. PEA is the most common arrest rhythm, next to ventricular fibrillation, and often occurs after prolonged ventricular fibrillation. Reversible causes include hypovolemia (most commonly the result of hemorrhage), hypoxia, cardiac tamponade, tension pneumothorax, hypothermia, massive pulmonary embolism, drug overdose, hyperkalemia, and acidosis. The survival to hospital discharge rate is less than 1%.

   a. **Clinical features.** There is no palpable pulse. However, it must be noted that the lack of a palpable pulse does not imply absolute absence of cardiac activity; invasive monitoring detects arterial pulse waveforms in 40%–50% of patients.

   b. **Evaluation**

     (1) **Diagnostic studies.** The ECG shows cardiac rhythm. Inefficient ventricular wall motion corresponding to the ECG cycle is noted in up to 80% of arrest victims using ultrasound. Invasive arterial monitoring may show a low-amplitude pulse waveform.

     (2) **Laboratory evaluation.** A serum electrolyte profile (especially the potassium level) and ABG determinations should be obtained.

c. Therapy. Reversible causes must be addressed. For acute therapy, the ACLS PEA algorithm is followed (see Figure 1–1).

    (1) Chest compressions should be initiated.

    (2) A **fluid bolus** (500 mL lactated Ringer's solution or normal saline) should be administered.

    (3) Epinephrine (1 mg every 3–5 minutes) should be administered. An escalating or high-dose protocol should be considered.

    (4) Bicarbonate administration may be appropriate (e.g., in hyperkalemia, bicarbonate-responsive acidosis, or tricyclic antidepressant overdose, or when urine alkalinization to enhance phenobarbital or aspirin elimination is necessary). Bicarbonate administration is controversial in patients who have been in sustained arrest or who have lactic acidosis because bicarbonate administration may cause a paradoxical decrease in cerebral intracellular pH.

d. Disposition. Patients are admitted to the intensive care unit (ICU).

3. Bradyasystole or **asystole** can result from profound myocardial injury (e.g., as a result of infarction, hypoxia, hyperkalemia, hypokalemia, acidosis, drug overdose, hypothermia, or trauma) and is responsible for 25%–56% of arrests. Survival to discharge rates are 0%–3% when bradyasystole is noted as the initial rhythm.

a. Clinical features. Physical examination reveals no pulse or heartbeat.

b. Evaluation. There is no detectable cardiac activity on the ECG monitor. **The diagnosis must be confirmed in two leads.**

c. Therapy. The ACLS asystole algorithm is shown in Figure 1–1.

    (1) Chest compressions should be initiated.

    (2) Immediate transcutaneous pacing should be considered.

    (3) Epinephrine (1 mg administered as an intravenous push for adults; 0.01 mg/kg for pediatric patients) should be repeated every 3–5 minutes.

    (4) Atropine (1 mg administered intravenously for adults; 0.02 mg/kg to a total dose of 0.04 mg for pediatric patients) should be repeated every 3–5 minutes.

    (5) Transvenous pacing should be considered.

d. Disposition. Patients are admitted to the ICU.

4. Atrial fibrillation is the most common arrhythmia and is frequently seen in elderly patients. Causes include coronary artery disease (CAD), CHF, cardiomyopathy, thyrotoxicosis, rheumatic heart disease, hypertension, alcohol ingestion, and pulmonary embolism. In atrial fibrillation, multiple atrial ectopic foci stimulate an irregular ventricular response. The enlarged and poorly contracting left atrium predisposes the patient to thrombus formation, emboli, and stroke.

a. Clinical features

    (1) Patient history. Atrial fibrillation may be chronic (and asymptomatic) in patients with long-standing arteriosclerotic heart disease. In paroxysmal situations, palpitations may be accompanied by weakness and near-syncope.

    (2) Physical examination. An irregularly irregular rhythm (approximately 80–180 beats/min) is detected. The heart rate in patients with chronic atrial fibrillation is usually 80–120 beats/min. A "pulse deficit" is not uncommon (i.e., electrical depolarization is seen on the monitor at a frequency greater than that of the palpable pulses).

b. Differential diagnoses include multifocal atrial tachycardia, paroxysmal supraventricular tachycardia, and atrial flutter.

c. Evaluation. An ECG shows a small, irregular baseline rhythm without discernible P waves. The QRS complex is narrow.

d. Therapy. Atrial flutter/atrial fibrillation is treated according to the ACLS algorithm shown in Figure 1–2. A slow response rhythm (less than 120 beats/min) usually requires no immediate therapy.

    (1) Anticoagulation therapy should be considered for patients who have been in atrial fibrillation for longer than 48 hours.

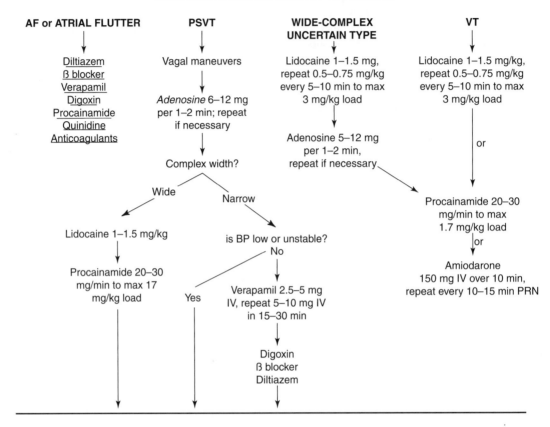

ABCs, oxygen 12-lead ECG, IV access, review history
if unstable →SYNCHRONOUS CARDIOVERSION (see below);
cardioversion seldom needed for HR <150 beats/min

| AF or ATRIAL FLUTTER | PSVT | WIDE-COMPLEX UNCERTAIN TYPE | VT |

SYNCHRONOUS CARDIOVERSION
Have suction and intubation kit ready
If awake, sedate with diazepam, midazolam, barbiturates
with or without morphine/fentanyl
VT/AF: 100J, 200J, 300J, 360J
PSVT/atrial flutter: 50J, 100J, 200J, 300J, 360J
Polymorphic VT: treat as VF 200J, 300J, 360J

FIGURE 1–2 Advanced cardiac life support (ACLS) algorithms for the treatment of tachycardias. *AF* = atrial fibrillation; *ABCs* = airway, breathing, circulation; *BP* = blood pressure; *ECG* = electrocardiogram; *HR* = heart rate; *IV* = intravenous; *PSVT* = paroxysmal supraventricular tachycardia; *VF* = ventricular fibrillation; *VT* = ventricular tachycardia. Reprinted with permission from the *Massachusetts General Hospital Medical Housestaff Manual 1996–1997*.

(2) **β Blockers** (e.g., esmolol, atenolol, metoprolol) or **calcium channel blockers** are preferred agents for rate control. Those agents are negative inotropes and can cause hypotension. Initiation of **digoxin therapy** (or the provision of additional digoxin to those patients who are already taking the drug) should be considered.

(3) **Sedation** and **countershock** beginning at 100 joules is indicated for unstable patients (i.e., those with chest pain, dyspnea, hypotension, CHF, or cardiac ischemia).

e. **Disposition.** Patients should be admitted to a telemetry unit or a cardiac care unit (CCU).

5. **Atrial flutter** is the result of an ectopic focus originating in a small area of the atrium. Causes include CAD, COPD, and rheumatic heart disease.

    a. Clinical features

        (1) Patient history. The patient usually has a history of heart palpitations, with or without symptoms.

        (2) Physical examination. The cardiac rate is approximately 150 beats/min (with a 2:1 block) and is usually regular. Rates of 75 beats/min occur with a 4:1 block. Rate and rhythm may be irregular, alternating between a 2:1 and 4:1 block.

    b. Evaluation. The ECG shows characteristic "sawtooth" flutter waves with an atrial rate between 250 and 350 per minute (see Figure 2–3). AV block is usually present.

    c. Therapy. The ACLS atrial flutter/atrial fibrillation algorithm is followed (see Figure 1–2).

        (1) β Blockers or **calcium channel blockers** should be administered as described for atrial fibrillation.

        (2) Cardioversion starting at 25–50 joules of synchronized energy is indicated for unstable patients. Higher energy may be required.

    d. Disposition. The patient should be admitted to a telemetry unit or the CCU.

6. Paroxysmal supraventricular tachycardia is a sudden increase in heart rate resulting from a reentrant signal that travels in a circular fashion through the AV node and an accessory pathway, resulting in sustained tachycardia. Causes include congenital conditions (e.g., mitral valve prolapse), Wolff-Parkinson-White (WPW) syndrome, hyperthyroidism, and arteriosclerotic heart disease.

    a. Clinical features

        (1) Patient history. There may be a history of heart palpitations, which may be accompanied by near-syncope.

        (2) Physical examination findings. The heart rate is 120–280 beats/min (typically 160–200 beats/min) and regular. The patient may present with angina, signs of CHF, or hypotension.

    b. Differential diagnoses include digitalis toxicity (i.e., paroxysmal supraventricular tachycardia with block), paroxysmal atrial fibrillation, ventricular tachycardia, and atrial flutter.

    c. Evaluation. The ECG usually shows a narrow QRS complex with flattened or notched P waves. In patients with WPW syndrome, a "delta" wave may be noted. P waves are seldom identified at heart rates greater than 200 beats/min.

    d. Therapy. The ACLS paroxysmal supraventricular tachycardia algorithm is followed (see Figure 1–2).

        (1) Vagal maneuvers (e.g., the **Valsalva maneuver, carotid massage**) may be attempted. Carotid massage is contraindicated in patients with a history of vascular disease or carotid bruits.

        (2) Adenosine, lidocaine, procainamide, or **verapamil** (depending on the QRS complex width) should be administered. Verapamil is contraindicated in wide-complex reentrant dysrhythmias.

        (3) Cardioversion beginning at 50 joules is indicated for unstable patients.

7. Ventricular tachycardia is defined as three or more consecutive premature ventricular contractions from an ectopic focus in the ventricle at a rate greater than 100 beats/min. Causes include MI, hypertrophic cardiomyopathy, drug toxicity, hypoxia, alkalosis, and electrolyte abnormalities.

    a. Clinical evaluation

        (1) Patient history. Ventricular tachycardia usually occurs in the setting of ischemic heart disease or MI.

        (2) Symptoms. Stable ventricular tachycardia may be asymptomatic. Unstable ventricular tachycardia may present with angina, hypotension, signs of CHF, or a decreased level of consciousness.

        (3) Physical examination findings. The pulse is regular with a rate of 150–200 beats/min, or absent.

    b. Differential diagnoses include paroxysmal supraventricular tachycardia with aberrant conduction.

   c. Evaluation. The ECG shows wide QRS complexes in a sustained pattern or in short bursts. Stat electrolyte and ABG determinations may be useful.

   d. Therapy. The ACLS ventricular tachycardia algorithm is followed (see Figure 1–2). Pulseless ventricular tachycardia should be treated in a manner similar to that of ventricular fibrillation.

     (1) Chest compressions are indicated.

     (2) Unsynchronized countershock beginning with 100 joules and increasing the level as needed to 360 joules is indicated for unstable patients.

     (3) Lidocaine (1–1.5 mg/kg every 5–10 minutes as needed, to a maximum dose of 3 mg/kg) should be administered to stable patients.

     (4) Procainamide (20–30 mg/min to a maximum dose of 17 mg/kg) should be administered.

     (5) Amiodarone (300 mg intravenously, repeat doses 150 mg) is also indicated.

     (6) Synchronized countershock is then instituted, beginning with 100 joules and increasing as needed to 360 joules.

   e. Disposition. Patients are admitted to the CCU.

 8. Polymorphic ventricular tachycardia (torsades de pointes) is ventricular tachycardia where the ECG demonstrates alteration in the amplitude and direction of electrical activity around the baseline. Polymorphic ventricular tachycardia is usually related to prolonged QT intervals and may be congenital (long QT syndrome), drug-induced (e.g., by procainamide, quinidine, cyclic antidepressants), or caused by an electrolyte imbalance.

   a. Clinical features. An irregular pulse greater than 150 beats/min is noted. The patient may present with palpitations, near-syncope, or syncope.

   b. Evaluation. The ECG shows an irregular rhythm with a wide QRS complex and independent or no P waves. The QRS complexes appear to gradually increase and decrease in amplitude. Stat electrolyte and drug levels should be considered.

   c. Therapy (see Figure 1–2)

     (1) Electrical ("overdrive") pacing is the treatment of choice. Sedation should be used in awake, stable patients.

     (2) Magnesium sulfate (1–2 g administered over 1–2 minutes and then the same dose repeated by infusion over 1 hour) is the drug of choice after pacing.

     (3) Unsynchronized countershock is appropriate for unstable patients.

   d. Disposition. Patients should be admitted to the CCU.

 9. Bradyarrhythmias

   a. Clinical features. The heart rate is less than 60 beats/min and may be regular or irregular.

     (1) Many athletes and other individuals have normal resting heart rates that are less than 60 beats/min and are asymptomatic. Treatment of bradycardia should be based on clinical symptoms.

     (2) Symptomatic bradycardia may be clinically manifested as a decreased level of consciousness, hypotension, chest pain, shortness of breath, pulmonary congestion, CHF, or acute MI.

   b. Evaluation. The ECG may show narrow-QRS sinus bradycardia, junctional rhythm, second-degree AV block, or third-degree AV block. Wide-QRS AV block bradycardia can also occur.

   c. Therapy is as described in the ACLS bradycardia algorithm (Figure 1–3).

     (1) Atropine (0.5–1.0 mg for adults; 0.01–0.02 mg/kg for pediatric patients) should be administered intravenously every 3–5 minutes to a total dose of 3 mg for adults and 0.04 mg/kg for children.

     (2) Transcutaneous pacing should be considered.

     (3) Dopamine (5–20 μg/kg/min) or **epinephrine** (2–10 μg/min for adults; 0.05–2 μg/kg/min for pediatric patients) should be considered.

   d. Disposition. The patient should be admitted to a telemetry unit or the CCU.

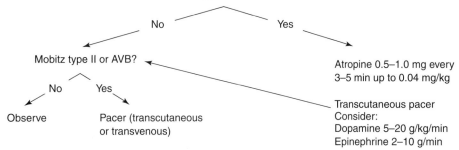

ABCs, oxygen, 12-lead ECG, IV access, review history

Treat the unstable patient immediately. Signs and symptoms of instability include ischemia, shortness of breath, decreased mental status, hypotension or shock, and CHF.

No — Yes

Mobitz type II or AVB?

No — Yes

Observe

Pacer (transcutaneous or transvenous)

Atropine 0.5–1.0 mg every 3–5 min up to 0.04 mg/kg

Transcutaneous pacer
Consider:
Dopamine 5–20 g/kg/min
Epinephrine 2–10 g/min

FIGURE 1–3 Advanced cardiac life support (ACLS) algorithm for bradycardia. *ABCs* = airway, breathing, circulation; *AVB* = atrioventricular block; *CHF* = congestive heart failure; *ECG* = electrocardiogram; *IV* = intravenous. Reprinted with permission from the *Massachusetts General Hospital Medical Housestaff Manual 1996–1997*.

B **Acute MI** is discussed in Chapter 2 II B 5.

C **Stroke** is discussed in Chapter 9 III A 4.

D **Electrocution**

1. Victims of electrocution may present with **cardiac arrest** due to depolarization of the myo-cardium by the external energy source. Ventricular fibrillation is common with low-voltage shock and asystole is common with high-voltage shock (e.g., lightning). **Respiratory arrest** may occur secondary to direct damage to the midbrain respiratory center or as a result of tetanic contraction of the respiratory musculature. **Associated conditions** that can complicate the resuscitation effort include fractures, myoglobinuria, head injury, and nerve injury.

2. The **extent of injury** is determined by:
   a. The **type of current** (an alternating current is more dangerous than a direct current, because alternating currents can induce tetany)
   b. The **duration of exposure**
   c. The **pathway of the current** (the hand-to-hand transthoracic path is associated with a higher mortality rate than the hand-to-foot path)

3. The **mortality rate** ranges from 15%–30%. Respiratory paralysis often outlasts transient asystole, leading to a second, hypoxic, arrest as the terminal event.

E **Near-drowning** is defined as temporary recovery after submersion injury.

1. Adverse consequences causing arrest are **hypoxemia, acidosis,** and **pulmonary edema** caused by alveolar damage.

2. Resuscitation is guided as usual with particular **emphasis on airway management.** Over-aggressive suctioning (to remove fluid from the airway) may cause aspiration and prolong definitive airway management. An orogastric tube may be placed after intubation to decrease the risk of further aspiration.

F **Hypothermia** is defined as a decrease in the core body temperature to below 35°C. Severe hypothermia is defined as a decrease in the core body temperature to below 30°C.

1. Patients may have **severe depression of cerebral and cardiac function,** appearing clinically dead. Resuscitation from this state is possible and so all appropriate efforts must be made to warm the patient and restore vital signs before declaring death (thus the phrase, "You are not dead until you are warm and dead").

   a. Symptoms of moderate hypothermia include lack of shivering, decreased respiratory rate, depressed mental status, muscular rigidity, bradyarrhythmias, and decreased reflexes.

   b. Symptoms of severe hypothermia may include hypotension, apnea, ventricular fibrillation, and asystole.

2. Resuscitation efforts follow the standard format. Warm, humidified oxygen should be provided. **Rapid core rewarming** is the key to resuscitation. Rewarming alternatives include warmed intravenous fluids provided centrally, peritoneal lavage with warm, potassium-free fluid, pleural lavage via a chest tube thoracostomy, and cardiopulmonary bypass. Selection of rewarming modality depends on the patient's condition and available alternatives. Defibrillation attempts may be ineffective until the core temperature is greater than 30°C.

G **Pregnancy** Cardiac arrest is rare during pregnancy. Causes of arrest include pulmonary embolism, trauma, CHF, MI, amniotic fluid embolism, and peripartum hemorrhage or hypovolemia. Initially, resuscitation of the pregnant patient should follow the same guidelines as if there were no pregnancy. **Special considerations** include the following:

1. Hemodynamic changes of pregnancy include an increase in maternal blood volume and cardiac output of up to 50%. Uterine blood flow accounts for 20% of cardiac output at term. Systemic peripheral vascular resistance is decreased.

2. Pulmonary changes that occur in pregnancy include a decrease in the functional residual capacity and decreased pulmonary vascular resistance.

3. The enlarged uterus compresses the inferior vena cava and impedes venous return in the supine position. **Positioning the patient on her left side and displacing the uterus from the inferior vena cava may resolve hypotension and hasten stabilization.**

4. In the setting of cardiac arrest unresponsive to standard therapy after 5 minutes, perimortem cesarean section should be performed immediately if the fetus is past the age of viability (if possible, ultrasound is used to assess fetal size and cardiac activity). Perimortem cesarean section may be lifesaving for both the fetus and the mother.

Study Questions

Directions: *Each of the numbered items or incomplete statements in this section is followed by answers or by completions of the statement. Select the ONE lettered answer or completion that is BEST in each case.*

1. A 56-year-old woman is found apneic and pulseless. Cardiac monitoring shows sinus tachycardia at a rate of 130 beats/min. What actions are the appropriate next step in the management of this patient?

- (A) Initiation of cardiopulmonary resuscitation (CPR) and administration of a 500-mL fluid bolus of normal saline
- (B) Intubation and the administration of amiodarone
- (C) Initiation of CPR and the administration of atropine
- (D) Initiation of CPR and unsynchronized countershock with 200 joules
- (E) Initiation of CPR and synchronized countershock with 50 joules

2. Which one of the following is the most common cause of airway obstruction?

- (A) Tracheal–laryngeal fracture
- (B) Foreign body
- (C) Pooled secretions
- (D) Prolapse of the tongue
- (E) Fractured mandible

3. A 27-year-old man with severe hypovolemia requires rapid fluid resuscitation. Which one of the following catheters would be ideal for this resuscitation effort?

- (A) 12-inch 8 French introducer
- (B) 5½-inch 9 French introducer
- (C) 2-inch 14-gauge catheter
- (D) 12-inch 16-gauge catheter
- (E) 5-inch, 16-gauge catheter

4. Rapid sequence induction (RSI) using lidocaine, thiopental, and succinylcholine is most appropriate for which one of the following patients?

- (A) A 67-year-old woman with sudden-onset hemiplegia who is nonverbal with pooled secretions in her oropharynx and who appears slightly cyanotic, with a blood pressure of 220/115 mm Hg and a pulse rate of 60 beats/min
- (B) A 24-year-old man who was thrown 25 feet from a motorcycle and who was unconscious in the field and is still unconscious, with a blood pressure of 86/46 mm Hg and a pulse rate of 110 beats/min
- (C) A 24-year-old woman with severe exacerbation of her asthma and a blood pressure of 170/100 mm Hg
- (D) A 92-year-old man with sudden-onset aphasia, pooled secretions, a blood pressure of 90/60 mm Hg, and a pulse rate of 110 beats/min
- (E) A 64-year-old man with rapid-onset tongue edema suspected to be caused by angioedema induced by therapy with a new angiotensin-converting enzyme (ACE) inhibitor

5. A 28-year-old woman who is 38 weeks pregnant is resuscitated by paramedics and brought to the emergency department (ED). The patient is hypotensive and groans spontaneously. What is the first step in treating this patient?

- (A) Administering a 500-mL fluid challenge
- (B) Performing a perimortem cesarean section

C Positioning the patient on her left side

D Administering 1 mg epinephrine intravenously

E Initiating rapid sequence induction (RSI)

6. A 50-year-old man presents to the emergency department (ED) complaining of "palpitations." In the triage area, he collapses after complaining of shortness of breath and substernal chest pain. Quick-look with a cardiac monitor reveals a regular, narrow QRS complex and a heart rate of 200 beats/min. A tentative diagnosis of paroxysmal supraventricular tachycardia is made. What is the most appropriate first intervention?

A Vagal maneuvers

B Adenosine, 6 mg administered intravenously

C Synchronized countershock at 200 joules

D Synchronized countershock at 50 joules

E Unsynchronized countershock at 200 joules

7. Which one of the following induction agents causes a dissociative state and is associated with relaxation of bronchial smooth muscle?

A Fentanyl

B Ketamine

C Etomidate

D Midazolam

E Thiopental

8. Which one of the following means of providing supplemental oxygen allows the most precise adjustment of oxygen concentration?

A Bag-valve-mask system

B Nonrebreather mask

C Standard (simple) face mask

D Venturi mask

E Nasal cannula

9. An elderly patient presents to the emergency department (ED) with severe pulmonary edema and an initial room-air oxygen saturation of 86%. Oxygen saturation increases to 98% with supplemental oxygen and bilevel positive airway pressure (BiPAP) via face mask; however, the patient is clearly too fatigued to continue spontaneous respirations much longer and intubation is required. When commencing rapid sequence induction (RSI), which one of the following actions is most appropriate?

A The patient should be preoxygenated for several minutes with vigorous bag-valve-mask assisted ventilation.

B The patient should be preoxygenated for several minutes with a tight-fitting nonrebreathing mask, unassisted bag-valve-mask ventilation, or by several full volume breaths via a bag-valve-mask just before intubation.

C A nasogastric tube should be placed to remove the gastric contents prior to intubation (to decrease the risk of aspiration).

D The Sellick maneuver should be performed once the decision to intubate has been made.

E The patient should be aggressively ventilated throughout the RSI protocol.

Answers and Explanations

1. The answer is A The patient is in pulseless electrical activity (PEA). The most common cause of reversible PEA is hypovolemia. In addition to establishing the ABCs (airway, breathing, and circulation), chest compressions and a fluid challenge (i.e., the administration of 500 mL of normal saline or lactated Ringer's solution) are indicated. Epinephrine may be indicated for the treatment of PEA following a fluid challenge. Amiodarone, atropine, and cardioversion have no role in the treatment of PEA.

2. The answer is D The tongue is the most common cause of airway obstruction because it easily prolapses into the posterior oropharynx. The head-tilt/chin-lift and jaw-thrust maneuvers move the tongue forward and prevent obstruction. Oropharyngeal airway (OPA) and nasopharyngeal airway (NPA) devices also relieve obstruction caused by the tongue. Foreign bodies and facial, mandibular, or tracheal–laryngeal fractures can also result in airway obstruction, but are not the most common causes. Pooled oral secretions are an indication that the patient has lost the ability to swallow (and, therefore, is incapable of clearing the airway).

3. The answer is B The flow through any catheter is limited by length and diameter. The most rapid rate of fluid infusion occurs with the catheter of the widest diameter and shortest length. Flow is limited by the catheter, not the size or location of the vein cannulated. The 8 French and 9 French introducer catheters have the fastest flow rates (247 mL/min and 243 mL/min, respectively). According to the Hagen-Poiseuille equation, doubling the length of the catheter will decrease the flow by one half; therefore, the best choice would be the shorter of the two (i.e., the 5½-inch 9 French introducer catheter).

4. The answer is A Lidocaine and thiopental are used in RSIs where there is concern for increased intracranial pressure (ICP) normally associated with intubation, as in the woman with sudden-onset hemiplegia. Thiopental is contraindicated for those who do not have adequate blood pressure, such as the motorcycle rider and the elderly man with sudden-onset aphasia. The asthmatic patient will probably not benefit from the addition of lidocaine to the sequence, but ketamine would be a good medicine. The patient with angioedema is a poor candidate for induction using paralytic agents, and fiberoptic intubation should thus be considered.

5. The answer is C Resuscitation of the pregnant patient must take into consideration the physiologic and anatomic changes of pregnancy. The most common cause of hypotension in late pregnancy is compression of the inferior vena cava by the gravid uterus, resulting in decreased venous return and reduced cardiac output. Positioning the patient to the left helps relieve this pressure on the inferior vena cava, which is located to the right of the aorta. Perimortem cesarean section is indicated following 5 minutes of cardiac arrest that is unresponsive to standard therapy. The need for intubation and fluid or pharmacologic intervention is assessed in the usual manner after repositioning of the patient.

6. The answer is D The patient presents with paroxysmal supraventricular tachycardia and is unstable, as evidenced by his shortness of breath, chest pain, and syncope. Unstable paroxysmal supraventricular tachycardia is treated with synchronized cardioversion starting at 50 joules. Unsynchronized countershock in this patient risks converting the rhythm to ventricular fibrillation. Vagal maneuvers followed by intravenous adenosine are appropriate first therapies for paroxysmal supraventricular tachycardia if the patient is stable.

7. The answer is B Ketamine is a phencyclidine (PCP) derivative that produces dissociative anesthesia, and also relaxation of bronchial smooth muscle. It is the only anesthetic agent that provides analgesia, sedation, and hypnotic properties. Fentanyl provides for analgesia and sedation, but has no inherent hypnotic properties.

8. The answer is D The Venturi mask allows adjustment of inspired oxygen via adjustment of the oxygen flow rate. The ability to precisely control the oxygen concentration can be useful when titrating to oxygen requirements, particularly in patients with chronic obstructive pulmonary disease (COPD) who retain carbon dioxide and are at risk of losing their remaining respiratory drive in the setting of high-flow oxygen. A nasal cannula allows adjustment of the concentration of delivered oxygen, but final inspired oxygen levels depend on many patient factors. Nonrebreather masks provide the highest inspired oxygen levels, but they are not adjustable.

9. The answer is B Before commencing with RSI, the patient should be preoxygenated for several minutes with a tightly fitting nonrebreather mask or unassisted bag-valve-mask ventilation, or asked to take several full-volume breaths via a bag-valve-mask device just prior to intubation. A frequent error committed by well-meaning participants involved in RSI is overzealous ventilation of the patient using a bag-valve-mask system. While there may be some severely hypoxic patients who require such vigorous "bagging," many patients do not need such extreme mechanical ventilation. The resultant gastric filling can increase the risk of vomiting and aspiration. Nasogastric intubation takes time, poses the risk of aspiration, and interferes with the administration of supplemental oxygen. The Sellick maneuver (i.e., application of pressure to the cricoid cartilage) should be performed when the patient is no longer able to protect his or her own airway (as the result of sedation medications or the administration of paralytic agents), not once the decision to intubate has been made. The point of RSI is not to ventilate the patient following paralysis. Preoxygenation should be sufficient.

PART **II**

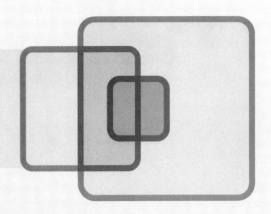

Medical Emergencies

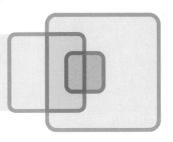

chapter 2

Cardiovascular Emergencies

ANTHONY J. DEAN · KATHLEEN M. BEAVER

I CHEST PAIN

A Discussion

1. **Visceral pain.** Visceral afferent fibers are present in the sympathetic and parasympathetic nerves of the chest. These nonmyelinated fibers provide sensation from the heart, pericardium, lungs, and all visceral structures embryologically derived from the foregut. **Pain** signals are **poorly localized** and **perceived as "dull" or "aching."**

2. **Somatic pain.** Somatic innervation gives rise to sensation from the mesodermal structures (e.g., the parietal pleura and peritoneum and muscular, skeletal, and dermal structures). Most fibers have precise somatotropic and dermatomal organization, giving rise to **pain perceived as well localized** and **"sharp."**

3. **Referred pain.** Both visceral and somatic afferent fibers share synaptic projections in the spinal cord and brain stem, which can cause visceral pain signals to be perceived in somatic structures. An example is the classic radiation of cardiac pain to the arms, neck, teeth, or jaw.

4. **"Atypical" chest pain** is a term often used to refer to chest pain that does not clearly fit in any category. The use of this term as shorthand for "nonsignificant chest pain" should be avoided, because many serious diseases present atypically.

B Clinical features

1. **History.** The history is the most important tool in determining the cause of a patient's pain.
   a. **Description of pain.** A description of the pain with regard to its onset, location, quality, duration, and radiation must be obtained.
      (1) The patient should be questioned regarding exacerbating and relieving factors, such as activity, position, exertion, swallowing (solids versus liquids), meals, respiration, and medications (especially analgesic and antacid use).
      (2) The distinction between visceral and somatic pain is clinically useful but not well defined. Deep skeletal structures such as joint capsules and vertebrae are innervated by poorly localized nonmyelinated fibers. Conversely, disease processes in visceral organs can irritate adjacent somatically innervated structures; for example, myocardial infarction (MI) can cause pericardial irritation, leading to the typical sharp pain of pericarditis.
   b. **Description of previous episodes.** A history of previous episodes of chest pain or trauma should be sought.
   c. **Determination of risk factors.** Many significant causes of chest pain have identifiable risk factors; therefore, the patient's family history, medical history, and social history (especially concerning the use of tobacco, cocaine, or alcohol) may reveal clues pertinent to the current episode.

2. **Symptoms**
   a. **Symptoms of acute, critical illness.** Recognition of the following symptoms mandates immediate intervention according to the ABC principle (airway, breathing, and circulation; see Chapter 1) prior to further evaluation or work-up.

(1) **Inability to speak**
(2) **Difficulty breathing**
(3) **Thready pulse**
(4) **Rapid** or **very slow heart rate**
(5) **Systolic blood pressure less than 100 mm Hg**
(6) **Diaphoresis**
(7) **Confusion**

b. **Autonomic symptoms** (e.g., **nausea, vomiting, diaphoresis, tachypnea, eructation**) are often associated with visceral chest pain as a result of neural connections in the brain stem and in autonomic ganglia.

c. **Palpitations, dizziness, fever, coughing,** or **weakness** may be seen, depending on the underlying cause of the chest pain.

C Differential diagnoses

1. **Life-threatening causes of chest pain**

a. **Myocardial ischemia.** The signs and symptoms of MI and stable and unstable angina are discussed in II.

b. **Pulmonary embolism** causes a spectrum of symptoms ranging from no chest pain at all, to sharp, pleuritic, or dull chest pain (see Chapter 3 VI). The traditional wisdom that pulmonary embolism always causes pleuritic chest pain (more accurately termed "respirophasic" pain—pain that changes with respiration) is based on studies of hospitalized patients, and even in this group, pleuritic chest pain is described only 75% of the time.

c. **Aortic dissection** is discussed in XII A.

d. **Cardiac tamponade** is discussed in IX C.

e. **Tension pneumothorax.** Patients usually present with dyspnea accompanied by the signs or symptoms of shock. In most cases, the complaint of pain occurs in the context of a known history of trauma. Still, tension pneumothorax evolving from spontaneous pneumothorax is a consideration in a patient with respiratory distress and chest pain.

f. **Acute esophageal perforation** can cause sharp pleuritic, poorly localized, midline pain anywhere from the base of the neck to the epigastrium. Pain is not invariably present initially, but with the development of mediastinitis over the following days, pain becomes more diffuse, constant, and severe, and is associated with systemic signs of infection.

2. **Serious but not immediately life-threatening causes of chest pain**

a. **Stable angina** is discussed in II A.

b. **Pneumothorax** (see also Chapter 3 X) can be traumatic or spontaneous (i.e., atraumatic). The former usually presents little diagnostic difficulty. Spontaneous pneumothorax is often associated with minimal symptoms and mild chest discomfort without significant dyspnea. In view of these nonspecific clinical findings, the emergency physician should have a low threshold for obtaining chest radiographs in patients with atypical chest discomfort.

c. **Pneumonia** is suggested by cough and fever with or without chest pain. The pain is classically sharp, localized, and pleuritic in nature.

d. **Abdominal processes.** Diseases of the stomach, liver, gallbladder, spleen, and kidneys can cause chest pain by one of several mechanisms.

(1) **Referred pain.** Pain fibers from the gallbladder can lead to the perception of pain in the right scapular region, and pain fibers from the spleen can lead to the perception of pain in the left scapular area. Painful processes affecting the central diaphragm can be referred to the third and fourth cervical dermatomes.

(2) **Pain originating from structures in direct proximity to the diaphragm** can be perceived as originating in the chest. Sources of this type of pain include **subdiaphragmatic abscesses** and **perforated peptic ulcers.**

(3) Extension of abdominal disease processes into the chest can lead to chest pain. Examples include diaphragmatic herniation of abdominal viscera and the development of pleural effusions or empyema secondary to a hepatic or subdiaphragmatic abscess.

3. **Chronic or benign causes of chest pain**
   a. **Pericarditis** is discussed in IX A.
   b. **Mitral valve prolapse** is discussed in VIII B 3.
   c. **Esophageal diseases** usually cause a poorly defined, burning, midsternal chest pain that can often be reproduced by asking the patient to swallow cold fluids or food. Pain of esophageal origin is referred in the same pattern as that of the heart, making for diagnostic difficulties. When there is doubt, the physician should assume that the pain is cardiac in origin and act accordingly pending further work-up.
   d. **Musculoskeletal disorders.** Patients describe well-localized pain that can be reproduced by palpation or specific movements. Causes include muscle strain, costosternal and costochondral inflammation, osteoarthritis of the spine, and bursitis, arthritis, or tendinitis of the shoulder girdle. Such conditions can coexist with serious causes of chest pain.
   e. **Pulmonary** and **abdominal processes** of a less life-threatening nature include viral pneumonitis, pleurisy, nonperforating peptic ulcer, biliary disease, chronic pancreatitis, and most forms of hepatitis.

D **Evaluation**   Most patients with chest pain should be placed on supplemental oxygen and monitored using a pulse oximeter, cardiac monitor, and blood pressure monitor until it is determined that they are not at risk for acute decompensation and do not require emergent intervention.

1. **Physical examination**
   a. As a part of the initial assessment of the ABCs, the vital signs should be noted prior to even obtaining the history.
   b. Initial attention to the cardiopulmonary examination should be followed by a comprehensive examination in all stable patients.

2. **Diagnostic tests**
   a. **Electrocardiography.** The electrocardiogram (ECG) gives direct and indirect information about many of the causes of chest pain. For this reason, an ECG should be obtained in all patients in whom the history and physical examination have not definitively ruled out a cardiopulmonary etiology. Conversely, a normal ECG does not exclude any cause of chest pain.
   b. **Radiography.** A chest radiograph, like electrocardiography, is a rapid, noninvasive, and inexpensive way of ruling out or identifying many of the diseases in the differential diagnosis [e.g., pneumothorax, pneumonia, congestive heart failure (CHF) and, indirectly, pulmonary embolus and aortic dissection]. A chest radiograph should be obtained unless the patient clearly has a disorder for which it is noncontributory.
   c. **Arterial blood gas (ABG).** An ABG is rarely diagnostic, but can be used as a measure of severity of illness or to assess acid–base status.
   d. **Pulse oximetry** provides instant information about a patient's oxygenation status.
   e. **Other laboratory studies** should be obtained as guided by the clinical evaluation (e.g., **cardiac enzyme studies** should be obtained in patients suspected of having ischemia).
   f. **Bedside echocardiography** is diagnostic of cardiac tamponade and can provide information about cardiac wall motion and valvular function.

E **Disposition**

1. **Admission**
   a. Patients with chest pain due to life-threatening causes require admission to an intensive care unit (ICU) and in some instances will require emergent cardiac catheterization or surgery. Early subspecialty consultation in the emergency department (ED) is indicated.

    b. Patients with serious but not life-threatening causes of chest pain will most likely require admission to the hospital for further evaluation and treatment. Discussion with the patient's primary physician provides additional historical information and ensures coordinated outpatient follow-up for those patients well enough for discharge.

  2. Discharge. Patients with benign or chronic causes of chest pain can, in most instances, be safely discharged with a prescription for analgesics and arrangements for outpatient follow-up.

II MYOCARDIAL ISCHEMIC DISEASE

Myocardial ischemic disease encompasses angina, MI, acute coronary syndrome, and cardiogenic shock.

A Angina

1. Discussion

  a. Definition. Angina means pain, understood to refer to pain of cardiac origin, and implies myocardial ischemia.

  b. Mechanisms. Ischemia results from an imbalance between myocardial oxygen demand and supply.

    (1) Decreased myocardial oxygen supply

      (a) Coronary artery occlusion resulting from **atherosclerosis** of coronary arteries is the most common cause of ischemic heart disease and is the focus of this section. Other causes of coronary artery occlusion include **coronary artery spasm, dissection, arteritis,** and **embolism.**

      (b) Decreased coronary artery perfusion pressure (e.g., as a result of hypotension, shock, or aortic regurgitation) can lead to decreased myocardial oxygen supply.

      (c) Anemia, hypoxia, and **carbon monoxide poisoning** are other causes of decreased oxygen delivery to the myocardium.

    (2) Increased myocardial oxygen demand can be due to many causes, including hypertension, hypertrophy, aortic stenosis, and emotional or physical stress.

  c. Pathogenesis of coronary occlusion

    (1) Atherosclerotic narrowing of the coronary arterial lumen occurs gradually and will usually give rise to a pattern of stable anginal symptoms related to exertion and recognized by the patient. Angina typically occurs with exercise when the artery is 75% occluded, and at rest when the artery is 90% occluded.

    (2) Acute coronary occlusion may be caused by thrombus formation or embolization. These acute events can cause unstable angina or MI.

    (3) Vasospasm, which can cause myocardial ischemia or infarct and usually occurs proximally in the artery at the site of an atherosclerotic plaque, can be a cause of Prinzmetal's (variant) angina.

2. Clinical features

  a. Patient history

    (1) Symptoms. Patients typically describe the pain of angina as "dull," "pressure-like," "heavy," "squeezing," and poorly localized. Patients may demonstrate Levine's sign (i.e., the clenching of a fist in front of the sternum to describe the pain). Associated symptoms include nausea, vomiting, diaphoresis, shortness of breath, syncope, and palpitations. Pain can radiate to the arms, neck, or jaw.

      (a) Anginal equivalent symptoms do not fit the strict definition of angina. Examples include jaw, neck, or epigastric pain, shortness of breath, and eructation. Patients may recognize their own anginal equivalent, and a high index of suspicion should be maintained for patients complaining of these symptoms.

      (b) Vague symptoms in elderly or diabetic patients (e.g., dizziness, syncope, confusion, symptoms of peripheral emboli, or unexplained hypotension) may represent silent ischemia or infarct. In patients older than 75 years, 50% of infarcts occur without chest pain.

(2) **Patterns.** Details of the history of chest pain should be obtained (see I B 1).

    (a) **Stable angina** occurs in a pattern of frequency, intensity, and associated level of exertion that is recognized as "usual" by the individual patient. The pain should also have an identifiable pattern of relief with rest and nitroglycerin.

    (b) **Unstable angina** is characterized by symptoms that are different from the "usual" pattern and is frequently a prelude to infarction. Patients with a first episode of angina, or without prior evaluation, have unstable angina.

    (c) **Prinzmetal's (variant) angina** often occurs with an explosive onset, waking patients from sleep.

(3) **Risk factors** must be elicited and include a personal history of ischemic heart disease, a family history of ischemic heart disease before age 55, smoking, hypertension, male sex, increasing age, and elevated serum cholesterol.

  b. **Physical examination findings** are rarely contributory.

    (1) The blood pressure and respiratory rate are typically elevated, but otherwise, the vital signs are usually normal.

    (2) The patient may be diaphoretic and pale, with cool, clammy extremities.

    (3) Signs of CHF may be present (see III B 2).

3. **Differential diagnoses** include those discussed in I C.

4. **Evaluation**

  a. **Electrocardiography.** An ECG should be performed to risk-stratify patients. The ECG is normal in 50% of patients with angina who are pain-free. In patients who are experiencing pain, acute ischemia may be represented by ST-segment and T-wave abnormalities.

    (1) Classically, ST-segment depression and T-wave inversion suggest nontransmural (subendocardial) ischemia (Figure 2–1), whereas Prinzmetal's angina and transmural ischemia cause ST-segment elevation similar to the pattern of acute infarction (Figure 2–2).

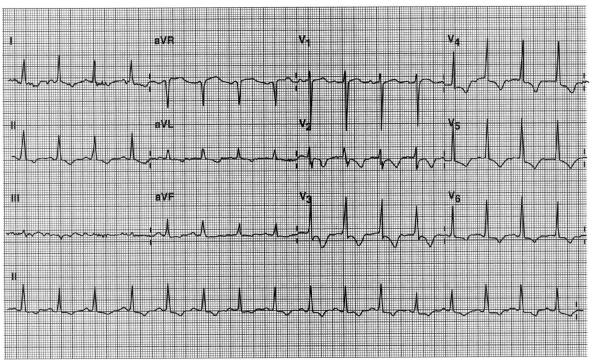

FIGURE 2–1 Electrocardiogram (ECG) strip showing anterior, septal, and lateral nontransmural (subendocardial) ischemia. Symmetrical T-wave inversion and ST-segment depression are noted in leads I, II, aVL, and V₂–V₆.

A

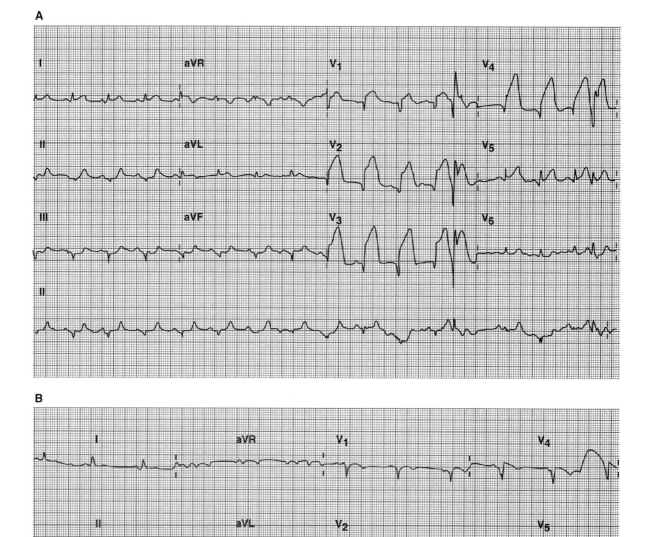

B

FIGURE 2–2 **(A)** Electrocardiogram (ECG) showing anterior septal myocardial infarction (MI). Transmural ischemia is evidenced by ST-segment elevation and hyperacute T waves seen in leads V_1–V_5. **(B)** ECG from the same patient, 24 hours later. Q-wave development, resolution of the ST-segment elevation, and T-wave inversion in leads V_1–V_5 are evident.

TABLE 2–1   Location of Cardiac Ischemia or Infarction as Suggested by Findings in Various Electrocardiogram (ECG) Leads

Location of Ischemia or Infarct	Leads in Which Abnormalities Are Seen
Inferior wall	II, III, aVF
Lateral wall	I, aVL, V_5, V_6
Anterolateral region	V_1–V_6, I, aVL
Anterior wall	V_1, V_2
Anteroseptal region	V_1–V_4
Right ventricle	V_3R–V_6R
Posterior wall	V_1, V_2, V_7–V_9

(2) The leads in which ST-segment abnormalities are seen suggest the area of ischemic myocardium (Table 2–1).

b. **Radiography.** A chest radiograph should be performed to search for signs of CHF or lung disease.

c. **Laboratory studies.** A blood sample should be evaluated for cardiac enzymes, electrolytes, and blood urea nitrogen (BUN) and creatinine levels. A complete blood count (CBC) and baseline coagulation studies should be performed as well.

5. **Therapy.** Patients should be placed on a monitor and receive oxygen, 3 L by nasal canula, and on an intravenous line with normal saline at a keep vein open (KVO) rate in the ED, after determining that immediate instability and deterioration are not present.

   a. **Stable angina.** A patient who has had an episode of stable angina, and is now pain-free, should be monitored for a period to ensure that there is no recurrence of pain. An ECG should be obtained, and some advocate checking cardiac enzyme levels [see II B 4 c (1)].

   b. **Unstable angina.** Goals in the treatment of patients with unstable angina are to prevent further coronary thrombosis, to minimize workload, to maximize oxygenation of the myocardium, and to control pain. In most cases, these goals can be accomplished with oxygen, aspirin, heparin, nitrates, and β blockers.

      (1) **Oxygen** should be provided by nasal cannula at a rate of at least 2 L/min.

         (a) It should be given in high concentrations by face mask if the patient is cyanotic or has a pulse oximetry reading of less than 95%.

         (b) If the patient has a history of chronic obstructive pulmonary disease (COPD), oxygen should not be withheld, but the patient should be monitored carefully for signs of respiratory depression (e.g., somnolence, confusion, lethargy).

      (2) **Aspirin** (325 mg) should be given. The patient should chew the tablets to accelerate the antithrombotic effect. Aspirin can be tolerated by patients with peptic ulcer disease unless they are actively hemorrhaging.

      (3) **Heparin** should be given in a bolus of 80 U/kg and started as an infusion at a rate of 15 U/kg/hour. The partial thromboplastin time (PTT) should be checked after 6 hours; the goal is an international normalized ratio (INR) of 1.5 to 2.5. Also consider enoxaparin (Lovenox) 1 mg/kg subcutaneously every 12 hours.

      (4) **Nitroglycerin** decreases cardiac preload and afterload and dilates the coronary arteries. Sublingual nitroglycerin is preferred to intravenous nitroglycerin initially because a therapeutic blood level can be obtained much more rapidly with sublingual administration.

         (a) **Sublingual.** If the patient is presently experiencing pain, 1/150 grain (400 μg) should be administered sublingually unless the patient's systolic blood pressure is less than 90 mm Hg.

(i) The dose should be repeated every 5 minutes until the pain is relieved, the systolic blood pressure decreases to below 90 mm Hg, or a total of three nitroglycerin tablets or sprays have been given, whichever occurs first.

(ii) Patients who have never taken nitroglycerin can be very sensitive to its effects. A lower dose can be given using 1/200 or 1/300 tablets or by breaking the 1/150 tablet in half with a fingernail.

(b) **Intravenous.** If pain persists, intravenous nitroglycerin should be started and titrated to maintain the systolic blood pressure at 90–100 mm Hg. While the intravenous dosage is being adjusted, it is often necessary to give additional sublingual doses to control blood pressure and/or pain.

(c) **Dermal.** Once the pain has been relieved, nitroglycerin paste is applied to the skin.

(5) **Morphine** should be given in 2- to 5-mg aliquots if the patient has persistent chest pain, elevated blood pressure, or both.

(6) **β Blockers** may be helpful, especially if the patient is tachycardic and hypertensive. β Blockers are contraindicated in patients with hypotension, severe asthma, emphysema, CHF, high-grade heart block, severe bradycardia, or peripheral vascular disease with peripheral cyanosis.

(a) **Esmolol** is a β_1-selective agent with a half-life of 9 minutes.

(b) **Metoprolol,** also a β_1-selective agent, can be given by intravenous push in three separate 5-mg doses, titrating for effect on blood pressure and heart rate.

(7) **Calcium channel blockers** are indicated in the treatment of Prinzmetal's angina, but are otherwise of controversial utility.

6. **Disposition**

a. **Admission.** Unstable angina requires admission to at least a telemetry unit. If the pain is ongoing or difficult to control, if there is significant ECG evidence of ischemia, or if the patient is in any other way unstable, admission should be to the coronary care unit (CCU).

b. **Discharge.** Stable angina does not require admission. Because it is unusual for patients with stable angina to present to the ED, it is advisable to consult with the patient's primary care physician to ensure that the evaluation is consistent with the patient's known disease, and to coordinate follow-up.

B Myocardial infarction

1. **Discussion**

a. **Incidence.** In the United States, approximately 1.5 million patients each year experience acute MI; half of these MIs are fatal. The mortality rate is much lower, about 7%, for those patients reaching the ED alive. Patients discharged with a missed MI have a 14% mortality rate.

b. **Pathogenesis.** The risk factors and pathogenesis of MI are the same as those of angina. A number of complications can occur with MI and contribute significantly to morbidity and mortality rates. Complications include:

(1) Ventricular dysfunction, leading to shock, CHF, or chronically impaired cardiac output

(2) Conduction system damage, leading to bradycardia, heart block, and bundle branch blocks

(a) Inferior wall MI frequently affects the sinoatrial (SA) node, atrioventricular (AV) node, or both.

(b) Anterior wall MI can damage the His-Purkinje system.

(3) Other dysrhythmias, caused by repolarization abnormalities and myocardial irritability

(4) Tissue necrosis, leading to papillary muscle rupture, acute valvular incompetence, and ventricular free wall or septal wall rupture. Most such complications are fatal, but may be present in patients in shock.

(5) Intracardiac thrombus formation, leading to systemic emboli and arterial insufficiency

(6) Acute pericarditis, which can occur at any time during the 2 months following MI

c. **Types**

(1) **Q-wave MI** is not synonymous with transmural infarction, although 80% of Q-wave MIs are transmural. Q-wave MI tends to develop after transmural ischemia and is indicated by ST-segment elevation and peaked T waves (see Figure 2–2). Q-wave MI is associated with more extensive immediate damage and complications.

(2) **Non–Q-wave MI** may be transmural, but is more commonly caused by incomplete coronary artery occlusion, leading to subendocardial ischemia. It is indicated by ST-segment depression and T-wave inversion (see Figure 2–1). The immediate mortality rate is lower than that of Q-wave MI, but the incidence of reinfarction is higher. Mortality rates for the two types equalize after 3 years.

2. **Clinical features**

a. **History.** The focus of the history is the same as that discussed in I B 1. A clear history of the duration of continuous pain prior to ED presentation is essential for making decisions concerning thrombolysis.

b. **Physical examination findings**

(1) Vital sign abnormalities are nonspecific but may reflect some of the acute complications noted in II B 1 b.

(2) Cardiac examination may reveal a third or fourth heart sound (S_3 or S_4) suggestive of decreased ventricular compliance, increased end-diastolic pressure, or early ventricular failure, or a systolic murmur indicative of either papillary muscle dysfunction or rupture or of interventricular septal rupture. The physician should search for signs of left- or right-sided CHF (see III B 3).

3. **Differential diagnoses** include those discussed in I C. Because of the potential need for anticoagulation and thrombolytic therapy, it is essential to rule out aortic dissection, tamponade, and acute pericarditis.

4. **Evaluation.** The patient should be monitored for cardiac arrhythmias and oxygenation status, and an intravenous line for the administration of normal saline at a KVO rate should be placed. Continuous blood pressure monitoring is contraindicated with thrombolytic therapy, unless the patient is unstable.

a. **Electrocardiography.** An ECG must be obtained immediately. The ECG abnormalities characteristic of infarction are (in decreasing order of specificity): ST-segment elevation, "hyperacute" T waves, Q waves, ST-segment depression, T-wave inversions, and conduction abnormalities. A normal ECG does not rule out MI.

(1) The **time course** of the MI is suggested by characteristic ECG changes (see Figure 2–2):

(a) Minutes after the onset of ischemia, peaked "hyperacute" T waves may develop.

(b) Minutes to hours after the onset of ischemia, ST segments become elevated in transmural ischemia.

(c) T-wave inversions and Q-wave development occur in the same leads over a period of hours to days.

(2) The **location** of either ischemia or infarction is suggested by the ECG leads in which abnormalities are seen (see Table 2–1, Figure 2–1, Figure 2–2).

(3) The ECG abnormalities of MI persist despite ED interventions, whereas those of ischemia subside with appropriate therapy (e.g., oxygen, pain relief).

b. **Cardiac ultrasonography** may reveal acute valvular dysfunction, wall motion abnormalities, or pericardial fluid collections.

c. **Laboratory studies**

(1) **Cardiac enzyme studies. Creatinine phosphokinase** is an enzyme released from damaged muscle. Elevations due to myocardial damage are distinguished by concomitant elevations of the MB isoenzyme fraction. Creatinine phosphokinase elevations are found in 50%, 75%, and 90% of MI patients at 3, 6, and 9 hours after the onset of pain, respectively.

TABLE 2–2   Time Course of Serum Markers in Acute Myocardial Infarction

Test	Onset	Peak	Duration
Creatinine	3–12 hours	18–24 hours	36–48 hours
Troponin	3–12 hours	18–24 hours	Up to 10 days
Myoglobin	1–4 hours	6–7 hours	24 hours
Lactate dehydrogenase	6–12 hours	24–48 hours	6–8 days

(2) **Assays for myoglobin, troponin,** and **lactate dehydrogenase** are now widely used (Table 2–2).

(3) **Other laboratory studies** are similar to those for patients with angina (see II A 4 c).

(4) **Time course of serum markers.** Time course of serum markers is used to diagnose an acute MI. Early onset of elevations of creatinine kinase (CK), both total and MB fraction, and troponin permits early detection of MI, while the short duration of the elevation of CK permits identification of infarct extensions. The long duration of troponin and lactate dehydrogenase permits the diagnosis to be established days after the acute event. Myoglobin is rarely used because it is not heart specific.

5. **Therapy.** Clinical assessment is ongoing in the ED to determine the efficacy of therapy.

   a. **Antianginal therapy** is initiated immediately (see II A 5 b).

   b. **Reperfusion therapy.** In a patient with ischemic chest pain, it is essential to rapidly decide whether the pain is due to angina or infarction and assess the indications and contraindications for reperfusion therapy [i.e., thrombolysis or percutaneous transluminal coronary angioplasty (PTCA)]. Minimizing the "door to drug" interval so that reperfusion therapy is initiated within 30 minutes of ED presentation is the goal.

      (1) **Thrombolysis**

         (a) **Indications**

            (i) Thrombolytic therapy is strongly indicated in eligible patients with signs and symptoms of acute MI, and in patients with ST-segment elevations of at least 0.1 mV in two ECG limb leads or 0.2 mV in two contiguous chest leads within 6 hours of the onset of symptoms.

            (ii) Thrombolytic therapy may be indicated in patients with nondiagnostic ECGs but with a clinical picture strongly suggestive of acute MI, or in patients with clinical and ECG findings as described in II B 5 b (1) (a) (i) that occur 6–24 hours after the onset of symptoms.

         (b) **Contraindications** for thrombolysis are listed in Table 2–3.

         (c) **Thrombolytic agents**

            (i) **Tissue plasminogen activator (t-PA)** is not antigenic and is associated with a lower incidence of hypotensive events than other thrombolytic agents, but is approximately six times more expensive than streptokinase (approximately $2500 per dose). The "front-loading" schedule is most often used: 15 mg initially over 2 minutes, 60 mg over the next 30 minutes, and 25 mg over the following hour for a total dose of 100 mg. Heparin (given in a bolus of 80 U/kg and started as an infusion at a rate of 15 U/kg/hour) is indicated after t-PA infusion.

            (ii) **Streptokinase** is the preferred thrombolytic agent in hypertensive women because it is associated with a lower incidence of hemorrhagic stroke, but otherwise, it has been found to be questionably less efficacious than t-PA. It is contraindicated in patients who have received the drug previously or have had a severe sore throat within the past 12 months. Streptokinase is usually given in a dose of 1.5 million U over 1 hour. Heparinization is not necessary.

TABLE 2–3   Contraindications to Thrombolytic Therapy

Absolute	Relative
Suspected aortic dissection or pericarditis	Cerebrovascular accident
Cerebrovascular accident	Conditions placing the patient at high risk of intracardiac
Cerebrovascular surgery within the previous 2 months	thrombus (e.g., atrial fibrillation, mitral valve stenosis)
Cerebrovascular neoplasm or aneurysm	Major surgery within the previous 2 months
Active bleeding in the gastrointestinal tract or other	Puncture of, or recent injury to, a noncompressible vessel
noncompressible site; hemorrhagic diathesis	within the previous 2 weeks
Major surgery within the previous 2 weeks	Uncontrolled hypertension
Pregnancy or 2 weeks postpartum status	Prolonged cardiopulmonary resuscitation
Allergy to thrombolytic agent	Metastatic cancer
Unstable angina	History of gastrointestinal bleeding
	Hemorrhagic retinopathy

      (d) Complications of thrombolytic therapy

          (i) Reperfusion arrhythmias of any kind can occur, but accelerated idioventricular rhythms and sinus bradycardia are characteristic. These arrhythmias do not require treatment unless they are causing hemodynamic instability.

          (ii) Reperfusion injury is thought to be responsible for the increase in mortality rate observed on the first day after MI in patients given thrombolytics. Evidence suggests that intravenous magnesium given before thrombolysis may be protective [see II B 5 c (4)].

    (2) PTCA is indicated when quickly available, especially in patients with MI who are in cardiogenic shock, who have contraindications to thrombolytic therapy, or who do not meet criteria for thrombolysis but have a high likelihood of infarction or intractable unstable angina. In most centers with active cath labs, PTCA has become the treatment of choice.

  c. Supportive therapy

    (1) Morphine should be given in 2- to 5-mg aliquots in patients who have persistent chest pain or elevated blood pressure.

    (2) β Blockers, administered intravenously, are indicated for all MI patients without overt CHF or other contraindications [see II A 5 b (6)].

    (3) Nitroglycerin [see II A 5 b (4)] is indicated for careful reduction of hypertension. Lowering the blood pressure decreases the workload of the heart, but also decreases coronary perfusion pressure. Elevations in blood pressure are better tolerated with lower heart rates. For these reasons, morphine and β blockers may be the first agents to consider in the treatment of MI accompanied by hypertension.

    (4) Magnesium sulfate has been shown to be of benefit in several, but not all, studies. Postulated benefits include repletion of intracellular magnesium, antiarrhythmic effects, vasodilatation, and protection against reperfusion injury. If magnesium sulfate is given, it should be given early, either at the same time or prior to the administration of thrombolytics. The dosage is 3 g intravenously over 30 minutes, followed by a continuous infusion of 18 g over the following 24 hours.

    (5) Angiotensin-converting enzyme (ACE) inhibitors have been shown to improve outcome; the earlier they are administered, the more beneficial they are. Captopril (6.25 mg by mouth) should be given if the patient's systolic blood pressure is greater than 100 mm Hg.

    (6) Antiplatelet medications include aspirin, clopidogrel, and glycoprotein (GP) IIb/IIIa receptor inhibitors. These medications may be indicated. Protocols and doses are still in flux; consultation with the cardiologist in charge is usually indicated.

   d. Treatment of complications. Complications are treated as they arise.

     (1) Dysrhythmias. The treatment of dysrhythmias is described in IV.

       (a) Lidocaine is not indicated for routine prophylaxis in patients with acute MI or for patients with nonsustained runs of ventricular tachycardia (i.e., runs lasting less than 30 seconds). Sustained ventricular tachycardia should be treated as discussed in IV B 2 b. Any ventricular dysrhythmia should prompt a search for recurrent ischemia or electrolyte imbalance.

       (b) Prophylactic pacemaker placement. Transvenous pacemakers were routinely advocated prior to the development of reliable external pacemakers. In a stable, conscious patient, the latter, tested for capture, should be placed prior to making definitive decisions regarding the need for a transvenous pacemaker. Prophylactic pacemaker placement is indicated for the following rhythms in patients with acute MI:

        (i) Bradycardia causing symptoms, hypotension, or both

        (ii) Second-degree Mobitz type II AV block or third-degree AV block (controversial in stable inferior MI)

        (iii) New bifascicular block or left bundle branch block with first-degree AV block

        (iv) Alternating bundle branch block

        (v) Persistent atrial flutter or ventricular tachycardia

        (vi) New left bundle branch block or right bundle branch block (controversial)

     (2) Papillary muscle rupture and **acute valvular incompetence.** These patients are usually in cardiogenic shock; treatment usually involves maximal afterload reduction.

  6. Disposition. Patients are admitted to an ICU or taken directly to cardiac catheterization.

C Cardiogenic shock

  1. Discussion

    a. Definition. Cardiogenic shock occurs when the heart is unable to maintain perfusion adequate for the metabolic demands of the tissues.

    b. Causes. The cause of cardiogenic shock is usually acute MI, especially after extensive infarction of the anterior ventricular wall. Complications of acute MI, such as papillary muscle rupture, septal rupture, or right ventricular infarct, can precipitate cardiogenic shock in patients with smaller infarcts. Other causes include valvular stenosis, myocarditis, and cardiomyopathy.

  2. Clinical features

    a. History. Most patients are unable to give a history but efforts should be made to gather information from fire-rescue personnel, family members, or other witnesses.

    b. Physical examination findings include hypotension and tachycardia. Diaphoresis, cool extremities, and poor capillary refill are usually present. Breath sounds may be clear initially, or rales from acute pulmonary edema may be present. An S_3 gallop or a murmur from a ruptured papillary muscle, acute mitral regurgitation, or septal rupture may be heard.

  3. Differential diagnoses include other causes of shock, cardiac tamponade, primary CHF, adult respiratory distress syndrome (ARDS), asthma, and pulmonary embolism. A cardiac etiology is suggested by a patient in shock with risk factors for ischemic heart disease and signs of acute CHF (see III B).

  4. Evaluation

    a. Electrocardiography. ST-segment elevation may be observed. Right-sided leads may show a right ventricular infarct pattern, which mandates therapy that differs from therapy for other causes of cardiogenic shock.

    b. Radiography. A chest radiograph may appear normal initially or show signs of acute CHF (see III D 2).

    c. Bedside echocardiography is useful for demonstrating poor left ventricular function, assessing valvular integrity, and ruling out other causes of shock, such as cardiac tamponade.

   d. Laboratory studies. Blood studies are not of use in making the initial diagnosis but must be included in the overall evaluation. Cardiac enzyme studies, a CBC and serum electrolyte panel, BUN and creatinine levels, and coagulation studies should be ordered.

5. **Therapy**
   a. **Emergent therapy** is aimed at hemodynamically stabilizing the patient with oxygen, airway control, and intravenous access. An effort should be made to maximize left ventricular function.
   b. **Volume expansion.** If there is no sign of volume overload or pulmonary edema, volume expansion with 100-mL boluses of normal saline every 3 minutes should be tried until either adequate perfusion is restored or pulmonary congestion occurs. Patients with right ventricular infarcts need significantly increased filling pressures to maintain adequate cardiac output.
   c. **Inotropic support**
      (1) Patients with mild hypotension (i.e., a systolic blood pressure of 80–90 mm Hg) and pulmonary congestion are best treated with **dobutamine** (2.5 µg/kg/min, titrating upward by 2–3 µg/kg/min at 10-minute intervals). Dobutamine provides inotropic support while only minimally increasing myocardial oxygen requirements.
      (2) Patients with severe hypotension (i.e., a systolic blood pressure less than 75–80 mm Hg) should be treated with **dopamine.**
         (a) This drug has varying effects dependent on dose. At doses of 2.5–10 µg/kg/min, it has positive inotropic and chronotropic effects. At dosages greater than 5.0 µg/kg/min, α-adrenergic stimulation gradually increases, causing peripheral vasoconstriction. At doses greater than 20 µg/kg/min, dopamine increases ventricular irritability without additional benefit.
         (b) A combination of dopamine and dobutamine is an effective therapeutic strategy for cardiogenic shock, minimizing the unwanted side effects of dopamine at high doses and providing inotropic support.
      (3) If additional support of blood pressure is needed, **norepinephrine,** which has much stronger α-adrenergic effects, can be tried. The starting dose is 0.5–1 µg/min.
      (4) Mechanical support (e.g., **aortic counterpulsation**) may be an option while arranging for more definitive management strategies.
   d. **Reperfusion therapy.** Reperfusion of the ischemic myocardium is the only effective therapy for patients with acute MI and cardiogenic shock. **Emergent PTCA** is the modality of choice.

6. **Disposition.** Facilities without angiographic support should consider transferring the patient to a facility with a cardiac catheterization laboratory and cardiac surgery services.

III   CONGESTIVE HEART FAILURE AND PULMONARY EDEMA

A Discussion

1. **Definition.** CHF is failure of the pumping organ in its role as a pump.
2. **Causes.** Most patients who present in acute CHF have chronic heart failure that has been exacerbated to a critical point of decompensation. It is important to identify the precipitating cause so that appropriate therapy can be carried out. Acute precipitating causes include:
   a. **Cardiac causes**
      (1) Myocardial disease (e.g., ischemia, infarction, dysrhythmia, and myocarditis). Ischemia is by far the most common cardiac precipitating cause.
      (2) Valvular disease (e.g., stenosis, infection, rupture)
      (3) Pericardial disease (e.g., infection, restrictive cardiomyopathy)
   b. **Noncardiac causes** (e.g., noncompliance with diet or medications) are the most common precipitators of acute CHF. Other etiologies include hypertension, fluid overload, systemic infections, and pulmonary embolism.

3. **Pathogenesis**
   a. **Normal physiology.** In healthy people, there are three mechanisms by which cardiac output can be physiologically adjusted.
      (1) **Frank-Starling mechanism.** Cardiac output is varied on a beat-to-beat basis according to the principles of the Frank-Starling mechanism. The myocyte generates a force proportional to its length in diastole, thereby providing instant correction for changes in the end-diastolic volume as a result of posture and activity.
      (2) **Neural, humoral,** and **endocrine mechanisms.** Cardiac output is adjusted over a period of minutes to hours via vagal and sympathetic innervation of the SA and AV nodes, circulating catecholamines, the actions of antidiuretic hormone (ADH) and atrial natriuretic peptide, and the renin-angiotensin-aldosterone system. These mechanisms adjust the chronotropic and inotropic state of the heart, the preload, and the afterload.
      (3) **Cardiac remodeling.** Over a period of weeks, the cardiac output can be adjusted by cardiac remodeling, which is growth or hypertrophy of cardiac muscle.
   b. **Pathophysiology.** Pathophysiologic effects occur when the cardiac output does not meet the body's metabolic needs. Some physiologic mechanisms cease to have any effect, while others become actively dysfunctional. Several processes at work in the heart in patients with heart failure are not present in the "healthy stressed" state.
      (1) Progressive attempts to recruit the Frank-Starling mechanism cause cardiac dilatation, which leads to an increase in ventricular wall tension. In diastole, this increase in ventricular wall tension impairs coronary blood flow, and in systole, it ultimately leads to inadequate contraction with declining ejection fraction.
         (a) This progressive failure of left ventricular function causes elevated pulmonary hydrostatic pressure, alveolar interstitial edema, and ultimately the accumulation of fluid in the alveoli (i.e., pulmonary edema).
         (b) Pulmonary edema leads to decreased lung compliance, increased work of breathing, and impaired gas exchange, giving rise to the symptoms of shortness of breath and dyspnea.
      (2) Myocardial hypertrophy causes decreased diastolic compliance, while increasing oxygen requirements. In patients with CHF, the hypertrophied myocardium lacks normal architectural organization, leading to the additional loss of efficient systolic function.
      (3) Downregulation of β receptors occurs with chronic heart failure, leading to decreased systolic function through the loss of contractility, and further loss of diastolic compliance, which is mediated by β receptors.

B **Clinical features**

1. **History.** The duration, pattern, and progression of the patient's symptoms should be investigated. The medication list is an accessible source of additional historic information.

2. **Symptoms.** The primary symptom is usually shortness of breath or difficulty breathing (dyspnea). Dyspnea on exertion typically progresses to paroxysmal nocturnal dyspnea, then to orthopnea, and finally, to dyspnea while at rest.
   a. Symptoms of chronic "forward failure" result from hypoperfusion and include fatigue, weakness, and anorexia.
   b. Symptoms of "backward failure" include shortness of breath, anorexia, abdominal swelling and discomfort, and peripheral edema.

3. **Physical examination findings**
   a. **Vital signs**
      (1) **Heart rate, blood pressure,** and **respiratory rate.** In patients with "compensated" CHF, the heart rate, blood pressure, and respiratory rate are elevated. As preterminal events, the patient's respiratory rate and then his or her heart rate start to decrease. A low heart rate can also be due to heart block, inferior wall MI, or both.

(2) **Temperature.** An accurate rectal temperature should be obtained if concomitant infection is suspected.

   b. **Pulmonary examination.** Wheezing and rhonchi are heard early; in patients with left-sided CHF, rales are heard later. The lungs will be clear in patients with right-sided failure unless there is concomitant lung disease. Dullness suggests an effusion or infiltrate.

   c. **Cardiac examination** is likely to reveal tachycardia, with or without an S_3 gallop. An S_4 suggests chronic hypertension, hypertrophy, diastolic dysfunction, or acute MI. Murmurs and rubs might indicate specific precipitating causes. Jugular venous distention is seen in patients with right-sided heart failure.

   d. **General examination.** Hepatic enlargement and abdominojugular reflux may be seen with right-sided heart failure. Extremities should be checked for cyanosis, edema, jaundice, and cachexia.

4. **Clinical appearance.** Patients can be classified according to their clinical appearance.

   a. Patients with a normal or low blood pressure, often with signs of hypoperfusion (e.g., peripheral cyanosis, chest pain, impaired mentation), are in cardiogenic shock.

   b. Patients with severe CHF talk in short sentences, with words or gasps. They are too sick to give a full history, but have normal or increased blood pressure.

   c. Patients with mild to moderate CHF are well enough to provide a history; they have a clear sensorium and speak in complete sentences.

C **Differential diagnoses** The list of precipitating causes found in III A 2 must be addressed. The following diagnoses should be differentiated from pulmonary edema.

1. **Exacerbation of COPD** is suggested by the patient's history, medication list, and body habitus.

2. **Right-sided MI** is a consideration in patients with chest pain, jugular venous distention, clear lung fields, and hypotension.

3. **Cardiac tamponade** is suggested by Beck's triad of jugular venous distention, hypotension, and pulsus paradoxus. Lung sounds are clear.

4. **Pulmonary embolus** is suggested by jugular venous distention, the presence of risk factors, a precipitous onset, and the absence of rales. The patient may complain of chest pain and have wheezes.

5. **Pneumonia** should be considered if there is a history of fever and productive cough.

D **Evaluation** is indicated to rule in or rule out the differential diagnoses (see III C), identify immediate precipitating causes, and detect underlying medical conditions. Treatment should not be delayed by tests if there is confidence in the clinical diagnosis. The patient should be placed on a cardiac monitor with a pulse oximeter and continuous blood pressure monitoring (the blood pressure should be checked every 5 minutes until the patient is stabilized).

1. **Electrocardiography.** An ECG should be obtained to identify infarction, ischemia, and arrhythmias.

2. **Radiography.** A chest radiograph may show signs of failure depending on the extent and duration of pulmonary capillary hydrostatic pressure elevations. The first finding is cephalization due to dilatation of the pulmonary vessels. As the left ventricular end-diastolic pressures increase, interstitial fluid accumulation is indicated radiographically by fluffy margins to vessels, peribronchial cuffing, and Curley A and B lines. With very high hydrostatic pressures, fluid is exuded into the alveoli, causing diffuse fluffy alveolar infiltrates.

3. **Laboratory studies**
   a. **Serum cardiac enzyme levels** should be obtained to evaluate the possibility of infarction.
   b. **CBC.** The CBC may show evidence of anemia or infection.
   c. **Serum electrolyte panel, serum BUN,** and **serum creatine levels.** These studies will identify electrolyte imbalances and renal insufficiency. Many patients with CHF have an elevated BUN:creatinine ratio despite volume overload.

    d. ABG. ABGs rarely yield useful information in the initial evaluation and deflect attention from therapy to tests, as well as distress a patient whose only efforts should be directed to breathing. The decision to intubate is made clinically.

    e. B-natriuretic peptide (BNP). BNP elevation is highly suggestive of CHF although many other diseases may result in increased levels.

E **Therapy**

1. **Goals of therapy.** The goals of therapy are to optimize oxygenation and reverse the vicious cycle of decompensation. Therapy aims to:

    a. Lower the preload, allowing for lower end-diastolic volumes and pressures (thereby decreasing pulmonary edema)

    b. Decrease the afterload, improving ejection fraction and the perfusion of tissues, and minimizing the work of the heart

2. **Treatment modalities.** In practical terms, the goals of therapy are accomplished via vasodilatation, blood pressure control, and diuresis. The ABCs are addressed first, and continue to be monitored throughout.

    a. Oxygen. Patients with mild CHF can be administered oxygen via nasal cannula, but patients with moderate or severe failure should be given oxygen by 100% nonrebreather mask. (Blunting of the hypoxic respiratory drive in a patient with chronic carbon dioxide retention is not a risk when acute pulmonary edema is present.)

    b. Nitroglycerin is a venous and arteriolar dilator, with greater effect on the venous system.

        (1) Sublingual nitroglycerin (1/150 grain every 5 minutes until the systolic blood pressure is less than 130 mm Hg or the symptoms are resolved) is administered first. Intravenous nitroglycerin is generally initiated if symptoms are not resolved with three sublingual tablets. Administration of sublingual nitroglycerin should continue as the intravenous nitroglycerin drip is being titrated up to rapidly create a "loading bolus" effect.

        (2) Nitroglycerin should be used with caution in patients with conditions requiring high filling pressures (e.g., inferior wall MI with right ventricular infarct, cor pulmonale, hypertrophic cardiomyopathy, tight mitral stenosis).

    c. Nitroprusside is also a balanced preload and afterload reducer, but with greater effect on afterload. It is slightly less convenient to use than nitroglycerin because it is light sensitive, but it has a similarly rapid onset and short half-life. It is indicated in patients in whom hypertension is the cause of their acute pulmonary edema and in those patients who need rapid pressure control but have conditions that require high filling pressures.

    d. Furosemide is a loop diuretic that helps relieve acute pulmonary edema by diuresis of sodium and water, and prior to that by venodilation and preload reduction. A dose of 40–100 mg is customary; patients already taking the drug usually require the higher doses.

    e. Morphine decreases sympathetic outflow; at the same time, it acts as a direct arteriolar and venous dilator. It is given as an intravenous push in 2- to 4-mg aliquots.

    f. β_2-Agonist nebulizer treatments. Albuterol and terbutaline cause peripheral vasodilatation and help reduce the increased airway resistance caused by interstitial pulmonary edema and the release of inflammatory mediators. These agents are not routinely indicated, but should be administered to patients with significant wheezing or history of airway disease.

    g. Rarely, digoxin, theophylline, milrinone, and **amrinone** can be considered in certain circumstances.

    h. Intubation. Almost all patients presenting with CHF and an elevated blood pressure respond to intensive therapy with the rapidly acting agents that are now available. However, those presenting in extremis or remaining hypoxic despite intensive therapeutic efforts will need to be intubated.

F **Disposition**

1. **Admission**

   a. Patients with moderate or severe CHF generally require admission to a monitored setting. The decision to admit a patient to an ICU depends on the patient's response to therapy in the ED, the patient's baseline condition, and the precipitating cause.

   b. Patients with chronic CHF in whom no precipitating cause can be identified should probably be admitted to the hospital because of the high prevalence of serious medical conditions (including cardiac ischemia) in this group.

   c. Patients who have not been previously diagnosed as having CHF but who present with symptoms of acute CHF are likely to have an acute ischemic event as the underlying cause. These patients should be treated and admitted to a monitored bed as per unstable angina or infarction.

2. **Discharge.** Patients with an acute exacerbation of chronic CHF can be discharged if a benign precipitating event can be identified (e.g., medication noncompliance) and the patient's condition improves with treatment. The patient should be able to follow the discharge plans, discussion of which is advisable with the patient's primary physician. Outpatient therapy with diuretics, ACE inhibitors, and/or other vasodilators should be initiated in concert with the private physician.

IV **RHYTHM DISTURBANCES**

Rhythm disturbances can be classified as belonging to one of three major groups: supraventricular dysrhythmias, ventricular dysrhythmias, and disorders of cardiac conduction. Table 2–4 contains a summary of the drugs often used to manage dysrhythmias in the ED.

A **Supraventricular dysrhythmias** arise in or above the AV node.

1. **Sinus arrhythmia** occurs in young, healthy patients and refers to the cyclic variations of heart rate induced by respiration. Heart rate increases with inspiration and declines with expiration.

2. **Sinus tachycardia** is a response to many pathologic processes, including fever, hypovolemia, hemorrhage, pain, hypoxia, and many drugs. It can also be a normal response to exertion or emotion.

   a. **ECG findings** include an atrial rate of greater than 100/min (even higher in infants and children) with a 1:1 ratio between atrial and ventricular contraction.

   b. **Therapy** consists of identification and treatment of the cause.

3. **Multifocal atrial tachycardia** and **wandering atrial pacemaker.** Multifocal atrial tachycardia is usually seen in association with chronic lung disease. Wandering atrial pacemaker is seen in very young patients and in athletes.

   a. **ECG findings** include P waves of three or more different morphologies, with different PR intervals. Multifocal atrial tachycardia is characterized by an atrial rate greater than 100/min, whereas wandering atrial pacemaker is characterized by an atrial rate of less than 100/min.

   b. **Therapy** is directed toward improvement of pulmonary function. If a high heart rate is contributing to the patient's distress and improvement of pulmonary function fails to reduce it, intravenous magnesium and diltiazem may be tried.

4. **Atrial flutter** is seen in association with disorders that cause myocardial injury or inflammation (e.g., ischemic heart disease, myocardial infarction) and pulmonary embolism.

   a. **ECG findings** include an atrial rate of 250–350/min. Classically, a ventricular rate of 150/min with a 2:1 AV block is seen (Figure 2–3), although 3:1 and 4:1 AV blocks are possible. Patients with accessory bypass tracts may have ventricular rates high enough to place the patient at serious risk of ventricular fibrillation (see IV B 4).

TABLE 2–4 Commonly Used Drugs in the Emergency Treatment of Dysrhythmias

Antiarrhythmic Agent	Mechanism	Primary ED Indications	Contraindications	Dose	Side Effects	Dosing Considerations
Type 1a (e.g., procainamide)	Blocks fast sodium channels, thus slowing conduction (may increase PR and QRS duration) Prolongs action potential (increases QT interval) Decreases automaticity Increases refractory period	V tach, V fib not responsive to lidocaine, wide-complex tachycardia, SVT	Shock, second- or third-degree AV block, severe renal failure	Up to 1 g given IV over 50 minutes; stop for significantly decreased blood pressure, QT or QRS widening, control of arrhythmia	Hypotension, pro-arrhythmic effects (i.e., torsades), nausea, vomiting, CNS effects, seizures	Decrease maintenance infusion by half in patients with renal failure
Type Ib (e.g., lidocaine)	Blocks fast sodium channels selectively in injured cells, especially at a fast heart rate May shorten action potential duration	Arrhythmias, especially associated with MI (i.e., V tach, V fib, frequent multiform PVCs); wide-complex tachycardia	AV block, bradycardia, accelerated idioventricular tachycardia	1.5 mg/kg IVP (over 2 minutes if conscious); if no effect, 0.75 mg IVP every 5 minutes twice; infusion with 2–4 mg/min	Dizziness, numbness, speech disturbance	Decrease maintenance infusion in patients with liver disease
Type II (e.g., esmolol)	Increases SA automaticity Decreases AV conduction Increases AV refractory period Selective β₁ blocker	SVT or A fib (to achieve rapid control of heart rate); control of heart rate and blood pressure when CHF is of concern (e.g., in patients with acute ischemia); aortic dissection; hypertensive crisis	Severe CHF, severe asthma, severe peripheral vascular disease, bradycardia, AV block, prior calcium channel blocker administration	0.5 mg/kg IV bolus, then 0.05 mg/kg/min infusion; if no effect, repeat bolus and increase infusion by 0.05 mg/kg/min every 5 minutes up to 0.2 mg/kg/min maximum	Hypotension, CHF, dizziness, weakness	Complicated mixing and dosing can cause logistical problems in ED
Type IV (e.g., diltiazem)	Blocks slow calcium channels to decrease AV conduction velocity, increase the refractory period, and relax smooth muscle cells	SVT, ventricular rate control of A fib or flutter	Second- or third-degree AV block IV digoxin, IV β blocker, WPW syndrome with wide-complex tachycardia, V tach, hypotension	0.25 mg/kg bolus, repeated twice if needed, then 10–20 mg/hour infusion	Hypotension	Liver and kidney excretion

Drug	Mechanism	Indications	Contraindications	Dose	Side effects	Comments
Adenosine	Significantly decreases AV node conduction	SVT; can be used in stable wide-complex tachycardia for diagnostic purposes	Sick sinus syndrome, second- or third-degree AV block, severe asthma	6 mg IVP, may repeat 12 mg twice; IVP must be rapid by proximal vein, followed by rapid 20-mL saline flush	Atrial standstill, hypotension, syncope, transient chest pain, nausea, cough, flushing	Decrease dose if patient takes dipyridamole, increase dose if patient takes theophylline
Atropine	Acetylcholine blocker, blocks effects of vagus on the heart; Increases SA automaticity; Increases AV node conduction	Symptomatic bradycardia, bradycardia with PVCs, cholinergic overdose	Narrow-angle glaucoma	1 mg IV, may repeat up to a total of 4 mg	Tachycardia, palpitations, hypertension, dry mouth, blurred vision	Use with caution in patients with MI; ineffective postcardiac transplant
Digoxin	Sodium-potassium pump inhibition leads to increased calcium and positive inotropy without increasing the heart rate; Vagotonic effects lead to decreased AV conduction, and increased AV refractory period; Inhibition of sympathetic outflow	Control of heart rate in SVT or A fib, especially with CHF	WPW syndrome with wide-complex tachycardia, AV block, hypokalemia, cor pulmonale	0.25 mg IVP, repeated in 30 minutes, then in 3 and 6 hours or until desired effect	Bradycardia	…
Magnesium sulfate	Intracellular calcium antagonist increases muscle relaxation and decreases neuromuscular irritability	SVT in digoxin toxicity, torsades de pointes, +/– in acute MI, arrhythmias with hypomagnesemia, eclampsia	Renal failure with hypermagnesemia	1–2 g over 2 minutes followed by 0.5–1 g/hour infusion for torsades; 1–3 g in 50 mL D5W IV over 15 minutes, then infusion for digoxin toxicity (SVT)	Hypotension, flushing	…

A fib = atrial fibrillation; AV = atrioventricular; CHF = congestive heart failure; CNS = central nervous system; D5W = 50% dextrose in water; ED = emergency department; IV = intravenous; IVP = intravenous push; MI = myocardial infarction; PVCs = premature ventricular contractions; SA = sinoatrial; SVT = supraventricular tachycardia; V fib = ventricular fibrillation; V tach = ventricular tachycardia; WPW = Wolff-Parkinson-White.

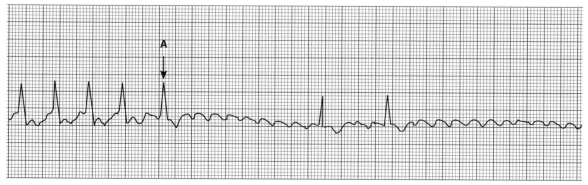

FIGURE 2–3 Rhythm strip from a patient with atrial flutter with 2:1 conduction. At point *A,* adenosine (12 mg) was administered, resulting in complete atrioventricular (AV) block and revealing flutter waves at a rate of 300/min.

    b. Therapy
        (1) Pharmacologic therapy. Diltiazem, verapamil, digoxin, β blockers, and procainamide can all convert the patient to sinus rhythm by slowing AV conduction (and therefore, the ventricular rate).
        (2) Direct current (DC) synchronized cardioversion at 25 to 50 joules converts 90% of patients to sinus rhythm and is indicated for unstable patients.

  5. Atrial fibrillation. Several medical conditions are often associated with atrial fibrillation, especially cardiac ischemia, pulmonary embolism, hypertension, COPD, alcohol intoxication, mitral valve disease (often in patients with a history of rheumatic heart disease), pericarditis, and thyrotoxicosis.
    a. Clinical findings. The pulse is irregularly irregular. CHF can occur, either as a result of a precipitating ischemic event or as a result of acute loss of the atrial contribution to ventricular filling (i.e., the "atrial kick").
    b. ECG findings include an irregularly irregular ventricular rhythm with fine fibrillatory waves that is seen best in the right chest leads. Ventricular rates are typically around 160/min. In patients who are not taking AV node blockers (e.g., digoxin), a slow ventricular response to acute atrial fibrillation indicates extensive heart disease.
    c. Therapy
        (1) Hemodynamically unstable patients are cardioverted first with 100 joules, then with 200 joules.
        (2) In hemodynamically stable patients, ventricular rate control is obtained using intravenous diltiazem and β blockers. Chemical cardioversion with procainamide can then be effected, barring any contraindications.
        (3) A patient with symptoms suggestive of atrial fibrillation that last for more than 2 days is at risk of intracardiac thrombus formation and systemic embolization with cardioversion. These patients need ventricular rate control and systemic anticoagulation therapy for 2 weeks prior to cardioversion.

  6. Supraventricular tachycardia
    a. Wide-complex supraventricular tachycardia cannot reliably be distinguished from ventricular tachycardia, and is therefore treated as ventricular tachycardia (see IV B).
    b. Narrow-complex supraventricular tachycardia
        (1) Reentrant supraventricular tachycardia
            (a) Cause. In the majority of patients with supraventricular tachycardia, the dysrhythmia is related to the mechanism of reentry. An abnormal loop of conductive tissue in the AV node or a bypass tract (see IV C 5) allows a circus rhythm to develop, with

ventricular depolarization occurring at a rate of 140–200/min. Reentrant supraventricular tachycardia can occur in patients with normal hearts, and also in association with MI, pericarditis, mitral valve prolapse, or one of the preexcitation syndromes (see IV C 5). The onset is usually sudden.

(b) **ECG findings.** Inverted, retrograde-conducted P waves are often buried in the QRS complex or found in the ST segment (Figure 2–4).

(c) **Therapy**

   (i) **Unstable patients. DC synchronized cardioversion** should be carried out, starting with 50 joules.

   (ii) **Stable patients**

   Vagal maneuvers (e.g., facial immersion in cold water, the Valsalva maneuver, carotid massage) can be attempted. Carotid massage is performed by applying steady pressure on the carotid for 10 seconds after first palpating for bilaterally intact carotid pulsations and auscultating for carotid bruits. If neither of these is present, the carotid on the side of the nondominant hemisphere should be massaged.

   Adenosine, diltiazem, verapamil, digoxin, or **β blocker** therapy can be tried if vagal maneuvers are unsuccessful. If adenosine is used, it is essential that it be administered rapidly through a large vein (antecubital or more proximal), followed by a saline flush.

(2) **Ectopic supraventricular tachycardia**

   (a) **Cause.** Ectopic supraventricular tachycardia is often caused by digoxin toxicity; in this situation, it is often associated with AV block. Ectopic supraventricular tachycardia also occurs with myocardial ischemia, lung disease, and alcohol abuse. The onset and resolution are usually gradual.

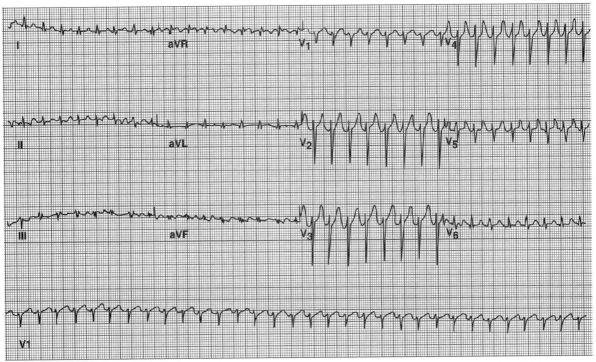

FIGURE 2–4   Electrocardiogram (ECG) from a patient with supraventricular tachycardia (heart rate = 190 beats/min).

(b) ECG findings. Ectopic supraventricular tachycardia is characterized on the ECG by P waves before each QRS complex.

(c) Therapy

    (i) If digoxin toxicity is suspected, treatment entails discontinuation of the drug and a stat drug level. If the patient is unstable, cardioversion is contraindicated, and digoxin-specific Fab may need to be given, in consultation with a toxicologist. Magnesium and Dilantin can also be used.

    (ii) In patients who have not been taking digoxin, treatment should be directed toward the underlying cause. Agents that decrease automaticity, AV conduction, or both (e.g., procainamide, β blockers, calcium channel blockers, digoxin) may also be administered.

7. Sinus bradycardia

  a. Causes. Sinus bradycardia occurs in three situations:

    (1) As a normal finding in athletes

    (2) Secondary to drug therapy with sympatholytics, AV blockers, or vagotonics (e.g., β blockers, digoxin, calcium channel blockers, narcotics, miotic glaucoma medications)

    (3) Secondary to pathologic processes, especially myocardial ischemia, but also hypothermia, hypothyroidism, and increased intracranial pressure

  b. ECG findings include normal-width QRS complexes preceded by P waves at a rate less than 60/min.

  c. Therapy consists of atropine for hemodynamically unstable patients followed by elective pacemaker placement, depending on the clinical circumstances. Patients with signs of hypoperfusion may need immediate external or internal pacing if atropine is ineffective. Epinephrine and dopamine can be used as adjunctive therapy if there is difficulty achieving pacemaker capture or if the hypotension persists.

8. Junctional arrhythmias arise at the AV node and occur in situations of impaired sinus node discharge, impaired AV node conduction, and increased nodal automaticity. All of these mechanisms are associated with digoxin toxicity and diseases of the myocardium, especially ischemia, cardiomyopathy, and myocarditis.

  a. Premature junctional beats usually occur in patients with myocardial ischemia or in those with digoxin toxicity. The ECG reveals normal-appearing QRS complexes that occur prematurely, with no antecedent P wave. Treatment is of the underlying disease, or with procainamide.

  b. Junctional rhythm is characterized by a regular narrow-complex QRS morphology, at a rate of about 40–60 beats/min. Usually there is no evidence of atrial activity, which is the reason the junctional pacemaker cells have taken control. If P waves are seen, unrelated to the QRS complexes, the patient is in third-degree AV block (see IV C 3; Figure 2–5).

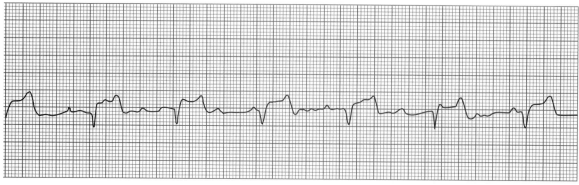

FIGURE 2–5 Rhythm strip from a patient with junctional rhythm at a rate of 60 beats/min and third-degree (complete) atrioventricular (AV) block.

    c. **Accelerated junctional rhythms** are characterized by normal-width QRS complexes at a rate of 60–100 beats/min and an absence of P waves.

    d. **Junctional tachycardia** is characterized by a rate greater than 100 beats/min.

B **Ventricular dysrhythmias** arise below the AV node.

  1. **Premature ventricular contractions (PVCs)** are often observed in people with healthy hearts. However, they are more common in cardiac disease, especially ischemic states. They are also seen in conditions of increased myocardial irritability, such as severe electrolyte or acid–base imbalances or toxicity from stimulants or digoxin. In the setting of acute MI, PVCs occur in most patients and are not predictive of which patients will develop ventricular fibrillation.

    a. **ECG findings** include premature, wide, bizarre-appearing QRS complexes, not preceded by a P wave. The QRS vector is usually opposite that of normally conducted complexes. There is typically a full compensatory pause, because the SA node is not reset by the PVC.

    b. **Therapy.** In the setting of acute MI, PVCs should prompt a search for recurrent ischemia or metabolic abnormalities that need to be treated. Suppression of PVCs or nonsustained ventricular tachycardia with antiarrhythmic agents is no longer advocated by authorities in cardiology.

  2. **Ventricular (wide-complex) tachycardia** usually occurs in patients with serious heart disease. Other causes include severe electrolyte and acid–base disorders and toxicity from drugs, especially stimulant drugs of abuse, tricyclic antidepressants, and digoxin.

    a. **ECG findings.** Even experienced cardiologists cannot reliably distinguish supraventricular tachycardia with aberrant conduction (wide-complex supraventricular tachycardia) from ventricular tachycardia on the basis of the ECG.

      (1) The ECG reveals a wide QRS complex (greater than 0.12 second, or 3 mm). The rhythm is usually regular (there may be beat-to-beat variation) and ranges from 100–200 beats/min. P waves independent of ventricular complexes (AV dissociation) may be noted, confirming the presence of ventricular tachycardia (Figure 2–6).

      (2) **Torsades de pointes** are runs of ventricular tachycardia, usually lasting 20–30 seconds, in which the amplitude of the QRS complexes waxes and wanes in any given lead. Torsades is associated with any condition that causes prolongation of cardiac repolarization, such as hypokalemia, bradycardia, or toxicity from antiarrhythmic agents.

    b. **Therapy**

      (1) Unstable patients should undergo DC cardioversion, starting at 50 joules. Pulseless ventricular tachycardia is treated like ventricular fibrillation, starting with 200 joules (see IV B 4).

      (2) Stable patients are treated with lidocaine or procainamide. If the wide-complex tachycardia is suspected to be supraventricular tachycardia with abnormal conduction, adenosine can be used for both diagnostic and therapeutic effect.

      (3) Torsades de pointes is treated with intravenous magnesium sulfate. Type Ic and type Ia antiarrhythmic agents are contraindicated.

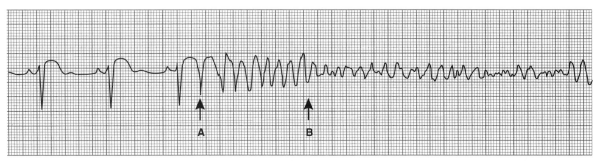

FIGURE 2–6 Electrocardiogram (ECG) from a patient with an acute myocardial infarction (MI). Ventricular tachycardia has developed at point *A,* rapidly degenerating into ventricular fibrillation (point *B*).

3. **Accelerated idioventricular tachycardia** is seen in association with acute MI. The QRS morphology is similar to that of ventricular tachycardia, but the rate is 40–100 beats/min. **Accelerated idioventricular tachycardia** should **not** be treated with lidocaine, because it may represent the only functioning pacemaker in the heart.

4. **Ventricular fibrillation** is caused by chaotically disorganized electrical activity. Because there is no concerted electrical activity, there is no cardiac contraction, and no perfusion.
   a. **ECG findings.** The ECG shows an irregular waveform of varying amplitude (see Figure 2–6).
   b. **Therapy.** The treatment is defibrillation, cardiopulmonary resuscitation (CPR), epinephrine, lidocaine, and procainamide, as per current Advanced Cardiac Life Support (ACLS) protocols.

C **Disorders of cardiac conduction** are traditionally divided into those occurring in the AV node ("AV blocks") and those occurring in one or more of the main conduction fascicles of the His-Purkinje system ("bundle branch blocks"). However, AV blocks can occur in the bundle of His and the proximal Purkinje system, as well as in the AV node.

1. **First-degree AV block** is really prolonged AV conduction, and is usually found in patients with cardiac ischemia, rheumatic fever, myocarditis, or toxicity from digoxin or other AV blockers. First-degree AV block is diagnosed by finding a prolonged PR interval (i.e., greater than 0.20 second) on the ECG.

2. **Second-degree (intermittent) AV block.** Only some P waves are transmitted. Traditionally, second-degree AV block is classified as type I or type II; however, pathologically, the important distinction to make is between those conduction disturbances that are high in the ventricular conduction system and those that are low in the conduction system. The former, "low-grade" blocks, are less likely than the latter, "high-grade" blocks, to progress to complete heart block, and if they do, the rescue pacemaker is usually high in the conduction system, allowing for coordinated ventricular depolarization at a physiologically acceptable rate.
   a. **Mobitz type I (Wenckebach) block.** The same conditions that can cause first-degree AV block can cause a Mobitz type I block.
      (1) **ECG findings.** The PR intervals become progressively longer until a P wave is completely blocked.
      (2) **Therapy.** If the patient is asymptomatic, no treatment is required. Symptomatic patients are treated as for bradycardia (see IV A 7 c).
   b. **Mobitz type II block** is also associated with the same clinical conditions as first-degree AV block.
      (1) **ECG findings.** Mobitz type II block is characterized by nonconducted P waves that are not heralded by progressive PR prolongation. It is often caused by disease of the distal bundle of His or proximal Purkinje system, so that there might be ECG evidence of concomitant fascicular or bundle branch blocks.
      (2) **Therapy.** For patients without antecedent MI, Mobitz type II block is treated as discussed in IV A 7 c. Most patients with MI require prophylactic pacemaker placement.

3. **Third-degree AV block (complete heart block)** is characterized by AV dissociation with no relation between P waves and QRS complexes (see Figure 2–5). The causes and treatment are similar to those of Mobitz type II block.

4. **Fascicular** and **bundle branch blocks** can be a sign of many forms of myocardial pathology, but are most significant when they develop in association with acute MI. In patients with acute MI, the development of fascicular or bundle branch blocks signals extensive myocardial damage, the potential for unstable heart blocks, and the possible need for pacemaker placement.
   a. **Left anterior hemiblock** is identified by the presence of a normal-width QRS complex and a leftward QRS axis of less than −45°.

    b. Left posterior hemiblock is suggested by a normal-width QRS complex and a rightward QRS axis of greater than 110°.

    c. Right bundle branch block is diagnosed by a prolonged QRS complex (i.e., greater than 0.12 second) and a triphasic QRS complex in lead V_1—the rSR' pattern—and a prominent S wave in V_6. Right bundle branch block is seen in ischemic and valvular heart disease, and may be idiopathic.

    d. Left bundle branch block causes a QRS complex of a duration greater than 0.12 second with wide, predominantly negative complexes in lead V_1 and positive complexes in V_6. Left bundle branch block is most commonly associated with ischemia, long-standing hypertension, cardiomyopathy, and severe aortic valve disease.

    e. Bifascicular blocks are identified by the presence of either left anterior or left posterior hemiblocks with right bundle branch block, or left bundle branch block alone.

5. Preexcitation syndromes are caused by abnormal bypass tracts between the atrial and ventricular conduction systems. These fibers can generate dysrhythmias by providing routes for the circus rhythms of reentrant tachycardias or by permitting abnormal retrograde conduction of ventricular impulses to the atria. **Wolff-Parkinson-White (WPW) syndrome** is the most common preexcitation syndrome; it is characterized by a high incidence of tachydysrhythmias—approximately 75% supraventricular tachycardias and 25% atrial fibrillation. Patients with WPW and atrial fibrillation may present with a rapid wide-complex ventricular response that can deteriorate to ventricular fibrillation if treated with AV nodal blockers (e.g., digoxin, calcium channel blockers, β blockers).

V IMPLANTED CARDIAC DEVICES

A Pacemakers

1. Discussion

    a. Components

      (1) Pulse generator. The pulse generator is a hermetically sealed titanium box that contains the **battery**, a **radiopaque unique identifying marker**, and **electronic circuits.** These circuits are designed to sense and analyze electrical activity and to generate pacing stimuli.

      (2) Leads. The pacemaker leads are composed of conductor wires surrounded by insulation. The conductor wires carry sensed and pacing signals. **Dual-chamber pacemakers** have two leads exiting the pulse generator, one of which is fixed in the right atrium and one in the right ventricle.

    b. Implantation of the pacemaker is through one of two approaches.

      (1) In most patients, the pacemaker is inserted in a pocket made under the skin of the chest wall. The lead wires are inserted transvenously (usually through the subclavian vein) into the heart, where they contact the endocardium. The leads are fixed to the myocardium with screws, tines, or prongs at the end of the lead. The screws are visible at the end of the lead on a chest radiograph.

      (2) Occasionally, the pacemaker is inserted in a pocket in the abdominal wall and the leads are tunneled up to the heart, where they contact the epicardium. This approach is usually reserved for patients with poor venous access.

    c. Functions. Pacemakers attempt to simulate normal cardiac electrical activity.

      (1) Pacing. The pacing function is accomplished via an electrode that contacts the myocardium. The stimulus is delivered from the pulse generator based on the parameters set by the implanting cardiologist. The ventricle, atrium, or both chambers may be paced.

      (2) Sensing. The sensing function allows the pacemaker to detect spontaneous depolarization of the myocardium and therefore inhibit delivery of a pacing stimulus. The pacemaker may be set to sense the ventricle, atrium, or both chambers (Figure 2–7).

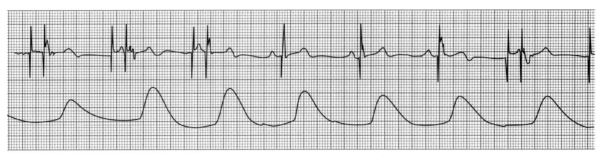

FIGURE 2–7 Rhythm strip showing functioning atrioventricular (AV) sequential pacemaker with intermittent appropriate atrial pacemaker suppression by native P waves.

(a) The electrical activity sensed is analyzed by the pulse generator, and a response occurs based on predetermined settings and thresholds. In dual-chamber pacemakers, any combination of sensing and pacing in both cardiac chambers is possible, thereby allowing the pacemaker to mimic normal sequential AV contraction.

(b) Programmable pacemakers that can respond to changing conditions and the patient's needs have been developed. Biosensors within the pacemaker can detect increases in physical exertion and increase the paced rate accordingly. Some pacemakers are equipped with antitachycardia functions, such as implantable defibrillators or over-drive pacing.

d. Identification

(1) All patients receive a **card** from the manufacturer following implantation of a pacemaker that provides information about the type of pacemaker.

(2) The **unique radiopaque identifier,** which provides information about the manufacturer and model, can be seen on a chest radiograph. Standard references containing telephone numbers of the various manufacturers should be available in every ED.

(3) All pacemakers have a three- to five-letter **code** that conveys the following information:

(a) **Chamber paced:** V = ventricle, A = atrium, D = dual

(b) **Chamber sensed:** V = ventricle, A = atrium, D = dual, O = none

(c) **Response to sensing:** I = inhibited, T = triggered, D = dual, O = none

(d) **Programmability:** R = rate responsive, P = simple programmable, M = multipro-grammable, C = communicating

(e) **Antitachycardia function:** P = pacing, S = shock, D = dual

2. Clinical features

a. In a patient with a pacemaker, symptoms such as **dizziness, syncope,** or **palpitations** should be considered to be pacemaker related, and therefore life threatening, until proven otherwise.

b. **Pacemaker syndrome,** characterized by **fatigue, palpitations,** and **shortness of breath,** is a problem unique to patients with VVT pacemakers. The syndrome is related to loss of AV synchrony, retrograde ventricle–atrium conduction, and the inability of the patient to increase heart rate and cardiac output in response to exertion.

c. **Fever** in a patient with an implanted pacemaker should raise the suspicion of pacemaker wire infection or endocarditis.

3. Differential diagnoses. Pacemaker malfunction can have several causes.

a. **Failure to pace**

(1) **Pulse generator malfunction.** The pulse generator can malfunction due to loosening of the leads within the set screws, end of battery life, or migration of the box within or alto-gether out of the pocket. Box migration can be caused by "twiddler syndrome" (i.e., moving, rotating, or wiggling of the box by the patient).

      (2) Lead malfunction can be caused by insulation fracture, conductor fracture, or lead migration away from or through the myocardium.

      (3) Failure to capture occurs when the pacemaker is sending pacing stimuli to the myocardium but the chamber is not depolarizing. Failure to capture can result from decreased pacing energy output or increased myocardial pacing thresholds (e.g., as a result of myocardial fibrosis, acute MI, electrolyte imbalance, or drugs).

   b. Sensing malfunction can be related to oversensing or undersensing.

      (1) Oversensing leads to inhibition of the pacing stimulus by a variety of mechanisms.

         (a) External causes include myopotential sensing from skeletal muscle, electrocautery devices, magnetic resonance imaging (MRI) machines, arc welding, bingo wands, and lithotripsy. Microwave ovens are no longer a risk for patients.

         (b) Far-field sensing occurs when the pacemaker oversenses cardiac electrical events.

            (i) Dual-chamber pacemakers can sometimes oversense so that a QRS complex is sensed by the atrial channel as a P wave, thus inhibiting atrial pacing.

            (ii) Crosstalk occurs when the atrial pacing spike is sensed as a ventricular event, thus inhibiting ventricular pacing, and is a problem associated only with dual-chamber pacemakers.

      (2) Undersensing leads to delivery of pacing stimuli to the myocardium despite native cardiac depolarization.

   c. Pacemaker-induced arrhythmia (endless-loop tachycardia) is another problem unique to dual-chamber models programmed for AV sequential pacing. Most newer pacemakers have been programmed with a sensing delay following a pacing stimulus in order to avoid such complications.

4. Evaluation. Patients must be placed on a cardiac monitor to provide continuous assessment of pacemaker function.

   a. Electrocardiography. The ECG should be evaluated for signs of acute ischemia or infarction.

   b. Radiography. A chest radiograph is useful for checking lead placement or for a fractured lead.

   c. Magnet interrogation. Interrogation of the pacemaker with a magnet may need to be arranged with a cardiologist. The magnet will turn off the sensing function of the unit, making automatic pacing evident. Magnet interrogation can help distinguish between oversensing and failure to pace.

5. Therapy

   a. Emergent therapy

      (1) Acute MI and **life-threatening arrhythmias** should be treated according to the usual guidelines with DC cardioversion or countershock. The leads or paddles must be placed as far from the pulse generator as possible.

      (2) Cardiac arrest is usually due to ventricular tachycardia or fibrillation rather than bradycardia or asystole; resuscitative measures should be directed accordingly.

   b. Correction of pacemaker failure. Pacemaker failure may occur post-MI or postresuscitation and can be treated by increasing the pacing output (if reprogramming is possible in the ED). A temporary transcutaneous pacemaker can be employed if necessary; the anterior lead should be placed as far from the pulse generator as possible.

   c. Treatment of infection. Infection of any of the components of the pacemaker is a serious complication that requires intravenous antibiotics and often necessitates removal of the pacemaker. Vancomycin is recommended for empiric antibiotic therapy pending cultures.

6. Disposition. Most patients will require admission for further observation and evaluation.

   a. Consultation with a cardiologist is essential if pacemaker malfunction is suspected.

   b. Patients with fever or leukocytosis should be admitted and cultures should be obtained to evaluate for pacemaker system infection or endocarditis.

B **Implantable cardioverter-defibrillator (ICD) systems**

1. **Discussion.** ICD systems have been available since 1980.

   a. **First-generation models** consisted of a pulse generator and a lead system that contained both sensing and shocking electrodes. They were designed to detect and treat ventricular fibrillation only. These devices were usually implanted in the abdominal wall and employed epicardial defibrillator leads and transvenous sensing electrodes.

   b. **Second-generation models,** of which close to 30,000 are in use, are designed to sense heart rate as well as fibrillation through sensing leads that are attached to the epicardium. The electrical therapy is still limited to shocks, but the device can be programmed to deliver high- or low-voltage cardioversion. These devices are "committed," in that once a treatable rhythm is detected, the device charges the capacitor and delivers the shock even if the rhythm has spontaneously converted in the interim.

   c. **Third-generation models** are multifunctional and programmable for delivery of electrical therapy for a variety of rhythm disturbances. These models can sense bradyarrhythmias as well as tachyarrhythmias and can perform cardiac pacing, overdrive pacing, and low- and high-energy cardioversion. Most third-generation models are "noncommitted" (i.e., they are able to take a "second look" so that a shock will be aborted if the patient's rhythm spontaneously reverts during charging). These devices can also perform telemetric functions and provide information regarding the arrhythmia that triggered the previously delivered shock.

2. **Clinical features**

   a. **History**

      (1) The patient should have a medic alert bracelet or an identification card containing information about the device.

      (2) The patient should be questioned regarding:

         (a) The number of times the device has delivered a shock

         (b) The patient's activity and symptoms at the time the shock was delivered

         (c) Recent changes in medications, most notably antiarrhythmic medications

   b. **Symptoms** such as fever, chills, pain in the generator pocket, shortness of breath, or chest pain should be elicited.

   c. **Physical examination** should be focused on evaluation of vital signs, the cardiovascular system, examination of the generator pocket, and evaluation for possible trauma secondary to shock delivery. Any erythema or drainage around the generator pocket is presumptive evidence of infection of the leads.

3. **Differential diagnoses.** Patients may present to the ED for several reasons. These include concerns about ICD discharge, as well as infection, thromboembolic events, pericarditis, arrhythmias not recognized by the device, and cardiac arrest.

   a. **Inappropriate shock delivery.** Questions regarding the appropriateness of recently delivered shocks is the most common cause of ED visits by patients with an ICD system. Shocks received following symptoms similar to prior symptoms for which the device was implanted are considered appropriate. Shocks delivered in unmonitored situations without symptoms are of unknown appropriateness. There are many potential causes of inappropriate shock delivery.

      (1) **False sensing (oversensing)** can be caused by supraventricular tachycardias, double counting (e.g., sensing T waves as QRS complexes), sensing of extraneous sources (e.g., pacemaker spikes, tapping on the chest wall, or vibrations), and muscular activity (e.g., shivering, diaphragmatic contractions, trauma).

      (2) **Unsustained tachyarrhythmias** may generate a shock. This is seen most often in patients with second-generation devices, which are not capable of aborting a shock stimulus despite spontaneous conversion of rhythm.

      (3) **Permanent pacemakers** can interfere with the sensing ability of the ICD system, resulting in inappropriate shocks.

      (4) Component failure is an uncommon cause of inappropriate shocks.

      (5) Worsening of arrhythmias can be a cause of increased frequency of shocks and must be investigated. Common causes include myocardial ischemia, electrolyte imbalances (e.g., hypokalemia), and drug toxicity.

  b. Infection can occur around any of the components. Infections are frequently indolent and must be suspected in patients with an ICD system who have elevations in body temperature. Endocarditis is a risk in any patient with indwelling transvenous lines.

  c. Thrombosis and **pulmonary embolism.** The intravascular lines also place patients at risk for thrombosis and pulmonary embolism.

  d. Pericarditis is most likely to occur in the early postoperative period following implantation but can occur at any time. Treatment is with nonsteroidal anti-inflammatory drugs (NSAIDs).

  e. Symptomatic arrhythmias or **cardiac arrest** results when the device malfunctions. There are several causes of device malfunction:

      (1) Accidental deactivation by electromagnetic fields can occur. MRI scanners, bingo wands, stereo speakers, and lithotripsy are potential deactivators. Microwave ovens are no longer a risk for patients with these devices.

      (2) Failure to sense can be due to lead fracture, lead migration, or component malfunction.

      (3) "Failure of therapy" is ventricular tachycardia or fibrillation that is recognized by the device but unsuccessfully treated by electrical shocks. Failure of therapy may be caused by increased defibrillation thresholds from acute MI, ischemia, or drug therapy. Lead migration or fracture may result in insufficient energy output.

4. Evaluation

  a. Electrocardiography. An ECG and cardiac monitoring are essential to evaluate for ischemia, infarct, or arrhythmia. ST-segment changes due to shocks should resolve within 15 minutes of stimulus discharge.

  b. Radiography. A chest radiograph will show leads and epicardial electrodes and is needed to assess for possible displacement. A radiograph of the pulse generator will reveal the radiopaque identifier if the model type is unknown.

  c. Laboratory studies. A serum electrolyte panel, CBC, and drug levels should be obtained. Cardiac enzyme elevations are to be expected following shock delivery to the myocardium and are not useful in distinguishing acute myocardial shock injury from infarct.

5. Therapy. Patients requiring emergency surgery should have the device detached prior to being transferred to the operating room.

  a. Inappropriate discharge. If the device is inappropriately discharging in the presence of sinus tachycardia, atrial fibrillation, or normal sinus rhythm, the device must be temporarily deactivated in the ED. A toroid, doughnut-shaped magnet can be used to inhibit the device from delivering a shock stimulus by placing it over the ICD externally.

      (1) Second-generation models. The pulse generator is palpated to check its position and the magnet is placed on the patient's skin, usually on the right upper corner of the device. A beeping tone, in sync with the QRS, indicates inhibition of the device and is followed in 30 seconds by a solid tone, which indicates deactivation. (If no tones are heard, the magnet should be placed over the left lower corner because the device may have been implanted upside down.) Reactivation is accomplished in reverse; the solid tone will be heard, followed by the beeping tone, indicating that the device is again armed.

      (2) Third-generation models cannot be deactivated by the magnet, but they can be inhibited by the presence of the magnet. It may be necessary to tape the magnet to the patient's skin to continue the inhibition. Unfortunately, third-generation models do not usually emit an audible tone to indicate inhibition.

  b. Cardiac arrest. Patients with ICD systems who present to the ED in cardiac arrest should be assumed to have received the full set of four shocks without success.

(1) Patients must be treated based on standard ACLS guidelines for cardiac arrest. Transcutaneous DC cardioversion or pacing is not contraindicated; however, the external paddles should be oriented perpendicular to the epicardial patches if possible, usually from sternum to apex on the chest wall. If defibrillation is unsuccessful, it should be attempted again after changing the paddle placement.

(2) Healthcare workers who perform CPR should be reassured that to date no one has been harmed by devices that discharge during CPR, although a small shock may be felt.

    c. **Infection.** Hospitalization is mandatory if systemic infection is suspected. Vancomycin is recommended for empiric antibiotic therapy pending cultures.

6. **Disposition.** In most patients with ICD systems, consultation with the patient's cardiologist should be obtained. The following patients should be admitted:

    a. Patients who have experienced two or more shocks in 1 week

    b. Patients whose device required deactivation in the ED

    c. Patients whose device is suspected of malfunctioning

    d. Patients who are found to have correctable problems contributing to the arrhythmia

VI   HYPERTENSION

A Overview

1. **Definition.** Hypertension, defined as a systolic blood pressure greater than 140 mm Hg or a diastolic pressure greater than 90 mm Hg, occurs in 20%–40% of the population.

2. **Types**

    a. **Primary (essential) hypertension** does not have a cause that can be found on evaluation. Most cases of hypertension are primary.

    b. **Secondary hypertension** occurs secondary to another disease process (e.g., a renal or endocrine disorder) in approximately 5%–10% of patients.

3. **Assessment of hypertensive patients in the ED.** Elevated blood pressure is a common abnormal vital sign noted in the ED setting.

    a. **Transient hypertension** in the ED is quite commonly associated with acute anxiety, pain, drug intoxication, or overdose and is not, in and of itself, a medical emergency. Treatment should be directed toward the underlying cause.

    b. **Uncomplicated hypertension** is frequently noted incidental to or in combination with many patient presentations to the ED. In most patients, the hypertension represents a chronic medical condition that requires long-term management. Isolated diastolic blood pressure elevations of less than 115 mm Hg, without evidence of acute end-organ damage, do not necessitate emergency medical treatment. Patients should be educated about their disease, encouraged to adhere to a low-sodium diet, and referred to a primary care physician for reevaluation.

    c. **Hypertensive urgency** and **hypertensive emergency** are characterized by diastolic blood pressure elevations of greater than 115 mm Hg and constitute medical emergencies. Although the degree of blood pressure elevation is useful in determining the need for emergent medical management, it should be remembered that, in the presence of signs of acute end-organ dysfunction, any elevation of blood pressure represents a medical emergency.

B Hypertensive urgency

1. **Discussion.** Hypertensive urgency has been defined as an elevation of the diastolic blood pressure to greater than 115 mm Hg without evidence of acute end-organ damage. Elevations beyond this point place the patient at risk for vascular endothelial damage and disruptions in cerebral blood flow autoregulation.

2. **Clinical features**
    a. **History.** Noncompliance with medication is usually the precipitating event. A history of illicit drug or alcohol use should be sought as well.
    b. **Symptoms** are nonspecific. Patients may present to the ED for problems unrelated to their hypertension. Headache is a common presenting complaint. Focal neurologic complaints, visual symptoms, and chest pain or shortness of breath imply hypertensive emergency, not urgency.
    c. **Physical examination findings.** Signs of chronic hypertension may include the following:
        (1) An elevated blood pressure
        (2) An S_4 or a prominent ventricular heave (or both) on cardiac examination
        (3) "Copper wiring" of arterioles and arteriovenous nicking on funduscopic examination

3. **Differential diagnoses.** Hypertensive urgencies must be differentiated from:
    a. **Transient, situational hypertension**
    b. **True hypertensive emergencies**
    c. **Pseudohypertension,** resulting from incorrect blood pressure cuff size or significant arteriosclerosis (leading to a noncompressible arterial system)

4. **Evaluation** must include an ECG, serum electrolyte panel, BUN and creatinine levels, and urinalysis to evaluate and exclude signs of acute end-organ damage.

5. **Therapy.** The goal of therapy is to reduce the patient's blood pressure within 24–48 hours.
    a. **Clonidine** is the most commonly used oral agent. It has an onset of action of approximately 30 minutes. Clonidine, 0.2 mg, can be given orally, with additional doses of 0.1 mg added every hour until the desired response is achieved or the maximum dose of 0.7 mg is reached. Because of its side effects of sedation and xerostomia, clonidine is not as useful in the ED as nifedipine.
    b. **ACE inhibitors, β blockers,** and **diuretics** are also useful in lowering the mean arterial pressure within 24 hours, especially if the patient has been prescribed one of these medications previously.

6. **Disposition.** Patients must be referred to their primary physician for reevaluation and should be discharged with a prescription for an antihypertensive medication.

C **Hypertensive emergency (malignant hypertension)**

1. **Discussion**
    a. **Definitions.** Hypertensive emergency is an uncommon complication of hypertension and is defined as decompensation of brain, heart, or kidney function in the face of severe hypertension. Malignant hypertension is defined as an elevated blood pressure complicated by papilledema. The actual pressure at which end-organ dysfunction ensues is variable but, with the exception of pregnancy, this life-threatening situation does not occur unless the diastolic pressure exceeds 115–130 mm Hg.
    b. **Pathophysiology.** Consistently high pressure at the arteriole level overwhelms the normal autoregulatory mechanisms leading to dilatation, increases in capillary pressures, and leakage of fluid into the perivascular space. Tissue perfusion is compromised, resulting in areas of local ischemia.
        (1) Endothelial damage, fibrinoid necrosis within vessel walls, rupture of the vessel, and tissue edema result in a microangiopathic hemolytic anemia.
        (2) Cerebral blood flow is especially compromised due to the limited space in the cranial vault. The sensitivity of brain tissue to increases in pressure causes cerebral edema, further compromising cerebral blood flow.

2. **Clinical features**
    a. **History** often reveals noncompliance with antihypertensive medications. Again, the use of illicit substances, especially cocaine, must be considered.

    b. Symptoms
        (1) Headache, nausea, vomiting, visual complaints, or any change in mental status should be taken as evidence of encephalopathy.
        (2) Cardiac symptoms (e.g., ischemic chest pain, dyspnea due to CHF) may be present.
    c. Physical examination findings
        (1) Funduscopic examination may reveal flame hemorrhages, exudates, and papilledema.
        (2) Cardiopulmonary examination may reveal evidence of acute CHF.
        (3) Neurologic examination may demonstrate alterations in mental status ranging from confusion and lethargy to coma. Focal findings may result from encephalopathy alone or be the result of concomitant cerebral vascular ischemia or hemorrhage, a common complication with dire consequences. Subarachnoid hemorrhage may be the result or the cause of malignant hypertension.

3. Differential diagnoses include hypertensive urgency, transient hypertension, and pseudo-hypertension.

4. Evaluation
    a. Laboratory studies
        (1) Serum electrolyte panel. A serum electrolyte panel may reveal evidence of hypokalemia, present in 50% of patients with malignant hypertension.
        (2) CBC. Microangiopathic hemolytic anemia with schistocytes on peripheral smear is a common finding.
        (3) BUN and creatinine levels. End-organ damage to the kidneys may be reflected by an increased serum creatinine level.
        (4) Urinalysis. Renal abnormalities may be reflected by hematuria and proteinuria. A urine drug screen can be useful when cocaine toxicity is suspected.
    b. Electrocardiography and **radiography.** An ECG and chest radiograph are useful for assessing the degree of cardiac ischemia or the presence of CHF.
    c. Computed tomography (CT). A CT scan of the head to look for intracranial bleeding is appropriate.

5. Therapy. Emergent treatment should be initiated as soon as the diagnosis is made.
    a. Goals of therapy. The goal of therapy is to decrease the blood pressure so that the mean arterial pressure (i.e., the diastolic pressure plus one third of the pulse pressure) is lowered by 20%–25%. Cerebral blood flow autoregulation is chronically altered in hypertensive states, and lowering the mean arterial pressure by more than 25% may result in a significant decrease in cerebral perfusion pressure, leading to cerebral ischemia.
    b. Pharmacologic agents. Oral agents are not useful in treating true hypertensive emergencies due to their delayed onset of action and the inability to closely titrate the medication based on effect.
        (1) Sodium nitroprusside, which has a rapid onset of action, consistency of effect over the dose range, and a duration of effect of only 1–3 minutes, is considered the drug of choice for non–pregnancy-related emergencies. The dosage range is 0.5–10 µg/kg/min. Cyanide or thiocyanate toxicity can develop in patients with hepatic or renal insufficiency and in those treated for more than 48 hours.
        (2) Nitroglycerin has a rapid onset of action, is also consistent over the dose range, and has a duration of minutes. In patients with hypertensive crisis complicated by angina or pulmonary edema, nitroglycerin is the drug of choice. The initial dose is 20–30 µg/min and can be titrated up based on the response to therapy.
        (3) Labetalol is both an α and a β blocker that is available for intravenous use. It has an onset of action of less than 15 minutes and a duration of action of 2–8 hours. A continuous intravenous infusion of 2 mg/min can be initiated; the maximum daily dose is 300 mg. Although labetalol is useful in hypertensive patients with acute MI, the drug is not yet considered first-line therapy for most hypertensive emergencies.

(4) **Nicardipine** is a calcium channel blocker with properties similar to those of nifedipine, except that it is not a negative inotropic agent and it can be given intravenously. The dosage range is 5–15 mg/hour. The onset of action is 15–30 minutes and the duration of action is 40 minutes.

(5) **Benzodiazepines** are useful for controlling the hypertension and other adrenergic symptoms of cocaine overdose.

(6) **Fenoldopam mesylate** is a pure dopaminergic agonist that causes vasodilatation in renal, mesenteric, and splanchnic beds. Fenoldopam has been shown in trials to have an efficacy close to that of nitroprusside without the associated problems.

6. **Disposition.** Patients require admission to the ICU for further observation and treatment.

VII SYNCOPE

A Discussion   Syncope is the basis of at least 1% of ED visits annually.

1. **Definition.** Syncope is a transient loss of consciousness from which the patient has spontaneously recovered.
   a. **Presyncope**, or **near syncope**, is a poorly defined term referring to symptoms of weakness, dizziness, or faintness, without complete loss of consciousness, which resolve spontaneously. The term can also be applied to symptoms preceding a full syncopal attack.
   b. Patients presenting with loss of consciousness followed by a partial recovery do not have true syncope, although the underlying mechanism may be similar to several of the causes of syncope.

2. **Causes.** The mechanism of syncope, in the vast majority of cases, is a shortfall in the supply of oxygen to the brain. This deficiency is usually due to disruption of cerebral circulation, rather than inadequate oxygenation of blood in the lungs.
   a. **Autonomic dysfunction.** Adequate cerebral perfusion depends on adequate venous return, adequate peripheral resistance (maintained by arteriolar constriction), and adequate cardiac output (maintained by cardiac inotropy and chronotropy). Impairment of any one of these components of the circulatory system, which are largely under autonomic control, can cause a critical fall in cerebral perfusion. Autonomic dysregulation is the most common single cause of syncope.
      (1) **Vasovagal syncope** usually occurs in the context of an emotionally disturbing situation, such as extreme fear or injury. The patient may report that the syncopal episode was preceded by nausea, warmth, dizziness, or "roaring in the ears," and that the episode resolved rapidly once the patient was placed in a recumbent position. A first episode of syncope is unlikely to be attributable to benign vasovagal causes in patients older than 35 years.
      (2) **Postural syncope**
         (a) **Benign postural syncope** occurs in a percentage of healthy people after prolonged standing. A typical scenario is syncope after prolonged standing during a religious ceremony. Patients are always more susceptible to autonomic syncope while standing, because the head is the hydrostatically lowest pressure zone of the body in a person who is standing erect.
         (b) **Pathologic postural syncope** differs from benign postural syncope in that patients tend to be elderly and often have systemic disorders responsible for central or peripheral neuropathies. Pathologic postural syncope usually occurs after the patient rises from a seated or lying position. On examination, symptoms can often be reproduced by asking the patient to stand up; orthostatic blood pressure measurements are often abnormal. Medications are a common cause and a careful history will often illicit the source of the problem.
      (3) **Carotid hypersensitivity** is associated with a history consistent with inadvertent carotid stimulation, such as a tight collar or head turning.

(4) Pain-induced syncope is often associated with severe pain, especially pain of a visceral origin (e.g., abdominal aortic aneurysm, ruptured ectopic pregnancy).

(5) Vasoactive drugs. A vast number of drugs have vasoactive effects (e.g., antihypertensives, sedative-hypnotics, opiates, neuroleptics, cholinergics).

b. Inadequate venous filling

(1) Hypovolemia. Syncope can be caused by inadequate intravascular volume, such as can occur with dehydration or hemorrhage. The patient shows signs of orthostatic hypotension.

(2) Mechanical obstruction of venous return to the heart (due to severe mitral or tricuspid valve stenosis or a ball-valve thrombus, atrial myxoma, pulmonary embolus, or prosthetic valve malfunction) may cause syncope.

(3) Situational causes are due to decreased venous return to the heart from Valsalva, which is exacerbated by increased vagal cardiopressor effects—for example, paroxysmal coughing ("tussive syncope"), voiding ("micturition syncope"), or defecation.

c. Inadequate pumping action of the heart

(1) Cardiac conduction problems

(a) Tachydysrhythmia, atrial or ventricular, is frequently associated with a history of palpitations or previous episodes. Syncope due to resolved ventricular tachycardia may be suggested by a prolonged QT interval or the murmur of hypertrophic cardiomyopathy (see X B 3 b).

(b) Bradydysrhythmia (usually characterized by a heart rate of less than 40 beats/min) can be due to injury to pacemaker cells or to the conduction system.

(i) AV nodal block can cause syncope with no prodromal symptoms. Complete AV block, persistent or intermittent, that leads to syncope is known as **Stokes-Adams syndrome.** The diagnosis is suggested by the absence of prodrome and an ECG showing bradycardia, new fascicular or Mobitz type II blocks, or bundle branch block.

(ii) Sick sinus (bradycardia–tachycardia) syndrome can cause syncope by sinus arrest following paroxysmal supraventricular tachycardia. A history of prodromal palpitations should be sought.

(2) Ischemic heart disease can cause syncope by damaging the conduction system or the myocardium. In patients older than 65 years, syncope becomes an increasingly common presentation of MI; these patients often do not experience chest pain.

d. Obstruction of pulmonary blood flow due to pulmonary embolism, pulmonary outflow tract obstruction, or chronic pulmonary hypertension should be suspected in patients with increased respiratory rates, increased heart rates, or decreased oxygenation.

e. Obstruction of cardiac outflow. Aortic outflow tract obstruction often causes syncope associated with exertion.

(1) Aortic stenosis can lead to syncope by both the mechanism of diminished arterial perfusion pressure and that of conduction system calcification (leading to heart block and arrhythmias).

(2) Hypertrophic cardiomyopathy can cause syncope via impairment of aortic outflow, but most commonly the syncope is related to ventricular arrhythmias associated with the cardiomyopathy.

f. Disturbances of arterial circulation

(1) Cerebrovascular insufficiency (due to embolic, atherosclerotic, or thrombotic phenomena) usually causes focal neurologic deficits rather than a loss of consciousness. Rarely, occlusion of the vertebrobasilar artery can lead to dysfunction of the reticular activating system, causing syncope.

(2) Subclavian steal is an unusual cause of syncope. It is suggested by syncope associated with exertion involving the upper extremities. An arterial blood pressure difference of 20 mm Hg or more is found between measurements taken in the left and right arm.

    g. Other causes

      (1) Hyperventilation is a common cause of presyncope and can cause syncope. A history of anxiety or precipitating emotional stress should be sought. Patients may complain of numbness, tingling in the lips, face, or extremities, and spasms or dysfunction of the hands or feet. A provocative test with the patient carefully monitored can be performed. Pulmonary embolism must be carefully excluded in any patient in whom hyperventilation is being considered as a cause of syncope.

      (2) Intracerebral vascular catastrophe. Subarachnoid hemorrhage or the sentinel bleed of a leaking saccular aneurysm can cause syncope, probably by autonomic mechanisms and cerebral vasospasm. However, intracerebral vascular catastrophe usually leads to coma, not syncope. Headache, photophobia, nausea, vomiting, neck pain, or meningeal signs suggest the diagnosis. A careful search for cranial nerve abnormalities might reveal signs of aneurysmal nerve compression.

      (3) Drugs can cause syncope by almost any of the mechanisms described. Any drug that has autonomic, vascular, cardiac, or CNS sedative or stimulant effects can cause or predispose to syncope.

      (4) Psychogenic syncope is a diagnosis of exclusion that cannot be reliably made with the time and resources available in the ED, especially since psychiatric or psychologic processes can precipitate organic causes of syncope.

B Clinical features

    1. History. The history of events surrounding the syncopal episode may suggest the cause.

      a. Palpitations, chest pain, or shortness of breath may suggest an arrhythmic event, ischemia, or a pulmonary etiology.

      b. A change in posture or prolonged standing immediately preceding the episode may reflect a postural cause or orthostatic syncope.

      c. Emotional upsets usually precede vasovagal syncope or syncope caused by hyperventilation.

      d. Recent changes in medications as well as a current drug history may reveal drugs likely to precipitate syncope (e.g., β blockers, antiarrhythmic agents, antidepressive agents, diuretics, other antihypertensive medications, alcohol, cocaine).

      e. The patient should be questioned regarding recent illnesses that may have resulted in dehydration.

      f. A past medical history of ischemic or valvular heart disease, pulmonary disease, or prior syncopal episodes may help determine the cause.

    2. Physical examination findings. The physical examination must be focused on the cardiovascular system to assess the probability of a life-threatening cause; however, abnormal findings are usually absent.

      a. Evaluation of vital signs with testing of blood pressure in all extremities and orthostatic vitals is mandatory.

      b. Rectal examination with Hemoccult testing may reveal gastrointestinal bleeding.

      c. Examination of the extremities may reveal evidence of thrombophlebitis as a source for pulmonary embolism.

      d. Neurologic examination may reveal subtle findings suggestive of cerebrovascular insufficiency.

C Differential diagnoses

    1. Hypoglycemia usually causes a gradual impairment of consciousness that is not reversed until dextrose is administered. Hypoglycemia should be considered a reversible cause of coma, rather than a cause of syncope.

    2. Seizures are a cause of spontaneously reversible loss of consciousness, and must be distinguished from syncope. If, in spite of the clues listed below, the diagnosis is still unclear, the disposition should be based on the diagnosis of both possible syncope and possible new-onset (atypical) seizure.

    a. Seizures usually have a postictal period of impaired consciousness that lasts at least 10 minutes. In syncope, there is a rapid and complete return to a clear sensorium.

    b. Patients are rarely limp during seizures. In syncope, there is usually a complete absence of motor activity. In the uncommon situation that transient tonic–clonic activity is witnessed during a syncopal episode, it will be described as following a short period of flaccid paralysis, whereas in seizures, convulsive motor activity occurs simultaneously with the loss of consciousness.

    c. Most patients with seizures have a known history of the problem.

D **Evaluation**   The cause of a given patient's syncope will be found in only 50% of patients despite extensive testing.

    1. **Electrocardiography.** An ECG is warranted in all patients without an unequivocal noncardiac diagnosis, and cardiac monitoring should be initiated in the ED in these patients.

    2. **Radiography.** A chest radiograph is indicated in any patient with abnormal vital signs, respiratory complaints, or suspected cardiac syncope.

    3. **Laboratory studies.** A CBC and serum electrolyte panel may reveal an anemia or electrolyte imbalance that may contribute to the cause of syncope.

    4. **Echocardiography** at the bedside can be useful in revealing cardiac tamponade, valvular abnormalities, abdominal aortic aneurysm, or ventricular wall motion abnormalities.

E **Disposition**

    1. **Admission**

      a. Patients with an identified serious cause of syncope will be admitted for urgent treatment or observation and monitoring.

      b. In the case of patients with an indeterminate cause of syncope (by far the largest group), clinical judgment is necessary to determine the likelihood of serious underlying illness. The following criteria—age greater than 55 years, history or risk factors for serious underlying illness or advanced atherosclerosis [e.g., a history of transient ischemic attacks (TIAs), cerebrovascular accident, or cardiac ischemia], or an adverse psychosocial profile—warrant a period of inpatient observation and work-up.

    2. **Discharge.** Patients with a clearly benign cause for their syncope can be discharged from the ED to follow up with their primary physician within several days.

VIII   **VALVULAR DISEASE**

A **Aortic valve disease**

    1. **Aortic stenosis**

      a. **Discussion**

        (1) **Cause.** Stenosis of the aortic valve develops due to **abnormal valvular architecture.** The ordinary dynamic stress of blood flow across the defective valve progressively traumatizes the valve, resulting in thickening, calcification, and narrowing of the valve orifice.

          (a) **Congenital.** A congenital bicuspid valve is the cause of aortic stenosis in 50% of symptomatic patients.

          (b) **Rheumatic endocarditis** leads to commissural fusion of valve leaflets, often affecting the mitral valve as well.

          (c) **Degenerative calcific aortic stenosis** occurs in elderly patients and appears to be part of the aging process. Degenerative calcific aortic stenosis is less likely to result in symptoms.

(2) Pathophysiology. The obstruction to ventricular outflow that results from the stenotic valve stimulates concentric hypertrophy of the left ventricle to overcome the systolic pressure gradient and maintain cardiac output. The increased muscle mass of the ventricle leads to increased myocardial oxygen demands. The hypertrophied hyperdynamic ventricle loses its ability to compensate for hemodynamic changes and eventually fails, leading to increased atrial pressures and pulmonary congestion. The ventricle also loses its ability to increase cardiac output, leading to syncope or angina with exertion.

b. Clinical features

(1) Symptoms usually do not occur until the valve orifice has narrowed to less than 1 cm². Patients may have been diagnosed previously or may present for the first time to the ED with dyspnea, angina, or syncope.

(2) Physical examination findings

  (a) The carotid arterial pulse is delayed and diminished in amplitude.

  (b) The point of maximal impulse (PMI) may be hyperdynamic and enlarged.

  (c) Auscultation of the heart reveals a harsh systolic murmur that occurs just after the S_1 and is transmitted to the carotid arteries. The S_2 may diminish as the disease progresses and the contribution of the aortic component (A_2) is lost.

c. Differential diagnoses. The murmur of aortic stenosis must be differentiated from other systolic murmurs such as occur with mitral regurgitation, tricuspid regurgitation, pulmonic stenosis, and hypertrophic cardiomyopathy. Significant aortic stenosis must be differentiated from insignificant flow murmurs.

d. Evaluation

(1) Electrocardiography. Most patients show electrocardiographic evidence of left ventricular hypertrophy.

(2) Radiography. A chest radiograph is usually normal until critical aortic stenosis develops. After critical aortic stenosis develops, the chest radiograph may reveal an increased cardiac silhouette and signs of CHF.

e. Therapy. Emergent management is guided by the presenting complaint. Valve replacement or repair will be necessary at some point in many of these patients.

f. Disposition. Patients with syncope, cardiac chest pain, CHF, or arrhythmias usually require admission to the hospital.

2. Aortic regurgitation

a. Discussion

(1) Causes include **infective endocarditis, aortic dissection, rheumatic heart disease,** and **congenital valve abnormalities.**

  (a) Acute aortic regurgitation is most often caused by infective endocarditis and aortic dissection.

  (b) Chronic aortic regurgitation may also result from infective endocarditis, but is more often secondary to rheumatic heart disease or congenital valve abnormalities. Rheumatic heart disease and congenital valve dysfunction usually cause both aortic stenosis and aortic regurgitation.

(2) Pathophysiology

  (a) Acute aortic regurgitation causes sudden increases in end-diastolic volumes and acute left ventricular failure with pulmonary edema.

  (b) Chronic aortic regurgitation. The left ventricle dilates and hypertrophies to accommodate the regurgitant volume while maintaining cardiac output. Increasing the end-diastolic volume (i.e., the preload) is the primary hemodynamic compensation for aortic regurgitation. Eventually, the left ventricle fails, leading to signs of CHF. Myocardial oxygen demands are increased due to increased muscle mass, and coronary blood flow is diminished as a result of low diastolic blood pressures, leading to cardiac ischemia.

b. **Clinical features**
  (1) **Symptoms.** As is the case with aortic stenosis, symptoms occur late in the course of the disease.
    (a) Patients may complain of an uncomfortable awareness of their heartbeat or palpitations, especially in bed, for years before exertional symptoms develop.
    (b) Chest pain may be present, either as a result of ischemia or as a result of chest wall discomfort from the hypertrophied hyperdynamic heart.
    (c) As the ventricle fails, symptoms of left-sided, then right-sided, heart failure develop.
    (d) Patients are at risk for sudden death due to arrhythmia.
  (2) **Physical examination findings** include:
    (a) A **widened pulse pressure**
    (b) A **"water-hammer" pulse** that rises quickly, then collapses in late systole
    (c) **Head bobbing,** due to the jarring of the entire body with systole
    (d) **Quincke's pulse,** observed following the application of light pressure to the tip of the nail, which reveals pulsatile flushing of the nailbed at the root
    (e) A **"pistol shot" sound** or **Duroziez's sign** (a to-and-fro murmur), observed during auscultation of femoral pulses
    (f) A **high-pitched, blowing, decrescendo diastolic murmur,** often accompanied by a loud systolic ejection sound or murmur due to the large volume of flow in early systole
    (g) The **Austin Flint murmur,** a soft middiastolic rumble produced by displacement of the anterior leaflet of the mitral valve by the regurgitant stream
c. **Differential diagnosis.** The murmur of aortic regurgitation may be confused with the Graham Steell murmur of pulmonic regurgitation.
d. **Evaluation**
  (1) **Electrocardiography.** The ECG is usually normal in patients with mild aortic regurgitation, but signs of left ventricular hypertrophy and ischemia may become evident as the disease progresses.
  (2) **Radiography.** A chest radiograph will usually show cardiac enlargement and pulmonary congestion. Dilatation of the ascending aorta and aortic knob may be seen.
  (3) **Echocardiography.** An echocardiogram reveals a hyperdynamic left ventricle, dilatation of the aortic annulus, and characteristic high-frequency fluttering of the anterior leaflet of the mitral valve during diastole. Failure of the aortic valve to close in diastole may also be noted.
e. **Therapy.** Emergent stabilization is based on symptoms. Nitrates should be considered in patients with ischemia, despite the characteristically poor response. Arrhythmias are poorly tolerated and should be treated emergently.
f. **Disposition** is the same as for aortic stenosis (see VIII A 1 f).

B **Mitral valve disease**

1. **Mitral stenosis**
  a. **Discussion**
    (1) **Cause.** Mitral stenosis occurs mostly in women and is almost always the result of earlier **rheumatic heart disease.** Approximately 40% of all patients with rheumatic heart disease develop mitral stenosis.
    (2) **Pathophysiology**
      (a) Stenosis of the mitral valve results in decreased left ventricle filling. As the valve orifice narrows, the atrium must generate more and more pressure to fill the ventricle, thus leading to marked atrial enlargement and elevated atrial pressures. The increase in atrial pressure is transmitted back to the pulmonary arterial system and eventually to the right side of the heart, leading to pulmonary hypertension and right-sided heart failure.

      (b) Cardiac output is maintained at the expense of dramatically increased pulmonary vascular pressures until late in the course of disease. Acute decompensation may be precipitated by conditions that increase the heart rate, such as fever, or conditions that increase circulating blood volume, such as pregnancy.

b. Clinical features

    (1) Symptoms develop after the hemodynamic compensatory changes begin to result in pulmonary hypertension.

      (a) Patients most commonly complain of **exertional dyspnea** and **cough** progressing to symptoms of CHF, then right-sided heart failure.

      (b) Hemoptysis can occur due to rupture of bronchial vessels but is rarely fatal.

      (c) Embolic phenomena are a common complication of mitral stenosis; patients may present with **symptoms of cerebral, extremity, renal,** or **pulmonary embolism.**

    (2) Physical examination findings

      (a) Patients have a normal or low blood pressure and a thin body habitus.

      (b) The carotid pulse is brisk but diminished. The jugular venous pulse reveals a prominent *a* wave later in the course of illness.

      (c) The first heart sound (S_1) is increased in intensity and, as pulmonary hypertension develops, the pulmonic component of the second heart sound (P_2) increases in intensity as well. An opening snap may be heard just after the second heart sound (S_2).

      (d) A low-pitched diastolic rumble can be heard at the apex after the opening snap. Soft systolic murmurs are often associated with pure mitral stenosis. In severe forms of the disease, a pansystolic murmur of functional tricuspid regurgitation may be heard.

c. Differential diagnosis. Mitral stenosis must be differentiated from primary pulmonary hypertension and causes of secondary pulmonary hypertension, such as lung disease and recurrent pulmonary embolism.

d. Evaluation

    (1) Electrocardiography. An ECG usually shows P mitrale (i.e., tall, notched P waves in lead II) and biphasic P waves in lead V_1 indicative of left atrial enlargement. Atrial fibrillation, which is poorly tolerated, may be seen.

    (2) Radiography. A chest radiograph reveals straightening of the left heart border, prominent pulmonary arteries and, later in the course of the illness, signs of CHF.

e. Therapy

    (1) CHF and arrhythmias should be treated.

    (2) Hemoptysis is best controlled by bed rest in an upright position and by diuretics. Both of these measures help decrease pulmonary venous pressure.

    (3) Patients with embolic phenomena should be anticoagulated.

f. Disposition is as noted in VIII A 1 f.

2. Mitral regurgitation

a. Discussion

    (1) Cause

      (a) Acute mitral regurgitation may be the result of **papillary muscle rupture in acute MI, infective endocarditis,** or **trauma.**

      (b) Chronic mitral regurgitation is most commonly caused by **rheumatic heart disease** in association with mitral stenosis. Mitral regurgitation may be due to **mitral valve prolapse, hypertrophic cardiomyopathy, congenital valve deformity,** or **connective tissue disease.**

    (2) Pathophysiology

      (a) Acute mitral regurgitation causes acute pulmonary edema due to the large volume of regurgitant blood flow and is a diagnosis to consider when a previously healthy person presents to the ED with pulmonary edema.

  (b) Chronic mitral regurgitation. The left ventricle dilates to increase the end-diastolic volume in order to maintain cardiac output as a greater percentage of the ejection fraction is ejected back into the left atrium. The left atrium also progressively dilates. As the chambers dilate, closure of the mitral valve orifice is disrupted even more as the posterior leaflet is pulled away from the orifice. This progressive course of events has led to the saying, "Mitral regurgitation begets mitral regurgitation." Enlargement of the atrium also begets atrial fibrillation, a common finding in patients with mitral regurgitation. Cardiac output is maintained until late in the course.

b. Clinical features

  (1) Symptoms

   (a) Acute mitral regurgitation is associated with **symptoms of acute pulmonary edema.** Acute mitral regurgitation may be catastrophic, leading to cardiogenic shock.

   (b) Chronic mitral regurgitation. Patients remain asymptomatic until the mitral regurgitation becomes severe. At this point, patients may complain of **fatigue, dyspnea,** or **palpitations.** Patients are at risk for systemic emboli from the damaged valve leaflets and may present with **symptoms of embolic events.**

  (2) Physical examination findings

   (a) Acutely, only a murmur may be heard in association with signs of CHF. The murmur is loud and holosystolic, but may be a decrescendo murmur in patients with sudden valve failure. Often the murmur can be heard through the back when auscultating breath sounds.

   (b) The S_1 may be absent or lost in the murmur and there is usually an S_3. A palpable systolic thrill and ventricular heave are usually present in patients with chronic mitral regurgitation.

c. Differential diagnoses. The murmur of mitral regurgitation must be differentiated from the murmurs of aortic stenosis, hypertrophic cardiomyopathy, and other systolic murmurs.

d. Evaluation

  (1) Electrocardiography. The ECG is normal in acute mitral regurgitation, but signs of left ventricular hypertrophy and atrial enlargement will be evident in chronic disease. Atrial fibrillation may be seen.

  (2) Radiography. A chest radiograph may reveal an increased cardiac silhouette and evidence of pulmonary vascular congestion. Pulmonary edema with a normal heart size would be expected in patients with acute mitral regurgitation.

  (3) Echocardiography may demonstrate erratic movement of the valve leaflets in papillary or chordae rupture. Chamber enlargement will be evident in patients with chronic mitral regurgitation.

  (4) Cardiac catheterization. Although cardiac catheterization is not an ED procedure, it may be necessary to diagnose acute mitral regurgitation emergently and evaluate for surgery.

e. Therapy

  (1) Cardiogenic shock should be treated as outlined in II C 5. Dopamine should be avoided because it increases afterload.

  (2) Counterpulsation devices may be necessary to stabilize the patient for catheterization and surgery.

  (3) Anticoagulant therapy may be a consideration if embolic events are suspected.

f. Disposition. Emergent surgical intervention may be indicated in patients with acute mitral regurgitation; consultation with a cardiothoracic surgeon should be considered.

3. Mitral valve prolapse (systolic click–murmur syndrome, floppy valve syndrome, Barlow's syndrome)

a. Discussion. Mitral valve prolapse varies from minimal prolapse of valve leaflets during systole to severe mitral regurgitation. (Mitral valve prolapse is the most common cause of isolated mitral regurgitation.) The cause of mitral valve prolapse is unclear, but the syndrome may be due to congenital collagen tissue disorders, Marfan's syndrome, or cystic medial necrosis.

b. **Clinical features**

   (1) **Symptoms.** Most patients with mitral valve prolapse remain asymptomatic. Some patients develop chest pain, often vague in nature, palpitations, lightheadedness, and syncope. Neurologic symptoms from embolic events are rare but possible. Severe mitral valve prolapse with mitral regurgitation results in symptoms similar to those described in VIII B 2 b (1) (b).

   (2) **Physical examination findings.** A midsystolic click followed by a crescendo–decrescendo murmur is best heard at the apex with the patient in the left lateral decubitus position. Orthostatic hypotension is a common finding.

c. **Differential diagnoses** include other causes of mitral regurgitation, such as hypertrophic cardiomyopathy and ischemic papillary muscle dysfunction [see VIII B 2 a (1)].

d. **Evaluation**

   (1) **Electrocardiography.** The ECG is usually normal but may show T-wave abnormalities in leads II, III, and aVF. An ECG will also reveal any rhythm disturbances that may be present.

   (2) **Radiography.** A chest radiograph is usually unremarkable.

   (3) **Echocardiography** may reveal prolapse of the valve leaflet during systole.

e. **Therapy**

   (1) Chest pain often responds to treatment with β blockers.

   (2) Patients with more severe forms of the syndrome may require treatment for arrhythmia.

   (3) Aspirin is recommended for patients who develop symptoms suggestive of transient neurologic events, and anticoagulation may be considered for patients with more severe symptoms.

f. **Disposition.** Uncomplicated mitral valve prolapse does not require admission.

C **Tricuspid valve disease**

1. **Tricuspid stenosis**

   a. **Discussion**

      (1) **Cause.** Tricuspid stenosis is most commonly caused by **rheumatic heart disease,** often in association with mitral valve disease. The second most common cause is **infective endocarditis.**

      (2) **Pathophysiology.** Stenosis of the tricuspid valve is well tolerated. The normal valve area is 7 cm²; adequate blood flow is possible through openings as small as 1.5 cm².

   b. **Clinical features**

      (1) **Symptoms** of right-sided heart failure may be noted, especially after surgical correction of mitral lesions.

      (2) **Physical examination findings** include **jugular venous distention** with **giant a waves,** along with **signs of right-sided heart failure.** The **diastolic murmur** of tricuspid stenosis is best heard along the left lower sternal border and may be obscured by an accompanying murmur of mitral stenosis. The murmur is increased in inspiration when venous return to the heart is increased, and the murmur is diminished during expiration and with performance of the Valsalva maneuver.

   c. **Differential diagnoses.** Constrictive cardiomyopathy, which can also result in jugular venous distention, must be ruled out. The murmur of tricuspid stenosis is often confused with or obscured by the murmur of mitral stenosis.

   d. **Evaluation**

      (1) **Electrocardiography.** An ECG will reveal evidence of right atrial enlargement with tall, peaked P waves in leads II and V_1.

      (2) **Radiography.** A chest radiograph may be unremarkable.

   e. **Therapy** entails fluid restriction, diuresis, and, if the stenosis is severe, surgical correction.

   f. **Disposition** is the same as that for aortic stenosis (see VIII A 1 f).

2. **Tricuspid insufficiency (tricuspid regurgitation)**
   a. **Discussion.** Tricuspid insufficiency is most commonly caused by a dilated right ventricle secondary to **left-sided heart failure** or **pulmonary hypertension.** It is also often the result of **infective endocarditis** arising from intravenous drug abuse. Tricuspid insufficiency is usually very well tolerated.
   b. **Clinical features**
      (1) **Symptoms.** Intravenous drug abusers with endocarditis may appear ill and feverish. Other patients with tricuspid insufficiency may present with symptoms of systemic venous congestion (especially patients with pulmonary hypertension).
      (2) **Physical examination findings** may include a blowing, holosystolic murmur along the left lower sternal border in addition to jugular venous distention and hepatomegaly with edema.
   c. **Differential diagnoses.** Acute bacterial endocarditis with tricuspid insufficiency, progressive heart failure due to cardiac disease, acute pulmonary embolism, and other causes of pulmonary hypertension must be considered.
   d. **Evaluation** should proceed as noted in the discussions of endocarditis (see XI D), CHF (see III D), and pulmonary embolism (see Chapter 3 VI D).
   e. **Therapy** should be directed toward the underlying cause (e.g., CHF, pulmonary hypertension, pulmonary embolism, endocarditis).
   f. **Disposition** is as noted in VIII A 1 f.

D **Pulmonic valve disease**

1. **Pulmonic stenosis**
   a. **Discussion.** Pulmonic stenosis is usually secondary to **congenital valve deformity.** The pulmonic valve is rarely affected by rheumatic heart disease or infective endocarditis.
   b. **Clinical features**
      (1) **Symptoms.** Patients note **progressive fatigue** from decreased cardiac output and may present with **syncope.**
      (2) **Physical examination findings** include evidence of systemic venous congestion. The murmur of pulmonic stenosis is a harsh, systolic ejection murmur often accompanied by a thrill at the upper left sternal border and a parasternal lift with a right ventricular heave on palpation. Severe pulmonic stenosis leads to tricuspid insufficiency, and the murmur of tricuspid insufficiency along with jugular venous distention may be evident.
   c. **Differential diagnoses.** Supravalvular obstruction from narrowing of the pulmonary arteries due to rubella embryopathy also presents a picture of right ventricular outflow obstruction. The murmur may be confused with the murmur of aortic stenosis.
   d. **Evaluation.** Chest radiographs and ECGs are not usually helpful in the diagnosis of pulmonic stenosis.
   e. **Therapy.** Fluid restriction and diuretics will alleviate the symptoms of systemic venous congestion.
   f. **Disposition** is as noted in VIII A 1 f.

2. **Pulmonic regurgitation**
   a. **Discussion.** Pulmonic regurgitation is almost exclusively the result of **pulmonary hypertension,** which in turn can be caused by mitral valve disease, COPD, or pulmonary embolism.
   b. **Clinical features**
      (1) **Symptoms.** Patients suffer from symptoms related to the underlying cause of the pulmonic regurgitation, which in and of itself is not clinically significant.
      (2) **Physical examination findings.** The Graham Steell murmur of pulmonic regurgitation is a high-pitched, diastolic, decrescendo blowing sound heard along the upper left sternal border.

c. **Differential diagnoses.** The murmur may be confused with that of aortic regurgitation.

d. **Evaluation.** An ECG may reveal signs of pulmonary hypertension with right axis deviation and right atrial hypertrophy. A chest radiograph is usually unremarkable.

e. **Therapy.** Because pulmonic regurgitation is usually well tolerated, no specific therapy or surgical correction is indicated.

f. **Disposition** is as noted in VIII A 1 f.

IX PERICARDIAL DISEASE

The pericardium is composed of a thin visceral layer adjacent to the epicardium and a loose parietal layer normally separated by approximately 15–50 mL of fluid. The parietal pericardium is composed of a dense collagen layer (approximately 1 mm thick) with very few elastic fibers. The parietal pericardium creates a minimally distensible sac that encases the heart.

A Acute pericarditis

1. **Discussion.** Pericarditis occurs when inflammation develops within the pericardium. Specific causes are listed in Table 2–5.

a. **Postcardiac injury pericarditis** often involves blood in the pericardial space.

(1) **Post-MI pericarditis.** Patients with post-MI pericarditis can develop one of two syndromes:

(a) **Acute fibrinous pericarditis** develops in 20% of patients with acute transmural infarctions within days of the infarction. This type of pericarditis is usually of short duration.

(b) **Dressler's syndrome** is a delayed complication of MI that occurs 1 week to several months after the acute event. Dressler's syndrome is less prevalent and may result from an autoimmune reaction that occurs when antimyocardial antibodies are produced following the infarction.

(2) **Postpericardiotomy syndrome** occurs after cardiac surgery.

(3) **Posttraumatic pericarditis** may be due to blunt or penetrating injury and is also thought to represent an autoimmune phenomenon due to circulating autoantibodies elicited after cardiac injury.

TABLE 2–5   Causes of Pericarditis

Noninfectious	Infectious	Hypersensitivity
Postcardiac injury	Viral	Drug-induced
Postmyocardial infarction	Coxsackie B virus infection	Procainamide
Postpericardiotomy	Echovirus infection	Hydralazine
Posttraumatic	HIV infection	Isoniazid
Uremic	Epstein-Barr virus infection	Rheumatic fever
Idiopathic	Bacterial	Kawasaki syndrome
Malignancy	*Mycobacterium tuberculosis* infection	Collagen vascular disease
Leukemia	β-Hemolytic *Streptococcus* infection	Rheumatoid arthritis
Lymphoma	*Streptococcus pneumoniae* infection	Systemic lupus
Metastatic carcinoma	Syphilis	erythematosus
Metastatic melanoma	Lyme disease	Scleroderma
Familial	Fungal	Dressler's syndrome
Radiation-induced	Histoplasmosis	
Cholesterol pericarditis	Protozoal	
Myxedema	Chagas' disease	
	Toxoplasmosis	

    b. Uremic pericarditis occurs in up to one third of patients with end-stage renal disease and is most frequently seen in those on hemodialysis. Patients are often asymptomatic with sero-sanguineous effusions.

    c. Idiopathic pericarditis is most common and frequently follows an upper respiratory infection.

2. Clinical features

    a. Symptoms

      (1) Chest pain is typically severe and retrosternal, and it worsens with inspiration and when the patient is in the supine position. It is characteristically referred to the back and trapezius ridge. Pain is usually improved by sitting forward.

      (2) Constitutional symptoms such as fever and malaise are present, as well as dyspnea and possibly dysphagia due to associated irritation of the distal esophagus.

    b. Physical examination may reveal the hallmark **pericardial friction rub,** described as a scratchy, leathery sound, with three components resulting from movement of the heart within the inflamed pericardium. Friction rubs tend to be intermittent over time and may change in intensity with position—they are heard best when the patient is leaning forward.

3. Differential diagnoses. Patients of all ages present to the ED with complaints of chest pain. The diagnosis of pericarditis must be differentiated from other causes of chest pain (see I C).

4. Evaluation

    a. Electrocardiography (Figure 2–8)

      (1) ST elevations in many leads are a classic finding that probably represents associated subepicardial inflammation. PR-segment depression accompanies the ST elevation in the early stages of the disease and is specific for pericarditis. After several days, T-wave inversion is seen following normalization of the ST-segment elevation.

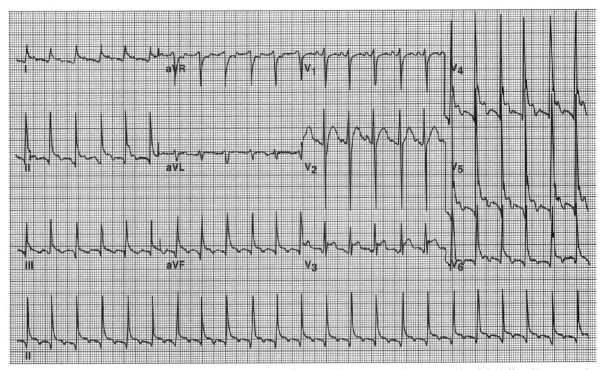

FIGURE 2–8 Electrocardiogram (ECG) from a 38-year-old man with fever and chest pain caused by acute pericarditis. Diffuse ST-segment elevations are evident and PR-segment depression is noted.

(2) Differentiating these changes from early repolarization may be difficult. It may be helpful to calculate the ratio of the ST-segment elevation to the total amplitude of the T wave. Early repolarization variants usually have an ST-segment: T-wave ratio of less than 0.25.

(3) ECG changes usually resolve, but in a few patients, they may persist for years.

   b. Radiography. A chest radiograph may show an enlarged cardiac silhouette resulting from an associated effusion, but usually the chest radiograph is unremarkable.

   c. Echocardiography is useful for demonstrating a pericardial effusion and excluding tamponade.

   d. Laboratory tests. The white blood cell (WBC) count, sedimentation rate, and serum cardiac enzyme level may all be elevated.

5. **Therapy** consists of bed rest until the fever and pain subside. Anti-inflammatory agents are useful in controlling the pain and specific therapy should be directed toward the underlying cause of the pericarditis, if it is known.

6. **Disposition.** Hospitalization is indicated for patients with intractable pain and for those in whom the diagnosis of myocardial infarction or ischemia cannot be excluded. Some authors recommend hospitalization of patients with moderate to large effusions to observe for signs of tamponade.

B **Pericardial effusion**

1. **Discussion.** Effusion within the pericardial sac develops in response to inflammation or injury. Most commonly an exudate, the fluid can also represent blood from an injury or a leaking thoracic dissection of the aorta. Causes are the same as those of pericarditis (see Table 2–5).

2. **Clinical features**

   a. Symptoms may be the same as in pericarditis, but most patients with small effusions are asymptomatic. Anxiety, dyspnea, or fatigue in patients with pericardial effusion may be early signs of tamponade.

   b. Physical examination findings include decreased heart sounds with or without a friction rub.

3. **Differential diagnosis.** Dilated cardiomyopathy may be difficult to distinguish from pericardial effusion on a chest radiograph. Differentiating a stable pericardial effusion from an evolving process that might result in cardiac tamponade is difficult and may require close observation in the hospital.

4. **Evaluation**

   a. Electrocardiography. An ECG may reveal low QRS voltage throughout or an alternating QRS amplitude, referred to as **electrical alternans,** caused by the swinging of the heart beat to beat within the pericardial effusion.

   b. Radiography. A radiograph may show an enlarged cardiac silhouette with a "water bottle" appearance. Lucent epicardial fat lines may be visible when displaced into the cardiac silhouette due to the fluid density surrounding the heart.

   c. Bedside echocardiography is useful for demonstrating an effusion and excluding tamponade.

5. **Therapy.** Emergent treatment may include pericardiocentesis and should be performed if symptoms of cardiac tamponade are present. Treatment of underlying conditions should be initiated in the ED.

6. **Disposition.** Patients with newly diagnosed pericardial effusions should be admitted to the hospital for close observation. Signs or symptoms of an enlarging effusion mandate admission to an ICU.

C **Cardiac tamponade**

1. **Discussion.** Tamponade can occur when the effusion surrounding the heart exerts pressure sufficient enough to impair diastolic filling of the ventricles. Cardiac tamponade is usually fatal if untreated.

   a. Factors contributing to the development of tamponade include the rate of fluid accumulation, the mass of the ventricular muscle, and the total intravascular blood volume.

    b. Causes. In patients who are seen in the ED, tamponade is usually a complication of **trauma.** However, other causes of tamponade include **malignant effusions, idiopathic pericarditis,** and **uremia.** Patients with acute pericarditis are at risk for cardiac tamponade if treated with anticoagulants.

2. Clinical features

    a. Symptoms include dyspnea, fatigue, possibly chest pain, and other symptoms associated with the various causes of pericarditis. Patients may be moribund due to hemodynamic compromise.

    b. Physical examination findings

        (1) Beck's triad of neck vein distention, hypotension, and muffled heart sounds is classic.

        (2) Pulsus paradoxus, which is a decrease in arterial systolic pressure with inspiration that is greater than normal (i.e., greater than 10 mm Hg), is an important finding but is not pathognomonic.

        (3) Kussmaul's sign (i.e., increased jugular venous distention with inspiration) is rare in tamponade.

        (4) Examination of the lungs often reveals normal breath sounds, and peripheral edema is usually absent.

3. Differential diagnoses. Tamponade must be distinguished from constrictive pericarditis and restrictive cardiomyopathy; however, emergently, tamponade must be assumed to be present in patients with hypotension and jugular venous distention.

4. Evaluation

    a. Electrocardiography. Electrical alternans is often noted.

    b. Radiography. Cardiomegaly without evidence of pulmonary vascular congestion may be seen.

    c. Bedside echocardiography can confirm the diagnosis and will reveal an effusion with a hyperdynamic heart that demonstrates diastolic collapse of the right ventricle and atrium.

5. Therapy entails immediate pericardiocentesis; removal of as little as 10 mL of fluid can be lifesaving. Volume expansion with intravenous fluids and inotropic medications such as dobutamine may improve the stroke volume and cardiac output in patients in cardiogenic shock when combined with therapeutic pericardiocentesis.

6. Disposition. Patients with traumatic cardiac tamponade may require emergent surgery. Patients who are not treated surgically require admission to an ICU for close observation and definitive treatment.

D **Constrictive pericarditis**

1. Discussion. Constrictive pericarditis occurs when diffuse thickening and scarring with fibrinous adhesions develops within the pericardium following acute pericarditis, leading to impaired ventricular filling. Ventricular filling is unimpeded during early diastole, but abruptly reduced when the elastic limit of the pericardium is reached. Causes are the same as those of pericarditis (see Table 2–5). Once caused predominantly by tuberculosis, chronic constrictive pericarditis now more commonly follows uremic pericarditis, postcardiac injury pericarditis, and viral pericarditis.

2. Clinical features

    a. Symptoms include dyspnea on exertion, mild orthopnea, fatigue, and weakness. Complaints referable to right-sided heart failure may predominate. Frank pulmonary edema does not occur.

    b. Physical examination findings

        (1) Jugular venous distention with Kussmaul's sign may be seen. A paradoxical pulse is occasionally found.

        (2) Cardiac examination may reveal a diastolic shock on palpation and a pericardial knock on auscultation. The knock, which represents the sudden deceleration in ventricular filling, is heard just after the S_2 and is higher in pitch than an S_3.

(3) Hepatomegaly with hepatic tenderness and ascites, often more prominent than peripheral edema, is common.

(4) A pericardial friction rub is not usually found.

3. **Differential diagnoses.** Constrictive pericarditis is often confused with CHF and may mimic tamponade, restrictive cardiomyopathy, or tricuspid and pulmonic valvular disease. The diagnosis is not one made in the emergent setting but should be suspected in anyone with evidence of elevated venous pressure without prior myocardial dysfunction or in anyone with a clinical picture of hepatic cirrhosis accompanied by distended neck veins.

4. **Evaluation**
   a. **Electrocardiography.** An ECG may show low QRS amplitude and atrial arrhythmias.
   b. **Radiography.** A chest radiograph reveals pericardial calcification (best seen on the lateral view) in 50% of patients. The cardiac silhouette is frequently normal in size, but some degree of cardiomegaly may be present.
   c. **Bedside echocardiography** is limited in its diagnostic utility but useful in excluding tamponade.

5. **Therapy.** Emergent treatment includes fluid restriction, diuretics, and, possibly, inotropic agents. Mild cases may be followed with medical therapy alone; however, pericardiectomy is the definitive treatment in patients with elevated central venous pressure.

6. **Disposition.** Patients with evidence of decompensation due to decreased cardiac output or CHF require admission for improved medical management. Patients in whom the diagnosis is suspected require cardiac catheterization because constrictive pericarditis is a potentially treatable disease.

X PRIMARY MYOCARDIAL DISEASES

A Myocarditis

1. **Discussion**
   a. **Definition.** Myocarditis is an inflammatory process of the myocardium that leads to patchy myocytolysis and interstitial destruction. Pathologically, myocarditis is characterized by focal inflammatory infiltration. The process frequently extends to the pericardium, causing a pericarditis.
   b. **Causes**
      (1) **Infectious causes**
         (a) **Viral causes** include infection with coxsackie B virus, echovirus, HIV, influenza B, parainfluenza, Epstein-Barr virus, and hepatitis B virus.
         (b) **Bacterial causes** include Lyme disease and infection with *Corynebacterium diphtheriae, Neisseria meningitidis, Mycoplasma,* β-hemolytic streptococci, and *Staphylococcus aureus.*
         (c) **Other infectious causes** include Chagas' disease and toxoplasmosis.
      (2) **Immunologic causes** include rheumatic fever, giant cell myocarditis, and Kawasaki syndrome.
      (3) **Toxic causes** include cyclic antidepressants, hydrochlorothiazide, vaccines, cocaine, and radiation.

2. **Clinical features**
   a. **Symptoms**
      (1) Constitutional symptoms such as fever, fatigue, myalgias, and headache often accompany cardiac-specific symptoms.
      (2) Chest pain, often vague or pleuritic and accompanied by palpitations, is a common complaint.
         (a) The pain may represent associated pericarditis.
         (b) Myocardial irritability, conduction system involvement, or both are common and may be perceived as palpitations.

        (3) Dyspnea may be present in more severe cases in which myocardial dysfunction has progressed to heart failure.

    b. Physical examination findings may be normal in patients with mild disease. In patients with more moderate illness, a muffled S_1 along with an S_3 and a mitral regurgitation murmur may be elicited. A pericardial friction rub may be heard with associated pericarditis. Severe disease results in progressive systolic dysfunction and typical signs of CHF.

3. Differential diagnoses

    a. Chest pain must be differentiated from that of acute myocardial infarct or ischemia and other causes of chest pain as discussed in I C.

    b. Palpitations must be differentiated from benign palpitations and other arrhythmias as discussed in IV.

    c. Dyspnea can be secondary to many primary pulmonary etiologies (e.g., pneumonia, pneumothorax, pulmonary embolism, obstructive lung disease). Patients with acute CHF, valvular disease, or pulmonary hypertension might also present with complaints of dyspnea.

4. Evaluation

    a. Electrocardiography. An ECG most commonly reveals nonspecific ST-segment and T-wave changes. Elevations of the ST segments, due to accompanying pericarditis, along with conduction disturbances (e.g., AV block, prolonged QRS duration) reflect more severe disease. Arrhythmias, ectopy, or both may be noted.

    b. Radiography. A chest radiograph is usually unremarkable unless the illness has progressed to heart failure, in which case pulmonary vascular congestion and cardiomegaly may be noted.

    c. Laboratory studies reveal elevations of the WBC count and sedimentation rate, as well as elevations in cardiac enzyme levels.

    d. Myocardial biopsy is diagnostic and may be indicated after initial emergency management to direct continued therapy.

5. Therapy. Emergent treatment is supportive and symptom directed. Antibiotics should be administered if an acute bacterial cause is suspected. Steroids remain experimental therapy, limited to the treatment of idiopathic disease, and are not part of the emergency management of myocarditis.

6. Disposition

    a. Patients with evidence of more severe disease accompanied by myocardial dysfunction, CHF, or significant arrhythmias, or those suspected of having bacterial myocarditis, should be admitted to a monitored setting.

    b. Most patients with idiopathic or viral myocarditis can be safely treated and followed as outpatients. Discussion of follow-up plans with a cardiologist or the patient's primary care physician is appropriate.

B **Cardiomyopathies** are the third most common form of cardiac disease in the United States, after ischemic and hypertensive heart disease.

1. Introduction

    a. Definition. This group of cardiac illnesses is characterized by primary abnormalities or dysfunction of the heart muscle. According to the World Health Organization (WHO) classification, only disease with no known cause is a true cardiomyopathy (once referred to as "idiopathic cardiomyopathy"). Therefore, the WHO definition excludes myocardial dysfunction due to hypertension, ischemia, or valvular heart disease from the definition of "cardiomyopathy."

    b. Cause. By definition, the cause of true cardiomyopathy is unknown; however, viral infections may account for a subgroup of illnesses currently thought to be idiopathic. Contrary to this strict definition, however, the term "cardiomyopathy" is used to refer to a number of disorders of cardiac function (Table 2–6).

TABLE 2–6   Classification of Cardiomyopathies

Dilated	Hypertrophic	Restrictive
Idiopathic	Asymmetric septal hypertrophy	Endomyocardial fibrosis
Secondary	Friedreich's ataxia	Löffler's endocarditis
Infective		Secondary
Viral myocarditis		Infiltrative/granulomatous
Protozoal		Familial storage diseases
Spirochetal		Amyloidosis
Bacterial		Progressive systemic sclerosis
Fungal		Fibroelastosis
Toxic		Radiation
Ethanol		
Cocaine		
Heavy metals		
Radiation		
Drugs		
Doxorubicin		
Nutritional/metabolic		
Collagen vascular diseases		
Infiltrative/granulomatous		
Amyloidosis		
Sarcoidosis		
Malignancy		
Hemochromatosis		
Peripartum heart disease		
Neuromuscular disorders		
Familial storage diseases		

2. **Dilated (congestive) cardiomyopathy**
   a. **Discussion.** Dilated cardiomyopathy is the most common type of cardiomyopathy.
      (1) **Causes** (see Table 2–6). Alcohol is the most common cause of dilated cardiomyopathy in the United States.
      (2) **Pathogenesis.** Systolic and diastolic dysfunction due to increased ventricular volume and pressure eventually leads to decreased cardiac output and overt heart failure. Cardiomegaly with chamber enlargement can result in arrhythmias and mural thrombi. Patients typically have a progressively downhill course; death usually occurs within 2 years of symptom onset unless cardiac transplantation is attempted.
   b. **Clinical features**
      (1) **History.** The patient should be questioned regarding a recent pregnancy, substance abuse, a recent viral illness, and systemic illness.
      (2) **Symptoms** suggestive of left- and/or right-sided heart failure predominate. Chest pain, often vague, may be present. Palpitations are common. Cerebral or systemic embolic phenomena secondary to mural thrombi occur with complaints of focal weakness, numbness, or a cold, painful extremity.
      (3) **Physical examination findings**
         (a) Evidence of cardiac enlargement with an enlarged PMI, an audible S_3 and S_4, and murmurs of mitral or tricuspid regurgitation (or both) are often present.
         (b) Findings of left- and right-sided heart failure may be evident.
         (c) Focal neurologic findings or a cold, pulseless extremity may be found when embolic phenomena occur.

    c. Differential diagnosis. The differential diagnosis includes ischemic or hypertensive heart disease, acute ischemia or infarct, decompensation of valvular disease, and other causes of pulmonary edema.

    d. Evaluation

        (1) Radiography. A chest radiograph reveals cardiomegaly with variable degrees of pulmonary congestion.

        (2) Electrocardiography. An ECG most commonly shows nonspecific changes and may reveal sinus tachycardia, atrial fibrillation, AV conduction abnormalities, or ventricular arrhythmias.

        (3) Bedside echocardiography will reveal chamber enlargement and decreased ventricular function.

    e. Therapy

        (1) CHF should be treated as discussed in III E 2.

        (2) Anticoagulation should be initiated if there are no contraindications.

        (3) Antiarrhythmic therapy may be necessary (see IV). Rapid atrial fibrillation can usually be controlled with intravenous diltiazem, digoxin, or both. Implantation of automatic defibrillators or surgical ablation of arrhythmic circuits is gaining favor for treatment of rhythm disturbances.

        (4) Nonemergent, longer term treatment includes discontinuing any offending agents (e.g., alcohol, drugs). Maximizing known disease-specific therapies, such as nutritional supplementation or therapies for infiltrative malignancies, is essential. Cardiac transplantation may be a consideration.

    f. Disposition depends on the severity of symptoms, but most patients present to the ED in a decompensated state and require admission.

3. Hypertrophic cardiomyopathy

    a. Discussion. Hypertrophic cardiomyopathy is characterized by muscular hypertrophy of a nondilated left ventricle. Most patients have regional variations in the extent of hypertrophy, but the majority demonstrate disproportionate septal hypertrophy.

        (1) Hypertrophy of the left ventricle results from cardiac muscle cell disorganization and variable myocardial fibrosis. Diastolic dysfunction occurs secondary to stiffness of the hypertrophied muscle, which leads to increased end-diastolic pressures and restricted ventricular filling.

        (2) Outflow obstruction due to systolic motion of the anterior leaflet of the mitral valve has been demonstrated in up to 25% of patients and is dynamic in nature depending on the end-diastolic volume, the heart rate, and the afterload.

    b. Clinical features

        (1) Symptoms vary depending on the extent of the disease and the patient's age and are related to the progressive diastolic dysfunction, not the presence or degree of outflow obstruction.

            (a) Sudden death may be the first clinical manifestation and is more common in children or young adults. Syncope and near-syncope can occur.

            (b) Dyspnea on exertion is a common complaint and an exercise history must be obtained.

            (c) Anginal chest pain is due to the increased oxygen requirements of the hypertrophied muscle that are not met by coronary blood flow.

            (d) Palpitations due to arrhythmia may be a complaint. Atrial arrhythmia is usually poorly tolerated due to the loss of atrial contribution to ventricular filling.

        (2) Physical examination findings are often benign and unrevealing.

            (a) Examination may reveal an audible S_4 as well as a double or triple atrial impulse palpable over the chest wall.

            (b) Cardiac examination reveals the **hallmark systolic murmur,** which is harsh, occurs after the S_1, and is diamond shaped in only 25% of patients. The murmur is best heard at the left sternal border and may be accentuated by performing a Valsalva maneuver. Passively raising the legs, squatting, or a sustained handgrip will decrease the intensity of the murmur. A blowing quality to the murmur may be heard at the apex and represents mitral regurgitation due to the poor apposition of the anterior mitral valve leaflet.

   c. **Differential diagnoses**

   (1) Differential diagnoses include aortic or mitral valvular disease, hypertensive heart disease, ischemic heart disease, and other causes of diminished diastolic compliance such as restrictive cardiomyopathy or constrictive pericarditis.

   (2) Athlete's heart syndrome, in which ventricular hypertrophy is physiologic, is often accompanied by similar physical examination findings, ECG abnormalities, and benign arrhythmias and may be confused with hypertrophic cardiomyopathy. However, a history consistent with that of an asymptomatic trained athlete is a clue to this diagnosis.

   d. **Evaluation.** The diagnosis of hypertrophic cardiomyopathy may be entertained in a patient with a history of exertional dyspnea, classic physical examination findings, and a family history of the disease; however, this diagnosis is not usually made based on the ED evaluation.

   (1) **Radiography.** A chest radiograph is initially normal but may show a mild to moderate increase in the cardiac silhouette. Pulmonary vascular congestion is unusual.

   (2) **Electrocardiography.** An ECG demonstrates left ventricular hypertrophy and left atrial enlargement. Broad, deep Q waves (septal Q waves) in multiple leads may mimic those that indicate an old MI. Atrial and ventricular rhythm disturbances are common.

   (3) **Bedside echocardiography** is the diagnostic modality of choice and is useful for distinguishing athlete's heart syndrome from hypertrophic cardiomyopathy.

   e. **Therapy**

   (1) Emergent management of the acutely symptomatic patient, especially one with chest pain, is with β blockers to decrease the force of ventricular contraction and increase diastolic filling time. Calcium channel blockers may be of benefit in decreasing ventricular wall stiffness, thereby decreasing ventricular filling pressures. Amiodarone is effective in reducing supraventricular as well as ventricular arrhythmias. Digoxin, nitrates, diuretics, and β agonists should be avoided.

   (2) Longer term therapy may include implantation of a dual-chamber pacemaker and surgical myomectomy.

   (3) Endocarditis prophylaxis is indicated as discussed in XI F 2.

   f. **Disposition.** Patients who present with syncope or chest pain require admission to a monitored setting for further evaluation and treatment. Patients in whom the diagnosis is suspected but who do not demonstrate acute signs and symptoms should be advised to avoid strenuous activity until more thorough evaluation can be performed by a cardiologist.

4. **Restrictive cardiomyopathies**

   a. **Discussion.** Restrictive cardiomyopathies are also pathophysiologically characterized by diastolic dysfunction, which results from noncompliance of the ventricles secondary to myocardial fibrosis, infiltration, scarring, or thrombus. The progressively rigid ventricle leads to impedance of filling, high filling pressures, and persistently elevated venous pressure.

   b. **Clinical features**

   (1) **Symptoms** relate to the persistently elevated venous pressures from a small, rigid ventricular cavity and include those of right- and left-sided heart failure.

   (2) **Physical examination findings** may include jugular venous distention, often with Kussmaul's sign, findings of right-sided heart failure, and findings of CHF. Heart sounds may be distant and an S_3 and an S_4 are common. A murmur of mitral regurgitation is also common.

   c. **Differential diagnoses** include constrictive pericarditis, cardiac tamponade, pulmonary hypertension, causes of right-sided heart failure (e.g., right ventricular infarct, valvular dysfunction), and causes of left-sided heart failure.

d. Evaluation

(1) Radiography. A chest radiograph may be unremarkable but may show evidence of pulmonary vascular congestion with a normal cardiac silhouette.

(2) Electrocardiography. An ECG usually reveals nonspecific changes and may show low QRS voltages, also a finding in constrictive pericarditis.

(3) Echocardiography typically reveals symmetric thickening of the ventricular walls with normal or mildly reduced systolic function.

e. Therapy.
Emergent treatment is symptom-directed and entails the judicious use of diuretics, vasodilators, and antiarrhythmics as necessary. Patients with amyloidosis may be sensitive to digoxin; therefore, this medication should be used with caution.

f. Disposition.
Again, the disposition depends on the severity of the presenting symptoms, but most patients will require admission for treatment of heart failure.

XI INFECTIOUS ENDOCARDITIS

A Discussion

1. Definition. Infectious endocarditis is an infection of the endothelial surface of the heart, most commonly affecting the heart valves.

2. Pathogenesis

a. Platelet and fibrin thrombi form on areas of endocardium with damaged endothelium. Endothelial damage can result from scarring (e.g., following rheumatic fever), turbulent blood flow (e.g., such as occurs with ventricular septal defect or patent ductus arteriosus), direct trauma (e.g., caused by pacemaker wires or pulmonary artery catheters), or cachectic states (e.g., malignancy).

b. Transient bacteremia occurs as a result of everyday activities (brushing teeth, chewing hard food, straining during defecation). Iatrogenic procedures can also induce a transient bacteremia.

(1) Bacteria in the bloodstream colonize the thrombus, where they multiply to form an infectious or inflammatory vegetation on the heart valve.

(2) Aggressive pathogens, such as *S. aureus,* can infect previously undamaged valves, often with rapid local tissue invasion and destruction, leading to symptoms of acute valvular dysfunction, heart failure, and shock.

3. Classification of infectious endocarditis. Infectious endocarditis is classified by course, predisposing factors, and the side of the heart affected. These classification systems are predictive of typical infecting organisms, clinical syndromes, and prognosis, and thus provide a basis for empiric therapy.

a. Classification by course

(1) Acute infectious endocarditis has a fulminant presentation, characterized by a high fever and systemic toxicity. Acute infectious endocarditis is usually caused by *S. aureus,* and is more often seen in younger patients. Untreated, it is fatal in days to weeks.

(2) Subacute infectious endocarditis has a more indolent course with nonspecific symptoms and signs. It is most often caused by *Streptococcus viridans* and enterococci (group D streptococci), which usually infect previously damaged valves.

(3) Chronic infectious endocarditis is now included as part of the subacute category.

b. Classification by predisposing factors

(1) Prosthetic valves are present in 10%–20% of patients with infectious endocarditis. In such patients, fever without a source mandates admission and empiric antibiotics pending the results of blood cultures.

(2) Intravenous drug abuse. Intravenous drug abusers are at high risk for infectious endocarditis, which is usually acute. In 50% of these patients, the right side of the heart is affected.

TABLE 2–7   Common Causes of Infectious Endocarditis

Predisposing Condition	Typical Pathogens
Prosthetic valve	
Less than 60 days postoperative	*Staphylococcus epidermidis, Staphylococcus aureus,* Gram-negative bacilli, fungi
More than 60 days postoperative	*Streptococcus viridans* (40%), *S. epidermidis* (30%), *S. aureus,* Gram-negative bacilli
Intravenous drug abuse	*S. aureus* (more than 50%), group D streptococci (enterococci), *Pseudomonas aeruginosa,* other Gram-negative bacilli, *S. viridans,* fungi
Prior history of valvular disease	*S. viridans* (40%), enterococci, *S. epidermidis, S. aureus*
No prior history of valvular disease	*S. aureus,* group A and group B streptococci

    (3) Prior valvular lesions. Approximately two thirds of patients with native valves who develop infectious endocarditis and do not use intravenous drugs have a prior valvular lesion. Most of these patients have a history of **rheumatic fever. Congenital heart disease** (including mitral valve prolapse and hypertrophic cardiomyopathy) and **degenerative problems** (e.g., calcific aortic stenosis) can also predispose to native valve endocarditis. In older patients, native valve infectious endocarditis typically has a subacute course.

    (4) No identifiable antecedent risk factors. In patients with infectious endocarditis without a prosthetic valve or a history of intravenous drug abuse, approximately one third will have no identifiable antecedent risk factors.

  4. Microbiology of infectious endocarditis. An understanding of the typical pathogens in various clinical settings provides the basis for empiric therapy. Table 2–7 lists typical pathogens in various clinical settings in order of frequency.

    a. The streptococci, staphylococci, and enterococci listed in Table 2–7 are responsible for more than 90% of cases of infectious endocarditis; however, almost any organism can cause infectious endocarditis.

    b. *S. aureus* usually causes fulminant disease, whereas *Staphylococcus epidermidis* and *S. viridans* typically have a more indolent presentation.

B Clinical features

  1. Symptoms are nonspecific. Fever is the most common symptom, occurring in 80% of patients. Other symptoms include chills, weakness, malaise, sweats, weight loss, neurologic symptoms (especially focal weakness and change of mental status), headache, pain (in the chest, back, abdomen, or joints), cough, shortness of breath, and hemoptysis.

  2. Physical examination findings are inconsistently present.

    a. In retrospective review, fever and heart murmur are present at some time during the course of 80%–90% of cases of infectious endocarditis.

    b. Signs of chronic infection, vasculitis, and circulating immune complexes occur in various combinations.

      (1) Osler's nodes are painful nodules on the fingers and toes.

      (2) Janeway lesions are nontender hemorrhagic nodules on the palms and soles.

      (3) Splinter hemorrhages and clubbing may be seen.

      (4) Petechiae can occur in any part of the body, but are most characteristically seen in the mouth, on the conjunctivae, and on the upper extremities.

      (5) Splenomegaly and cachexia may be noted.

    c. Emboli can give rise to signs caused by occlusive and septic phenomena.

      (1) Embolic occlusion can cause infarction in any organ without rich collateral circulation, especially the kidneys (causing flank pain and hematuria), the brain (giving rise to neurologic findings in 33% of patients with infectious endocarditis), and the heart. Less commonly, occlusion of large arteries (e.g., the femoral artery) can be caused by fungal emboli.

    (2) Septic emboli can cause pneumonia with multiple infiltrates in patients with right-sided infectious endocarditis. In patients with left-sided infectious endocarditis, foci of infection in the brain (abscesses), meninges (meningitis), heart (myocarditis, myocardial abscesses, pericarditis), kidneys (pyelonephritis), and arteries (mycotic aneurysms) may be seen.

  d. Local tissue destruction of valves and myocardium can cause signs and symptoms of heart failure, acute valvular insufficiency, myocarditis, heart blocks, dysrhythmias, and myocardial abscesses.

C **Differential diagnoses** The diagnosis of infectious endocarditis should be considered in all febrile patients when the source of the fever cannot be identified, especially if the patient has predisposing factors or a heart murmur. Early subacute infectious endocarditis is frequently misdiagnosed as a urinary tract infection (UTI) or viral syndrome. Other considerations include Lyme disease, malignancy (predisposing to nonbacterial endocardial thrombosis), disseminated gonococcemia or meningococcemia, acute rheumatic fever, valvular myxoma, and collagen vascular disease [especially systemic lupus erythematosus (SLE)].

D **Evaluation** The diagnosis is made by blood culture. Other tests are of limited utility in the ED.

1. **Blood cultures.** Detection of bacteria becomes almost impossible after administration of antibiotics. For this reason, and because infectious endocarditis is a disease with high morbidity and mortality rates if inadequately treated, it is necessary for the emergency physician to ensure that optimal blood cultures are obtained.

  a. It is essential to obtain three blood samples for culture, from three different sites. At least 10 mL of blood for both the aerobic and anaerobic bottle should be collected from each site.

    (1) If the patient is taking antibiotics, as many as six sets of cultures may be necessary.

    (2) A request for fungal cultures should be made if the patient is an intravenous drug abuser or immunocompromised.

  b. Iodine or povidone–iodine solution is applied in concentric circles, working outward from the planned venipuncture site. The solution is allowed to dry. The area is then cleansed with alcohol, which is also allowed to dry.

  c. Blood culture bottles are prepared, one aerobic and one anaerobic for each site. The stoppers are cleansed with alcohol swabs. (The stoppers are not sterile, even with protective caps.)

  d. Sterile gloves are worn while palpating the vein. The blood is drawn through a 20-gauge needle. In view of the risks of needle stick, it is currently recommended that the phlebotomy needle not be changed prior to the inoculation of the blood culture bottles (first anaerobic, then aerobic).

2. **Other tests**

  a. **CBC.** A CBC will reveal an increased WBC count with a left shift in patients with acute infectious endocarditis. In patients with subacute infectious endocarditis, the WBC count is usually normal, with a mild normochromic normocytic anemia. The erythrocyte sedimentation rate is usually elevated.

  b. **Urinalysis** is abnormal in the majority of cases, showing some combination of proteinuria, hematuria, and pyuria.

  c. **ECGs, chest radiographs,** and **blood chemistries** may reveal signs of damage to the heart, lungs, or kidneys, respectively; however, these test results are nonspecific, and may actually detract attention from the correct diagnosis.

  d. **Echocardiography.** Routine echocardiography, even in the hands of a cardiologist, is only 50%–80% sensitive in detecting valvular vegetations. Transesophageal echocardiography is reportedly more sensitive. Both modalities can be used to rule in, but not rule out, the diagnosis.

E **Therapy** The following regimens for empiric therapy are based on American Heart Association (AHA) recommendations.

1. **Prosthetic valve endocarditis.** In all cases, patients with prosthetic valve endocarditis are treated with **vancomycin** and **gentamicin.**

2. **Native valve endocarditis**
   a. **Sick or unstable patients.** Patients with acute infectious endocarditis are often thought to have undifferentiated sepsis at the time of their ED presentation. If endocarditis is recognized as a possible cause for the patient's clinical presentation, the patient should be treated with **nafcillin** and **gentamicin,** unless he or she is an intravenous drug abuser in an area of methicillin-resistant *S. aureus,* in which case **vancomycin** and **gentamicin** are indicated.
   b. **Patients with a subacute presentation and a strong suspicion for native valve endocarditis.** Intravenous drug abusers should be treated as described in XI E 2 a. Other patients are treated with **penicillin** and **gentamicin.** (In patients who are allergic to penicillin or nafcillin, vancomycin should be substituted.)
   c. **Patients with a subacute presentation and a low suspicion for native valve endocarditis.** These patients should undergo three or more blood cultures over 6 hours, with or without initiating antibiotic therapy, as determined in consultation with the admitting physician or the patient's private physician.

F **Prevention** Infectious endocarditis is more easily prevented than cured.

1. **Conditions requiring antibiotic prophylaxis.** Patients with the following conditions should receive endocarditis prophylaxis prior to undergoing invasive, potentially contaminating procedures.
   a. **Valvular disease.** Any patient with a ventricular murmur identified on physical examination should receive prophylaxis. Patients with a history of previous endocarditis, rheumatic fever, mitral valve prolapse with a holosystolic murmur, or hypertrophic cardiomyopathy should also receive prophylaxis.
   b. **Congenital heart disease** (except atrial septal defect)
   c. **Endovascular foreign bodies or shunts** (e.g., prosthetic valves, arteriovenous dialysis shunts, pacemakers, ventriculoatrial shunts)
2. **Prophylactic regimens** and some of the ED procedures that necessitate them are summarized in Table 2–8.

TABLE 2–8 Common Endocarditis Prophylaxis Regimens

Procedure	Targeted Organism	Antibiotic
Ear, nose, and throat procedures (e.g., nasal packing, incision and drainage of abscesses)	*Streptococcus viridans*	
Low to moderate risk*		Ampicillin, erythromycin, or clindamycin
High risk†		Vancomycin OR ampicillin + gentamicin
Gastrointestinal or genitourinary procedures	Enterococci	
Minor procedures (e.g., urethral catheterization anoscopy)		Ampicillin
Major procedures (e.g., preoperative for abdominal or genitourinary surgery)		Ampicillin + gentamicin OR vancomycin + gentamicin
Dermal procedures (e.g., incision and drainage of abscesses)		
Low to moderate risk*	*Staphylococcus aureus*	First-generation cephalosporin or nafcillin
High risk†	*S. aureus, Staphylococcus epidermidis*	Vancomycin + gentamicin

*For example, suspicion of native valve endocarditis, no history of infectious endocarditis, or mild to moderate murmur.
†For example, history of infectious endocarditis or prosthetic valve.

G **Disposition** Diagnosis is not possible in the ED. Therefore, clinical judgment is required to weigh the likelihood of infectious endocarditis against the risks and expenses of unnecessary treatment. The diagnosis must at least be considered in any patient with a fever. Risk of infection is increased if the patient has a murmur of undetermined etiology, or any of the predisposing conditions listed in XI A 3 b.

1. **Admission**
   a. Patients with prosthetic valves are at risk for devastating complications if endocarditis is misdiagnosed, so those with unexplained fever should have blood cultures and be admitted for empiric treatment.
   b. Clinical assessment of intravenous drug abusers with fever has been shown to be unreliable in ruling out dangerous bacteremic states. It is prudent to obtain blood samples for culture and admit these patients to the hospital.
   c. Patients with a high likelihood of infectious endocarditis or those who are deemed unlikely to comply with follow-up arrangements should be admitted for observation and transesophageal echocardiography studies, pending culture results.

2. **Discharge.** Patients who may have infectious endocarditis, but in whom the diagnosis is unlikely, can be discharged after blood cultures are obtained if the physician is reasonably sure that the patient will comply with follow-up arrangements.

XII   VASCULAR DISEASE

A **Thoracic aortic dissection**

1. **Discussion**
   a. **Cause.** Causes include the following:
      (1) **Hypertension,** the most common cause of thoracic aortic dissection
      (2) **Congenital conditions** (e.g., Marfan's syndrome, Ehlers-Danlos syndrome, Turner's syndrome)
      (3) **Pregnancy** (the most common cause of dissection in women younger than 40 years)
      (4) **Trauma**
   b. **Pathogenesis.** The affected aorta is usually not aneurysmal. The aging process combined with dynamic stress of persistently elevated pressures results in loss of structural integrity with weakening of the medial and intimal layers. Tears in the intima most commonly occur either just distal to the aortic valve or at the level of the ligamentum arteriosum. Blood then dissects between the layers of the arterial wall forming a false lumen, reentering the true lumen through another intimal tear.
      (1) Dissection can proceed proximally, distally, or in both directions, accounting for the various associated problems such as acute aortic valve insufficiency, coronary artery occlusion, and neurologic deficits due to affected carotid arteries.
      (2) Occasionally, the vessel can rupture outward into the pleural space, esophagus, or pericardium, causing massive hemorrhage, cardiac tamponade, or both.

2. **Clinical features**
   a. Patients complain of severe pain, often radiating to the back or abdomen, and usually of sudden onset. Pain may be described as ripping or tearing and may be associated with diaphoresis, nausea, and vomiting. A family history of aneurysms may be elicited.
   b. Physical examination often reveals hypertension.
      (1) A systolic blood pressure difference of more than 15 mm Hg between measurements taken in each arm or a unilateral absence of pulses suggests dissection.
      (2) Hypotension suggests rupture of the dissection, possibly into the pleural space (causing a hemothorax) or into the pericardium (causing tamponade).
      (3) Cardiac examination may reveal a musical, diastolic murmur of aortic insufficiency.

(**4**) Neurologic deficits are common and are due to cerebral or spinal ischemia from decreased blood flow or occlusion of affected arteries.

3. **Differential diagnoses.** The chest pain of thoracic aortic dissection must be differentiated from that of acute MI and esophageal rupture.

4. **Evaluation**
   a. **Electrocardiography.** An ECG will demonstrate left ventricular hypertrophy and may be helpful in differentiating thoracic aortic dissection from acute MI, but up to 40% of patients with thoracic aortic dissection may have evidence of ischemia or infarction on ECG.
   b. **Radiography.** A chest radiograph is abnormal in 80% of patients and may show mediastinal widening, obliteration of the aortic knob, tracheal displacement to the right, a double density appearance of the aorta, or pleural effusion (usually on the left).
   c. **Laboratory studies.** Blood tests are of little value emergently, but a CBC, BUN and creatinine level, serum electrolyte panel, coagulation studies, and type and cross match should be sent.
   d. **Transesophageal echocardiography** or **CT** of the chest helps establish the diagnosis, but **aortography** is the gold standard and is needed in preparation for surgical repair.

5. **Therapy** initially entails controlling the blood pressure and heart rate.
   a. Afterload reduction with nitroprusside must be combined with a β blocker to control heart rate and decrease the shearing forces in the aorta. Esmolol is often used, because this agent can be given intravenously and closely titrated to effect along with the nitroprusside.
   b. Labetalol, with both α and β blocker activity, has been advocated as a single agent, but lacks the flexibility of nitroprusside and esmolol administration.

6. **Disposition.** Surgery is indicated for patients with a dissection involving the ascending aorta and aortic arch, ruptured dissections, aortic regurgitation, cerebral complications, and uncontrollable pain. Distal descending aortic dissections can be treated medically with antihypertensive medications and observation.

B **Peripheral artery disease**

1. **Chronic arterial insufficiency**
   a. **Discussion.** Chronic arterial insufficiency is usually caused by advanced atherosclerosis, but may be caused by Buerger's disease and vasculitis (especially SLE). Advanced atherosclerosis is more likely to affect the aortic arch, the bifurcation of the common carotids, the infrarenal aorta, the common iliac bifurcation, the bifurcation of the common femorals, the adductor canal, and the trifurcation of the popliteal arteries. The upper extremities are usually spared.
   b. **Clinical features**
      (**1**) **History.** Arterial insufficiency often occurs in patients with "panatherosclerosis." A history of myocardial ischemia, cerebrovascular disease, or renal insufficiency should be sought. Chronic arterial insufficiency shares the risk factors of smoking, hypertension, diabetes, hypercholesterolemia, and obesity with these disorders.
      (**2**) **Symptoms.** Pain on exertion, referred to as claudication ("limping"), progresses to pain at rest and then to cellular injury and frank gangrene.
         (**a**) Occlusion in the aortoiliac region ("inflow disease") is suggested by Leriche's syndrome: buttock or thigh claudication accompanied by impotence in men.
         (**b**) Occlusion in the infrainguinal region ("outflow disease") causes symptoms in the calf and foot.
      (**3**) **Physical examination findings**
         (**a**) Cool, shiny, atrophic skin with thickened nails, poor capillary refill, and cyanosis is seen. As the ischemia progresses, muscle atrophy occurs. Ulcers develop over the bony prominences of the toes, the metatarsophalangeal joints, and the heels.
         (**b**) Pulses should be palpated and evaluated for strength and symmetry. If not palpable, they should be sought by Doppler. In healthy patients, the Doppler signal has a sharp,

"whipping," triphasic sound, which becomes progressively less distinct as the occlusion worsens.

(c) The **ankle–arm index** is the ratio between the systolic blood pressures as measured in the posterior tibial and brachial arteries. The ankle–arm index should be about 100%; a value less than 50% indicates severe disease.

(d) **Buerger's sign** indicates advanced disease. With the patient supine, the extremity becomes white and painful when the foot is elevated 12 inches. When the extremity is placed in a dependent position, the foot regains color abnormally slowly, and then an intense hyperemia ("dependent rubor") occurs.

c. Differential diagnoses

(1) Chronic arterial insufficiency must be distinguished from acute arterial occlusion (see XII B 2) on the basis of the patient history.

(2) Poorly defined pain of the hips and pelvis, sometimes associated with exertion ("pseudo-claudication"), can be a sign of spinal cord disease.

(3) Lower extremity ulcerations caused by venous insufficiency have a different location and appearance [see XII B 3 c (2) (b)]. Other causes of lower extremity ulcerations include diabetes, vasculitis, vasospasm, pyoderma gangrenosum, carcinoma, spider bites, and infections.

d. Disposition

(1) Chronic arterial insufficiency that has progressed to loss of motor or sensory function must be treated as an acute occlusion (see XII A 2 e).

(2) Patients with chronic arterial insufficiency (diagnosed on the basis of the history) require no further ED evaluation and should be referred to their family doctor for continued treatment. Smokers should be warned about the dire consequences of continuing to smoke.

2. Acute arterial occlusion

a. Discussion. Acute arterial occlusion can be caused by emboli or in situ thrombosis.

(1) **Embolic disease.** Embolism is suggested by a precipitous onset, asymmetrical extremity examination, or sharp demarcation of ischemia, in the context of dysrhythmias, recent MI, or ventricular aneurysm.

(a) **Sources of emboli**

(i) The **heart** is the source of 85% of emboli, at least 66% of which originate in the ventricles (even in the presence of atrial fibrillation). Ventricular thrombi are associated with MI and ventricular aneurysm.

(ii) Approximately 15% of emboli are **arterioarterial,** originating from ruptured atheromatous plaques (**atheroemboli),** or **mural thrombi,** which typically form in arterial aneurysms. Atheroemboli tend to be small and can occur in showers, leading to focal, asymmetric areas of ischemia and necrosis in regions dependent on a single end-arterial arcade—typically the digits (e.g., "blue toe syndrome").

(b) **Sites.** The most common site of embolic occlusion is the femoral bifurcation. A bounding "water hammer" pulse can be heard at that site initially; the water hammer pulse then disappears as the thrombus propagates proximally.

(2) **In situ thrombosis** is usually seen as an acute deterioration of limb function in patients with chronic arterial insufficiency. These patients have usually developed extensive collateral circulation so that symptoms are less severe, and signs of chronic disease are present bilaterally.

b. Clinical features are summarized by the **"six Ps": pain, pallor, pulselessness, paresthesia, paralysis,** and **poikilothermia.** A thorough extremity examination should be performed.

c. Differential diagnoses are the same as for chronic arterial insufficiency. A search for a possible cardiac source should be made.

d. Evaluation. As soon as acute arterial occlusion or limb-threatening chronic ischemia has been clinically identified, a vascular surgeon should be consulted. Preoperative laboratory studies, including a CBC, coagulation studies, blood type and screen, an ECG, and a chest radiograph, should be obtained. There are several options for vascular imaging.

(1) **Ultrasound** can demonstrate an intra-arterial clot. If ultrasound is available in the ED, definitive information about femoral thromboembolism may be available, precluding the need for time-consuming radiologic studies. Duplex ultrasound provides color representation of blood flow.

(2) **Angiography** provides definitive anatomic information about the vascular tree, and is essential for most decisions about vascular bypass. However, it is time consuming, invasive, and subject to several complications, including allergic reactions, intrinsic endothelial toxicity from radiocontrast agents, direct arterial damage, and renal failure.

(3) **CT** is indicated to evaluate the possibility of abdominal aorta or popliteal artery aneurysm.

e. **Therapy**
   (1) **Supportive measures**
       (a) **Aspirin.** The patient should be administered aspirin (325 mg, to be chewed) immediately to inhibit propagation of the platelet-rich "white thrombus" characteristic of arterial occlusion.
       (b) **Heparin.** The patient should be administered heparin as per the protocol described in XII C 1 e (1).
   (2) **Definitive therapy.** If complete occlusion is suspected (on the basis of loss of sensation or motor function), emergency revascularization is required within 4 hours if the limb is to be salvaged. Options include the administration of thrombolytic agents, Fogarty catheter embolectomy, endarterectomy, PTCA, bypass grafting, and primary amputation. Which therapy is used depends on the time course, site, and cause of the occlusion, as well as surgical preferences.

f. **Disposition.** Patients with limb-threatening chronic arterial insufficiency or acute arterial occlusion must be admitted to the hospital for emergency revascularization. Patients with acute partial occlusion may be admitted and observed at the discretion of the vascular surgeon.

3. **Arterial trauma** is an obvious consideration whenever a patient presents with blunt or penetrating extremity trauma and any or all of the "six Ps" of acute insufficiency. However, arterial trauma can also occur without any immediate sign of arterial insufficiency. Arterial trauma must be considered with trauma in the proximity of a major neurovascular bundle, even in the presence of normal pulses and perfusion. The decision regarding whether to perform emergent arteriography or to observe the patient expectantly is usually made in consultation with a vascular or trauma surgeon.

C **Venous disease**

1. **Deep venous thrombosis (DVT) of the lower extremities**
   a. **Discussion**
      (1) **Normal physiology.** The anatomy and physiology of the venous system are such that blood is returned to the heart passively.
          (a) **Venous valvular competence.** Venous valves work as a "water ladder," returning blood in a series of steps, pumped by the motion of surrounding muscles. Any process injuring the valves puts an additional stress on those that remain, causing them to fail sooner. Most of the blood in the superficial veins of the lower extremities passes via valved perforating veins through the muscles to the deep system (i.e., the tibial, peroneal, popliteal, and femoral veins). The rest passes via the lesser saphenous vein into the popliteal vein at the knee, or the greater saphenous vein to the femoral vein at the foramen ovale. At both of these junctions, there are also valves.
          (b) **Coagulation.** The ideal coagulation system rapidly arrests hemorrhage with specificity of action (i.e., clotting is tied temporally and spatially to sites of hemorrhage), forms blood clots that permit blood-borne agents of inflammation and healing access

to the site of injury, and initiates clot lysis as soon as tissue repair is completed. Physiologically, these functions are accomplished by means of a dynamic equilibrium between procoagulant/thrombotic and anticoagulant/thrombolytic agencies. The former predominate in health, but the balance is tipped in favor of procoagulant forces at any site of acute injury.

   (i) **Procoagulant mechanisms** are effected primarily through endothelial cells, platelets, and the clotting cascades.

   (ii) **Anticoagulant mechanisms.** Agents include **antithrombin III,** which inactivates factors XIIa, XIa, Xa, IXa, and IIa in a reaction catalyzed by heparin, and **proteins C and S,** which act together to inhibit factors VIIIa, Va, and IIa. **Thrombolysis** (fibrinolysis) is mediated primarily by plasmin, which is formed from plasminogen by tissue plasminogen activator (t-PA) and urokinase. **Active blood flow** dilutes and removes activated clotting factors, platelets, and platelet aggregates and provides access to coagulation inhibitors.

(2) **Pathophysiology.** Dysfunction of the venous valves leads to stasis of blood and endothelial injury, two of the three components of **Virchow's triad: stasis, hypercoagulability,** and **endothelial injury.** Pathologic clotting occurs when procoagulant forces predominate in intravascular sites where there is no acute injury. Disruption of thrombolysis can occur as a result of decreased levels of plasminogen activators, or abnormal configurations of fibrin or plasmin. Conditions that predispose to DVT are summarized in Table 2–9.

(3) **Types of DVT**

   (a) **Distal DVT.** Most venous thromboses of the lower extremities are thought to originate in the veins of the calf. Distal DVT does not pose a significant risk of pulmonary embolus.

   (b) **Proximal DVT.** Twenty percent of calf thromboses extend to the popliteal, femoral, or iliac veins. DVT in these locations mandates therapy because pulmonary embolism occurs in as many as 50% of these patients.

TABLE 2–9 Clinical Conditions Associated with Deep Venous Thrombosis (DVT)

Predisposing Condition	Examples
Medical conditions associated with significant inflammation	Acute MI, DIC, ulcerative colitis
Surgical conditions	Burns, multiple trauma, CNS trauma, orthopedic surgery
Hypercoagulable states	Antithrombin III deficiency, protein C deficiency, dysfibrinogenemia, lupus anticoagulant
Venous stasis	Rheologic (e.g., polycythemia vera) Immobilization (e.g., illness, long journeys) Local (e.g., chronic venous insufficiency) Systemic (e.g., CHF)
Endothelial injury	Vasculitis, especially SLE
Drug therapy	Oral contraceptives, estrogens
Other conditions	Previous DVT, age, obesity, cerebrovascular accident, blood type A, pregnancy, malignancy, intravenous drug abuse, sepsis

CHF = congestive heart failure; CNS = central nervous system; DIC = disseminated intravascular coagulation; MI = myocardial infarction; SLE = systemic lupus erythematosus.

(c) **Phlegmasia alba dolens** is an advanced and clinically identifiable syndrome of DVT in which iliofemoral thrombosis is so severe as to cause massive edema of the extremity. The leg is pale, cool, and in jeopardy.

(d) **Phlegmasia cerulea dolens** is a syndrome in which occlusion has progressed from the iliofemoral system to include all of the collateral veins of the lower extremity. Arterial ischemia and cyanosis are present. The patient and the limb are in immediate jeopardy.

b. **Clinical features**

(1) **Symptoms** include pain, tenderness, and leg swelling. Of these, the most specific symptom is swelling. With such nonspecific symptoms, DVT must be considered in every patient with nontraumatic leg pain.

(2) **Physical examination findings** are similarly nonspecific, and include leg swelling, edema, tenderness in the calves and thighs, and fever. Homans' sign and palpable "cords" are neither sensitive nor specific.

(a) A ballpoint pen should be used to mark both legs at the same point, at midcalf and midthigh (usually approximately 7 cm below and 22 cm above the tibial tubercle). The circumference of the legs should be compared at these points. A difference of more than 1.5 cm is usually considered significant.

(b) The location of leg tenderness cannot reliably distinguish proximal from distal thrombosis, although pain in areas distant from the anatomic location of deep veins suggests an alternative diagnosis.

c. **Differential diagnoses** include cellulitis, a ruptured popliteal (Baker's) cyst, lymphedema, chronic venous insufficiency (with or without acute phlebitis), superficial thrombophlebitis, arterial insufficiency, and musculoskeletal disorders, including trauma, arthritis, and tendonitis. The most difficult distinction is between chronic postphlebitic inflammation and recurrence of acute DVT; the two can rarely be differentiated without diagnostic testing.

d. **Evaluation**

(1) **Modalities**

(a) **Duplex ultrasound** combines ultrasonographic images of the veins with color representations of blood flow. Clots are imaged directly or indirectly at sites of impaired flow. Sensitivity is around 92%, with a specificity of 98% for femoral vein thrombi.

(b) **Doppler testing** measures venous flow of blood, the effect of respiration, and distal and proximal compression. Sensitivity and specificity are 85%–90% for proximal DVT. The test is noninvasive, can be performed in the ED, and can diagnose superficial thrombophlebitis. Its main disadvantage is that it is highly operator dependent.

(c) **Venography** is often considered the gold standard for diagnosis of DVT because of its high degree of sensitivity and specificity. It is the only modality that reliably demonstrates DVT in the calf. However, venography is time consuming, technically difficult (5% of studies are "inadequate"), invasive (2%–4% of studies actually cause venous thrombosis), and in most institutions, available only on a limited basis.

(d) **Impedance plethysmography (IPG)** measures the volume of venous blood in an extremity as reflected by its electrical impedance. This test is approximately 92% sensitive and specific for proximal DVT. Severe arterial insufficiency and an increased central venous pressure are conditions that interfere with the test.

(e) **Laboratory studies** prior to treatment are limited to a CBC, platelet count, and coagulation studies [e.g., prothrombin time (PT), PTT]. Therapy should not be withheld pending laboratory test results unless coagulopathy is suspected on clinical grounds.

(2) **Approach to the patient**

(a) In most institutions, diagnostic testing is not readily available at all times. In patients without contraindications to heparin who are clinically suspected of DVT, anticoagulation therapy should be initiated and the patient should be admitted for inpatient work-up.

(b) Patients who are clinically suspected of having DVT but have contraindications to anticoagulation require a diagnostic study emergently to establish the diagnosis and determine the relative risk of heparin therapy versus surgical intervention. If emergent testing is performed, the results generally put the patient in one of the four following categories:

  (i) An unequivocally positive result is indication for starting heparin therapy or intervening surgically.

  (ii) A patient with a venogram showing calf DVT or with a negative IPG or duplex scan does not usually require anticoagulation, but needs repeat noninvasive testing in 3–7 days to monitor for proximal extension.

  (iii) An unequivocally negative result rules out DVT.

  (iv) If noninvasive testing is equivocal, or suspected of being false positive, the patient will need a venogram, and is then treated accordingly.

e. Therapy. Therapeutic options include the following:

  (1) Heparin is given in an initial bolus of 80 U/kg, followed by an infusion of 15 U/kg/hour. The PTT should be checked in 6 hours and the heparin rate adjusted to 1.5 to 2.5 times control. As an alternative, consider enoxaparin (Lovenox) 1 mg/kg subcutaneously every 12 hours.

  (2) Surgical therapy is indicated for those with contraindications to anticoagulation. A filter or "umbrella" can be placed in the inferior vena cava fluoroscopically, without the need for general anesthesia. Thrombectomy is indicated for patients with phlegmasia cerulea dolens.

  (3) Thrombolytic therapy for proximal DVT of the lower extremities is controversial, but recommended by some for the treatment of phlegmasia cerulea dolens and acute-onset DVT in young patients.

f. Disposition. Patients with a possible or established diagnosis of DVT must be admitted to the hospital. Patients in whom proximal DVT has been ruled out, but distal DVT is still possible, can be discharged with arrangements made for repeat diagnostic studies in 5–7 days; however, it is essential that the patient be compliant and motivated.

2. DVT of the upper extremities

a. Discussion. Thrombosis of the axillary or subclavian veins represents less than 2% of the cases of DVT. It is often associated with anatomic obstructions at the thoracic inlet. Other causes include excessive muscular activity of the arms (i.e., "effort thrombosis") and trauma (including intravenous catheters and drug abuse). Pulmonary embolism can occur in 10%–15% of cases.

b. Clinical features. Symptoms and signs are similar to those of lower extremity DVT. Distended superficial veins are more easily identifiable, and strongly suggest the diagnosis if they fail to collapse when the patient's arm is raised. Prominent superficial veins of the shoulder suggest that the thrombosis is chronic.

c. Differential diagnoses include cellulitis and lymphedema. Precipitating causes, including occult cancer, should be considered.

d. Evaluation is made by venography, IPG, or duplex scanning. Venography is frequently the modality of choice because of the definitive anatomic information it provides and the opportunity it affords to administer thrombolytic agents directly to the clot.

e. Therapy. Axillary and subclavian vein thrombosis is usually an isolated event (i.e., not associated with preexistent venous insufficiency), and reestablishing venous patency is usually sufficient to prevent recurrence. For these reasons, and to avoid chronic and debilitating swelling of the upper extremity, thrombolytic therapy is generally advocated, barring contraindications.

3. Other venous system diseases

a. Varicose veins (i.e., swollen, usually nontender, superficial veins) can be primary or secondary. Primary varicose veins are associated with female sex and increasing age. Secondary varicose veins can be caused by any process that causes sustained venous hypertension. Common causes include valvular incompetence, pregnancy, and DVT. Varicose veins are rarely of clinical significance except as a cause of hemorrhage from minor trauma to the overlying skin. Hemorrhage can be controlled by application of an elastic bandage or sutures.

b. Superficial thrombophlebitis (i.e., thrombosis and inflammation of a superficial vein) is usually a diagnosis that can be made on clinical grounds. In the presence of varicose veins, superficial thrombophlebitis is generally a benign disease, and can be treated with elevation, local heat, and NSAIDs for pain. In the absence of varicose veins, it is frequently a sign of DVT, occult malignancy, or both. DVT must be ruled out prior to discharge; occult malignancy can be worked up on an outpatient basis.

c. Chronic venous insufficiency refers to the skin and tissue changes seen with chronic venous hypertension.

  (1) Discussion. With loss of venous valvular function, a state of chronic venous hypertension develops in the veins of the legs, causing direct endothelial injury. The endothelial injury leads to a vicious cycle of capillary leakage, increased interstitial oncotic pressure, and further edema. Impaired diffusion and perfusion of metabolic substrates with concomitant accumulation of waste products cause cellular injury and death. Chronic fibrosis further impedes cellular nutrition, while skin breakdown causes bacterial invasion and cellulitis, propagating the injury.

  (2) Clinical features

   (a) Symptoms start at the ankles and progress proximally. The patient complains of a swelling, burning sensation of the skin, and later, venous ulceration. Venous claudication, a bursting pain in the calves with exercise, is relieved by raising the leg. (This is in contrast to arterial claudication, where the leg is held dependently for relief.)

   (b) Physical examination findings include hyperpigmented skin with pitting or brawny edema and loss of skin appendages, eventually progressing to beefy ulceration. Findings predominate on the ankle, anterior to the medial malleolus.

  (3) Therapy ultimately requires prolonged outpatient follow-up. In the ED, depending on the severity of the disease, a patient may need compression stockings or an Unna boot; admission may be necessary for some patients, especially if cellulitis is present.

  (4) Disposition. Admission is indicated if there is ischemia, significant necrosis, signs of systemic toxicity, or obvious inability of the patient to care for himself or herself. If the patient is to be discharged, cellulitis must be treated if present, and the patient must be educated about meticulous elevation of the extremity at all times while not active.

Study Questions

Directions: *Each of the numbered items or incomplete statements in this section is followed by answers or by completions of the statement. Select the ONE lettered answer or completion that is BEST in each case.*

1. A 26-year-old man is brought to the emergency department (ED) because he felt dizzy, weak, and faint while playing soccer. The patient says that he has not experienced chest pain or shortness of breath, and denies antecedent drug use. His medical history is unremarkable. Review of systems reveals a recent decrease in exercise tolerance due to dyspnea. Which one of the following statements regarding this case is true?

  A The cause of this patient's near-syncope is most likely benign and he should be advised to follow up with his family doctor within 1 week.

  B A urine drug screen will most likely reveal recent cocaine use, which could cause a toxic cardiomyopathy and precipitate the near-syncopal episode.

  C A murmur may be present on physical examination and can be expected to increase in intensity with squatting.

  D Electrocardiographic findings of left ventricular hypertrophy along with physical examination findings of cardiac enlargement in this patient would suggest the diagnosis of athlete's heart syndrome.

  E Despite an unremarkable physical examination, this patient should undergo emergent echocardiography and may require admission to the hospital for further evaluation.

2. Which of the following symptoms is present in mild to moderate mitral stenosis?

  A Fatigue
  B Exertional dyspnea
  C Chest pain
  D Peripheral edema
  E Dysphagia

3. Which one of the following measures is most appropriate for the treatment of cardiogenic shock due to acute myocardial infarction (MI)?

  A Oxygen, nitrates, and heparin
  B Dopamine and intravenous nitroglycerin
  C Emergent percutaneous transluminal coronary angioplasty (PTCA) following hemodynamic stabilization
  D Streptokinase, heparin, and intravenous fluids

4. Which one of the following signs or symptoms is characteristic of mitral regurgitation?

  A Head bobbing
  B A palpable systolic thrill and a ventricular heave
  C Jugular venous distention with cannon *a* waves
  D Ascites
  E Diminished carotid upstroke

5. Which one of the following statements regarding syncope is true?

  A The diagnosis is confirmed electrocardiographically in 50% of patients.
  B Patients usually report a prodrome of palpitations or chest pain when the cause of the syncope is a conduction disturbance.

C) Patients may give a history of recent medication change.

D) Patients may have subtle focal findings on neurologic examination.

E) Admission to a monitored setting is required.

6. Which one of the following signs or symptoms is characteristic of aortic regurgitation?

  A) Florid congestion of the cheeks

  B) A widened pulse pressure

  C) Kussmaul's sign

  D) A third heart sound (S_3)

7. Which one of the following statements regarding thoracic aortic dissection is true?

  A) The patient will most likely be hypotensive on initial presentation.

  B) ST-segment elevation in the anterior leads is a typical electrocardiogram (ECG) finding.

  C) Patients are likely to describe chest pain that is ripping, is severe, worsens with inspiration, and radiates to the right shoulder.

  D) Radiographic findings include a widened mediastinum with possible obliteration of the aortic knob.

  E) Nitroprusside and dopamine are the therapeutic agents of choice.

8. A 58-year-old woman presents to the emergency department (ED) after falling on an icy sidewalk. Her left ankle is painful and swollen. The patient denies any medical problems, stating that she is "never sick." Her blood pressure is 165/108 and her heart rate is 80 beats/min. The most reasonable approach for the ED physician to take would be to treat the patient's ankle injury and

  A) administer nifedipine (10 mg) to lower her blood pressure and discharge her from the ED after her blood pressure has decreased by 20% with the recommendation that she be reevaluated by her family physician in 2 days

  B) initiate intravenous antihypertensive medication

  C) refer the patient to a nephrologist for evaluation of probable secondary hypertension

  D) discharge her from the ED with a prescription for an antihypertensive medication

  E) advise her to follow up with her family doctor

9. Which one of the following statements regarding mitral stenosis is true?

  A) It is sometimes heralded by the development of hemoptysis, which is often fatal.

  B) Patients have an enlarged point of maximal impulse (PMI) due to left ventricular hypertrophy.

  C) Lifelong anticoagulation therapy is usually necessary.

  D) It develops in 40% of patients following rheumatic heart disease.

  E) It causes atrial enlargement and the development of atrial fibrillation, which is usually well tolerated.

10. Which one of the following statements regarding Dressler's syndrome is true?

  A) It occurs within 1–4 days of acute myocardial infarction (MI).

  B) It is commonly associated with a bloody pericardial effusion.

  C) It occurs from 1 week to several months following acute MI.

  D) It is a life-threatening emergency and should be treated with emergency pericardiocentesis.

  E) It results in an increased risk for thoracic aortic dissection.

Answers and Explanations

1. The answer is E This patient most likely has hypertrophic cardiomyopathy, which can cause syncope or near-syncope. Patients with hypertrophic cardiomyopathy who develop syncope or near-syncope may be experiencing arrhythmias and should be admitted for further evaluation. A murmur, which increases in intensity with maneuvers that decrease preload (e.g., the Valsalva maneuver or standing up) and decreases in intensity with maneuvers that increase preload (e.g., squatting), can be heard in 25% of patients. Athlete's heart syndrome is a physiologic response to intensive physical training and is not associated with symptoms.

2. The answer is B Dyspnea on exertion is a common complaint early in the course of mitral stenosis. The dyspnea results from increased pulmonary capillary pressures. Fatigue, due to decreased cardiac output, and peripheral edema, due to right-sided heart failure, develop late in the course of illness. Dysphagia due to compression of the esophagus by an enlarged left atrium may also be a late finding. Chest pain is uncommon.

3. The answer is C Cardiogenic shock is most often a complication of transmural, anterior wall MI. Dobutamine, dopamine, or counterpulsation devices, if necessary, should be used to achieve hemodynamic stabilization; emergent percutaneous transluminal coronary angioplasty is then performed.

4. The answer is B Mitral regurgitation results in dilatation and hypertrophy of the left ventricle, which on physical examination can be felt by palpation as a thrill and a heave. Cannon *a* waves with jugular venous distention are caused by atrial contraction against a stenotic mitral valve or closed tricuspid valve. Diminished carotid upstroke would be expected in disorders that decrease cardiac output. Head bobbing is associated with aortic regurgitation and ascites due to severe right-sided congestive heart failure (CHF) and would not be characteristic of mitral regurgitation.

5. The answer is C A common cause of syncope is a change in medication. Electrocardiography is only useful when the syncope is cardiac in origin, and despite extensive evaluation, a definitive diagnosis is made in only approximately 50% of patients with syncope. The end result of most causes of syncope is a decrease in cerebral oxygen; most patients will have a normal physical examination on presentation to the emergency department (ED). Conduction disturbances frequently cause syncope without prodromal symptoms. Admission to a monitored setting is required if the cause of syncope is serious. In most situations, clinical judgment is necessary to determine the likelihood of serious underlying illness.

6. The answer is B In aortic regurgitation, a widened pulse pressure is noted as the forceful ejection of blood in systole rapidly falls off due to regurgitation through the aortic valve in diastole. Kussmaul's sign, increased jugular venous distention with inspiration, would not be expected. A third heart sound (S_3) is usually heard in mitral regurgitation, but not aortic regurgitation. "Mitral facies," florid congestion of the cheeks, may be seen with mitral stenosis.

7. The answer is D Thoracic aortic dissection is most commonly a complication of hypertension. Patients most commonly present with hypertension and complain of pain radiating to the back. An ECG will reveal left ventricular hypertrophy; ST-segment elevations may be present but are not helpful in making the diagnosis. A chest radiograph is abnormal in 80% of patients and will reveal widening of the mediastinum, obliteration of the aortic knob, displacement of the trachea to the right, and/or a double-density appearance of the aorta. Treatment consists of lowering the blood pressure and the heart rate, usually by administering intravenous nitroprusside combined with a β blocker, and immediate consultation with a cardiothoracic surgeon.

8. The answer is E This patient may have undiagnosed essential hypertension, or her blood pressure may be transiently elevated as a result of pain and anxiety. The best course of action is appropriate management of the patient's ankle injury, including pain medication if indicated, referral of the patient to her family doctor for reevaluation, and repeat blood pressure checks along with hypertension and diet education.

9. The answer is D Mitral stenosis develops in 40% of patients following rheumatic heart disease. Hemoptysis, caused by rupture of bronchial vessels, is rarely fatal but may be observed. Atrial fibrillation, a source of emboli, is poorly tolerated. Patients with atrial fibrillation require lifelong anticoagulation therapy, but not all patients with mitral stenosis do. Left ventricular hypertrophy is not a finding in patients with pure mitral stenosis.

10. The answer is C Dressler's syndrome is a delayed complication of MI that occurs 1 week to several months following MI. Bloody pericardial effusions are more commonly associated with uremia or trauma.

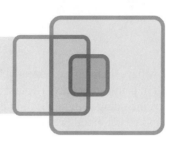

chapter **3**

Pulmonary Emergencies

PETER E. SOKOLOVE · EDWARD A. PANACEK

I **ACUTE RESPIRATORY FAILURE**

A **Discussion**

1. **Definition.** Acute respiratory failure is defined as an acute impairment in oxygen or carbon dioxide exchange that results in, or has the potential to result in, patient morbidity or mortality. **Impaired gas exchange** [e.g., as a result of shunting, alveolar hypoventilation, ventilation–perfusion ($\dot{V}/\dot{Q}$) mismatch, or decreased pulmonary diffusion capacity] leads to **hypoxia** [i.e., a decreased arterial oxygen tension (Pao_2)]. **Impaired ventilation** causes **hypercapnia** [i.e., an elevated carbon dioxide tension (Pco_2)]. Because the baseline respiratory status may vary greatly among patients, it is difficult to characterize acute respiratory insufficiency by purely numeric criteria.

   a. Generally, a patient who acutely develops a Po_2 below 60 mm Hg on room air or a Pco_2 greater than 50 mm Hg with an arterial blood pH less than 7.35 is considered to be in respiratory failure.

   b. Some patients [e.g., those with chronic obstructive pulmonary disease (COPD)] chronically have an elevated Pco_2 but a normal arterial blood pH. In these patients, respiratory failure is defined as a Pco_2 higher than baseline with a concurrent decrease in serum pH.

2. **Causes.** There are many causes of acute respiratory failure, including most pulmonary diseases as well as many cardiac diseases. Most commonly, one should consider airway obstruction, asthma, COPD, congestive heart failure (CHF), noncardiogenic pulmonary edema, pulmonary emboli, massive pleural effusion, pneumonia, hemothorax, pneumothorax, toxic inhalation, advanced lung cancer, and neurologic or muscular disorders that result in impaired respiratory abilities.

B **Clinical features**

1. **Symptoms**

   a. Cardiovascular. Dyspnea is the most common symptom of acute respiratory failure.

   b. Neurologic

      (1) Confusion, agitation, and **disorientation** can occur with marked hypoxia.

      (2) Lethargy or **somnolence** is commonly seen in patients with marked hypercapnia.

      (3) Generalized seizures or **coma** may result from profound central nervous system (CNS) hypoxia.

   c. Other signs of respiratory failure include **cyanosis, diaphoresis,** and **severely labored breathing** (including the use of accessory muscles). Children may demonstrate nasal flaring, audible grunting, or retractions (i.e., intercostal, subcostal, suprasternal).

2. **Physical examination findings**

   a. Tachycardia, tachypnea, and **mild hypertension** are usually present.

   b. Bradypnea may be seen in patients with hypercapnia. **Wheezing, rales,** or **decreased breath sounds** may be noted on pulmonary examination, depending on the underlying disease.

C **Evaluation** In a patient with suspected acute respiratory failure, patient evaluation and treatment are begun simultaneously.

1. **Patient history and physical examination.** A brief, focused history and physical examination, including vital signs, will often reveal the cause of respiratory failure prior to obtaining any diagnostic studies.

2. **Diagnostic tests**
   a. **Chest radiographs** are helpful for determining the underlying cause of the acute respiratory failure. Radiographs should be obtained rapidly at the patient's bedside.
   b. **Arterial blood gas (ABG).** An ABG should be obtained in all patients with suspected acute respiratory failure. The most important elements of the ABG are the P_{O_2}, P_{CO_2}, and pH.
   c. **Pulse oximetry** may provide an immediate measurement of the patient's oxygen saturation.
   d. **Ancillary tests** may be indicated, depending on the cause of the respiratory failure [e.g., an electrocardiogram (ECG) for a patient with suspected CHF, a $\dot{V}/\dot{Q}$ scan or pulmonary angiogram for a patient with suspected pulmonary embolism, a urine toxicology screen for a patient with suspected narcotic overdose].

D **Therapy**

1. **Airway, breathing, circulation (ABCs)**
   a. **Airway.** Airway management, usually **orotracheal intubation,** is required for patients who do not have an intact airway or who are unable to protect their airway.
   b. **Breathing.** After an airway has been established, ensuring adequate oxygenation and ventilation is the mainstay of treating respiratory failure.
      (1) **Oxygenation.** Patients should be administered supplemental oxygen in order to maintain a serum oxygen saturation of at least 90%.
         (a) In **intubated patients,** it is best to start with an inspired oxygen concentration (F_{IO_2}) of 100% and then reduce this percentage, depending on the ABG results.
         (b) In **nonintubated patients,** supplemental oxygen can be administered in various ways, including via **nasal cannula** or **face mask.** Although the concentration of oxygen delivered by each of these methods is variable, it is best to start with a method that delivers a high oxygen concentration (e.g., a nonrebreather face mask).
      (2) **Ventilation** should be addressed in addition to oxygenation. Patients with a P_{CO_2} greater than 50 mm Hg and an arterial blood pH below 7.30 require intubation and mechanical ventilation if their condition cannot be quickly improved.
         (a) Following intubation, ventilator settings for respiratory rates and tidal volumes should generally be adjusted to gradually normalize the blood pH. In general, the initial respiratory rate should be 12–16 breaths/min, with a tidal volume of 10–12 mL/kg.
         (b) As a general rule, oxygenation is more important than ventilation. For this reason, it is acceptable to have a mild respiratory acidosis (e.g., a pH less than 7.35) if necessary to maintain adequate oxygenation or to minimize peak airway pressures.
   c. **Circulation.** The placement of **two peripheral intravenous lines** allows the administration of fluids and medications to the patient.

2. **Specific therapy** that addresses the cause of the acute respiratory failure should be undertaken after the ABCs have been addressed. In some cases, aggressive treatment of the underlying condition may reverse the respiratory failure and eliminate the need for intubation (e.g., nitroglycerin and diuretics for CHF, inhaled β_2 agonists for asthma or COPD, chest tube placement for a large pneumothorax or hemothorax).

E **Disposition** All patients with acute respiratory failure should be admitted to an intensive care unit (ICU). Patients who are clinically stable but have the potential for developing respiratory failure should be admitted to an ICU or another closely monitored setting.

II ASTHMA

A Discussion

1. **Definition.** Asthma is defined as the presence of intermittent symptoms from airway hyperactivity and reversible airway obstruction. Airway obstruction is usually caused by smooth muscle contraction and airway inflammation.
   a. **Extrinsic asthma** is immunologically mediated and tends to develop in childhood.
   b. **Intrinsic asthma** has no identifiable cause and tends to worsen with age.
2. **Incidence.** Asthma affects approximately 5% of adults in the United States; approximately 1.5 million patients seek care for asthma in the emergency department (ED) each year.

B Clinical features

1. **Symptoms**
   a. **Wheezing, dyspnea,** and **coughing** are most common. In cough-variant asthma, coughing, which is often worse at night, is the prominent feature.
   b. **Pleuritic chest pain** is noted in some patients.
   c. **Accessory muscle use** may be seen in patients having moderate to severe attacks.
   d. **Altered mental status, severely labored breathing,** or **extreme fatigue** are signs of **impending respiratory arrest.**
2. **Physical examination findings**
   a. **Tachypnea** and **tachycardia** are common.
   b. Pulmonary examination often demonstrates **wheezing,** a **prolonged expiratory phase,** and **decreased breath sounds.** When airflow is very low, wheezing may be absent.

C Differential diagnoses include CHF ("cardiac asthma"), upper airway obstruction, foreign body aspiration, pulmonary embolism, an anaphylactic reaction, pneumonia, croup, bronchiolitis, COPD, and toxic inhalation.

D Evaluation

1. **Pulmonary function tests.** The **peak expiratory flow rate (PEFR)** can be used to evaluate the degree of obstruction.
2. **Pulse oximetry** can be used to evaluate the degree of hypoxia.
3. **Chest radiographs** should be ordered for patients with hypoxia, fever, a focal lung examination, or symptoms not responsive to bronchodilator therapy.
4. **ABG.** ABGs should not be ordered routinely; they should be reserved for patients with severe attacks or suspected respiratory failure. Because a patient having an asthma exacerbation is breathing quickly, his or her arterial carbon dioxide tension ($Paco_2$) should be less than 40 mm Hg (respiratory alkalosis). A normal or elevated $Paco_2$ in a patient with an asthma exacerbation represents impending or actual respiratory failure.
5. **Theophylline levels** should be obtained in patients taking this medication. Theophylline toxicity is seen as serum levels exceed 20 µg/mL.

E Therapy

1. **Oxygen** is indicated for all asthma patients to keep the oxygen saturation greater than 95%.
2. **Pharmacologic therapy**
   a. **Standard (first-line) agents**
      (1) **Inhaled β_2 agonists** act as bronchial smooth muscle relaxants. Nebulized **albuterol** (2.5 mg) or **metaproterenol** (10 mg) is administered every 15–20 minutes; in patients with severe

attacks, these agents may be administered continuously. Albuterol is preferred because its higher selectivity for β_2 receptors minimizes cardiac effects.

(2) **Corticosteroids** suppress the inflammatory component of asthma and are considered first-line agents for the treatment of patients with asthma that does not respond rapidly to inhaled β_2 agonists.

    (a) Oral **prednisone** (60 mg in adults, 2 mg/kg in children) may be administered. **Methylprednisolone** (125 mg in adults, 2 mg/kg in children) may be administered intravenously if the patient is unable to tolerate oral prednisone secondary to vomiting or respiratory distress.

    (b) Patients who have been administered steroids in the ED who are subsequently discharged to home should continue to take oral steroids for 5 days (e.g., prednisone, 40–60 mg once daily for adults or 1 mg/kg/day for children) to reduce the rate of asthma relapse. Patients who are steroid dependent or who have used steroids recently should be gradually tapered off the steroids over 10–14 days, rather than discontinuing steroids after 5 days.

(3) **Anticholinergic agents** relax bronchial smooth muscle, particularly in the more proximal airways. Although these agents are most useful in the treatment of COPD, they may also be used for patients with asthma exacerbations that do not rapidly respond to inhaled β_2 agonists.

    (a) Metered-dose or nebulized **ipratropium bromide** can be administered (500 μg every 15 minutes) for up to three doses.

    (b) **Ipratropium** and **albuterol solutions** may be mixed together and administered in the same hand-held nebulizer.

b. Second-line agents

(1) **Magnesium sulfate** (2–4 g intravenously over 20 minutes) should be considered in adults with severe asthma exacerbations that are not responding to previous therapy.

(2) **Epinephrine** (0.3 mg subcutaneously in adults or 0.01 mg/kg in children, up to 0.3 mg) or **terbutaline** (0.25 mg subcutaneously in adults or 0.01 mg/kg/dose for children, maximum dose = 0.4 mg) can be considered for young patients with severe asthma that does not respond to first-line agents. Epinephrine should not be used during early pregnancy.

(3) **Theophylline** has fallen out of favor due to its high rate of toxicity and is no longer recommended in the acute management of asthma, except for selected patients already taking the medication.

c. Other pharmacologic options

(1) **Inhaled general anesthetics** are potent bronchodilators. Their use in the treatment of asthma is reserved for patients with severe asthma exacerbations in whom previous therapy has not resulted in adequate oxygenation or ventilation.

(2) **Ketamine** is a dissociative anesthetic agent that also causes bronchodilation and can be used for severe, refractory asthma.

    (a) An initial bolus of 1–2 mg/kg is administered intravenously over 30–60 minutes, followed by an intravenous ketamine drip (1 mg/kg/hour).

    (b) Ketamine is contraindicated in patients with ischemic heart disease, increased intracranial pressure, severe hypertension, or preeclampsia.

(3) **Heliox,** a mixture of 60%–70% helium and 30%–40% oxygen, can be administered via face mask or nebulizer to patients with severe, refractory asthma. In nonintubated patients, heliox decreases the work of breathing by improving laminar gas flow. In intubated patients, heliox results in improved oxygenation and decreased peak airway pressures.

3. Intubation and mechanical ventilation. Intubation is indicated for patients with impending respiratory failure. Orotracheal intubation is preferred over nasotracheal intubation because orotracheal intubation allows for the placement of a larger endotracheal tube, which decreases the work of breathing (by lowering airway resistance) and facilitates the management of pulmonary secretions.

  a. Rapid sequence induction (RSI; see Chapter 1 III B 3 c) should be considered for asthmatic patients requiring intubation.

    (1) Ketamine (2 mg/kg intravenously), because of its bronchodilation properties, is a good choice of induction agent.

    (2) Benzodiazepines, rather than opiates, should be used for sedation in intubated patients with asthma because opiates may induce histamine release from mast cells, exacerbating the bronchospasm.

    (3) Pancuronium or **vecuronium** may be administered to induce muscle paralysis if ventilation is difficult following intubation.

  b. Complications

    (1) Barotrauma is a common complication of mechanical ventilation in patients with asthma. To avoid this complication, the tidal volume should be decreased to 10 mL/kg and the ventilator should be adjusted to increase the time allowed for expiration to minimize peak airway pressures.

    (2) Hypotension that develops rapidly after intubation and mechanical ventilation usually results from the auto–positive end-expiratory pressure (auto-PEEP) phenomenon or a tension pneumothorax.

      (a) Auto-PEEP phenomenon. Air trapping in the lungs can lead to increased intrathoracic pressure, which may result in decreased venous return and a resultant decrease in cardiac output. If air trapping is suspected as the cause of hypotension, the respiratory rate on the ventilator should be decreased to allow adequate time for exhalation.

      (b) Pneumothorax. A tension pneumothorax may develop as a result of air trapping and increased airway pressures, leading to kinking of the mediastinal vessels, a decrease in venous return to the heart, and decreased cardiac output. If a tension pneumothorax is suspected as the cause of hypotension, immediate needle decompression of the affected side should be undertaken, followed by chest tube placement.

F Disposition

1. **Admission.** In a patient with asthma, evidence of pneumonia is generally an indication for hospital admission.

2. **Discharge**

  a. Patients may be discharged to home if they have made significant clinical improvement, have a PEFR greater than 60% of the predicted value (or equal to their baseline PEFR), have a normal respiratory rate, and are able to walk without recurring symptoms.

  b. Patients with a PEFR that is 35%–60% of the predicted value may be discharged if they are otherwise stable, compliant, and have a good follow-up system.

III CHRONIC OBSTRUCTIVE PULMONARY DISEASE

A Discussion

1. **Definition.** COPD is a syndrome characterized by chronic dyspnea and expiratory airflow obstruction as a result of increased resistance or decreased airway caliber throughout the small bronchi and bronchioles. There are two types of COPD.

  a. Emphysema is permanent, abnormal enlargement of the terminal bronchioles accompanied by destruction of the bronchoalveolar lining.

  b. Chronic bronchitis is defined by a productive cough on most days for at least 3 months per year for at least 2 consecutive years.

2. **Incidence.** COPD is the fifth leading cause of death in the United States.

3. **Causes.** Smoking is the leading cause of COPD. Cystic fibrosis, α_1-antitrypsin deficiency, and some occupational exposures predispose to the development of COPD.

B **Clinical features**   Exacerbations are what bring most patients with COPD to the ED.

1. **Symptoms**
   a. **Wheezing, dyspnea on exertion,** and **cough** are the most common symptoms. Wheezing may not be audible if the patient's airflow is very poor.
   b. **Accessory muscle use** may be seen in patients with moderate to severe COPD exacerbations.
   c. **Pursed-lip breathing** may be present.
   d. **Altered mental status, severely labored breathing,** and **extreme fatigue** signal impending respiratory arrest.

2. **Physical examination findings. Signs of right-sided CHF (cor pulmonale)** may be present and include jugular venous distention, peripheral edema, and hepatomegaly.

C **Differential diagnoses** include CHF, upper airway obstruction, foreign body aspiration, pulmonary embolism, an anaphylactic reaction, pneumonia, asthma, toxic inhalation, and pneumothorax.

D **Evaluation**   The evaluation of a patient with COPD exacerbation is similar to that for patients with asthma.

1. **Pulmonary function testing.** The PEFR can assist in monitoring response to treatment; however, it is not as useful as an evaluation tool for patients with COPD (as compared with those with asthma) because acute bronchospasm contributes less to dysfunction in patients with COPD.

2. **Pulse oximetry** can be used to evaluate the degree of hypoxia.

3. **Chest radiographs** should be considered for patients with hypoxia, fever, a focal lung examination, or symptoms not responsive to bronchodilator therapy.

4. **ABG.** An ABG should be obtained on patients who do not respond to bronchodilator therapy or in whom acute or serious respiratory failure is suspected. When interpreting the ABG, it is important to remember that COPD patients may retain carbon dioxide on a chronic basis. If a patient has an elevated P_{CO_2} in the face of a normal blood pH, then this usually represents chronic carbon dioxide retention rather than acute respiratory failure. However, if the P_{CO_2} is elevated and the blood pH is low, the patient is probably in respiratory failure.

5. **Laboratory studies**
   a. The **hematocrit** may be elevated secondary to increased erythrocytosis.
   b. The **serum bicarbonate level** may be elevated, suggesting that a secondary metabolic alkalosis is compensating for the chronic respiratory acidosis.

E **Therapy**

1. **Oxygen** should be administered to all COPD patients. Some COPD patients with a chronically elevated P_{CO_2} have lost their sensitivity to hypercarbia, and thus depend on the hypoxic drive to stimulate their respirations. If an excessive concentration of oxygen is administered to these patients in an attempt to normalize their oxygen saturation, it may depress their respiratory drive and lead to hypoventilation and respiratory failure. Therefore, the minimum amount of oxygen that is needed to maintain the oxygen saturation at 90% should be administered.

2. **Pharmacologic therapy**
   a. **Inhaled β_2 agonists** are first-line agents for the treatment of acute exacerbations of COPD. Dosage and administration is the same as that for patients with asthma [see II E 2 a (1)].
   b. **Inhaled anticholinergic agents** are the second-line agents for the treatment of acute COPD exacerbations. Dosage and administration is the same as that for patients with asthma [see II E 2 a (3)].

  c. Corticosteroids should be considered for patients with COPD who do not respond rapidly to inhaled β_2 agonists or anticholinergics. The dosing and administration is the same as that for patients with asthma [see II E 2 a (2)].

  d. Theophylline is often used in the chronic management of COPD, but may not be helpful in acute COPD exacerbations. Theophylline should be considered only for patients with severe exacerbations who are already taking theophylline.

 3. Intubation and mechanical ventilation are generally indicated for patients with impending respiratory failure. Unlike asthmatic patients, COPD patients with mild acute elevations in Pco_2 and a decreased blood pH can sometimes be managed without intubation, as long as they do not demonstrate CNS or cardiovascular dysfunction, and are not severely fatigued.

  a. Noninvasive positive-pressure ventilatory support can often assist ventilation and improve a patient's clinical condition enough to obviate intubation. Positive pressure is delivered through either a nasal or face mask using a ventilator or a bilevel positive airway pressure (BiPAP) system.

  b. Ketamine is **not a preferred induction agent** in these patients, because many of them have concomitant ischemic heart disease.

F **Disposition** Patients with COPD exacerbations are more likely to be admitted than patients with an asthma exacerbation because reversible disease accounts for a smaller part of their clinical presentation.

 1. Admission. Pneumonia, CHF, or other existing comorbid conditions are indications for hospital admission.

 2. Discharge. Patients may be discharged to home if they have made a significant clinical improvement and are near their baseline respiratory status. Oxygen saturation must be over 90% in discharged patients.

IV NONCARDIOGENIC PULMONARY EDEMA (NCPE)

NCPE is also known as adult respiratory distress syndrome (ARDS).

A **Discussion**

 1. Definition. NCPE is a form of pulmonary edema resulting from an abnormal increase in the permeability of pulmonary vascular membranes.

 2. Causes of NCPE include sepsis, aspiration of gastric contents, near-drowning, thermal injury, trauma, high-altitude pulmonary edema, radiation, multiple transfusions, eclampsia–preeclampsia, and selected drug reactions or overdoses, including narcotic and aspirin overdose.

 3. Pathogenesis. NCPE is not related to cardiac, hydrostatic, or hemodynamic edema. The proposed mechanism for the edema is damage to the vascular endothelium as a result of complement cascade activation or direct damage by bacterial endotoxin. Pulmonary surfactant is disrupted and lung compliance is decreased.

B **Clinical features**

 1. Symptoms. Dyspnea with **rapidly progressive tachypnea** is common.

 2. Physical examination findings include **bilateral rales.**

C **Differential diagnoses** NCPE is most commonly confused with CHF or pneumonia. Asthma, COPD, pulmonary embolism, an anaphylactic reaction, and foreign body aspiration should also be considered.

D **Evaluation** It is most important to assess the respiratory status of a patient with NCPE.

1. **Chest radiographs, ABGs,** and an **ECG** should be obtained for all patients suspected of having NCPE.
   a. The chest radiograph demonstrates bilateral patchy alveolar infiltrates and a normal heart size. In severe cases, the infiltrates may progress to a "white out" of the lungs.
   b. The ABG demonstrates hypoxia and an increased alveolar–arterial (A-a) gradient.

2. **Laboratory tests.** Pertinent laboratory tests include a **complete blood count (CBC), urinalysis,** an **electrolyte panel,** and **blood urea nitrogen** (BUN) and **creatinine levels.**

E Therapy

1. **Supplemental oxygen** should be administered to maintain the oxygen saturation above 90%. In intubated patients, the FIO_2 should be kept below 50%, if possible, because of the potential for pulmonary oxygen toxicity.

2. **Intubation and mechanical ventilation** are indicated for patients who, despite supplemental oxygen, have inadequate oxygenation or ventilation. **PEEP** should be added if adequate oxygenation cannot be maintained with an FIO_2 of less than 50%. The minimal amount of PEEP to maintain adequate oxygenation should be used because high levels of PEEP can result in pneumothorax or hypotension secondary to a decreased preload.

3. **Treatment of the underlying disorder** should be undertaken (e.g., antibiotics for sepsis, alkalinization and dialysis for aspirin overdose).

4. The use of **corticosteroids, nonsteroidal anti-inflammatory drugs (NSAIDs),** and **anticoagulants** is being investigated for the future treatment of NCPE.

F Disposition

1. **Admission.** The vast majority of patients with NCPE will need to be admitted to the hospital, and should be sent to a monitored bed.
   a. Many patients who develop NCPE do so as a result of medical conditions that often require hospitalization in and of themselves (e.g., sepsis, near-drowning, thermal injury, trauma, aspirin overdose).
   b. NCPE may be rapidly progressive, and patients may have a rapid deterioration in their respiratory status. Intubated or critically ill patients require ICU admission.

2. **Discharge.** Overdose patients who are not hypoxic and are asymptomatic after 6–12 hours of observation are usually discharged home.

V HEMOPTYSIS

A Discussion

1. **Definition.** Hemoptysis is the expectoration of blood from the respiratory tract when the source of the bleeding is below the level of the larynx. The degree of hemoptysis can range from blood-tinged sputum to massive hemoptysis. **Massive hemoptysis** is defined as the expectoration of more than 100 mL of blood per hour or more than 300–500 mL over 24 hours.

2. **Causes.** The most common cause of minor hemoptysis is chronic bronchitis. Other causes of hemoptysis in general include pneumonia, tuberculosis, fungal infection, bronchiectasis, cystic fibrosis, pulmonary parasitic disease (e.g., ascariasis), lung abscess, bronchial malignancy, CHF, mitral stenosis, pulmonary embolism, pulmonary arteriovenous malformation, pulmonary hypertension, Wegener's granulomatosis, Goodpasture's syndrome, foreign body aspiration, and trauma. All of these conditions can be aggravated by a coagulopathy or thrombocytopenia.

3. **Pathogenesis.** Death from hemoptysis results from suffocation, secondary to impaired gas exchange, rather than from exsanguination.

B **Clinical features**   The clinical presentation of hemoptysis depends on the underlying cause as well as the amount of bleeding.

1. **Symptoms.** Patients may complain of a cough, chest pain, dyspnea, or systemic symptoms.

2. **Physical examination findings.** Patients may appear well with normal vital signs, or they may demonstrate respiratory distress. Findings on pulmonary examination depend on the cause of hemoptysis but may include rhonchi in patients with bronchitis, rales in patients with CHF, decreased breath sounds in patients with pneumonia, or a pleural rub in patients with pulmonary infarction.

C **Evaluation**   It is important to first assess whether the bleeding represents true hemoptysis, or if the patient is actually bleeding from the stomach (hematemesis), the nose, or the oropharyngeal cavity.

1. A **CBC** and **chest radiograph** should be obtained in all patients with hemoptysis.

2. **Other laboratory studies.** Unless the patient is believed to have very minor hemoptysis secondary to bronchitis and is in no respiratory distress, it is prudent to obtain the following:
   a. **Prothrombin time (PT)** and **partial thromboplastin time (PTT)**
   b. **Electrolyte panel**
   c. **BUN** and **creatinine level**
   d. **Glucose level**
   e. **Blood type** and **screen** (type and cross if the hemoptysis is massive)
   f. **Urinalysis**
   g. **ECG**

3. **Specific tests** may be ordered depending on the suspected disease process. For example:
   a. If pulmonary embolism is suspected, pertinent studies include **pulse oximetry** or **ABG, lower extremity Doppler ultrasound, V/Q scanning,** or **pulmonary angiography.**
   b. If malignancy is suspected, **bronchoscopy** or a **chest computed tomography (CT) scan** would be appropriate.
   c. If mitral stenosis is suspected, an **echocardiogram** should be ordered.
   d. If tuberculosis is suspected, a **purified protein derivative (PPD) skin test, sputum acid-fast bacillus stain,** or **mycobacterial culture** may be requested.

D **Therapy**

1. **ABCs.** The management of hemoptysis begins with addressing the patient's airway, breathing, and circulation status.
   a. **Airway.** The patient should be intubated if he or she is having difficulty maintaining airway patency secondary to bleeding. Oral intubation with a large endotracheal tube is best for ease of suctioning.
      (1) If the patient is bleeding from the left lung, the right mainstem bronchus can be selectively intubated in order to maximize ventilation. This can be accomplished by advancing the tube 4–5 cm beyond the usual position.
      (2) If massive bleeding is occurring from the right lung, then selective intubation of the left mainstem bronchus is desirable but more difficult. If one rotates the endotracheal tube 90° counterclockwise from the usual position and alters its concavity to face the left during intubation, there is an increased likelihood of left mainstem bronchus intubation.
      (3) Alternatively, a double-lumen endotracheal tube can be used to separately intubate the left and right mainstem bronchi.
   b. **Breathing.** Supplemental oxygen should be given to maximize oxygenation. The spread of blood can be minimized and ventilation improved by having the patient lie on the affected side, if known.
   c. **Circulation.** Intravenous access should be obtained to administer crystalloid or blood products as needed. The patient's vital signs should be monitored closely.

2. **Localization and control of the bleeding.** Once the ABCs have been addressed, localization and control of the bleeding are necessary.
   a. Anemia, thrombocytopenia, and coagulopathy should be corrected.
   b. Consultation with various specialists may be advisable:
      (1) A pulmonologist may be called upon to perform bronchoscopy in an attempt to localize and control the bleeding.
      (2) An angiographer may be helpful if arterial embolization is needed.
      (3) A cardiothoracic surgeon should be consulted if surgical resection is being considered.
3. **Treatment for the cause of the hemoptysis** should be attempted.

E Disposition
1. **Discharge.** Patients who meet the following criteria can be considered for discharge from the hospital, provided that they see a primary care physician for close follow-up care:
   a. Minor degree of hemoptysis
   b. Normal vital signs and near-normal hematocrit
   c. No additional hemoptysis over 2–3 hours of observation
   d. No other acute medical condition that requires hospitalization
2. **Admission.** All other patients should be admitted for further care and evaluation. Patients with unstable vital signs, life-threatening hemoptysis, respiratory compromise, or potential respiratory compromise should be admitted to the ICU.

VI   PULMONARY EMBOLISM

A Discussion
1. **Definition.** Pulmonary embolism occurs when a venous thrombus (or, occasionally, another substance, such as fat or amniotic fluid) embolizes to the lung, causing occlusion of a pulmonary artery. Pulmonary emboli may be small, involving only a branch of the pulmonary artery, or large, causing an occlusion of both pulmonary arteries (a saddle embolus).
2. **Incidence.** Pulmonary embolism is the third most common cause of death in the United States. Because the symptoms, history, and physical examination findings are often nonspecific, this disease is underdiagnosed.
3. **Predisposing conditions** include heart disease (e.g., acute myocardial infarction, CHF, arrhythmia), venous stasis, pregnancy, obesity, prolonged immobilization, trauma, deep venous thrombosis, and conditions that lead to a hypercoagulable state (e.g., malignancy, oral contraceptive use, protein C or S deficiency). Risk factors are identifiable in approximately 90% of patients with pulmonary embolism.

B Clinical features
1. **Symptoms**
   a. The **classic triad** of **pleuritic chest pain, dyspnea,** and **hemoptysis** is present in less than 25% of patients.
   b. Other symptoms include **coughing** and **apprehension, diaphoresis,** a **low-grade fever,** or **symptoms of deep venous thrombosis.** Patients with a large pulmonary embolism may present with **syncope** or **cardiopulmonary arrest.**
2. **Physical examination findings**
   a. **Pulseless electrical activity (PEA)** is often seen in patients with pulmonary embolism and cardiopulmonary arrest.
   b. **Tachypnea** is seen in approximately 70% of patients with pulmonary embolism. **Tachycardia, rales,** and an **accentuated second heart sound (S_2)** are also common signs of pulmonary embolism. An S_3 or S_4 gallop may also be observed.
   c. **Lower extremity edema** may be observed.

C **Differential diagnoses** include myocardial infarction, pneumonia, pleurisy, spontaneous pneumothorax, pericarditis, aortic dissection, esophageal perforation, costochondritis, asthma, COPD, rib fracture, and hyperventilation syndrome.

D **Evaluation**

1. **Laboratory studies.** A CBC, electrolyte panel, BUN and creatinine level, glucose level, PT/PTT, D-dimer, and urinalysis should be performed for patients with suspected pulmonary embolism. In women of reproductive age who have not had a hysterectomy, urine pregnancy test results should be obtained.

2. **Chest radiograph.** A chest radiograph should be obtained for all patients with suspected pulmonary embolism. The chest radiograph is usually not completely normal but the findings are not specific for pulmonary embolism; therefore, chest radiographs are most helpful for excluding other diseases (e.g., pneumothorax, pneumonia, CHF). Specific signs associated with pulmonary embolism include Westermark's sign and Hampton's hump.
   a. **Westermark's sign** is a prominent central pulmonary artery with diminished distal pulmonary vessels in one lung field.
   b. **Hampton's hump** is a triangular or "wedge-shaped" pleural-based density that points toward the hilum, commonly seen at the costophrenic angle on the posterior-anterior (PA) view.

3. **ECG.** An ECG should be obtained in order to evaluate for cardiac ischemia, and to assist in the diagnosis of pulmonary embolism. A completely normal ECG is found in only 5%–15% of patients with pulmonary embolism.
   a. **Sinus tachycardia** and **nonspecific ST-T–wave changes** are the most common abnormalities in patients with pulmonary embolism.
   b. Approximately 25% of patients with pulmonary embolism have some evidence of **right-sided heart strain,** such as right bundle branch block, right axis deviation, p-pulmonale, or a right ventricular strain pattern.
   c. The **classic finding** of a prominent S wave in lead I along with a Q wave and an inverted T wave in lead III ($S_1 Q_3 T_3$) is more specific to the diagnosis of pulmonary embolism, but is seen in only 12% of patients.

4. **ABG.** An ABG may demonstrate hypoxia, hypocapnia, or an elevated A-a gradient. An abnormal ABG may help make the diagnosis of pulmonary embolism, but a normal ABG does not rule out the disorder, because 5%–15% of patients with pulmonary embolism will have a normal ABG.

5. **$\dot{V}/\dot{Q}$ scan.** Because the chest radiograph, ECG findings, and ABG are not sufficient to exclude the diagnosis of pulmonary embolism, a $\dot{V}/\dot{Q}$ scan is usually obtained in the ED. The result of the $\dot{V}/\dot{Q}$ scan is reported as **normal, low probability, intermediate** (or **indeterminate**) **probability,** or **high probability.** The applicability of the $\dot{V}/\dot{Q}$ scan result depends on the clinical context and the degree of clinical suspicion for pulmonary embolism (Table 3–1).

6. **Noninvasive studies to evaluate the lower extremities** [e.g., **impedance plethysmography (IPG), Doppler ultrasound**] should be obtained in patients who have nondiagnostic $\dot{V}/\dot{Q}$ scans.

7. **Spiral CT.** Rapid CT evaluation is slowly becoming the most common and reliable method of diagnosing a pulmonary embolism.

8. **Pulmonary angiography** is the gold standard for the diagnosis of pulmonary embolism.
   a. Pulmonary angiography, an invasive test, is particularly risky for elderly patients with severe underlying cardiopulmonary disease. Serial outpatient IPG testing may be a reasonable alternative to pulmonary angiography in some patients.
   b. Pulmonary angiography is generally indicated for patients in whom the clinical suspicion for pulmonary embolism is high, but the $\dot{V}/\dot{Q}$ scan is nondiagnostic and the lower extremity study is negative.

TABLE 3–1 Evaluation and Treatment of Patients Suspected of Having Pulmonary Embolism on the Basis of Ventilation–Perfusion ($\dot{V}/\dot{Q}$) Scanning Results and Clinical Suspicion

Clinical Suspicion for Pulmonary Embolism	$\dot{V}/\dot{Q}$ Scanning Results			
	NORMAL	LOW PROBABILITY	INTERMEDIATE PROBABILITY	HIGH PROBABILITY
Low	No treatment	No treatment	NIS(+): treat NIS(−): no treatment	NIS(+): treat NIS(−): PA
Medium	NIS(+): treat NIS(−): no treatment	NIS(+): treat NIS(−): no treatment	NIS(+): treat NIS(−): PA, consider serial IPG	NIS(+): treat NIS(−): PA
High	NIS(+): treat NIS(−): no treatment	NIS(+): treat NIS(−): PA, consider serial IPG	NIS(+): treat NIS(−): PA, consider serial IPG	Treat

IPG = impedance plethysmography; NIS = noninvasive study of the lower extremities; PA = pulmonary angiography.

E **Therapy**   Patients with pulmonary embolism may range from being mildly symptomatic to being in full cardiopulmonary arrest.

1. **ABCs.** Initial evaluation and support of airway, breathing, and circulation is the highest priority.
   a. **Supplemental oxygen** should be administered to all patients with suspected pulmonary embolism.
   b. Hypotension that is refractory to **crystalloid** should be treated with **pressors** (e.g., intravenous dopamine, 5 μg/kg/min titrated to maintain adequate blood pressure).

2. **Anticoagulation. Intravenous heparin** should be used for anticoagulation in most patients with pulmonary embolism. A loading dose of 5000–10,000 U (100 U/kg) is administered via an intravenous bolus, followed by a maintenance infusion of 1000 U/hour (18 U/kg/hour).
   a. Heparin therapy should be initiated prior to making a final diagnosis in patients with high clinical probability for pulmonary embolism.
   b. **Contraindications**
      (1) **Absolute contraindications** include active bleeding, intracranial lesions, or severe uncontrolled hypertension.
      (2) **Relative contraindications** include recent stroke or major surgery, advanced liver or kidney failure, bacterial endocarditis, or a bleeding diathesis.

3. **Thrombolytic therapy** [e.g., with **streptokinase, tissue plasminogen activator (t-PA),** or **urokinase**] should be considered in patients with pulmonary embolism who are hemodynamically unstable.

4. **Inferior vena cava (Greenfield) filters** may be placed by a vascular surgeon or invasive radiologist in patients who are diagnosed with pulmonary embolism but have contraindications to anticoagulation therapy. They may also be used in patients who experience recurrent pulmonary embolism despite appropriate anticoagulation.

5. **Surgical embolectomy** to remove pulmonary emboli is controversial and has largely been replaced by the use of thrombolytic therapy in hemodynamically unstable patients.

F **Disposition**

1. **Admission.** All patients suspected of having pulmonary embolism require admission to a telemetry bed for monitoring and anticoagulation therapy. Patients who demonstrate hemodynamic instability or potential respiratory compromise should be admitted to the ICU.

2. **Discharge.** If clinical suspicion and diagnostic tests suggest that the patient does not have pulmonary embolism, he or she may be discharged unless another condition that requires hospital admission is responsible for his or her symptoms.

VII PLEURAL EFFUSIONS

A Discussion

1. **Definition.** A pleural effusion is present when fluid in the pleural space is visible on a chest radiograph. Normally, the pleural space contains only a minimal amount of fluid that is not apparent radiographically.

2. **Causes**
   a. **Intrathoracic causes** of pleural effusion include pulmonary infection (e.g., parapneumonic effusion, empyema), CHF, malignancy, pulmonary embolism, esophageal perforation, aortic dissection, collagen vascular disease, sarcoidosis, superior vena cava obstruction, and traumatic vascular disruption.
   b. **Systemic causes** include nephrotic syndrome, cirrhosis, pancreatitis, intra-abdominal abscess, myxedema, and severe malnutrition.

B Clinical features

1. **Symptoms.** Pleural effusions may develop gradually and are **commonly asymptomatic.** Symptomatic patients may complain of **dyspnea, pleuritic chest pain,** or **cough.**

2. **Physical examination findings.** Pulmonary examination reveals **decreased breath sounds** and **dullness to percussion.** A **friction rub** is sometimes heard. The patient's respiratory status may be impaired, depending on the size of the effusion.

C Evaluation

1. **Chest radiograph.** A chest radiograph may reveal the presence of an effusion, whether the effusion is free-flowing or loculated, and the cause of the effusion (e.g., malignancy, CHF, pneumonia).
   a. **PA view.** A **blunted costophrenic angle** on the PA chest radiograph indicates that at least 175 mL of fluid is present.
   b. **Lateral decubitus view.** The lateral decubitus view may help determine whether the effusion is free-flowing or loculated.

2. **Laboratory studies.** Routine laboratory analysis includes a CBC, an electrolyte panel, and BUN, creatinine, and glucose levels.

3. **Pulse oximetry** should be used to evaluate for hypoxia.

4. **Pleural fluid analysis.** Thoracentesis should be performed in patients with previously undiagnosed effusions or large effusions that compromise oxygenation or ventilation.
   a. As much as 1500 mL of pleural fluid can be withdrawn and sent for laboratory analysis. Pleural fluid should be sent for **cell count and differential; pH determination; lactate dehydrogenase (LDH), protein,** and **glucose levels;** and **Gram staining, bacterial culture,** and **cytology. Amylase** should be ordered if pancreatitis or esophageal rupture is suspected to be the cause of the effusion. If the pleural fluid is serosanguineous or bloody, a **pleural fluid hematocrit** should be ordered.
   b. Pleural effusions are classified as either **exudates** or **transudates** according to pleural fluid characteristics (Table 3–2).
      (1) Transudates are generally caused by CHF.
      (2) Exudates generally have less benign causes (e.g., infection, cancer, trauma).

5. **Other tests** may be indicated depending on the suspected cause of the pleural effusion (e.g., aortic angiography for suspected dissection, Gastrografin swallow for suspected esophageal perforation).

TABLE 3–2   Classification of Pleural Effusions

Characteristic	Transudate	Exudate
Pleural fluid protein:serum protein ratio	<0.5	>0.5
Pleural fluid LDH:serum LDH ratio	<0.6	>0.6
Protein level	<3 g/dL	>3 g/dL
LDH level	<200 IU/mL	>200 IU/mL
Specific gravity	<1.016	>1.016

LDH = lactate dehydrogenase.

D Therapy

1. **Large effusions.** If the effusion is very large, patients should first be treated for impairment of oxygenation, ventilation, and circulation. Therapeutic thoracentesis should then be performed.

2. **Small effusions.** For smaller, non–life-threatening pleural effusions, treatment focuses on the underlying disease process. A diagnostic thoracentesis is usually performed after admission in well-appearing patients, unless an empyema, esophageal perforation, or a hemothorax is suspected. Each of these requires emergent placement of a chest tube and additional diagnostic studies.

E Disposition

1. **Admission.** The need for hospital admission is determined by the presence of respiratory or circulatory impairment, as well as the underlying cause of the pleural effusion. Most patients are admitted to the hospital for further evaluation of their medical condition, and for observation following thoracentesis.

2. **Discharge.** If a patient is well appearing, has no impairment in respiration or circulation, and has undergone thoracentesis (if the effusion is small and transudative), the patient may be discharged to home for outpatient follow-up after 4–6 hours of observation in the ED, provided that a repeat chest radiograph rules out a pneumothorax.

VIII   PNEUMONIA

A Discussion

1. **Definition.** Pneumonia is defined as an infection of the pulmonary parenchyma.
   a. **Typical pneumonia** refers to pneumonia caused by bacteria; common causative organisms include *Streptococcus pneumoniae*, *Haemophilus influenzae*, *Staphylococcus aureus*, *Klebsiella pneumoniae*, anaerobes, and *Pseudomonas*.
   b. **Atypical pneumonia.** Common causative organisms include *Mycoplasma pneumoniae*, viruses, *Chlamydia pneumoniae*, *Mycobacterium tuberculosis*, *Pneumocystis carinii*, and *Legionella*.

2. **Incidence.** Pneumonia accounts for 10% of all hospital admissions and is a leading cause of death in the United States.

3. **Causes.** The causative agent of pneumonia depends, in part, on host factors.
   a. **Community-acquired pneumonia** is usually caused by *S. pneumoniae*, *M. pneumoniae*, viruses, *C. pneumoniae*, *H. influenzae*, and, occasionally, *Legionella* or *S. aureus*.
   b. **Nosocomial pneumonia** is usually caused by Gram-negative bacilli, *S. aureus*, or anaerobic oral flora. Less often, *S. pneumoniae* or *Legionella* is involved.
   c. Patients with a history of travel, specific exposures, or certain risk factors may develop pneumonia caused by other agents (Table 3–3).

TABLE 3–3 Causes of Pneumonia in Patients with Selected Risk Factors

Risk Factor	Common Organisms
Age	
Infants (1–4 months)	Chlamydia trachomatis, Streptococcus pneumoniae, Haemophilus influenzae
Infants and children younger than 5 years	Viruses, S. pneumoniae, H. influenzae
Older children and young adults	Atypical organisms (e.g., Mycoplasma or viruses) and S. pneumoniae
Elderly	S. pneumoniae, influenzavirus, Legionella
Health status	
Healthy patients	S. pneumoniae, Mycoplasma, viruses
Debilitated patients (e.g., those in hospitals and nursing homes), neutropenic patients, patients with cystic fibrosis	Gram-negative organisms, especially Pseudomonas
Patients with periodontal disease	Oral anaerobes
HIV-positive patients	Pneumocystis carinii, Mycobacterium avium-intracellulare, Mycobacterium tuberculosis, S. pneumoniae, H. influenzae, Coccidioides immitis, Histoplasma
Patients with sickle cell disease	S. pneumoniae, H. influenzae
Living conditions	
Patients in dormitories and barracks	Mycoplasma pneumoniae, Chlamydia, M. tuberculosis, viruses
Exposures	
Contaminated water from air conditioning units	Legionella
Cows	Coxiella burnetii
Birds	Chlamydia psittaci
Geographical area	
Southeast Asia	M. tuberculosis, Paragonimus, Pseudomonas pseudomallei
Ohio and Mississippi valleys	Histoplasma, Blastomyces
Southwestern United States	Coccidioides immitis

4. **Predisposing conditions** include those that impair host defense mechanisms.
    a. Failure of the gag or cough reflex may be secondary to **altered mental status, seizures, sedative use,** or **stroke. Endotracheal** and **nasogastric tubes** bypass these protective mechanisms and therefore also predispose to the development of pneumonia.
    b. Mucociliary clearance is affected by **smoking, smog inhalation, alcohol use, COPD,** and **viral infection.** Patients with **cystic fibrosis** and **chronic bronchitis** produce thick sputum that is difficult to expectorate.
    c. Cellular defense mechanisms can be impaired in patients with **AIDS, diabetes, asplenia, sickle cell disease, uremia,** or **malignancy. Chemotherapy** and **corticosteroid use** can also impair cellular defense mechanisms.

B Clinical features

1. **Symptoms**
    a. The clinical presentation of a patient with pneumonia depends, in part, on whether the patient suffers from typical or atypical pneumonia. However, there is considerable clinical overlap.
        (1) **Typical pneumonia** is characterized by the abrupt onset of a **high fever, shaking chills, purulent sputum,** and significant respiratory complaints (e.g., **cough, dyspnea, pleuritic chest pain**). **Chest retractions** and **diaphoresis** may be evident.

(2) **Atypical pneumonia** usually has an insidious onset accompanied by **mild respiratory complaints, low-grade fevers,** and **scant sputum.**

b. Some patients may present predominantly with **abdominal complaints** (e.g., upper abdominal pain and vomiting), either from irritation of the diaphragm as a result of lower lobe infection or from the swallowing of purulent secretions.

c. In elderly patients, the presentation of pneumonia may be more subtle (e.g., **weakness, fatigue,** or a **change in behavior**).

2. **Physical examination findings**
   a. **Vital signs.** Fever, tachypnea, and tachycardia may be present.
   b. **Pulmonary examination** may reveal decreased or bronchial breath sounds, rales, dullness to percussion, increased tactile fremitus, and egophony.
   c. **Cyanosis** (if the patient is very hypoxic) may be noted.

C **Differential diagnoses** include asthma, COPD, upper respiratory infection, bronchitis, pneumothorax, pulmonary embolism, foreign body aspiration, and an allergic reaction.

D **Evaluation**

1. **Pulse oximetry** is used to evaluate for hypoxia.

2. **Chest radiograph.** A chest radiograph is used to diagnose pneumonia, and the radiographic pattern may be a clue to the causative organism.
   a. Classically, lobar infiltrates are seen with *S. pneumoniae* and *Klebsiella* infection. *Klebsiella* typically involves the right upper lobe and may cause bulging of the interlobar fissures.
   b. Patchy infiltrates, often multilobar and bilateral, are seen with *S. aureus* and *H. influenzae* infection.
   c. Interstitial infiltrates are seen with *Mycoplasma, Legionella,* and viral infections.
   d. Cavitation and pulmonary abscesses can be seen with infections caused by anaerobic organisms, *S. aureus, Klebsiella, Pseudomonas,* and *M. tuberculosis.*
   e. Pleural effusions are most commonly seen with *H. influenzae, Mycoplasma,* and *S. pneumoniae* infection.

3. **Sputum Gram stain.** A sputum Gram stain is often helpful in identifying the causative organism, but its sensitivity is only 40%–60%. A good lower respiratory sputum sample should contain more than 25 leukocytes per high-power field and fewer than 10 squamous cells per high-power field.

4. **Sputum cultures** should be sent if an adequate specimen is available and for patients admitted to the hospital.

5. **ABG.** An ABG does not need to be obtained routinely, but may be useful in assessing patients with severe respiratory failure caused by the pneumonia.

6. **Special tests** can be helpful in the diagnosis of certain types of pneumonia.
   a. Acute and convalescent *Legionella* antibody titers and **sputum direct fluorescent antibody** should be sent for patients with pneumonia thought to be caused by *Legionella.*
   b. **Sputum acid-fast bacillus stain** and **culture** should be sent for patients with suspected pulmonary tuberculosis.
   c. Acute and convalescent **serum titers** as well as **cold agglutinins** may be helpful in the diagnosis of *M. pneumoniae* infection. Acute and convalescent titers may also be helpful in diagnosing *Chlamydia* pneumonia.
   d. The diagnosis of *P. carinii* pneumonia can be made by special **immunofluorescent stains of sputum** from induced specimens or bronchoscopy.
   e. **Counterimmune electrophoresis** can help diagnose *S. pneumoniae, H. influenzae, Klebsiella,* and *Pseudomonas* as the cause of pneumonia.

E **Therapy**

1. **ABCs.** Therapy begins with airway management, supplemental oxygen in all patients, mechanical ventilation in patients with respiratory failure, and cardiovascular stabilization.

2. **Antibiotic therapy** should be initiated early. Empiric choices depend on the patient's age, underlying medical conditions, specific exposures, clinical and radiographic presentation, and the results of sputum Gram staining. Recommended antibiotic regimens for the outpatient and inpatient treatment of common causes of pneumonia are given in Tables 3–4 and 3–5, respectively.

F **Disposition**

1. **Admission**
   a. Patients who are intubated or have the potential for respiratory failure should be admitted to the ICU.
   b. Patients should be admitted to the hospital for intravenous antibiotic therapy if they meet any of the following criteria:
      (1) They have a serious underlying disease (e.g., COPD, AIDS, asplenia).
      (2) They are older than 65 years or younger than 6 months.
      (3) They show signs of toxicity or significant volume depletion.
      (4) They are dyspneic or hypoxic on room air.
      (5) An empyema or abscess has developed.
      (6) Dense multilobar involvement is present.
      (7) Their living conditions are poor.

2. **Discharge.** Otherwise healthy adults who are not hypoxic and are well appearing may be discharged to home. Outpatient therapy with oral antibiotics should be initiated, and close follow-up is necessary.

TABLE 3–4 Outpatient Treatment of Community-Acquired Pneumonia*

Patient Profile	Drug	Dosage
Children	Erythromycin-sulfisoxazole	1.25 mL/kg/day divided every 6 hours
	Amoxicillin	40 mg/kg/day divided every 8 hours
	Trimethoprim-sulfamethoxazole	1 mL/kg/day divided every 12 hours
	Amoxicillin-clavulanic acid	40 mg/kg/day divided every 8 hours
Healthy young adults	Erythromycin	500 mg four times daily
	Trimethoprim-sulfamethoxazole	Double strength twice daily
	Azithromycin	500 mg (initial dose), followed by 250 mg daily for 4 more days
	Clarithromycin	500 mg twice daily
Debilitated adults (smokers, alcoholics, patients >65 years)	Trimethoprim-sulfamethoxazole	Double strength twice daily
	Azithromycin	500 mg (initial dose), followed by 250 mg daily for 4 more days
	Amoxicillin-clavulanic acid	500 mg three times daily
Patients with *Pneumocystis carinii pneumoniae*	Trimethoprim-sulfamethoxazole	Double strength, two tablets every 6 hours for 21 days

*10 days of treatment unless stated otherwise.

TABLE 3–5   Inpatient Treatment of Community-Acquired Pneumonia

Suspected Cause	Antibiotic Regimen
Typical organism	Cefuroxime
Atypical organism	Cefuroxime + erythromycin
Aspiration	Cefuroxime + penicillin or clindamycin
Gram-negative organism	Ceftazidime + antipseudomonal aminoglycoside
(e.g., *Klebsiella, Pseudomonas*)	Ticarcillin or mezlocillin + antipseudomonal aminoglycoside
Pneumocystis carinii	Sulfamethoxazole–trimethoprim or pentamidine; consider prednisone for severe cases
Mycobacterium tuberculosis	Isoniazid + rifampin + pyrazinamide + ethambutol or streptomycin

IX   MYCOBACTERIAL PULMONARY DISEASE

A Discussion

1. **Causes.** *M. tuberculosis* and *M. avium-intracellulare* are the most common causes of mycobacterial pulmonary disease in humans.

2. **Incidence**
   a. **Tuberculosis.** The number of tuberculosis cases was decreasing at a rate of 5% per year until the mid-1980s, when the number of cases stabilized and then began to rise again. A higher incidence of tuberculosis is seen among individuals who are:
      (1) HIV-positive
      (2) Foreign-born
      (3) Residents of nursing homes, prisons, or shelters
      (4) Homeless
      (5) Intravenous drug users
   b. **Pulmonary infection with *M. avium-intracellulare*** is seen predominantly in AIDS patients, although it is also seen in patients with COPD.

3. **Pathogenesis.** Tuberculosis is transmitted via infectious droplets.
   a. Following primary infection, host defenses stop replication of the organism in 2–10 weeks. The patient then enters a **latent period,** during which he or she is clinically well, not infectious, and the chest radiograph is without infiltrate.
   b. **Reactivation** of pulmonary tuberculosis occurs when cell-mediated immunity wanes. There is increased risk of reactivation with HIV infection, corticosteroid therapy, chemotherapy, malignancy, renal failure, diabetes, malnutrition, and other causes of immune suppression.

B Clinical features

1. **Symptoms**
   a. **Pulmonary symptoms.** Patients with active pulmonary tuberculosis or *M. avium-intracellulare* infection typically complain of a **chronic cough** that is usually nonproductive or productive of scant sputum. **Hemoptysis** may be present, and can range from blood-tinged sputum to massive bleeding [as a result of arteriolar rupture following erosion by a tuberculous cavity (Rasmussen's aneurysm)].
   b. **Systemic symptoms** are common with active tuberculosis, and may include **fever, night sweats, weight loss,** and **anorexia.**

2. **Physical examination findings** may include **fever, tachypnea, lymphadenopathy,** or **generalized wasting.** Pulmonary examination may demonstrate **decreased breath sounds, rales,** or **bronchial breath sounds,** or it may be normal.

C **Differential diagnoses** include bacterial pneumonia, a lung abscess or tumor, and other atypical pneumonias.

D **Evaluation**

1. **Patient history and physical examination.** Emphasis should be placed on determining if the patient has risk factors for tuberculosis.

2. **Pulse oximetry** should be used to determine if the patient is hypoxic.

3. **Chest radiograph**
   a. Reactivation of tuberculosis usually appears as an infiltrate in the upper lobes or superior segment of the lower lobes, often with cavitary lesions.
   b. The chest radiograph may also demonstrate a diffuse, patchy, interstitial, and alveolar pattern that represents endobronchial spread of tuberculosis.
   c. Patients with AIDS may have atypical chest radiographs, with infiltrates in the middle or lower lobes or mediastinal lymphadenopathy without any infiltrate. In approximately 10% of patients, the chest radiograph is completely normal. It is not possible to radiographically distinguish between *M. tuberculosis* and *M. avian-intracellulare* infection.

4. **Intradermal skin tests** (e.g., the PPD test) may be helpful; however, many patients with active pulmonary tuberculosis or AIDS will have false-negative skin results as a result of anergy.

5. **Sputum analysis.** Sputum should be obtained for acid-fast bacillus stain and culture, although a single acid-fast bacillus smear will be positive in only approximately 30% of tuberculosis cases.

6. **Blood cultures** should be considered in critically ill or complicated patients.

E **Therapy**

1. **Isolation.** If a patient is suspected of having pulmonary tuberculosis, he or she should be asked to wear a surgical mask and placed in respiratory isolation for the protection of ED personnel and other patients. Any AIDS or immunocompromised patient with pneumonia should be considered to have tuberculosis until proven otherwise. Health care workers should wear a particulate respirator-type mask while in the patient's room. All respiratory isolation precautions should be instituted as soon as possible, usually prior to obtaining a chest radiograph.

2. **Supplemental oxygen** should be administered if the patient is hypoxic.

3. **Antibiotic therapy.** Because the exact regimen varies depending on the patient's clinical situation, it is advisable to discuss treatment for mycobacterial disease with an infectious disease consultant.
   a. **Tuberculosis.** Patients with tuberculosis should usually be treated with isoniazid, rifampin, pyrazinamide, and either ethambutol or streptomycin for at least 6 months.
   b. *M. avium-intracellulare* infection is treated with clarithromycin and ethambutol.

F **Disposition** The criteria used to decide whether a patient with pulmonary mycobacterial infection requires hospital admission are generally the same as those for patients with other types of pneumonia.

1. **Admission.** Patients who are admitted to the hospital for known or suspected tuberculosis should be placed in respiratory isolation initially.

2. **Discharge.** Patients should be provided with a number of surgical masks and instructed to wear a mask if they will be in contact with other individuals. Patients should follow up within 1 week with a primary care provider. In order to be discharged, patients should meet the following criteria:
   a. Well appearing
   b. Asymptomatic or minimally symptomatic
   c. Not hypoxic on room air
   d. Absence of significant hemoptysis

    e. Willing to comply with medical treatment and follow-up visits

    f. Acceptable living conditions

X   PNEUMOTHORAX

A   **Discussion**   Pneumothorax is defined as an accumulation of free air in the pleural space.

1. **Simple pneumothorax**
   a. **Spontaneous pneumothoraces** can be secondary (i.e., occurring with underlying pulmonary disease) or primary (i.e., occurring in the absence of underlying pulmonary disease).
      (1) Primary spontaneous pneumothoraces are more common in men (85%) and are often recurrent.
      (2) Risk factors for spontaneous pneumothorax include smoking, changes in ambient pressure (e.g., during scuba diving or aviation), inherited conditions (e.g., Marfan's syndrome, mitral valve prolapse, α_1-antitrypsin deficiency), and underlying pulmonary disease (e.g., asthma, COPD, pneumonia, tumors).
   b. **Traumatic pneumothoraces** may be caused by blunt or penetrating chest trauma. Iatrogenic causes of pneumothorax (e.g., central venous pressure line placement) are also included in this category.

2. **Tension pneumothorax** is a complication of pneumothorax that can occur if air continues to enter the pleural space but is unable to escape. Accumulating air collapses the lung and results in shifting of the mediastinum away from the pneumothorax, leading to kinking of the mediastinal vessels, a decrease in venous return to the heart, decreased cardiac output, and, ultimately, shock.

B   **Clinical features**

1. **Simple pneumothorax**
   a. **Symptoms.** Patients commonly complain of the sudden onset of **pleuritic chest pain** with **dyspnea** and **tachypnea.**
   b. **Physical examination findings**
      (1) **Tachycardia** may result from impaired venous return.
      (2) **Decreased breath sounds** on the involved side of the chest and **hyperresonance to percussion** are evident on pulmonary examination.
      (3) **Crepitus** may be palpable in the neck or chest as a result of subcutaneous emphysema.

2. **Tension pneumothorax.** Patients with a tension pneumothorax are in severe respiratory distress, and may be unconscious. Physical examination findings include **hypotension, jugular venous distention, tracheal deviation** away from the side of the pneumothorax, and **decreased breath sounds and chest movement** on the affected side. Tracheal deviation is a late sign of tension pneumothorax and may not always be present.

C   **Differential diagnoses** include pulmonary embolism, pneumonia, pericarditis, acute myocardial infarction, pleurisy, aortic dissection, esophageal perforation, costochondritis, and rib fracture.

D   **Evaluation**

1. **Simple pneumothorax.** If a simple pneumothorax is suspected, **pulse oximetry** should be used to evaluate oxygenation. A **chest radiograph** should be obtained to diagnose the pneumothorax as well as to look for the underlying cause.

2. **Tension pneumothorax.** Diagnosis of a tension pneumothorax is based on **history** and **physical examination.** If a tension pneumothorax is suspected, it should be treated immediately, rather than waiting to obtain a chest radiograph.

E **Therapy**

1. **Oxygen** should be administered to all patients with pneumothorax. In addition to improving oxygenation, high oxygen concentrations increase the rate of resorption of air from the pleural space.

2. **Definitive therapy** for pneumothoraces is the release of air from the pleural space.

   a. **Tension pneumothorax.** If a tension pneumothorax is suspected, immediate **needle thoracostomy** should be performed, followed by **chest tube placement.** A needle thoracostomy is performed by placing a large-bore needle into the pleural space through the anterior second intercostal space along the midclavicular line. An alternative site is the fourth or fifth intercostal space in the midaxillary line.

   b. **Traumatic pneumothoraces** should be treated by placing a **large-bore thoracostomy tube** on the affected side in the fifth intercostal space along the anterior axillary line or midaxillary line.

   c. **Spontaneous pneumothoraces.** The management of spontaneous pneumothoraces depends on the size of the pneumothorax, the presence of respiratory impairment, and the underlying cause of the pneumothorax.

      (1) **Secondary spontaneous pneumothoraces** are treated by placing a **small-bore chest tube** for drainage.

      (2) **Primary spontaneous pneumothoraces** are managed variably.

         (a) A **chest tube** should be placed if the pneumothorax involves more than 20% of the hemithorax or is recurrent.

         (b) In a minimally symptomatic patient with a primary spontaneous pneumothorax that involves less than 20% of the hemithorax, **other techniques** may be attempted to avoid chest tube insertion.

            (i) **Needle aspiration.** Simple aspiration of the pneumothorax may be attempted by placing a 16-gauge needle through the second intercostal space anteriorly along the midclavicular line. A three-way stopcock is placed between the needle and the syringe. Air is drawn into the syringe and then released through the stopcock. If a repeat chest radiograph shows that this technique has failed to largely resolve the pneumothorax, a chest tube should be placed.

            (ii) **One-way catheter insertion.** A small catheter with a one-way valve (e.g., a Cook catheter) may also be used to treat small pneumothoraces. A one-way valve allows air to escape from the pleural space, while preventing air from entering from outside of the body. The catheter is placed in the same location as that used for needle aspiration. Patients can be discharged home with the catheter in place.

F **Disposition**

1. **Admission**

   a. **All patients with tension pneumothorax** should be admitted to the ICU following chest tube placement.

   b. **Patients with traumatic pneumothorax** should be cared for in the ICU or another closely monitored setting, largely depending on the other associated injuries.

   c. **Patients who have had a chest tube placed for a spontaneous pneumothorax** may be admitted to a medical ward, provided that the repeat chest radiograph shows resolution of the pneumothorax.

2. **Discharge.** Patients who have undergone successful needle aspiration or one-way catheter insertion in the ED to treat a small primary pneumothorax may be discharged to home, provided they are asymptomatic and without evidence of hypoxia. These patients should undergo a repeat evaluation and chest radiograph in 24 hours.

Study Questions

Directions: *Each of the numbered items or incomplete statements in this section is followed by answers or by completions of the statement. Select the ONE lettered answer or completion that is BEST in each case.*

QUESTIONS 1–2

A 30-year-old woman with a history of asthma presents to the emergency department (ED) complaining of shortness of breath. She is afebrile and has diffuse wheezing on pulmonary examination. Although she is mildly tachypneic, she appears well, is not cyanotic, and is not in respiratory distress. On arrival, her peak expiratory flow rate (PEFR) is 250 L/min.

1. What is the best initial therapy for this patient?
   - A Nebulized albuterol
   - B Subcutaneous epinephrine
   - C Nebulized albuterol and epinephrine
   - D Nebulized albuterol and theophylline

2. The patient improves slightly after two treatments. She still has mild wheezing, feels mildly dyspneic, and has a PEFR of 280. What is the agent of choice in this situation?
   - A Nebulized albuterol
   - B Nebulized albuterol and oral prednisone
   - C Intravenous methylprednisolone
   - D Subcutaneous epinephrine

3. A patient in respiratory failure has just been intubated. The ventilator should be set to deliver a tidal volume of
   - A 1–2 mL/kg
   - B 5–10 mL/kg
   - C 10–12 mL/kg
   - D 20–25 mL/kg

4. A patient presents to the emergency department (ED) with massive hemoptysis. He has a history of cancer of the left lung. Management of this patient might include which one of the following measures?
   - A Positioning the patient with his right side down
   - B Obtaining intravenous access pending hematocrit results
   - C Selectively intubating the right mainstem bronchus
   - D None of the above

5. When should a chest radiograph be ordered for a patient with asthma?
   - A When the patient presents with diffuse wheezing
   - B When the patient has a history of coughing
   - C When the initial physical examination findings include tachypnea
   - D When pulmonary examination reveals decreased breath sounds and egophony at the left lung base

6. A patient with chronic obstructive pulmonary disease (COPD) presents to the emergency department (ED) with mild respiratory distress. Which set of arterial blood gas (ABG) findings is suggestive of respiratory failure in this patient?

A. pH = 7.41, oxygen tension (P_{O_2}) = 70 mm Hg, carbon dioxide tension (P_{CO_2}) = 51 mm Hg
B. pH = 7.40, P_{O_2} = 70 mm Hg, P_{CO_2} = 52 mm Hg
C. pH = 7.28, P_{O_2} = 70 mm Hg, P_{CO_2} = 60 mm Hg
D. pH = 7.40, P_{O_2} = 75 mm Hg, P_{CO_2} = 60 mm Hg

7. Which one of the following findings is consistent with a diagnosis of noncardiogenic pulmonary edema (NCPE)?

A. Peripheral edema
B. Patchy alveolar infiltrates on chest radiograph
C. Jugular venous distention
D. A normal alveolar–arterial (A-a) gradient

8. Which one of the following symptoms is most suggestive of hypercapnia?

A. Agitation
B. Somnolence
C. Dyspnea
D. Disorientation

9. Which one of the following medications is contraindicated in the treatment of a 50-year-old asthmatic patient with a history of ischemic heart disease?

A. Ipratropium bromide
B. Ketamine
C. Albuterol
D. Heliox

10. Which one of the following statements regarding tension pneumothorax is true?

A. The patient may be asymptomatic.
B. Tracheal deviation is an early and unmistakable sign.
C. A chest radiograph should be ordered prior to initiating treatment.
D. The patient may present with pulseless electrical activity (PEA).

11. The evaluation of a patient with chronic obstructive pulmonary disease (COPD) who is experiencing an acute exacerbation but does not demonstrate signs of respiratory failure should always include

A. pulmonary function testing and pulse oximetry
B. pulmonary function testing and arterial blood gas (ABG) data
C. pulmonary function testing, pulse oximetry, and chest radiographs
D. pulmonary function testing, ABG data, and chest radiographs

12. Which one of the following statements regarding the treatment of patients with noncardiogenic pulmonary edema (NCPE) is true?

A. The inspired oxygen concentration (F_{IO_2}) should be at least 90%.
B. Positive end-expiratory pressure (PEEP) may improve oxygenation.
C. Corticosteroids should be administered routinely and immediately.
D. PEEP should not be used because it may result in pneumothorax.

13. A 50-year-old previously healthy patient presents to the emergency department (ED) because he is experiencing mild, left-sided chest pain. The patient says that he has been having this pain for the past 3 months. A chest radiograph demonstrates a left pleural effusion of moderate size. A lateral decubitus view demonstrates that the effusion is free-flowing, and the patient is not in respiratory distress. The best initial management of this patient would include

- (A) chest tube placement
- (B) thoracentesis
- (C) the administration of 100% oxygen and overnight observation
- (D) Gastrografin swallow

14. A 72-year-old patient is brought to the emergency department (ED) from a nursing home and is diagnosed with pneumonia. When selecting an antibiotic regimen, it is important to provide adequate coverage for which one of the following organisms?

- (A) *Legionella*
- (B) *Mycoplasma*
- (C) *Pseudomonas*
- (D) *Coccidioides*

15. A 47-year-old man comes to the emergency department (ED) complaining of a cough and fever. The nurse informs the emergency physician that the patient is homeless and an intravenous drug user. He has a temperature of 101°F and all of his other vital signs are normal. Which one of the following actions should the emergency physician take first?

- (A) She should perform a thorough history and physical examination.
- (B) She should send the patient to radiology for a chest radiograph.
- (C) She should contact the ED social worker.
- (D) She should put on a respiratory mask prior to entering the patient's room.

Answers and Explanations

1–2. The answers are 1—A, 2—B Albuterol is a selective β_2 agonist that is used as first-line treatment for asthma exacerbations. Epinephrine can be considered for young patients with severe asthma who do not respond to first-line agents. Theophylline should not be used routinely in the treatment of asthma, except for selected patients already on this medication.

If the patient is clinically improving but is still symptomatic and has an abnormal PEFR despite initial albuterol therapy, steroid therapy should be initiated while the patient continues to receive nebulized albuterol. Because this patient is not in severe respiratory distress or vomiting, oral prednisone is the appropriate steroid. Methylprednisolone could be administered intravenously if the patient were unable to tolerate oral steroids. Epinephrine is not indicated because the patient is improving and is not having a severe asthma exacerbation.

3. The answer is C As a general rule, a tidal volume of 10–12 mL/kg will provide adequate ventilation for intubated patients.

4. The answer is C The goal of therapy for a patient with massive hemoptysis is to stabilize the patient's respiratory and hemodynamic status while preventing the spread of blood throughout the lungs. If intubation is needed, it is best to selectively intubate the right mainstem bronchus, because this will allow ventilation of the unaffected lung. Because this patient is most likely bleeding from the left side, he should be positioned so that he is lying on his left side, not his right side. Intravenous access should be obtained immediately in all patients with massive hemoptysis, regardless of the patient's hematocrit.

5. The answer is D A chest radiograph should be considered for patients with asthma who have hypoxia, fever, symptoms not responsive to bronchodilator therapy, or a focal lung examination. Wheezing, coughing, and tachypnea are common in the initial presentation of asthmatic patients, and they may resolve with the administration of β_2 agonists. A chest radiograph is warranted if these signs or symptoms persist despite therapy.

6. The answer is C An increased P_{CO_2} accompanied by a decreased serum pH is characteristic of respiratory failure in a patient with COPD. Patients with COPD may have a chronically elevated P_{CO_2}, but their blood pH should be normal (between 7.35 and 7.45). A P_{CO_2} greater than 50 mm Hg is considered to be elevated; therefore, all of the ABG findings show an elevated P_{CO_2}. However, only one set of data shows a decrease in serum pH as a result of the elevated P_{CO_2} (i.e., an acute respiratory acidosis), a sign that the patient is in respiratory failure.

7. The answer is B In patients with NCPE, the chest radiograph demonstrates bilateral patchy alveolar infiltrates and a normal heart size. Patients with NCPE develop pulmonary edema as a result of increased permeability of the pulmonary vascular membrane; therefore, signs of congestive heart failure (CHF), such as jugular venous distention and peripheral edema, are absent. The accumulation of fluid leads to hypoxia and an increased A-a gradient.

8. The answer is B Somnolence and lethargy are commonly seen in patients with hypercapnia. Agitation, dyspnea, disorientation, and confusion are usually seen in hypoxic patients.

9. The answer is B Ketamine, an anesthetic agent that is sometimes used in the treatment of severe, refractory asthma, can result in myocardial ischemia or infarction if administered to patients with ischemic heart disease.

10. The answer is D Patients with a tension pneumothorax are critically ill, are in severe respiratory distress, and may be unconscious. They may demonstrate jugular venous distention, hypotension, and decreased breath sounds on the affected side. Tracheal deviation away from the affected side may be seen, but is a late and unreliable sign of tension pneumothorax. If the patient progresses to cardiopulmonary arrest, PEA is commonly seen. Treatment of these patients should be initiated immediately on the basis of the clinical diagnosis alone.

11. The answer is A All patients with COPD who present to the emergency department (ED) with an acute exacerbation should undergo pulmonary function testing, to determine the peak expiratory flow rate (PEFR), and pulse oximetry, to evaluate the degree of hypoxia and obstruction, unless the patient is in respiratory failure. ABG data should not be ordered routinely for all patients with COPD, only for those patients who may be in respiratory failure. A chest radiograph is also not routine, but should be considered in selected patients (e.g., those who are unable to cooperate for an adequate PEFR measurement).

12. The answer is B Although high levels of PEEP may result in barotrauma, PEEP may improve oxygen saturation and is an important component of the treatment of patients with NCPE. Oxygen should be administered to maintain the oxygen saturation above 90%, but generally, the F_{IO_2} is approximately 50%. The F_{IO_2} should be minimized to avoid pulmonary oxygen toxicity. The use of corticosteroids and other anti-inflammatory agents in the treatment of patients with NCPE is currently controversial.

13. The answer is B Thoracentesis is the procedure of choice for diagnosing and draining pleural effusions. Chest tubes are used for treating large pneumothoraces, hemothoraces, and empyemas. The administration of 100% supplemental oxygen may cause resorption of air from the pleural space, but not pleural fluid. A Gastrografin swallow should be performed on patients with suspected esophageal perforation, but this patient does not seem to have any signs of that disorder.

14. The answer is C Patients who reside in nursing homes, are hospitalized, are neutropenic, or have cystic fibrosis are at increased risk for pneumonia caused by Gram-negative organisms, especially *Pseudomonas.*

15. The answer is D Because this patient is complaining of cough and fever, it is possible that he has pneumonia. However, homelessness and intravenous drug use are both risk factors for tuberculosis, and this diagnosis should be considered as well. In order to prevent exposure to tuberculosis, the emergency physician should wear a particulate respirator-type mask, and a surgical mask should be placed on the patient prior to beginning clinical evaluation.

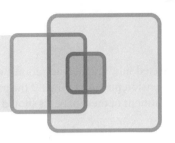

chapter **4**

Gastrointestinal Emergencies

RICHARD C. URGO • AMARJIT SINGH

I **ABDOMINAL PAIN**

A **Discussion**

1. Abdominal pain is the presenting complaint in approximately 5% of emergency department (ED) visits. Of these patients, 15%–30% will have a condition requiring surgery.

    a. In patients complaining of abdominal pain, the most common discharge diagnosis is abdominal pain of unknown etiology (40% of patients).

    b. The next most common diagnosis is gastroenteritis (approximately 7% of patients).

    c. Pelvic inflammatory disease (PID), urinary tract infection (UTI), nephrolithiasis, and appendicitis are the next four most common diagnoses in patients with abdominal pain.

2. **Types of abdominal pain.** Knowledge of the sources of abdominal pain is important in forming a differential diagnosis list.

    a. Visceral pain is crampy and poorly localized and originates from a solid or hollow viscus.

    b. Somatic pain arises from inflammation of the parietal peritoneum and is sharp and well localized. Early in the course of disease, patients typically experience visceral pain, but as the disease process progresses, the adjacent peritoneum becomes irritated and, therefore, the pain becomes more localized.

    c. Referred pain is pain felt at a distance from the disease process and is explained by the embryologic origins of the structures involved. For example, the diaphragm is innervated by C3–5, so diaphragmatic irritation is felt in those dermatomes (i.e., the shoulder).

B **Evaluation**

1. **Patient history**

    a. Characterization of the pain. Any change in the character of the pain over time should be noted because changes may give a clue regarding the organ involved. For example, appendicitis often begins as a poorly localized cramping pain that becomes sharp and localizes in the right lower quadrant.

    (1) Location

    (a) Epigastric pain is associated with pancreatitis, peptic ulcer disease, myocardial infarction (MI), aortic aneurysms, and gastritis.

    (b) Right upper quadrant pain is consistent with hepatitis and cholecystitis.

    (c) Right lower quadrant pain may be seen in patients with appendicitis, Crohn's disease, diverticulitis, or gynecologic disorders.

    (d) Left lower quadrant pain is associated with diverticulitis and gynecologic disorders.

    (2) Quality

    (a) A **cramping pain** suggests obstruction of a hollow viscus, such as occurs in cholecystitis, small bowel obstruction, or renal colic.

    (b) A **burning pain** is characteristic of gastroesophageal reflux and peptic ulcer disease.

    (c) Sharp, localized pain suggests peritoneal irritation.

    (3) Radiation
- **(a) Left shoulder.** Pain may radiate to the left shoulder in patients with a perforated peptic ulcer, subphrenic abscess, splenic rupture, or mononucleosis.
- **(b) Chest.** Pain may radiate to the chest in patients with gastroesophageal reflux disease (GERD), peptic ulcer disease, or a hiatal hernia.
- **(c) Back.** Radiation of pain to the back is seen primarily in association with pancreatitis, abdominal aneurysms, and acute aortic dissection.

    (4) Timing
- **(a)** An **abrupt onset** of pain occurs with the perforation of a hollow viscus.
- **(b)** A **waxing and waning** pain is indicative of obstruction (e.g., small bowel obstruction, cholecystitis).

    (5) Provocative and palliative factors
- **(a) Movement.** Patients with peritonitis find any movement painful.
- **(b) Position.** Patients with pancreatitis often find that leaning forward improves the pain.
- **(c) Food** may exacerbate the pain (as in pancreatitis and cholecystitis) or alleviate the pain (as in peptic ulcer disease).
- **(d) Medications.** Antacids usually relieve the pain of peptic ulcer disease.

b. Associated symptoms. The order of appearance of associated symptoms may yield clues to the diagnosis. For example, vomiting always precedes hematemesis in patients with a Mallory-Weiss tear of the esophagus.

    (1) Gastrointestinal symptoms
- **(a) Vomiting**
  - **(i) Bilious** or **feculent vomitus** suggests a bowel obstruction.
  - **(ii)** "**Coffee grounds**" or **frank blood** in the vomitus suggests peptic ulcer disease, a Mallory-Weiss tear, or bleeding esophageal varices.
- **(b) Anorexia** and **nausea** are important to note because the diagnosis of appendicitis is practically excluded if anorexia is not present.
- **(c) Diarrhea**
  - **(i) Bloody diarrhea** suggests inflammatory bowel disease, diverticulitis, or an invasive gastroenteritis.
  - **(ii) Melena** is consistent with an upper gastrointestinal source of bleeding.
- **(d) Constipation** or **obstipation** suggests obstruction.
- **(e) Fever, sweats,** and **chills** are noted in an infectious process.
- **(f) Weight loss** may be seen with cancer, inflammatory bowel disease, or ischemic bowel syndromes.

    (2) Gynecologic or **urologic symptoms** should be noted because these symptoms may point away from a gastrointestinal process.

c. Past history
- **(1) Surgical history.** Previous surgery should heighten suspicion for a bowel obstruction.
- **(2) Medication history.** Nonsteroidal anti-inflammatory drug (NSAID) use is associated with peptic ulcer disease. Any history of steroid use should be noted because symptoms may be masked, making the diagnosis much more difficult.
- **(3) Medical history.** A medical history should be taken, inquiring about any condition that can cause pain (e.g., diabetes, sickle cell anemia, porphyria, peptic ulcer disease, hepatitis, gallbladder disease). The patient should be queried regarding previous, similar episodes of pain.
- **(4) Gynecologic history.** A gynecologic history should be taken, including inquiring about the last menstrual period.
- **(5) Social factors**
  - **(a) Alcohol abuse** raises the possibility of pancreatitis, hepatitis, cirrhosis, gastritis, and peptic ulcer disease. **Alcohol use** increases the probability of peptic ulcer disease.
  - **(b) Smoking** also increases the probability of peptic ulcer disease.

2. Physical examination

a. General appearance. Patients who are lying very still may have peritonitis, whereas a patient who is writhing in pain should be suspected of having pancreatitis or renal colic.

b. Head, ears, eyes, nose, and throat (HEENT). The sclera and oropharynx should be evaluated for jaundice, which suggests biliary pathology. The mucosa will be dry if dehydration is present.

c. Chest

   (1) An irregularly irregular heartbeat usually represents atrial fibrillation, which should increase suspicion for mesenteric ischemia.

   (2) The lungs should always be auscultated because a lower lobe pneumonia may present as abdominal pain.

   (3) Gynecomastia may be noted in men with liver disease.

d. Extremities. The extremities should be examined for edema and palmar erythema, which suggest liver disease.

e. Skin. The skin should be inspected for spider angiomas, which appear in patients with liver disease.

f. Abdomen. Serial abdominal examinations should not be neglected because time is a key diagnostic aid.

   (1) Appearance

      (a) Surgical scars may be noted. In patients who have had abdominal surgery, the incidence of bowel obstruction from adhesions increases.

      (b) Distention may result from a bowel obstruction or ascites.

      (c) Peristalsis may be visible in a patient with a bowel obstruction or volvulus.

      (d) Cullen's sign (ecchymosis of the umbilicus) and **Grey-Turner's sign** (flank ecchymosis) are consistent with retroperitoneal hemorrhage from pancreatitis or trauma.

      (e) Caput medusae (dilated veins around the umbilicus) are seen in some patients with liver disease.

   (2) Auscultation

      (a) Short, high-pitched rushes of bowel sounds are consistent with a bowel obstruction.

      (b) Hypoactive or **absent bowel sounds** may be heard late in an obstruction or they may be caused by an ileus from another intra-abdominal process.

   (3) Palpation

      (a) Masses

         (i) In patients with an abdominal aortic aneurysm, a pulsating mass may be palpated in the epigastrium.

         (ii) In patients with acute cholecystitis, a tender right upper quadrant mass may be detected (Murphy's sign).

      (b) Organomegaly may be noted.

      (c) Peritoneal signs are indicative of peritoneal irritation and suggest that a condition requiring surgical intervention is present.

         (i) Rebound tenderness is pain elicited by the withdrawal of the examining hand.

         (ii) Guarding. The patient may resist palpation to prevent pain (voluntary guarding). Involuntary guarding is a muscle spasm of the abdominal wall in response to peritoneal irritation.

         (iii) Rovsing's sign is referred pain felt in the right lower quadrant when the examiner palpates the left lower quadrant. It is one of the signs of peritonitis and appendicitis.

   (4) Percussion

      (a) The liver span should be percussed. Shifting dullness and a fluid wave are indicative of ascites.

      (b) Areas of tenderness should be percussed to elicit tenderness. Percussion tenderness is a very sensitive sign of peritoneal irritation.

    g. Rectum. A rectal examination is essential and may demonstrate focal tenderness or a mass. Gross or occult blood must be noted.

    h. Genitals

        (1) In women, a pelvic examination is mandatory in order to evaluate gastrointestinal pathology and to rule out a disorder of the reproductive organs.

        (2) In men, the genitals should be examined to rule out epididymitis and torsion, which can cause referred abdominal pain.

        (3) In men and women, the inguinal and femoral regions should be examined to exclude an occult hernia.

    i. Back. The back should be percussed to reveal costovertebral angle tenderness, which is suggestive of pyelonephritis or nephrolithiasis.

3. Laboratory studies should be guided by the history and physical examination findings.

    a. Urinalysis should be performed, and women of childbearing age should be tested for pregnancy (usually with a urine pregnancy test).

    b. Blood work

        (1) Complete blood count (CBC). The white blood cell (WBC) count is a nonspecific gauge of inflammation and may be normal in spite of a serious medical or surgical condition.

        (2) Electrolytes may be abnormal due to vomiting or diarrhea.

        (3) Hemoglobin. The hemoglobin level is an important parameter when evaluating hemorrhage, but it may not be decreased immediately after acute blood loss.

        (4) Amylase and **lipase.** The amylase level is usually elevated in pancreatitis but may also be elevated in other conditions, such as perforated peptic ulcer, bowel necrosis, salivary gland disease, and a ruptured ectopic pregnancy. The lipase level is more specific for pancreatitis than the amylase level.

        (5) Liver enzyme [e.g., aspartate aminotransferase (AST), alanine aminotransferase (ALT), alkaline phosphatase (AP), γ-glutamyl transferase (GGT)] and **bilirubin levels** should be ordered when hepatic or biliary disease is suspected.

        (6) Coagulation studies. A prothrombin time (PT) and partial thromboplastin time (PTT) should be ordered in patients with a suspected surgical abdomen or evidence of upper or lower gastrointestinal bleeding.

4. Diagnostic imaging studies

    a. Radiography

        (1) Abdominal films may demonstrate cholelithiasis, nephrolithiasis, pancreatic calcification, or an appendicolith. They may show air–fluid levels or dilated bowel in a bowel obstruction. They may demonstrate calcification of the aorta in an abdominal aortic aneurysm.

        (2) Chest films may show free air, a pleural effusion, or a pulmonary process causing referred abdominal pain.

    b. Ultrasonography. Bedside ultrasonography is gaining acceptance and verification as research has demonstrated its usefulness for detecting cholelithiasis, abdominal aortic aneurysm, intra-abdominal fluid, and hydronephrosis. Formal ultrasonography can provide additional information in these areas, and is also useful for identifying pelvic pathology.

    c. Contrast imaging, computed tomography (CT), angiography, and **nuclear medicine studies** are useful in certain circumstances and should be employed following consultation with a specialist.

C Therapy   General supportive measures include the following:

1. Intravenous access should be obtained and the patient hydrated as necessary. **The patient should not receive anything by mouth.**

2. Pharmacologic management of symptoms may involve the use of **antiemetics** (e.g., droperidol, prochlorperazine), **antispasmodics** (e.g., dicyclomine), **antacids,** or **pain medication.**

    a. Adequate analgesia should be given to patients with renal colic or pain of aortic origin.

    b. Pain management in patients with possible or clear peritoneal signs is problematic. Most data indicate that narcotic analgesia given in moderate doses will not mask true peritoneal signs and may improve the reliability of the physical examination in patients with peritoneal signs. Humane application of analgesia should not be withheld from any patient without good cause.

II   ESOPHAGEAL DISORDERS

Esophageal problems present with one of three predominant symptoms: pain, dysphagia, or bleeding.

A **Esophageal pain**

  1. Gastroesophageal reflux disease (GERD)

    a. Discussion

      (1) Incidence. Ten percent of the population experiences reflux symptoms daily, and thirty-three percent experience symptoms at least once a month.

      (2) Pathogenesis. The reflux is caused by a decrease in the lower esophageal sphincter pressure. Pregnancy and drugs that cause smooth muscle relaxation (e.g., β agonists, calcium channel blockers) may worsen the condition.

    b. Clinical features. The reflux of acidic gastric contents into the esophagus causes a **retrosternal, burning pain** that may radiate to the neck or jaw.

      (1) The pain is often exacerbated by bending over, lying down, or consuming large meals.

      (2) It may be relieved by drinking liquids, taking antacids, standing, or sitting up.

    c. Differential diagnoses. Pain from GERD can be indistinguishable from **chest pain of cardiac origin;** therefore, a cardiac cause must be ruled out. The resolution of symptoms after a trial of oral antacids in the ED does not exclude a cardiac cause because cardiac pain may also respond to antacids. Esophageal and cardiac disease are also often coincident.

    d. Evaluation is primarily done on an outpatient basis and may include an upper gastrointestinal series, acid reflux testing, endoscopy, and manometry.

    e. Therapy entails the following supportive measures:

      (1) Elevating the head of the bed 6 inches and avoiding recumbency after eating

      (2) Eating smaller meals and avoiding fatty foods, chocolate, caffeine, and alcohol

      (3) Smoking cessation

      (4) Weight reduction (in obese patients)

      (5) Over-the-counter antacids, histamine-2 (H_2) antagonists (e.g., ranitidine, cimetidine), or other agents (e.g., omeprazole, metoclopramide)

    f. Disposition. Patients at risk for coronary disease should be admitted. If a cardiac cause can be excluded, the patient may be safely discharged and further evaluated as an outpatient.

  2. Esophagitis

    a. Discussion

      (1) Infectious esophagitis occurs more commonly in immunocompromised patients (e.g., AIDS patients, patients with diabetes mellitus, patients receiving chemotherapy). Commonly implicated organisms include *Candida* and **herpes simplex virus (HSV).**

      (2) Pill esophagitis occurs after taking oral medication. The tablet adheres to the esophageal wall and dissolves, leading to local inflammation and irritation. Medications frequently responsible include **doxycycline** (the most common offender), **potassium chloride, quinidine, NSAIDs,** and **ferrous sulfate.**

    b. Clinical features. Infectious esophagitis presents as odynophagia (pain with swallowing). The pain is retrosternal and may be aching, burning, or stabbing in character.

      (1) *Candida* **esophagitis.** The pain is usually mild. Oral candidiasis is often present (especially in patients with AIDS).

(2) **Herpes esophagitis.** The onset of pain is typically abrupt, and there may be a history of recent upper respiratory tract infection. Herpes esophagitis is associated with ulcerative lesions (distinct from the heaped plaques associated with oral candidiasis). Immunocompetent patients frequently demonstrate skin or oral lesions, but immunocompromised patients often do not.

  c. **Differential diagnoses**

    (1) **Cardiac disease** must always be excluded.

    (2) **Oropharyngeal odynophagia** can be caused by pharyngitis, retropharyngeal abscess, peritonsillar abscess, or epiglottitis and must be distinguished from esophageal odynophagia.

  d. **Evaluation**

    (1) *Candida* esophagitis may be confirmed in the ED using an air-contrast barium swallow, which will reveal ulceration and plaques.

    (2) Evaluation should include a soft tissue film of the neck if a retropharyngeal abscess or epiglottitis is suspected.

    (3) Esophagoscopy is the definitive study.

  e. **Therapy**

    (1) *Candida* **esophagitis.** Treatment is with oral ketoconazole or fluconazole. Granulocytopenic patients are at risk for dissemination; therefore, treatment with intravenous amphotericin B is warranted for these patients.

    (2) **Herpes esophagitis** is self-limited in immunocompetent patients. Oral or intravenous acyclovir is indicated for immunocompromised patients.

    (3) **Pill esophagitis.** Symptoms resolve without any specific treatment. The medication should be discontinued if possible. If it is not possible to discontinue the medication, the patient should take the pills with plenty of water and remain in an upright position (sitting or standing) immediately after taking the medication.

  f. **Disposition.** Immunocompetent patients with mild symptoms may be empirically treated with ketoconazole and should be referred for outpatient follow-up. Patients who are unable to maintain adequate oral fluid intake or those at risk for disseminated infection should be admitted.

3. **Boerhaave's syndrome** is rupture of the esophagus during forceful emesis.

  a. **Clinical features.** The patient reports an episode of severe, violent emesis and complains of chest pain.

  b. **Evaluation**

    (1) **Physical examination**

      (a) **Hamman's sign** is a crunching sound heard on auscultation of the heart. The crunching sound is due to mediastinal emphysema.

      (b) **Crepitation** may be found in the neck and signifies subcutaneous emphysema.

      (c) **Signs of septic shock** may be seen in late presentations.

    (2) **Diagnostic imaging**

      (a) **Chest radiographs** may demonstrate mediastinal air, subcutaneous emphysema, a widened mediastinum, pneumothorax, or air–fluid levels.

      (b) **Water-soluble contrast swallow** will show extravasation.

  c. **Therapy** entails fluid resuscitation, antibiotics, and surgical repair. A chest tube may be needed if a pneumothorax is present.

4. **Motility disorders** (see II B 1 b, 2 b) may produce esophageal pain.

B **Esophageal dysphagia**

1. **Discussion.** Dysphagia is defined as difficulty swallowing. It may or may not be accompanied by pain. Causes of esophageal dysphagia include:

  a. **Obstructive disorders** (e.g., aortic aneurysm, carcinoma, webs, and rings)

  b. **Motor disorders** (e.g., achalasia, diffuse esophageal spasm, scleroderma)

2. **Clinical features**
   a. **Obstructive disorders.** Patients tend to have greater dysphagia for solids than for liquids.
   b. **Motor disorders.** Patients tend to have equal dysphagia for both solids and liquids. Dysphagia resulting from a motor disorder is often associated with pain.

3. **Differential diagnoses**
   a. **Cardiac disorders** must be excluded if the patient is experiencing esophageal pain.
   b. **Oropharyngeal dysphagia** is defined as difficulty passing food from the mouth to the esophagus and must be differentiated from esophageal dysphagia.
      (1) **Common causes** include **cerebrovascular accident, multiple sclerosis, myasthenia gravis,** and **amyotrophic lateral sclerosis.**
      (2) **Clinical features** may include drooling, coughing, choking, nasal regurgitation, or aspiration.

4. **Evaluation**
   a. **Radiography.** A chest radiograph may demonstrate an aortic aneurysm, a tumor, a foreign body, or a dilated esophagus with an air–fluid level (characteristic of achalasia).
   b. **Other studies** are carried out on an outpatient basis and may include endoscopy, a barium swallow, manometry, and motility studies.

5. **Therapy**
   a. **Supportive therapy.** Intravenous hydration may be necessary.
   b. **Definitive therapy**
      (1) **Obstructive disorders**
         (a) **Medical treatment.** Acute esophageal obstruction may be treated medically with **glucagon, calcium channel blockers** (e.g., nifedipine) to induce smooth muscle relaxation, and **antispasmodics** (e.g., diazepam).
         (b) **Acute endoscopy** may be indicated if medical treatment fails to resolve the problem and complete esophageal obstruction persists.
      (2) **Motility disorders** can be treated with nitrates, calcium channel blockers, and anticholinergic drugs.

6. **Disposition.** Most patients can be discharged for an outpatient work-up. Dehydration is the major indication for admission.

C Esophageal bleeding An esophageal source is responsible for approximately 25% of cases of upper gastrointestinal tract bleeding. Of these, 80% are due to esophageal varices and 20% are due to Mallory-Weiss tears.

1. **Esophageal varices**
   a. **Discussion.** Varices are dilated submucosal veins that result from portal hypertension, which is most commonly caused by cirrhosis of the liver. The mortality rate for patients with esophageal varices approaches 50%.
   b. **Clinical features.** Patients with esophageal varices commonly present with **painless** and **massive hematemesis.** The **stigmata of chronic liver disease** (e.g., spider angiomas, palmar erythema, ascites, gynecomastia) are typically present as well.
   c. **Therapy**
      (1) **Supportive therapy.** Measures include:
         (a) **Administration of intravenous fluids** through two large-bore intravenous lines
         (b) **Administration of packed red blood cells (RBCs)** and **fresh frozen plasma** to correct any coagulopathy
         (c) **Nasogastric suction** to monitor bleeding
         (d) **Vasopressin,** which constricts the mesenteric arteries, thereby decreasing the portal pressure and slowing the bleeding
            (i) The **dose** is 20 U over 20 minutes followed by an infusion of 0.2–0.6 U/hour.

(ii) **Complications** result from coronary artery vasoconstriction and include MI, arrhythmias, and congestive heart failure (CHF).

(e) **Octreotide,** a synthetic somatostatin compound indicated for terminating upper gastrointestinal hemorrhage that, unlike vasopressin, does not induce vasoconstriction

    (i) **Dose.** Octreotide is usually administered as an intravenous infusion at a rate of 50–100 µg/hour.

    (ii) **Complications** of octreotide include hypoglycemia, hyperglycemia, and thrombocytopenia.

(2) **Definitive therapy**

(a) **Sengstaken-Blakemore tube.** The Sengstaken-Blakemore tube is an orogastric tube equipped with inflatable gastric and esophageal balloons. Inflation of the balloons applies direct pressure to the bleeding varices, controlling the hemorrhage.

    (i) Endotracheal intubation should be performed prior to Sengstaken-Blakemore tube placement.

    (ii) Sengstaken-Blakemore tube placement controls hemorrhage in 85% of patients but is associated with a 65% rebleed rate.

(b) **Endoscopic sclerotherapy** is associated with a 98% success rate.

(c) **Portosystemic shunt surgeries** are associated with a 75% mortality rate when performed during an active bleed; therefore, they are usually performed electively after the acute bleed has been controlled.

2. **Mallory-Weiss tears**

a. **Discussion.** Mallory-Weiss tears are partial-thickness lacerations of the gastroesophageal junction that result from forceful emesis.

b. **Clinical features.** There is a history of vomiting in 85% of patients. Many patients also have a history of alcohol abuse.

c. **Evaluation** includes nasogastric suction to rule out continued bleeding and a hemoglobin level.

d. **Therapy.** The bleeding usually stops spontaneously without causing significant blood loss. When necessary, the condition can be treated with endoscopic sclerotherapy or coagulation or with vasopressin.

e. **Disposition.** Most patients can be discharged.

III   GASTROINTESTINAL FOREIGN BODIES

The ingestion of foreign bodies is responsible for approximately 1500 deaths each year in the United States. Groups at risk include children, alcoholics, the mentally impaired, the demented, denture wearers, and prisoners.

A   Esophageal foreign bodies

1. **Discussion.** Eighty percent of patients with esophageal foreign bodies are children. The child is typically brought to the ED by a caretaker after a witnessed ingestion. If the ingestion was not witnessed, the diagnosis can be difficult to make.

2. **Clinical features**

a. **Symptoms**

(1) **Adults** typically complain of a foreign body sensation in the throat or chest. The patient may appear anxious and experience retching or vomiting, choking, or coughing.

(2) **Children.** Symptoms include refusal to eat, increased salivation, pain on swallowing, vomiting, choking, and referred respiratory symptoms (e.g., stridor, cough, wheezing).

b. **Physical examination** may reveal signs of infection. **Fever** and/or **subcutaneous emphysema** in the neck is consistent with esophageal perforation.

3. **Evaluation**
   a. **Laryngoscopy.** Direct or indirect laryngoscopy should be performed if the patient feels that the foreign body is in the throat or if respiratory symptoms are present.
   b. **Radiography**
      (1) Radiographs can be used to pinpoint the location of radiopaque objects (e.g., coins).
         (a) Coins in the esophagus align themselves in the frontal plane and are, therefore, seen face-on in an anterior-posterior view.
         (b) Coins in the trachea align themselves in the sagittal plane and are seen edge-on in an anterior-posterior view.
      (2) Pneumomediastinum or air in the soft tissues suggests perforation.
   c. **Endoscopy** also allows localization of the object and may be therapeutic.
   d. **Esophagraphy.** An esophagram should be performed only after consulting with a specialist because the contrast material may interfere with later attempts at endoscopy. Gastrografin, rather than barium, should be used if a perforation is suspected.

4. **Therapy**
   a. **Coins** and small smooth objects often pass through the gastrointestinal tract without difficulty. Coins are best removed by endoscopy. They can also be removed, by experienced physicians, using a Foley catheter guided by fluoroscopy.
   b. **Button batteries** cause chemical corrosion and perforation of the esophagus and must be endoscopically removed as soon as possible.
   c. **Sharp objects** must be removed by endoscopy.
   d. **Food impactions** can be treated expectantly if the patient is managing his or her secretions adequately. Medical interventions include the following:
      (1) **Glucagon** (1 mg intravenously) may relieve the impaction. A second, 2-mg dose can be administered in 20 minutes if the first dose is ineffective.
      (2) **Nitroglycerin** (administered sublingually) may also assist in relieving the impaction.
      (3) **Nifedipine** (10 mg sublingually) relaxes the lower esophageal sphincter and may allow passage of the food bolus.
      (4) **Diazepam** may be used as a last resort.
      (5) **Endoscopy** should be performed if the bolus has not passed after 12 hours.

5. **Disposition.** All patients need follow-up to rule out underlying esophageal pathology.

B **Nonesophageal foreign bodies**

1. **Discussion.** Once a foreign object has passed beyond the esophagus and into the stomach, 95% are eliminated without complications.

2. **Clinical features.** Typically, nonesophageal foreign bodies are asymptomatic unless perforation or impaction has occurred. Under these circumstances, the patient presents with signs of peritonitis or obstruction.

3. **Evaluation.** Abdominal radiographs should be obtained to localize the object.

4. **Therapy**
   a. **Peritonitis or obstruction.** Any patient with evidence of obstruction or perforation requires consultation with a surgeon.
   b. **Sharp objects** that are in the stomach should be removed endoscopically because they have a 15%–35% chance of perforating the bowel if they are not removed. If the sharp object has passed the pylorus, consultation with a surgeon is required.
   c. **Other objects** can be managed on an outpatient basis.
      (1) The stools should be checked for passage of the object, which usually occurs in 48–72 hours but may take as long as 6–14 days. A repeat radiograph should be obtained in 1 week if the object has not yet passed in the stool. If the object does not pass within 2 weeks, surgical removal is necessary.

(2) The patient should be advised to return immediately to the ED if he or she experiences fever, abdominal pain, or vomiting.

IV PEPTIC ULCER DISEASE

A **Discussion** Peptic ulcers are localized erosions of the gastric or duodenal mucosa that produce pain and can perforate into a blood vessel (causing hemorrhage) or into the peritoneal cavity. Peptic ulcers are the most common cause of upper gastrointestinal hemorrhage (40% of cases).

1. **Prevalence.** The prevalence of peptic ulcer disease is 1.7%. Approximately 350,000 new cases are diagnosed annually in the United States.

2. **Risk factors** include smoking, alcohol use, aspirin or other NSAID use, a family history of peptic ulcer disease, male gender, and age.

3. **Etiology.** *Helicobacter pylori,* a helical, Gram-negative bacterium, has been found to be responsible for over 90% of duodenal ulcers and 65%–70% of gastric ulcers.

B **Clinical presentation** Patients with peptic ulcer disease present to the ED for one of three reasons: pain, hemorrhage, or perforation.

1. **Pain.** Most frequently, the patient complains of a burning or gnawing epigastric pain that does not radiate. Physical examination may demonstrate epigastric tenderness but no peritoneal signs. The pain is typically relieved by over-the-counter antacids or H_2 blockers.
   a. **Gastric ulcer pain** usually occurs immediately after eating.
   b. **Duodenal ulcer pain** occurs between meals and may awaken the patient from sleep. It is often worse immediately before a meal and is relieved by eating.

2. **Hemorrhage** is the presenting complaint in 20% of patients with peptic ulcer disease.
   a. **Patient history.** The patient may have a history of epigastric pain.
   b. **Signs and symptoms.** Twenty percent of patients present with **melena,** thirty percent with **hematemesis,** and fifty percent with both.
   c. **Physical examination.** Epigastric tenderness may be present. Rectal examination will most likely be positive for occult blood, if not grossly melanotic.

3. **Perforation** occurs in 5%–10% of patients with peptic ulcer disease.
   a. **Signs and symptoms.** Patients present with the abrupt onset of **severe epigastric pain** that may be associated with **vomiting** and **diaphoresis.**
   b. **Physical examination** reveals a diffusely tender abdomen with rigidity, rebound, guarding, and hypoactive bowel sounds.

C **Differential diagnoses**

1. **Pain.** Differential diagnoses for the pain of peptic ulcer disease include pancreatitis, cholelithiasis, abdominal aortic aneurysm, superior mesenteric artery syndrome, and cardiac causes.

2. **Hemorrhage.** Differential diagnoses for upper gastrointestinal hemorrhage include esophageal varices, gastritis, and Mallory-Weiss tears.

3. **Perforation.** Differential diagnoses include perforation of other organs, ruptured abdominal aortic aneurysm, and ruptured ectopic pregnancy.

D **Evaluation**

1. **Uncomplicated peptic ulcer disease.** In patients who are experiencing only pain, the **hemoglobin level** should be evaluated to rule out anemia due to chronic blood loss.

2. **Hemorrhage.** In hemorrhaging patients, the evaluation should include a **CBC, PT,** and **blood typing and cross matching.** A nasogastric tube should be placed to monitor for continued bleeding.

3. **Perforation**
   a. **Radiography.** A chest radiograph will reveal free air in 75% of patients. The radiographic yield is enhanced by instilling 100–200 mL of air via a nasogastric tube and keeping the patient in an upright position for at least 10 minutes prior to taking the radiograph.
   b. **Upper gastrointestinal series.** In some patients, an upper gastrointestinal series is necessary to demonstrate the perforation.

E **Therapy**

1. **Uncomplicated peptic ulcer disease.** If *H. pylori* has been confirmed to be the etiologic agent, antibiotic therapy is indicated. Treatment with an antacid is initiated, and the patient is advised to avoid alcohol, caffeine, and NSAIDs.

2. **Hemorrhage.** Eighty percent of patients will cease bleeding spontaneously, but the mortality rate is still seven percent overall.
   a. **Supportive therapy**
      (1) **Fluid resuscitation** should be carried out through two large-bore intravenous lines.
      (2) **Administration of blood products** (e.g., packed RBCs to correct anemia, fresh frozen plasma for coagulopathy, or platelets for thrombocytopenia) may be necessary.
      (3) **Intravenous administration of H_2 blockers** is often initiated, although there are no studies demonstrating that these agents have a beneficial effect in either stopping the bleeding or preventing rebleeding.
      (4) **Administration of octreotide** or **vasopressin** may be useful for terminating the hemorrhage.
   b. **Definitive therapy**
      (1) **Endoscopy** with **electrocautery** or **sclerotherapy** is the therapy of choice.
      (2) **Angiographic embolization** or **surgery** may be required.

3. **Perforation.** Therapy entails **nasogastric suction, intravenous fluids, antibiotics** (e.g., cefoxitin), and **surgery.**

F **Disposition**

1. Patients with no evidence of active bleeding, a normal hemoglobin, and normal vital signs may be discharged with a prescription for an H_2 blocker and instructions to follow up with a primary care physician.

2. Patients with anemia or active bleeding should be admitted to the hospital after consultation with a surgeon or gastroenterologist.

3. Patients with hemodynamic instability should be admitted to the intensive care unit (ICU) and a gastroenterologist should be consulted immediately.

4. Patients with perforation must be evaluated by a surgeon.

V   **GASTROENTERITIS OF INFECTIOUS ORIGIN**

A **Discussion**

1. **Definitions**
   a. **Diarrhea** is the excretion of more than 250 g of stool per day.
   b. **Dysentery** is diarrhea that contains blood, mucus, and pus.
   c. **Gastroenteritis** is acute enteritis (i.e., inflammation of the intestines manifested as diarrhea) accompanied by nausea and vomiting.
   d. **Food poisoning** is a gastroenteritis that occurs suddenly and is often associated with abdominal pain and cramping. It is caused by ingestion of food containing preformed toxins.

2. **Etiology.** Gastroenteritis is caused by viruses in 50%–70% of cases, bacteria in 15%–20% of cases, and parasites in 10%–15% of cases.

B **Clinical features**

1. **Viral gastroenteritis**

    a. **Norwalk agent.** The Norwalk agent is a parvovirus-like pathogen that is spread by the fecal–oral route and is often responsible for epidemic outbreaks of gastroenteritis. The diarrhea is more prominent than the vomiting, and symptoms last 24–48 hours.

    b. **Rotavirus** is a major cause of gastroenteritis in children, but adults can also contract the virus. Infection is characterized by vomiting that lasts 24–36 hours and diarrhea that lasts 4–7 days.

2. **Bacterial gastroenteritis**

    a. **Invasive organisms** induce bloody diarrhea by invading the intestinal mucosa.

    (1) *Campylobacter* gastroenteritis. *Campylobacter* species are the most common cause of bacterial gastroenteritis in the United States. They are Gram-negative organisms that cause an acute dysentery (i.e., diarrhea containing blood, pus, and mucus). The diarrhea can last for weeks, but most patients are ill for less than 1 week.

    (2) **Salmonellosis.** *Salmonella* is most often contracted from the ingestion of contaminated poultry products. It produces an acute gastroenteritis characterized by fever, abdominal pain, and diarrhea that may be bloody. Salmonellosis usually lasts less than 5 days.

    (3) **Shigellosis.** *Shigella* produces a gastroenteritis similar to that produced by *Salmonella*, but bloody diarrhea is a less prominent feature. The gastroenteritis resolves within 1 week.

    (4) *Vibrio parahaemolyticus* **gastroenteritis.** The most common route of infection is the ingestion of inadequately cooked seafood. Diarrhea lasting 24–48 hours is the predominant symptom.

    b. **Toxigenic organisms** produce a toxin that induces diarrhea. These organisms do not invade the mucosa; therefore, the diarrhea is not bloody.

    (1) **"Traveler's diarrhea"** is most commonly caused by enterotoxigenic *Escherichia coli* (ETEC). ETEC produces a toxin that induces a mild diarrhea that typically lasts less than 1 week.

    (2) **Staphylococcal food poisoning.** *Staphylococcus aureus* produces a toxin in certain foods that are allowed to stand at room temperature (e.g., mayonnaise-based salads, cream-filled doughnuts). Ingestion of the toxin induces a gastroenteritis characterized by violent vomiting and diarrhea that lasts less than 24 hours.

    (3) *Bacillus cereus* **gastroenteritis.** *B. cereus* produces a heat-stable toxin that can produce either an emetic syndrome similar to that produced by *S. aureus* or a diarrheal syndrome that is characterized by diarrhea and abdominal cramps lasting 24–36 hours.

    (4) **Pseudomembranous enterocolitis.** *Clostridium difficile* can cause diarrhea as a result of alterations in the intestinal flora following antibiotic therapy. The organism produces an enterotoxin that causes the enteritis.

3. **Protozoal diarrhea**

    a. **Giardiasis** (see Chapter 6 VIII A 2 j) is characterized by flatulence and loose, foul-smelling stools. *Giardia* cysts are usually acquired by ingestion of lake or stream water.

    b. **Cryptosporidiosis** is characterized by a profuse, nonbloody diarrhea that lasts less than 3 weeks in immunocompetent individuals but may become chronic in immunocompromised patients.

C **Differential diagnoses** include inflammatory bowel disease and, if pain is a prominent symptom, appendicitis, diverticulitis, small bowel obstruction, mesenteric infarction, and gynecologic disorders.

D **Evaluation** It is not usually possible, or necessary, to identify the causative organism in the ED. Rather, the focus should be on identifying whether the organism is invasive or toxigenic.

1. **Patient history**

    a. The patient should be asked about the **onset of symptoms.** A sudden onset of nausea, violent vomiting, and diarrhea suggests a toxigenic cause, whereas a more gradual onset suggests an invasive cause.

    b. The **duration of symptoms** can also provide valuable information. Toxigenic gastroenteritis from a preformed toxin (i.e., food poisoning) typically lasts less than 24 hours.

    c. A history of **foreign travel, camping,** or **exposure to children in day care** should be sought.

    d. The patient should be asked about the **nature of the stool.** Blood, pus, or mucus in the feces is diagnostic of invasive diarrhea.

2. **Physical examination**

    a. **Fever** is an uncommon manifestation of a toxigenic gastroenteritis and therefore points to an invasive cause.

    b. **Abdominal tenderness** may be prominent in an invasive gastroenteritis but is minimal in a toxigenic gastroenteritis.

3. **Laboratory studies.** If the patient is only mildly ill and there is no suspicion of invasive disease, then no further evaluation is necessary. However, if it is still unclear whether the cause is invasive or toxigenic, laboratory studies may be appropriate.

    a. **Fecal analysis.** Finding leukocytes in the stool sample is diagnostic for an invasive diarrhea. Patients with a history of antibiotic use within the preceding 2 weeks should have a stool sample sent for a *C. difficile* toxin assay.

    b. **Blood work.** The CBC is usually normal in toxigenic gastroenteritis but demonstrates an elevated WBC count and a left shift in patients with an invasive gastroenteritis.

E **Therapy**

1. **Rehydration** and **correction of electrolyte imbalances** is indicated for dehydrated patients.

    a. **Intravenous rehydration** may be necessary for some patients.

    b. **Oral rehydration.** Patients who are able to tolerate oral fluids should be instructed to drink cold fluids containing sugars (e.g., fruit juice, nondiet soft drinks, Rehydralyte, Gatorade) because sugars assist in electrolyte absorption. Milk should be avoided because many patients experience a transient lactase deficiency during a case of gastroenteritis.

2. **Antiemetics** (e.g., prochlorperazine) may be useful.

3. **Antidiarrheals** (e.g., loperamide, diphenoxylate) may be used in toxigenic gastroenteritis but are **contraindicated in invasive gastroenteritis.**

4. **Empiric antibiotic therapy** is indicated for patients with invasive gastroenteritis, especially if the patient appears ill. Antibiotics are **contraindicated in toxigenic gastroenteritis.**

    a. **Ciprofloxacin** is the current drug of choice because it has good activity against the most common infectious agents. The dose is 500 mg twice a day for 3–4 days.

    b. **Metronidazole** or **oral vancomycin** is used to treat pseudomembranous enterocolitis.

F **Disposition**

1. Patients who can tolerate oral hydration can be discharged with follow-up.

2. Patients who are severely dehydrated or severely ill should be admitted.

VI INTESTINAL DISORDERS

A **Inflammatory bowel disease**

1. **Crohn's disease (regional enteritis)**

    a. **Discussion.** Crohn's disease is a granulomatous inflammatory condition that can affect any portion of the digestive tract but most often involves the large and small bowel.

       (1) **Incidence and prevalence.** Men are more frequently affected than women, and the disease is more common in Jewish people. There are two peaks of incidence, between the ages of 12 and 30 years and 50 and 60 years.

       (2) **Etiology.** The cause is unclear, but infectious agents, immunologic factors, and genetic factors have all been implicated.

(3) **Pathogenesis.** Crohn's disease is characterized by areas of transmural inflammation interspersed with areas of normal bowel. The transmural nature of the inflammation predisposes to the formation of fistulae and strictures. Complications include bowel perforation, obstruction, hemorrhage, and abscess formation.

b. **Clinical features** include **fever, weight loss, diarrhea** (possibly bloody), and **cramping abdominal pain** that may be worse after meals.

  (1) **Symptoms of complications** may be masked if the patient is taking steroids.

  (2) **Symptoms of hepatobiliary, renal, rheumatic, ocular,** and **cutaneous manifestations** may be noted:

    (a) Biliary abnormalities (e.g., fatty liver, sclerosing cholangitis, cirrhosis, cholelithiasis)

    (b) Nephrolithiasis (resulting from calcium oxalate stones)

    (c) Arthritis and ankylosing spondylitis

    (d) Uveitis and episcleritis

    (e) Erythema nodosum and pyoderma gangrenosum

c. **Differential diagnoses** include ulcerative colitis, lymphoma, gastroenteritis, and appendicitis.

d. **Evaluation**

  (1) **Known diagnosis.** In patients with known Crohn's disease, studies should be performed to rule out complications suggested by the history and physical examination findings.

    (a) **Blood work.** A CBC may reveal evidence of hemorrhage, infection, or abscess. Electrolyte levels can be used to assess dehydration and secondary aberrations.

    (b) **Liver studies** are indicated to evaluate suspected biliary pathology.

    (c) **Radiographs.** An abdominal series can help rule out obstruction. A chest radiograph may reveal free air resulting from a perforation.

  (2) **Suspected diagnosis.** In patients who are suspected of having Crohn's disease, a **contrast study** or **colonoscopy** is indicated. These studies are usually performed on an outpatient basis.

e. **Therapy**

  (1) **Complications** such as perforation or obstruction must be treated.

  (2) **Uncomplicated exacerbations** are ideally managed in consultation with the patient's gastroenterologist. Treatment measures include administration of **antibiotics** (e.g., metronidazole), **steroids** (e.g., prednisone; 40–60 mg orally four times daily), **sulfasalazine** (3–4 g four times daily), and **loperamide** or **diphenoxylate.**

  (3) **Severe exacerbations** are treated with **bowel rest** and the intravenous administration of **fluids, antibiotics,** and **steroids** (e.g., hydrocortisone; 100 mg every 8 hours) if the patient is currently taking steroids or **adrenocorticotropic hormone (ACTH)** if the patient is not currently taking steroids.

f. **Disposition**

  (1) **Admission.** Indications for admission in patients in whom the diagnosis of Crohn's disease has been established include:

    (a) Complications (e.g., obstruction, perforation)

    (b) Systemic symptoms (e.g., fever, weight loss)

    (c) Severe symptoms (e.g., pain, bloody diarrhea)

    (d) Dehydration

  (2) **Discharge.** Patients with a definitive diagnosis who are discharged require careful instructions to return if the symptoms worsen or complications develop. Follow-up is essential. Patients in whom the diagnosis is suspected (on the basis of the history and examination), but who do not require hospitalization, must be referred for follow-up to obtain a definitive diagnosis.

2. **Ulcerative colitis**

a. **Discussion.** Ulcerative colitis is a chronic inflammatory condition affecting the mucosa and submucosa of the large bowel and rectum.

(1) **Incidence and prevalence.** Women are affected more than men. Peak incidence occurs between the ages of 15 and 30 years and 50 and 65 years.

(2) **Pathogenesis.** Complications include perforation, obstruction, hemorrhage, and toxic megacolon. Toxic megacolon occurs secondary to the loss of muscle tone in the affected portion of the colon.

b. **Clinical features** include **watery diarrhea** containing blood, pus, and mucus; **crampy abdominal pain; fever;** and **weight loss.** In a patient with toxic megacolon, there may be a history of decreased stool output and the abdomen is distended, tender, and tympanitic. Symptoms of complications may be masked if the patient is taking steroids.

c. **Differential diagnoses** include Crohn's disease, colon cancer, and diverticulitis.

d. **Evaluation**

(1) **Known diagnosis.** In patients in whom a diagnosis of ulcerative colitis has been made, studies should be performed to rule out complications.

(a) **Radiography.** Dilatation of the large bowel to greater than 6 cm is evident on abdominal films in patients with toxic megacolon.

(b) **Other studies** should be ordered according to the clinical picture.

(2) **Suspected diagnosis.** Patients in whom ulcerative colitis is suspected require **sigmoidoscopy,** usually on an outpatient basis.

e. **Therapy**

(1) **Toxic megacolon.** Therapeutic measures include placement of a **nasogastric tube** for proximal decompression, administration of **intravenous fluids and electrolytes,** administration of **antibiotics** (e.g., ampicillin and clindamycin or metronidazole), and administration of **steroids** (e.g., hydrocortisone, 100 mg administered intravenously every 8 hours). **Surgical consultation** is advisable.

(2) **Exacerbations** are managed essentially the same as for Crohn's disease [see VI A 1 e (3)].

f. **Disposition** is as for Crohn's disease (see VI A 1 f).

B **Bowel obstruction**

1. **Discussion.** An obstruction of the normal flow of intestinal contents can occur in either the large or small bowel.

a. **Causes** include adhesions from prior surgery (the most common cause), hernias, cancer, inflammatory conditions (e.g., Crohn's disease, diverticulitis), foreign bodies, volvulus (i.e., twisting of the large bowel around its mesentery), and intussusception (i.e., invagination of one segment of the intestine into another).

b. **Pathogenesis.** Obstruction leads to third-spacing of fluid into the bowel wall and lumen, which can lead to hypovolemia and electrolyte abnormalities. If the circulation to a segment of the bowel is compromised, the bowel is said to be strangulated. Strangulation usually results from the twisting of the bowel on its mesentery and can lead to gangrene and perforation.

2. **Clinical features**

a. **Patient history.** The patient may describe **obstipation** (i.e., a lack of stool or flatus). Obstipation may not be a clinical feature if the patient presents early in the course of obstruction or if only a partial obstruction is present.

b. **Symptoms**

(1) The patient complains of **cramping epigastric or periumbilical pain** that **waxes and wanes.**

(2) **Vomiting** tends to be a prominent feature in patients with a proximal obstruction, but may be absent in patients with a distal obstruction. The vomitus may become bilious and then feculent over time.

c. **Physical examination findings**

(1) The **abdomen tends to be diffusely tender** and without peritoneal signs. Peritoneal signs suggest that strangulation or perforation has occurred.

    (2) Abdominal distention tends to be more prominent with distal obstructions.

    (3) Intermittent, high-pitched bowel sounds may be auscultated.

3. Differential diagnoses include paralytic ileus (due to electrolyte abnormalities, trauma, uremia, or peritonitis), cholecystitis, pancreatitis, appendicitis, perforated peptic ulcer, and mesenteric ischemia.

4. Evaluation

    a. Blood work

        (1) An elevated WBC count with a left shift is suggestive of strangulation.

        (2) Electrolytes, blood urea nitrogen (BUN), and creatinine levels should be ordered to rule out an electrolyte abnormality and to further assess hydration status.

        (3) The amylase level may be elevated in the presence of strangulated or gangrenous bowel.

    b. Abdominal radiographs

        (1) Distention of the large or small bowel or both may be evident.

            (a) Valvulae conniventes, which are numerous, narrowly spaced, and cross the entire lumen, are seen in the small intestine.

            (b) Haustra, which are less numerous, widely spaced, and do not cross the entire lumen, are seen in the large intestine.

        (2) Air–fluid levels in a **stepladder pattern** are consistent with small bowel obstruction.

        (3) A **dilated, looped large bowel** is characteristic of a sigmoid volvulus.

        (4) A **distended colon** in the left lower quadrant and absence of right-sided gas may indicate a cecal volvulus.

        (5) The **"string-of-pearls" sign** (i.e., a line of small pockets of air in the fluid-filled lumen) may be observed.

        (6) Free air indicates that perforation has occurred.

    c. Other studies such as a **barium enema, upper gastrointestinal series,** or **colonoscopy** may be required in the ED or on an outpatient basis.

5. Therapy

    a. Supportive therapy

        (1) A nasogastric tube should be placed to decompress the bowel proximal to the obstruction.

        (2) Intravenous fluid hydration is indicated and electrolyte abnormalities should be corrected. Bladder catheterization may be used to monitor fluid status.

    b. Definitive therapy

        (1) Intussusception is usually diagnosed and treated with a barium or air enema.

        (2) Small bowel obstruction may be managed expectantly or with surgical intervention.

        (3) Nonstrangulatory sigmoid volvulus is managed with decompression and detorsion using a rectal tube.

        (4) Cecal volvulus usually requires surgery.

6. Disposition. The patient should be admitted.

C Diverticular disease

1. Discussion. Diverticula are herniations of the colonic mucosa through the muscularis propria. They are most frequently found in the sigmoid colon.

    a. Incidence. The incidence of diverticula is 30% in patients older than 50 years and increases to 50% in patients 70 years and older.

    b. Etiology and pathogenesis. Diverticula are thought to be caused by a low-fiber diet, which leads to less stool mass. The diminished stool mass causes muscular hypertrophy as the colon attempts to move the stool along. Ultimately, the intraluminal pressure in the colon is increased, promoting herniation of the mucosa.

        (1) Pain is thought to result from the increased muscular contractions made necessary by the increased intraluminal pressure.

      (2) Diverticulitis is an inflammatory condition resulting from microperforation of the diverticulum, which is often caused by feces lodging in the diverticulum.

      (3) Bleeding. Diverticula form near the perforating vessels of the colon. Bleeding results when the vessel ruptures into the diverticulum. Seventy percent of bleeding diverticula are found in the right colon.

2. Clinical features. Diverticula are most often asymptomatic, but 20%–30% of patients eventually manifest some symptoms.

    a. Diverticular pain. The pain is a **dull, crampy left lower quadrant pain** that is **often relieved by the passage of stool or flatus.** A firm and tender cord, representing the hypertrophied sigmoid colon, may be palpable.

    b. Diverticulitis

      (1) Symptoms include **left lower quadrant pain that is worse with bowel movements** and may radiate to the back, **fever,** and, possibly, **dysuria** (resulting from bladder irritation).

      (2) Physical examination findings. A **mass** may be noted on palpation of the left lower quadrant. Rectal examination may reveal a palpable mass or tenderness.

    c. Bleeding. Massive, painless hemorrhage is characteristic.

3. Differential diagnoses

    a. Pain and diverticulitis. Differential diagnoses include irritable bowel syndrome, Crohn's disease, ulcerative colitis, gynecologic disorders (e.g., PID, ovarian torsion), nephrolithiasis, UTI, colon cancer, and abdominal aortic aneurysm.

    b. Bleeding. Differential diagnoses include arteriovenous malformation, upper gastrointestinal hemorrhage, and cancer.

4. Evaluation

    a. Pain. A CBC should be ordered to rule out diverticulitis. Sigmoidoscopy or barium enema may be done on an outpatient basis to confirm the diagnosis.

    b. Diverticulitis

      (1) Laboratory studies

        (a) Blood work. The WBC count is usually increased with a left shift.

        (b) Urinalysis may show microscopic hematuria.

      (2) Radiography. Abdominal films may demonstrate an ileus or an obstruction. A chest radiograph may show free air in the event of a perforation.

      (3) Other studies. A **barium enema** or **CT scan** may be needed when the diagnosis is not clear.

    c. Bleeding diverticula

      (1) Nasogastric lavage should be performed to rule out an upper gastrointestinal source of hemorrhage.

      (2) Anoscopy or **sigmoidoscopy** can be used to rule out a hemorrhoidal source of bleeding.

      (3) Other studies. If the bleeding continues, the patient may require angiography, a tagged RBC study, or colonoscopy.

5. Therapy

    a. Uncomplicated diverticular disease. A high-fiber diet increases stool bulk, which decreases the intraluminal pressure and relieves the symptoms. An antispasmodic agent (e.g., dicyclomine) may also be helpful.

    b. Diverticulitis. Supportive measures include bowel rest and intravenous hydration. Antibiotic therapy (e.g., cefoxitin and an aminoglycoside or ciprofloxacin and metronidazole) is indicated. Surgery may be necessary if the patient has evidence of perforation, obstruction, or abscess.

    c. Bleeding diverticula

      (1) Fluid resuscitation. Two large-bore intravenous lines should be placed, along with a Foley catheter to monitor the resuscitation effort.

(2) Blood products should be administered.

(3) Vasopressin or **angiographic embolization** may be necessary for patients with persistent bleeding.

6. **Disposition**

a. **Uncomplicated diverticula.** The patient should be carefully instructed to return if there is a worsening of the pain or the onset of fever. Follow-up sigmoidoscopy is necessary to rule out cancer and ulcerative colitis.

b. **Diverticulitis**

(1) **Patients with mild disease** can be treated with oral antibiotics (trimethoprim–sulfamethoxazole and metronidazole) on an outpatient basis.

(2) **Patients with more severe disease** should be admitted for intravenous antibiotic administration.

(3) **Patients with suspected perforation, obstruction,** or **abscess** require immediate surgical consultation.

c. **Bleeding diverticula**

(1) **Patients with significant blood loss** or **continuing hemorrhage** should be admitted to the ICU.

(2) **Patients with stable vital signs** and **no evidence of continuing bleeding** can be admitted to a general medicine unit.

VII ANORECTAL DISORDERS

A Hemorrhoids

1. **Discussion**

a. **Definition.** Hemorrhoids are dilatations of the veins of either the internal or external hemorrhoidal plexus. Internal hemorrhoids are found above the dentate line. There are four classifications of internal hemorrhoids:

(1) **First-degree:** simple internal hemorrhoids

(2) **Second-degree:** prolapsed internal hemorrhoids that reduce themselves spontaneously

(3) **Third-degree:** prolapsed internal hemorrhoids that must be reduced manually

(4) **Fourth-degree:** prolapsed internal hemorrhoids that cannot be reduced

b. **Incidence.** Sixty to seventy percent of the population will experience a hemorrhoid at some time.

c. **Etiology.** Contributing factors are thought to be constipation, diarrhea, and straining at stools.

2. **Clinical features**

a. **History and symptoms.** Patients may report itching, pain, and blood on the toilet paper or in the toilet bowl.

(1) Internal hemorrhoids present with painless rectal bleeding. They are painless because they originate above the dentate line.

(2) External hemorrhoids present with rectal bleeding that becomes very painful if the vein becomes thrombosed.

b. **Physical examination findings.** External and prolapsed internal hemorrhoids are visible on examination. Nonprolapsed internal hemorrhoids may be palpated as a hard mass on rectal examination if they are thrombosed.

3. **Differential diagnoses** include other causes of rectal bleeding, such as diverticular disease, arteriovenous malformations, cancer, and anal fissures.

4. **Evaluation.** Internal hemorrhoids are visualized using anoscopy.

5. Therapy

    a. Conservative measures include a high-fiber diet, adequate fluid intake, stool softeners, sitz baths, topical analgesia (via an ointment or suppository), and application of hydrocortisone cream (either topically or via a suppository) to relieve itching.

    b. An external thrombosed hemorrhoid may be resected in the ED. The area around the vein should be infiltrated with a local anesthetic. An elliptical incision is made in the hemorrhoid and the clot is completely expressed. A gauze compress is inserted into the wound, and the buttocks are taped together for 8 hours to form a pressure dressing. The packing may be removed by the patient while in a sitz bath.

6. Disposition

    a. **External hemorrhoids** usually resolve in 1–3 weeks with conservative therapy. Incision and clot removal provides instantaneous relief.

    b. **Internal hemorrhoids.** Patients should be referred to a surgeon if surgical treatment appears to be necessary.

B Anal fissures

1. Discussion. Anal fissures, the most common cause of anal pain, are linear tears distal to the dentate line. Ninety percent occur in the posterior midline and most of the remaining ten percent are found in the anterior midline. Any other location should raise the suspicion of Crohn's disease or ulcerative colitis.

2. Clinical features include burning or stinging pain associated with defecation and minimal rectal bleeding. The tears are visible on examination of the anus.

3. Therapy involves a high-fiber diet and showers or sitz baths after bowel movements. Patients with a chronic fissure or with a fissure in an unusual location (i.e., not the midline) should be referred to a surgeon.

C Anorectal abscesses

1. Discussion

    a. A **perianal abscess** is a tender, red, fluctuant mass located near the anus. There is no induration or palpable mass on rectal examination.

    b. An **ischiorectal abscess** is deeper, has more lateral swelling, and may demonstrate induration on rectal examination.

    c. **Intersphincteric, intermuscular,** and **supralevator abscesses (deep abscesses)** are swollen and tender on rectal examination. Deep abscesses are usually associated with fever, chills, and the sense of rectal fullness or heaviness.

2. Clinical features. The pain tends to be steady, throbbing, and worse with bowel movements.

3. Evaluation. Patients with systemic signs and symptoms should have a WBC count and blood cultures sent.

4. Therapy

    a. **Perianal** and **ischiorectal abscesses** in patients with no evidence of deep abscess can be drained in the ED. The abscess is incised and packed with gauze, which should be removed in 48 hours. Follow-up care involves sitz baths and antibiotics (if the patient is immunocompromised or has systemic symptoms, or if evidence of cellulitis is present).

    b. **Deep abscesses.** Consultation with a surgeon is necessary.

D **Anorectal fistulae** are abnormal tracts from the anal canal. Clinical manifestations may include a bloody or foul-smelling discharge, recurrent inflammation, or recurrent abscesses. Anorectal fistulae most often result from the external drainage of an anorectal abscess but may also result from diverticulitis, appendicitis, or inflammatory bowel disease. Patients should be referred to a surgeon for treatment.

VIII   HEPATITIS, PANCREATITIS, CHOLECYSTITIS, AND APPENDICITIS

A **Hepatitis**

1. **Discussion.** Hepatitis is most often caused by viruses, but it can also be caused by medications, toxins, and other infectious agents.

   a. **Hepatitis A virus (HAV)** is an RNA virus that is transmitted by the fecal–oral route. The incubation period is 2–6 weeks. The infection is self-limited and remains anicteric in 50% of patients. There is no chronic form or carrier state.

   b. **Hepatitis B virus (HBV)** is a DNA virus that is spread parenterally (i.e., via blood transfusion, intravenous drug abuse) or sexually. The incubation period is 1–6 months. Ten percent of patients eventually develop chronic hepatitis or a carrier state.

   c. **Hepatitis C virus (HCV)** is a DNA virus that, until a screening test became available, was responsible for 90% of transfusion-related cases of hepatitis. HCV has an incubation period of 2 weeks to 6 months. The disease tends to be milder than that caused by HBV, but 50% of patients eventually develop chronic hepatitis.

   d. **Hepatitis D virus (HDV, the delta agent)** is a defective virus that can only replicate in the presence of an acute or chronic HBV infection. HDV causes severe hepatitis in patients with an existing chronic HBV infection.

   e. **Hepatitis E virus** is a waterborne RNA virus that is endemic to Mexico, Asia, and Africa. It tends to cause fulminant hepatitis in pregnant women.

2. **Clinical features**

   a. **Prodromal phase.** The prodromal phase occurs after the incubation period and is characterized by nonspecific symptoms such as anorexia, low-grade fever, and malaise.

   b. **Icteric phase.** Some patients then enter the icteric phase, which is characterized by jaundice, dark urine, and pale stools. The liver is usually enlarged and tender.

   c. **Extrahepatic manifestations** (e.g., urticaria, arthralgia, arthritis) may be seen in patients infected with HBV.

   d. **Fulminant hepatic failure.** Encephalopathy, coagulopathy, and jaundice are seen in a minority of patients who present in fulminant hepatic failure.

3. **Evaluation**

   a. **Laboratory studies**

      (1) **Liver enzyme studies.** ALT and AST levels are typically 10 times greater than their normal values. Elevations two to three times greater than normal with a more significant increase in AST than in ALT suggest alcohol-induced liver damage. Significant elevation of the AP level is suggestive of biliary obstruction.

      (2) **Serum protein, albumin,** and **glucose levels** and the **PT** are a better index of liver damage than liver enzyme studies.

      (3) **Ammonia level.** Patients with mental status changes should have a baseline ammonia level sent.

   b. **Ultrasonography.** A right upper quadrant ultrasound should be ordered if there is suspicion of biliary obstruction.

   c. **Serologic studies** are required to identify the causative agent, but these studies and results are not generally available in the ED.

4. **Therapy.** Asymptomatic patients do not require treatment.

   a. **Supportive measures**

      (1) **Intravenous rehydration** is indicated for dehydrated patients.

      (2) **Antiemetics** may be given for vomiting. Theoretically, metoclopramide is the agent of choice because phenothiazines may promote cholestasis.

      (3) **Vitamin K** should be given if the PT is elevated.

b. Prophylaxis should be considered for household and sexual contacts.
   (1) Hepatitis A. Immune globulin is administered intramuscularly within 2 weeks of exposure.
   (2) Hepatitis B. Immune globulin should be administered and vaccination started within 1 week of exposure to HBV.
   (3) Hepatitis C and **non-A, non-B,** and **non-C hepatitis** can also be prevented by administering appropriate immune globulin.

5. Disposition
   a. Most patients can be treated as outpatients. Patients should be given a prescription for an antiemetic and be instructed to abstain from alcohol. Medication to attenuate alcohol withdrawal symptoms may be appropriate for some patients. Personal hygiene must be stressed to prevent spread of the infection to others.
   b. Indications for admission include intractable vomiting, dehydration, electrolyte derangement, a PT 3 seconds greater than normal, and encephalopathy.

B **Acute pancreatitis**

1. Discussion
   a. Etiology. Acute pancreatitis is most frequently caused by alcohol abuse. Alcohol abuse and cholelithiasis together account for 80% of all cases. Other causes include trauma, infection, drug reactions, hyperparathyroidism, and hyperlipidemia.
   b. Pathogenesis. Inflammation of the pancreas is thought to result from the inappropriate intrapancreatic activation of pancreatic proteolytic enzymes. Activation of these enzymes leads to coagulation necrosis of the pancreas and can progress to retroperitoneal hemorrhage or abscess formation.

2. Clinical features
   a. Symptoms include nausea, vomiting, and epigastric pain that often radiates to the back and may be relieved by leaning forward.
   b. Physical examination findings include:
      (1) Epigastric tenderness, which may or may not be associated with rebound tenderness and involuntary guarding, depending on the severity of the inflammation
      (2) Diminished bowel sounds
      (3) Fever
      (4) Jaundice (may be prominent in the case of a common bile duct stone)
      (5) Grey-Turner's sign (flank ecchymosis) or **Cullen's sign** (periumbilical ecchymosis), if retroperitoneal hemorrhage has occurred

3. Differential diagnoses include cholelithiasis, ascending cholangitis, peptic ulcer disease, abdominal aortic aneurysm, and MI.

4. Evaluation
   a. Laboratory studies
      (1) Serum amylase is almost always elevated in acute pancreatitis but may not be elevated in patients with preexistent chronic pancreatitis. If the serum amylase level is greater than 1000 IU/dL, one should suspect gallstone pancreatitis.
      (2) Serum lipase. An elevated lipase level is very specific (99%) for pancreatitis.
   b. Diagnostic imaging studies
      (1) Radiography
         (a) Abdominal plain films may demonstrate:
            (i) Calcification of the pancreas in patients with chronic pancreatitis
            (ii) Blurring of the psoas shadow
            (iii) The **"cutoff" sign** (i.e., abrupt ending of the transverse colon gas shadow at the pancreas)
            (iv) The **"inverted three" sign** (i.e., localized ileus of the duodenum and jejunum)
         (b) Chest radiograph. A left pleural effusion may be seen.

    (2) **Ultrasonography** may show pancreatic edema, a pseudocyst, or an abscess. It can also be used to rule out biliary pathology and an aortic aneurysm.

    (3) **CT** is the study of choice for imaging the pancreas and detecting complications such as pseudocysts.

  c. **Ranson's criteria** are prognostic indicators. Patients who fulfill less than three criteria have less than a 1% risk of mortality; the mortality rate increases to 100% if more than six criteria are met.

    (1) **Criteria at admission**

      (a) Age greater than 55

      (b) WBC count greater than 16,000/mm^3

      (c) Glucose level greater than 200 mg/dL

      (d) Lactate dehydrogenase (LDH) level greater than 350 IU/L

      (e) AST level greater than 250 U/L

    (2) **Criteria at 48 hours**

      (a) A drop in hematocrit greater than or equal to 10%

      (b) An increase in BUN greater than or equal to 5 mg/dL

      (c) Serum calcium less than 8 mg/dL

      (d) Arterial oxygen tension (PO_2) less than 60 mm Hg

      (e) Third-spacing of more than 6 L of fluid

      (f) Base deficit of greater than 4 mEq/L

5. Therapy

  a. **Nasogastric suction** (and possibly **antiemetics**) are indicated if the patient is vomiting.

  b. **Intravenous fluid hydration** should be initiated, and a Foley catheter placed to monitor fluid status.

  c. **Analgesics** may be necessary. Meperidine is preferred because it may cause less contraction of the sphincter of Oddi.

  d. **Antibiotics** should be administered only if there is evidence of infection.

6. Disposition

  a. Patients with very mild pancreatitis and no evidence of biliary disease can be discharged if they are able to tolerate oral liquids. Outpatient therapy entails oral analgesics and a clear liquid diet.

  b. Patients with hemodynamic instability or evidence of hemorrhagic pancreatitis warrant an ICU admission. Surgical consultation should be obtained for patients with severe pancreatitis.

C Cholecystitis

1. Discussion. Cholecystitis is inflammation of the gallbladder that results from the impaction of a gallstone in the cystic duct.

  a. **Incidence.** Gallstones are present in 15%–20% of the population, but in the majority of cases, they remain asymptomatic.

  b. **Risk factors** for gallstones include age, female sex, obesity, oral contraceptive use, family history of gallstones, diabetes mellitus, Crohn's disease, rapid weight loss, Asian race, and sickle cell anemia.

2. Clinical features

  a. **Symptoms.** Patients complain of a **constant, cramping right upper quadrant** or **epigastric pain** that may radiate to the scapula. The pain may be postprandial, particularly after consuming a high-fat meal. The pain may be accompanied by **nausea** and **vomiting.**

  b. **Physical examination**

    (1) **Right upper quadrant tenderness** with or without rebound tenderness is present.

    (2) **Murphy's sign,** an abrupt halt in inspiration when the examiner palpates the right upper quadrant, may be present.

    (3) The **gallbladder may be palpable.**

    (4) **Fever** may be present.

        (5) Jaundice suggests a common duct stone but may be present even if there is no stone in the common duct.

  3. Differential diagnoses

    a. Cardiac causes. MI or angina must always be considered.

    b. Biliary colic results from stone impaction in the cystic duct but resolves before progressing to cholecystitis. It is characterized by a constant epigastric or right upper quadrant pain that lasts less than 4–6 hours. There is no fever, and the WBC count, liver chemistries, and bilirubin levels are normal.

    c. Ascending cholangitis is a bacterial infection of the biliary system that results from the impaction of a gallstone in the common bile duct. It is characterized by **Charcot's triad** (right upper quadrant pain, fever and chills, and jaundice). Severe cases are characterized by the **pentad of Reynold,** which is Charcot's triad plus mental status changes and hypotension.

    d. Hepatitis. AST and ALT elevations are usually more prominent in hepatitis than in cholecystitis.

    e. Pancreatitis is discussed in VIII B.

    f. Peptic ulcer disease is discussed in IV.

    g. Mesenteric ischemia is discussed in X A.

  4. Evaluation

    a. Laboratory studies

      (1) CBC. The WBC count is elevated with a leftward shift.

      (2) Liver enzyme studies. AST and ALT are mildly elevated. The AP level is mildly elevated; a significant elevation suggests a common bile duct stone.

      (3) Bilirubin. The bilirubin level is usually only slightly elevated unless a common bile duct stone is present. The direct (conjugated) fraction is higher than the indirect (unconjugated) fraction.

      (4) Amylase. The amylase level is often elevated, but an elevation greater than three times normal should cause one to consider pancreatitis.

    b. Diagnostic imaging studies

      (1) Radiography. Plain films are useful to rule out other diagnoses such as bowel obstruction or perforation. Approximately 15% of gallstones are radiopaque.

      (2) Ultrasonography can detect gallstones, thickening of the gallbladder wall, or pericholecystic fluid, all of which suggest the diagnosis. Emergency bedside ultrasound is usually limited to evaluation for the presence or absence of cholelithiasis.

      (3) A **hepatobiliary radionuclide scan** should be performed if the ultrasound examination is equivocal. Nonvisualization of the gallbladder is consistent with cholecystitis, but false positives can occur.

  5. Therapy

    a. Cholecystitis is treated with nasogastric suction, bowel rest, and intravenous hydration. Surgical consultation is advisable. Antibiotics are not routinely indicated and should be used only after consulting with the surgeon.

    b. Biliary colic can be treated with antispasmodics (e.g., dicyclomine). The patient should be referred to a surgeon and instructed to return if he or she notices fever, persistent pain, acholic (light) stools, or darkening of the urine.

    c. Ascending cholangitis should be treated similarly to cholecystitis, but antibiotic therapy against Gram-negative enteric organisms should be initiated.

  6. Disposition. Patients with uncomplicated biliary colic may be discharged, but all other patients should be admitted.

D **Appendicitis**

  1. Discussion. Appendicitis is an acute inflammation of the appendix that is caused by the obstruction of its lumen.

    a. Incidence. The annual incidence is 1 in 1000, with the peak incidence occurring between the ages of 10 and 19.

    b. Etiology. The most common cause of obstruction of the lumen is a fecalith. Less common causes include lymphoid hypertrophy, cancer, and parasites.

    c. Pathogenesis. Obstruction of the lumen leads to distention, inflammation, bacterial overgrowth, and ischemia. If left untreated, the ischemia will progress to gangrene and, ultimately, perforation.

2. Clinical features

    a. Symptoms. The presentation tends to be atypical in pediatric and geriatric patients; therefore, higher morbidity and mortality rates due to delayed diagnosis are seen in these populations.

        (1) Pain. The pain begins epigastrically or periumbilically and then localizes to the right lower quadrant. In pregnant women, the pain localizes to the area of the appendix, which rises as the pregnancy progresses. The pain is typically described as crampy or gassy and may be confused with that of indigestion.

        (2) Anorexia is present in 92% of patients.

        (3) Nausea and **vomiting** are present in 78% of patients and invariably follow the onset of pain.

    b. Physical examination findings

        (1) Low-grade fever is present in only 21% of patients.

        (2) Right lower quadrant tenderness is classically located at **McBurney's point** (two thirds of the distance along the line drawn from the umbilicus to the anterior-superior iliac spine). Later in the course of the illness, the patient will have **involuntary guarding** and **rebound tenderness** in the right lower quadrant due to local peritonitis. In the event of perforation, the patient may present with an **acute surgical abdomen** (i.e., rigidity, rebound, involuntary guarding), fever, chills, and vomiting.

        (3) Rovsing's sign is right lower quadrant pain elicited by palpation in the left lower quadrant.

        (4) The **psoas sign** is pain elicited by extending the patient's right hip while the patient is lying on his or her left side.

        (5) The **obturator sign** is pain elicited by internal rotation of the right hip while the hip and knee are held in flexion.

        (6) Right-sided tenderness or a **mass** may be demonstrated by rectal or pelvic examination.

3. Differential diagnoses include mesenteric lymphadenitis, Crohn's disease, gastroenteritis, cecal diverticulitis, UTI, nephrolithiasis, and gynecologic conditions (e.g., PID, ovarian torsion, tuboovarian abscess, ectopic pregnancy).

4. Evaluation

    a. Laboratory studies

        (1) CBC. The WBC count is usually only moderately elevated, typically in the 10,000–16,000/mm^3 range.

        (2) Urinalysis may show some RBCs as a result of ureteral irritation.

    b. Diagnostic imaging studies

        (1) Radiography. Abdominal films may demonstrate a right lower quadrant ileus, a fecalith, or loss of the psoas shadow. A barium enema can be used to demonstrate nonfilling of the appendix, but false positives do occur.

        (2) Ultrasonography has a sensitivity of 75%–89% and a specificity of 86%–100% when performed by an experienced sonographer.

        (3) Directed appendix CT scanning is often diagnostic and has become the standard of care in evaluating most patients with suspected appendicitis.

5. Therapy. The patient should have nothing by mouth. Intravenous hydration should be initiated, and the patient should be seen by a surgeon immediately.

6. Disposition. Appendicitis is primarily a clinical diagnosis. If the diagnosis is unclear, the patient should be either admitted or kept in the ED for serial abdominal examinations.

IX HERNIA

A Discussion

1. **Definition.** A hernia is the protrusion of a viscus through an opening into an abnormal location. Hernias are present in approximately 5% of the population. Approximately 75% are inguinal, 10% are incisional, 5% are umbilical, and 5% are femoral.
    a. **Inguinal hernias**
        (1) **Indirect inguinal hernias** are the most common type of hernia in both men and women. They occur when the bowel travels down a patent processus vaginalis into the inguinal canal. The bowel may progress into the scrotum.
        (2) **Direct inguinal hernias.** The bowel protrudes through a defect in the abdominal wall in Hesselbach's triangle. The incidence increases with advancing age and physical exertion.
    b. **Incisional hernias** occur at sites of previous abdominal surgery.
    c. **Umbilical hernias** are 10 times more common in women than in men and they are often associated with pregnancy or with ascites.
    d. **Femoral hernias.** The bowel protrudes into the femoral canal. Over 80% of femoral hernias occur in women and they are thought to be related to pregnancy and physical exertion.

2. **Complications**
    a. **Incarceration.** An incarcerated hernia is one in which the protruding abdominal contents cannot be returned to the abdominal cavity. Left untreated, an incarcerated hernia can progress and become strangulated. Thirty to forty percent of femoral hernias become incarcerated or strangulated.
    b. **Strangulation.** A strangulated hernia is one in which the tissue becomes necrotic due to obstruction of its blood supply. Indirect inguinal hernias are more likely than direct inguinal hernias to become strangulated.

B Clinical features

1. **Uncomplicated hernias**
    a. **Symptoms.** The patient may complain of a bulge or mass that grows and shrinks over time. The hernia may spontaneously reduce or be reducible by the patient.
    b. **Physical examination findings.** The patient should always be examined in both recumbent and standing positions.
        (1) **Palpation.** The hernia may not be visible or palpable without provocative maneuvers (e.g., coughing or a Valsalva maneuver).
            (a) **Femoral hernias** may be palpable below the inguinal ligament.
            (b) **Inguinal hernias**
                (i) **Direct inguinal hernias** are palpable in Hesselbach's triangle superior to the inguinal ligament. In men, the examining finger should be placed in the inguinal canal by invaginating the scrotum, allowing palpation of the direct hernia at the floor of the inguinal canal.
                (ii) **Indirect inguinal hernias** can be palpated by moving the examining finger down the inguinal canal.
        (2) **Auscultation.** Bowel sounds may be heard in the area of the mass.

2. **Incarceration.** An incarcerated hernia cannot be reduced with gentle pressure by either the patient or physician. Otherwise, the findings are the same as for uncomplicated hernias.

3. **Strangulation**
    a. **Symptoms.** The patient may demonstrate symptoms of bowel obstruction (i.e., vomiting, obstipation, abdominal tenderness).
    b. **Physical examination findings.** The hernia will usually be tender to palpation. Fever is a consistent finding in patients with necrosis of the bowel.

C **Differential diagnoses** include hydrocele, lipoma, lymphadenopathy, abscess, and tumor.

D **Evaluation**   In patients who have a tender, irreducible mass or symptoms of strangulation, additional studies, including abdominal films, a WBC count, and amylase levels, should be performed.

E **Therapy**

1. **Relief of obstruction.** Patients with symptoms of strangulation or small bowel obstruction should be treated for bowel obstruction (see VI B 5).

2. **Reduction** is achieved through the application of continuous gentle pressure, often in conjunction with postural positioning. Pain or anxiolytic medications are often administered. **The abdomen is no place for dead bowel.** If necrosis or signs of acute strangulation are present, it is inappropriate to attempt to reduce the hernia.

3. **Surgery.** Patients with irreducible hernias require surgical consultation.

F **Disposition**   Patients with reducible hernias may be discharged with instructions to avoid strenuous activities and to return to the ED if any symptoms of incarceration or strangulation develop. Surgical follow-up is mandatory.

X   VASCULAR DISORDERS

A **Mesenteric ischemia**

1. **Discussion.** Mesenteric ischemia is inadequate oxygen delivery to some portion of the intestinal tract, which can ultimately result in necrosis and perforation. Mesenteric ischemia is associated with a mortality rate of 80%.

   a. **Etiology.** Ischemia can result from embolism, thrombosis, or low flow states. Acute ischemia is due to embolic obstruction of the superior mesenteric artery in most cases.

   b. **Risk factors** include atrial fibrillation and atherosclerosis. The mean age of occurrence is 60–80 years.

2. **Clinical features**

   a. **Patient history.** The patient may have a history of **"abdominal angina,"** a crampy, dull periumbilical pain commencing 15–30 minutes after eating and resolving over hours. The patient may have developed a fear of eating because of the pain and may have experienced weight loss.

   b. **Symptoms**

      (1) **Severe periumbilical pain.** Mesenteric ischemia most often presents as the acute onset of severe periumbilical pain "out of proportion" to physical findings.

      (2) **Vomiting** and **diarrhea** may be present.

   c. **Physical examination findings.** Occult blood may be present on rectal examination, but hematochezia is not common.

3. **Differential diagnoses.** The list of differential diagnoses is long and includes essentially every other cause of abdominal pain.

4. **Evaluation**

   a. **Laboratory studies** are nonspecific.

      (1) The hemoglobin may be elevated due to hemoconcentration.

      (2) The WBC count is usually elevated.

      (3) The amylase level may be mildly elevated.

      (4) Metabolic acidosis may be present, but this is usually a late sign.

   b. **Diagnostic imaging findings**

      (1) **Radiography.** Plain films are usually normal but may demonstrate an ileus. Gas in the portal system is a very late sign and an ominous finding.

      (2) **Angiography** is the definitive diagnostic study.

5. **Therapy.** Acute measures include intravenous fluid resuscitation. Consultation with a surgeon is imperative.

B **Abdominal aortic aneurysm**

1. **Discussion.** An abdominal aortic aneurysm is not a gastrointestinal emergency but may easily be misdiagnosed as a gastrointestinal problem. The mortality rate is 1%–5% if elective repair of an abdominal aortic aneurysm is performed, but it increases to 75% after rupture occurs.

   a. **Definition.** An aneurysm is defined as dilatation of a blood vessel by 50% or more. Given an average normal aortic diameter of 2 cm, a diameter greater than or equal to 3 cm is an aneurysm.

   b. **Incidence.** Abdominal aortic aneurysms are found in 2%–5% of the population older than 65 years.

   c. **Risk factors** include age greater than 65 years, male sex, smoking, chronic obstructive pulmonary disease (COPD), hypertension, atherosclerotic peripheral vascular disease, a family history, and collagen vascular diseases (e.g., Ehlers-Danlos syndrome, Marfan syndrome).

   d. **Complications.** The risk of rupture is directly related to the size of the aneurysm. Aneurysms 4–5 cm in diameter are associated with a 3%–12% chance of rupturing in 5 years, whereas larger aneurysms are associated with a 25%–41% chance of rupture.

2. **Clinical features**

   a. **Symptoms** may be produced by expansion of the aneurysm or by rupture.

      (1) **Pain.** Abdominal, back, or flank pain is usually the chief complaint. The pain is not affected by movement and may radiate to the testicle or leg.

      (2) **Syncope** may be the presenting symptom.

      (3) **Lower extremity claudication** or **neurologic symptoms** may be noted.

   b. **Physical examination findings**

      (1) A **pulsatile abdominal mass** is usually palpable. Because the aortic bifurcation occurs at the level of the umbilicus, the mass will be palpated above the umbilicus.

      (2) An **abdominal bruit** may be audible.

      (3) **Decreased pulses** may be noted in the lower extremities. In the case of rupture, **hypotension** may be present.

3. **Differential diagnoses**

   a. **Renal colic** is the most common misdiagnosis. The patient may even have microscopic hematuria due to irritation of the ureter. Abdominal aortic aneurysm must be ruled out in any patient older than 60 years with symptoms of renal colic and no history of nephrolithiasis. Twenty-five percent of patients with an abdominal aortic aneurysm have hematuria.

   b. **Diverticulitis**

   c. **Pancreatitis**

   d. **MI**

   e. **Musculoskeletal back pain**

4. **Evaluation**

   a. **Laboratory studies.** The blood should be typed and cross matched. Serum BUN and creatinine levels should be obtained. A CBC and PT should be sent. Electrocardiographic monitoring should be established.

   b. **Diagnostic imaging studies**

      (1) **Radiography.** Plain abdominal films show calcification of the aorta in 60% of cases. Plain films should never be used to exclude abdominal aortic aneurysm as the diagnosis.

      (2) **Ultrasonography** is 100% sensitive in detecting an abdominal aortic aneurysm but is not helpful in assessing leaking or rupture.

      (3) **CT** is the most accurate study to assess rupture, but it takes time to perform and requires that the patient leave the ED. A CT scan is helpful to the surgeon if the patient is stable enough to tolerate the study.

(4) **Angiography** is useful for defining the anatomy but is not as sensitive as CT for the detection of an abdominal aortic aneurysm.

5. **Therapy**
   a. **Asymptomatic patients.** An ultrasound study should be performed. If the aneurysm is less than 4 cm in diameter, and has no evidence of dissection or rupture, the patient can be discharged with follow-up. Patients with larger aneurysms should be seen by a surgeon.
   b. **Symptomatic patients without hemodynamic catastrophe**
      (1) Two large-bore intravenous lines should be established for the administration of crystalloid and blood products.
      (2) Hypertension should be pharmacologically managed, ideally with short-acting titratable agents.
      (3) Surgical and interventional radiology consultation should be arranged.
   c. **Unstable patients** need emergent surgery, which should not be delayed to obtain radiologic studies. The patient should be aggressively resuscitated while awaiting surgical intervention.

Study Questions

Directions: *Each of the numbered items or incomplete statements in this section is followed by answers or by completions of the statement. Select the ONE lettered answer or completion that is BEST in each case.*

1. What is the most common cause of upper gastrointestinal bleeding?
   - (A) Mallory-Weiss tear
   - (B) Esophageal varices
   - (C) Peptic ulcer
   - (D) Arteriovenous malformation
   - (E) Aortoenteric fistula

2. A 2-year-old boy presents to the emergency department (ED) after ingestion of a calculator battery. A chest radiograph demonstrates that the battery is in the esophagus. What would be the most appropriate next course of action?
   - (A) Observation
   - (B) Having the patient drink a glass of milk
   - (C) Intravenous administration of glucagon
   - (D) Sublingual administration of nifedipine
   - (E) Endoscopy

3. What is the most common cause of small bowel obstruction?
   - (A) Adhesions
   - (B) Cancer
   - (C) Foreign bodies
   - (D) Crohn's disease
   - (E) Hernia

4. In women, the most common type of hernia is
   - (A) indirect inguinal
   - (B) direct inguinal
   - (C) incisional
   - (D) umbilical
   - (E) femoral

5. Which one of the following statements regarding cholecystitis is true?
   - (A) It is caused by impaction of a gallstone in the cystic duct.
   - (B) It is characterized by Charcot's triad.
   - (C) Antibiotic therapy should be started as early as possible.
   - (D) Jaundice is not a sign of cholecystitis.
   - (E) Eighty-five percent of gallstones are visible on plain films.

6. Which one of the following statements about the emergency department (ED) management of hepatitis is true?
   - (A) Patients with severely elevated liver enzymes should be admitted.
   - (B) Vitamin K should be administered if the patient's partial thromboplastin time (PTT) is elevated.
   - (C) Prochlorperazine is the antiemetic of choice.

D Most patients can be referred for outpatient evaluation.

E Discharged patients should be instructed to avoid dairy products.

7. Abdominal aortic aneurysm is most commonly misdiagnosed as

A pancreatitis

B nephrolithiasis

C myocardial infarction (MI)

D lower back strain

E diverticulitis

8. A 10-year-old boy presents with illness for the past 2 days. Which of the following symptoms is least likely to be a sign of appendicitis?

A Vomiting

B Anorexia

C Fever

D Abdominal pain

E Nausea

9. A 58-year-old man with rectal bleeding is brought to the emergency department (ED) by his wife. His vital signs suggest early hypovolemia. He passes a large amount of further bright red blood per rectum in the ED. He has no abdominal pain or tenderness on examination. Which of the following plans would be most optimal for this patient?

A Nasogastric suction, placement of two large-bore intravenous lines, and an operation

B Administration of dobutamine and endoscopy

C Placement of a Foley catheter and further observation only

D Administration of intravenous fluids, antibiotics, and packed red blood cells (RBCs)

E Administration of IV fluids, packed RBCs, and endoscopy

Answers and Explanations

1. **The answer is C** Peptic ulcers are the most common cause of upper gastrointestinal hemorrhage, followed by gastritis, esophageal varices, and Mallory-Weiss tears. Regarding peptic ulcers, duodenal ulcers are a more common cause than gastric ulcers of upper gastrointestinal hemorrhage.

2. **The answer is E** Button batteries (e.g., calculator batteries) can cause perforation of the esophagus; therefore, they must be removed. Endoscopy is the appropriate method of extraction. Glucagon and nifedipine can be used to dislodge a food bolus. Milk is not indicated in foreign-body ingestions.

3. **The answer is A** Adhesions from prior surgery are the most common cause of small bowel obstruction.

4. **The answer is A** Indirect inguinal hernias are the most common type of hernia in both men and women. Eighty percent of femoral hernias occur in women, but only five percent of all hernias are femoral hernias.

5. **The answer is A** Cholecystitis is caused by the impaction of a gallstone in the cystic duct. Jaundice may be present, despite the fact that there is no obstruction of the common bile duct. Antibiotic therapy is not indicated for patients with uncomplicated cholecystitis. Charcot's triad is associated with ascending cholangitis, which results from bacterial infection of the biliary tree after impaction of a gallstone in the common bile duct. Only 15% of gallstones are radiopaque.

6. **The answer is D** Most patients who are clinically diagnosed as having hepatitis in the ED can be discharged and referred for outpatient evaluation. Elevated liver enzyme levels alone are not an indication for admission. Indications for admission include intractable vomiting, dehydration, electrolyte derangements, elevation of the prothrombin time (PT) by greater than 3 seconds, and hepatic encephalopathy. Administration of vitamin K is indicated when there is an elevation of the PT, not the PTT. Prochlorperazine is a phenothiazine and may promote cholestasis; therefore, metoclopramide is the antiemetic of choice. Dairy products are not contraindicated in patients with hepatitis, but should probably be avoided by patients recovering from a bout of acute gastroenteritis because these patients may experience a transient lactase deficiency.

7. **The answer is B** The most common misdiagnosis of an abdominal aortic aneurysm is nephrolithiasis causing renal colic. Any patient over the age of 60 with symptoms suggestive of renal colic, but no history of renal colic, should be suspected of having an abdominal aortic aneurysm. In patients with rupturing abdominal aortic aneurysm, 25% will have hematuria, contributing to misdiagnosis. Pancreatitis, MI, diverticulitis, and musculoskeletal back pain are other differential diagnoses for abdominal aortic aneurysm.

8. **The answer is C** Only 21% of patients with acute appendicitis have a fever. Abdominal pain is present in over 99% of patients, anorexia in 92%, nausea in over 75%, and vomiting in over 50%.

9. **The answer is E** Antibiotics are not indicated in the treatment of bleeding diverticula. They are indicated in the treatment of diverticulitis, which is caused by microperforation of the diverticulum. Nasogastric suction is indicated to rule out an upper gastrointestinal source of bleeding. An operation is not indicated at this time, but two large-bore intravenous lines should always be placed in patients with acute bleeding for the administration of fluids and blood products. A Foley catheter is needed to monitor the adequacy of the fluid resuscitation effort, and endoscopy or other diagnostic procedures is indicated in the setting of continued significant hemorrhage.

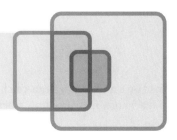

chapter 5

Urogenital Emergencies

KATHERINE C. CLARK · EDWARD J. MLINEK, JR.

I   URINARY TRACT INFECTIONS (UTIs)

A Discussion   UTIs are commonly evaluated in the emergency department (ED).

1. **Causes.** Most UTIs are caused by pathogens that normally inhabit the perineum and gastro-intestinal tract.
   a. *Escherichia coli* is responsible for 80%–90% of UTIs.
   b. *Klebsiella, Proteus, Enterobacter,* and *Pseudomonas* species account for 10%–20% of cases.
   c. Group D *Streptococcus, Chlamydia,* and *Staphylococcus* are responsible in fewer than 5% of cases.

2. **Predisposing factors**
   a. **Women** are affected more often than men because the shorter female urethra facilitates bacterial access to the bladder.
      (1) **Sexual intercourse** and the **use of nonoxynol-9–containing spermicides** predispose to the development of UTIs.
      (2) **Pregnancy** is associated with a high incidence of asymptomatic bacteriuria that may progress to pyelonephritis.
      (3) **Postmenopausal state.** Postmenopausal women are predisposed to UTIs because estrogen deficiency increases *E. coli* colonization of the bladder.
   b. **Men**
      (1) **Predisposing conditions** (e.g., anatomic abnormalities, tumors, calculi, prostatitis) are found in up to 80% of men with UTIs.
      (2) **Catheterization** accounts for many cases of UTIs in men.
      (3) **Uncircumcised men** (and women who have intercourse with uncircumcised men) are more prone to UTIs.

B Clinical features

1. **Symptoms.** Presenting symptoms may include **urinary urgency, frequency, nocturia, dysuria, a sensation of incomplete voiding,** and **suprapubic pain.** Patients with upper tract involvement may also have **fever, chills, nausea,** and **vomiting.**

2. **Physical examination findings. Flank pain, mild suprapubic midline tenderness,** and **costovertebral angle tenderness** may be associated with pyelonephritis and cystitis.

C Differential diagnoses

1. **Vaginitis** resulting from *Candida albicans, Trichomonas vaginalis,* or *Gardnerella* infection must be considered.

2. **Urethritis** is a particularly important consideration in men who present with urethral discharge. The most common pathogens are *Chlamydia trachomatis* and *Neisseria gonorrhoeae.*

3. **Prostatitis** (see VI D)

D **Evaluation**

1. **Urinalysis** should be performed on a midstream clean-catch specimen. Patients with certain clinical conditions (e.g., vaginal discharge, menstruation, obesity) may need to be catheterized to obtain a urine specimen.

   a. **Microscopic analysis**

      (1) **Hematuria** may represent lower or upper tract involvement.

      (2) **Bacteriuria.** More than 10–15 organisms per high-power field on a centrifuged specimen is suggestive of UTI. Finding any bacteria on an uncentrifuged specimen correlates with a positive urine culture (see I D 2).

      (3) **Pyuria** is defined by the presence of more than 10 white blood cells (WBCs) per high-power field on a centrifuged specimen.

   b. **Dipstick analysis**

      (1) **Leukocyte esterase test.** The leukocyte esterase test is a reliable screen for pyuria, although false-negative results may occur with low-level pyuria.

      (2) **Detection of nitrites** is indicative of infection with a Gram-negative organism.

2. **Urine cultures**

   a. **Indications.** Urine cultures are not routinely ordered, but may be indicated in neutropenic patients with fever, patients who have pyelonephritis or indwelling catheters, patients who fail to respond to therapy, and patients who experience relapses.

   b. **Interpretation.** The growth of 10^5 colonies/mL of urine is considered a positive culture. If urine culture yields 10^2–10^5 colonies/mL of urine in a symptomatic patient, treatment is required.

3. **Complete blood count (CBC).** The CBC may reveal leukocytosis in patients with suspected pyelonephritis. The leukocyte count is not elevated in patients with cystitis.

E **Therapy**

1. **Cystitis.** Specific regimens are given in Table 5–1.

   a. **Uncomplicated cases.** In patients without constitutional symptoms or complicating medical conditions and a short duration of symptoms, uncomplicated cystitis can be treated with a 1- to 3-day course of **oral trimethoprim–sulfamethoxazole** or a **fluoroquinolone.**

TABLE 5–1   Antibacterial Regimens for the Treatment of Lower Urinary Tract Infections (UTIs)

Type of Infection	Drug	Dosage	Dosage Frequency and Duration
Uncomplicated cystitis	Trimethoprim–sulfamethoxazole	160/800 mg	Twice daily for 3 days
	Trimethoprim–sulfamethoxazole	160/800 mg	One dose of two tablets
	Ciprofloxacin	250 mg	Twice daily for 3 days
	Norfloxacin	400 mg	Twice daily for 3 days
	Ofloxacin	200 mg	Twice daily for 3 days
Complicated cystitis	Trimethoprim–sulfamethoxazole	160/800 mg	Twice daily for 7–10 days
	Ciprofloxacin	500 mg	Twice daily for 7–10 days
	Ofloxacin	300 mg	Twice daily for 7–10 days
Uncomplicated cystitis in pregnancy	Amoxicillin	250–500 mg	Three times daily for 7–10 days
	Nitrofurantoin	50–100 mg	Four times daily for 7–10 days
	Cefpodoxime	100 mg	Twice daily for 7–10 days
Asymptomatic bacteriuria in pregnancy	Nitrofurantoin	50–100 mg	Four times daily for 3 days
	Cefpodoxime	100 mg	Twice daily for 3 days

    b. Complicated cases. In patients with complicating medical conditions, a longer duration of symptoms, or a relapse of infection, 7–10 days of therapy with **oral trimethoprim–sulfamethoxazole** or a **fluoroquinolone** is required.

    c. Pregnant patients. Uncomplicated cystitis and asymptomatic bacteriuria in pregnant women can be treated with **oral amoxicillin, nitrofurantoin, or cefpodoxime.**

2. Pyelonephritis

    a. Outpatient treatment. Mild cases of upper tract infection in young, otherwise healthy patients may be treated on an outpatient basis following an initial dose of intravenous antibiotics, hydration, and a short observation period.

        (1) **Parenteral antibiotics** should be given prior to discharge. **Ceftriaxone** (1–2 g), **gentamicin** (1.0 mg/kg) **with ampicillin** (1–2 g), or **trimethoprim–sulfamethoxazole** (160/800 mg) may be used.

        (2) **Oral antibiotics.** A 10- to 14-day course of **trimethoprim–sulfamethoxazole** (160/800 mg, twice daily by mouth) or a **fluoroquinolone** (e.g., ciprofloxacin, 500 mg twice daily) is required.

    b. Inpatient management entails the intravenous administration of the same **antibiotics noted in I E 2 a (1),** aztreonam (0.5–2 g two to four times daily), **imipenem** (600 mg three to four times daily), or **ciprofloxacin** (200–400 mg intravenously twice daily).

F Disposition

1. Admission to the hospital is indicated for the following patients:

    a. Those with clinical toxicity (e.g., fever, vomiting)

    b. Those who are unable to tolerate oral medications or fluids

    c. Those with known anatomic abnormalities that predispose to the development of UTIs

    d. Elderly, pregnant, or very young patients with pyelonephritis or suspected urosepsis

2. Discharge. Most patients are treated as outpatients. Prior to discharge, patients should be advised regarding the prevention of UTIs. Commonly accepted means of preventing UTIs include:

    a. Practicing postcoital voiding

    b. Urinating frequently and completely

    c. Increasing fluid intake

    d. Practicing local hygiene (including wiping from front to back)

II NEPHROLITHIASIS

A Discussion

1. Types of renal calculi (stones)

    a. Calcium oxalate and **calcium phosphate** stones account for 70%–80% of all renal calculi.

    b. Struvite (magnesium–ammonium phosphate) stones account for 10%–15% of all renal calculi.

    c. Uric acid stones account for 5%–10% of all renal calculi.

    d. Cystine and **xanthine** stones account for a small number of renal calculi.

2. Sites of calculus obstruction

    a. Ureteropelvic junction

    b. Pelvic brim. The ureter crosses the iliac vessels and narrows to 4 mm in diameter at the pelvic brim.

    c. Ureterovesical junction. At the ureterovesical junction, the most common site of obstruction, the ureter narrows to 1–5 mm in diameter.

    d. Renal pelvis. Struvite stones commonly form large **staghorn calculi,** which are too large to enter the ureter and, instead, fill the renal pelvis.

3. **Predisposing factors**
    a. **Certain clinical conditions** may predispose to stone formation (e.g., inflammatory bowel disease, immobilization, gout, hyperparathyroidism). Struvite stones are associated with **chronic infection** of the urinary tract by **urea-splitting bacteria** (e.g., *Proteus, Pseudomonas, Klebsiella*).
    b. **Dietary conditions.** Excess dietary oxalate, vitamin C abuse, or excess dietary purine can predispose the patient to the development of renal calculi.
    c. **Medications**
        (1) **Acetazolamide, antacids,** and **ascorbic acid** may predispose to the development of calcium stones.
        (2) **Hydrochlorothiazide** therapy can lead to the development of uric acid stones.
        (3) **Allopurinol** therapy has been associated with the development of xanthine stones.

B **Clinical features**

1. **Symptoms**
    a. **Pain.** The sudden onset of **acute, severe, intermittent, colicky pain** is most commonly observed. Intense episodes are followed by asymptomatic periods. The pain is located in the **flank** or **abdominal area** and radiates to the corresponding testicle or labia. The patient is in obvious distress and is unable to find a comfortable position.
    b. **Nausea, vomiting,** and **diaphoresis** are commonly present.

2. **Physical examination findings**
    a. **Tachycardia, tachypnea,** and **hypertension** are commonly observed secondary to pain.
    b. **Costovertebral angle tenderness** and **abdominal tenderness** without peritoneal findings are often present.
    c. **Fever** may be present if there is concomitant infection.

C **Differential diagnoses** include appendicitis, cholecystitis, diverticulitis, salpingitis, pelvic inflammatory disease (PID), tubo-ovarian abscess, ovarian cyst or torsion, ectopic pregnancy, abdominal aortic aneurysm, and pyelonephritis.

D **Evaluation**

1. **Laboratory studies**
    a. **Urinalysis**
        (1) **Hematuria** is usually present.
        (2) **Urinary leukocytes.** If leukocytes are found in the urine, a urine culture must be performed.
        (3) **Urinary crystals** may help identify the stone type.
        (4) **Urine pH.** A urine pH greater than 7.6 may indicate the presence of a UTI caused by urea-splitting bacteria, which may suggest that struvite calculi have formed.
    b. **CBC.** A CBC may reveal leukocytosis stemming from pain or infection.

2. **Radiographs.** A kidney-ureter-bladder (KUB) view should be obtained. Ninety percent of renal stones (calcium, struvite, and cystine stones) are radiopaque on a supine plain film of the abdomen.

3. **Intravenous pyelography (IVP),** which gives an indication of renal function and may reveal the stone location and size, is currently the test of choice for diagnosing renal calculi. Prior to performing IVP, blood urea nitrogen (BUN) and creatine levels should be obtained, and dye allergies and pregnancy should be ruled out.

4. **Computed tomography (CT).** A spiral CT with a new-generation scanner may prove useful in diagnosis of urolithiasis and in ruling out associated hydronephrosis. Tomography may also be required to identify or localize the calculus.

5. **Ultrasound** is useful in pregnant patients and those with a dye allergy, but is less sensitive for diagnosing stones smaller than 5 mm in diameter.

E Therapy

1. **Parenteral analgesia** with **narcotics** or a **nonsteroidal anti-inflammatory drug (NSAID)** is required. Physicians should be aware of patients in search of narcotics. These patients often have a history of renal stones, report an allergy to contrast dye (so that objective testing is impossible), and claim an allergy to all nonnarcotic analgesics.

2. **Antibiotic therapy.** Intravenous antibiotics are warranted if infection is present.

3. **Intravenous hydration** with an isotonic fluid (e.g., normal saline or lactated Ringer's solution) is necessary to compensate for the diuresis that occurs following relief of obstruction.

4. **Antiemetics** may be needed.

F Disposition

1. **Admission**
   a. Patients with **uncontrolled pain, persistent emesis,** or **concomitant infection** should be admitted to the hospital.
   b. Patients who have only **one kidney** should be admitted.
   c. Patients with **large** or **proximal stones** may require admittance to the hospital.
      (1) **Stone size**
         (a) 90% pass if less than 4 mm
         (b) 50% pass if 4–6 mm
         (c) 10% pass if greater than 6 mm
      (2) **Stone location.** The more proximal the stone is, the less likely it is that the stone will pass.

2. **Discharge.** Patients should be discharged with a prescription for an oral analgesic (e.g., acetaminophen with codeine) and instructions to strain the urine in an effort to recover passed stones for analysis. They should be advised to follow up with a urologist or primary care physician within 5 days and to return to the ED if symptoms of increased pain, vomiting, or fever occur. The recurrence rate is 30% within 1 year and 60% within 7 years without treatment of the underlying disorder.

III URINARY RETENTION

Urinary retention is the inability to void, resulting in bladder distention.

A Obstructive

1. **Causes**
   a. **Prostate enlargement.** Urinary retention in adult men is often due to an enlarged prostate gland. **Benign prostatic hypertrophy (BPH)** is the most common cause, followed by **prostatitis** and **prostate cancer.**
   b. **Urethral strictures** (see VI A 8)
   c. **Urethral foreign bodies** (see VI A 7)
   d. **Paraphimosis** and **phimosis** (see VI A 1–2)

2. **Clinical features**
   a. **Symptoms.** Urinary symptoms include **hesitancy, frequency, nocturia, urgency,** and a decrease in the amount and force of the urine stream, resulting in **"dribbling."**
   b. **Physical examination findings** include increased pain to suprapubic palpation and dullness to percussion over the distended fluid-filled bladder.

3. **Differential diagnoses** include neurogenic causes, drug-induced retention, urinary retention secondary to pain, psychogenic causes, renal failure, abdominal aortic aneurysm, bowel obstruction, and a gravid uterus.

4. **Evaluation**
   a. **Physical examination** readily identifies an obstructive etiology. A rectal examination should be performed to search for prostatic enlargement (a sign of BPH) or nodularity (a sign of cancer).
   b. **Urinary catheterization.** A postvoid residual of more than 300 mL of urine confirms the diagnosis.
   c. **Laboratory studies**
      (1) **Urinalysis** should be performed to rule out infection.
      (2) **Renal** and **electrolyte panel.** BUN, creatinine, and electrolyte levels should be assessed to rule out renal insufficiency.

5. **Therapy**
   a. **Acute relief.** Catheterization with a 16-French Foley catheter or a 16-French coudé catheter should provide acute relief.
   b. **Definitive therapy.** The source of the obstruction should be treated. Suprapubic cystostomy or filiforms with followers, performed by a urologic surgeon, may be necessary.

6. **Disposition.** Most patients with a mechanical obstruction may be discharged home with an indwelling catheter and a leg bag. Follow-up with a urologist should be arranged prior to discharge.

B **Neurologic**

1. **Causes.** Urinary retention may occur secondary to spinal cord trauma or compression, neuropathy (e.g., multiple sclerosis, diabetes mellitus, Guillain-Barré syndrome, tabes dorsalis), or viral infection.

2. **Clinical features**
   a. **Spinal cord injury** or **spinal shock**
      (1) **Areflexia (atonic) bladder** is seen with spinal pathology at or below the second lumbar vertebra.
      (2) **Reflex (hypertonic) bladder** is seen with pathology above the second lumbar vertebra.
   b. **Spinal cord compression.** Back pain, gait disturbance, and hyperreflexia accompanying urinary retention may be indicative of spinal cord compression (e.g., by a tumor, herniated disk, or abscess).
   c. **Other neurologic disorders** have characteristic associated motor, sensory, and reflex findings.

3. **Differential diagnoses** are the same as those for obstructive retention.

4. **Evaluation.** A CT scan or magnetic resonance imaging (MRI) scan should be obtained to evaluate spinal cord trauma, spinal shock, or suspected compressive etiologies.

5. **Therapy**
   a. **Acute relief**
      (1) **Atonic bladder** may be relieved with **self-catheterization** or **urecholine therapy.**
      (2) **Hypertonic bladder** may be relieved with **self-catheterization** or **flavoxate or oxybutynin therapy.**
   b. **Definitive therapy** depends on the underlying cause. Consultation with a specialist (e.g., a neurosurgeon, orthopedic surgeon, or neurologist) may be necessary.

C **Pharmacologic**

1. **Causes** include **antihistamines, antidepressants,** and **α-adrenergic medications,** including over-the-counter preparations.

2. **Differential diagnoses** include urethral obstruction, neurogenic retention, urinary retention secondary to pain, psychogenic causes, renal failure, abdominal aortic aneurysm, bowel obstruction, and a gravid uterus.

3. **Evaluation**

      a. Patient history. A thorough patient history, including recently prescribed medications, suggests the etiology.

      b. Physical examination should rule out other causes.

  4. Therapy. Catheterization will provide acute relief. The offending medication should be discontinued following consultation with the patient's primary care physician.

IV   RENAL FAILURE

A **Acute renal failure** is a sudden decline in renal function resulting in azotemia with an accumulation of nitrogenous waste products (creatinine and urea) over hours to weeks. Acute renal failure causes derangements in electrolyte, volume, and metabolic status. Patients in acute renal failure may be either **oliguric** (i.e., producing less than 500 mL urine/day) or **nonoliguric** (i.e., producing more than 500 mL urine/day). **Anuria** is defined as the production of less than 100 mL urine/day.

  1. Causes. There are three general mechanisms of acute renal failure.

    a. Prerenal causes. Acute renal failure results from **hypoperfusion of the renal parenchyma.**

      (1) True intravascular volume depletion (e.g., from hemorrhage, severe dehydration, or overzealous diuresis) can lead to acute renal failure.

      (2) Peripheral vascular changes leading to vasodilatation or **a decreased cardiac output** may result from cardiac pump failure, sepsis, or anaphylaxis, leading to acute renal failure.

    b. Renal (intrinsic) causes involve direct injury to the renal parenchyma.

      (1) Tubule injury [e.g., from acute tubular necrosis (ATN)] is the most common cause of acute renal failure in adults. ATN can occur secondary to ischemia, toxins (e.g., intravenous contrast dye or aminoglycoside antibiotics), or rhabdomyolysis; fortunately, in many cases, the damage is reversible.

      (2) Interstitial injury (e.g., from acute interstitial nephritis) is most often caused by an adverse drug reaction and is often associated with systemic manifestations, such as fever, rash, and joint pain.

      (3) Glomerular injury (e.g., from glomerulonephritis) is also an intrinsic cause of acute renal failure.

    c. Postrenal causes (i.e., obstructive nephropathy) must be bilateral in order to induce renal failure (unless the patient has only one kidney). The obstruction may be intrinsic or extrinsic in origin, and located anywhere along the urinary tract from the urinary meatus to the renal collecting system.

  2. Clinical features. No specific constellation of symptoms is typical of acute renal failure.

    a. Patients may be asymptomatic or have complaints of fatigue, weakness, or shortness of breath.

    b. Sometimes, patients present with complaints related to secondarily involved organ systems.

      (1) Central nervous system (CNS) symptoms include **confusion, a diminished level of consciousness,** and **altered mental status.**

      (2) Cardiovascular symptoms include **symptoms associated with congestive heart failure (CHF) or pulmonary edema** secondary to volume overload, **hypertension,** and **arrhythmias** secondary to hyperkalemia.

      (3) Hematologic symptoms. Anemia may be seen, but is more common in chronic renal failure.

      (4) Metabolic symptoms include **acidosis** and **uremia.**

  3. Differential diagnoses include chronic renal failure (see IV B).

  4. Evaluation

    a. Patient history and physical examination. A thorough history and physical examination may offer insight into the cause of the acute renal failure (e.g., dehydration, drug toxicity), as well as reveal any associated sequelae (e.g., CHF, ascites, edema, altered mental status).

b. Laboratory studies

    (1) Hematologic analysis should include:

        (a) A **CBC** (anemia is more commonly associated with chronic renal failure)

        (b) An **electrolyte panel** (to screen for acidosis and hyperkalemia)

        (c) BUN and **creatinine levels** (to assess renal function)

        (d) Glucose, calcium, and **phosphorus levels**

    (2) Urinalysis findings are summarized in Table 5–2.

c. Electrocardiography. An electrocardiogram (ECG) is appropriate if hyperkalemia is present.

5. Therapy

  a. Emergent therapy. Potentially life-threatening complications (e.g., hyperkalemia, hypertensive crisis) should be treated accordingly. **Dialysis,** performed under the supervision of a nephrologist, is warranted for patients with acidosis, hyperkalemia, volume overload, or uremia.

  b. Definitive therapy. The cause of the acute renal failure should be treated accordingly.

    (1) Prenal causes

        (a) Intravascular volume levels should be restored by administering **isotonic fluids.**

        (b) The cause of the intravascular volume depletion should be treated.

        (c) Low-dose dopamine (1–3 µg/kg/min) enhances renal blood flow and should be considered in this setting.

    (2) Renal causes

        (a) Although of unproven value, consideration must be given to the use of **diuretic agents** (furosemide and mannitol) with **low-dose dopamine** to enhance urine output. Mannitol may lead to volume overload in an anuric patient and should not be used in this setting.

        (b) If the patient has rhabdomyolysis, aggressive **saline diuresis** with **alkalinization of the urine** to attain a pH greater than 6.5 should be instituted.

    (3) Postrenal causes. Elimination of the obstruction with a Foley catheter (for outlet obstruction) or with urethral stents (for urethral blockage) may be required. Consultation with a urologist may be advisable.

B **Chronic renal failure** is defined as a reduction of renal function [as measured by the glomerular filtration rate (GFR)] over months to years to less than 20% of normal.

  1. Causes include diabetes mellitus, hypertension, glomerulonephritis, and hereditary disease.

  2. Clinical features

TABLE 5–2   Urinalysis Findings in Patients with Acute Renal Failure

	Prerenal Cause	Renal (Intrinsic) Cause	Postrenal Cause
Microscopic analysis	Unremarkable	Granular, hyaline, and cellular casts; red blood cell casts; proteinuria	Unremarkable
Urine sodium	<40 mEq/L	>40 mEq/L	Nondiagnostic
Urine specific gravity	>1.020	<1.010	<1.010
Urine osmolality	>500 mOsm/kg H_2O	<300 mOsm/kg H_2O	Nondiagnostic
Urine creatinine:serum creatinine ratio	>40:1	<20:1	<20:1
Serum urea nitrogen:serum creatinine ratio	>20:1	≈10:1	<10:1
Fractional excretion of sodium (FENa)*	<1%	>2%	>2%

$$*FENa = \frac{Urine\ Na/Serum\ Na}{Urine\ Cr/Serum\ Cr} \times 100$$

a. **CNS symptoms** include **fatigue, lethargy, seizures, coma,** and **dementia.**

b. **Cardiopulmonary symptoms** are **those of CHF, pulmonary edema, pericarditis,** and **hypertension.**

c. **Gastrointestinal symptoms** include **nausea, vomiting, anorexia,** and **symptoms of peptic ulcer disease.**

d. **Neuromuscular symptoms** include **peripheral neuropathy, myoclonus,** and **asterixis.**

e. **Dermatologic symptoms** include **pallor** (secondary to anemia) and **pruritus.**

f. **Hematologic symptoms** include **those of normocytic normochromic anemia** and **defective hemostasis.**

g. **Metabolic symptoms** include **hyperkalemia, hyperphosphatemia, hypocalcemia (osteodystrophy), metabolic acidosis, hyperuricemia, hyperamylasemia,** and **hypertriglyceridemia.**

3. **Differential diagnoses** include acute renal failure. The following clues, in addition to a thorough review of the patient's medical records and family history, may help to differentiate the two:

a. Long-standing anemia is seen more often with chronic renal failure.

b. The associated metabolic and electrolyte disturbances of renal failure are less clinically dramatic in patients with chronic renal failure.

c. The finding of small kidneys on a KUB radiograph, ultrasound, or CT scan is more consistent with chronic renal failure.

4. **Therapy.** Chronic renal failure is treated with **dialysis** (hemodialysis or peritoneal dialysis) or **renal transplantation.**

V GENITAL LESIONS (Table 5–3)

A Primary syphilis

1. **Cause.** Syphilis is caused by *Treponema pallidum* infection.

2. **Clinical features**

a. **Lesion.** The typical lesion of primary syphilis is called a **chancre,** which forms at the site of inoculation (e.g., the genitalia, anus, rectum, mouth, or perioral region). The painless

---

TABLE 5–3 Summary of Genital Lesions

	Lesion	Lymphadenopathy	Average Incubation	Typical Patient Profile
Primary syphilis	Painless ulcer (chancre)	Regional, painless	21 days (10–90 days)	Man, 20–39 years of age
Genital herpes	Painful vesicles and ulcerations	Unilateral, tender	6 days (2–20 days)	Young, sexually active adult
Chancroid	Painful ulcer	Buboes	4–7 days	Young men
Lymphogranuloma venereum (LGV)	Painless ulcer	Suppurative, painful buboes	Primary stage: 3–12 days Secondary stage: 10–30 days	Man or woman, 20–30 years of age
Condylomata acuminatum	Filiform, sessile, or cauliflower-like masses	None	Weeks to years	Young, sexually active adult
Molluscum contagiosum	Umbilicated papules	None	2–3 months	Child or adult
Pediculosis pubis	Brown or white specks	Associated with secondary infection of excoriations	Life span ≅20 days	Young adult

papular lesion erodes to form an ulcer with a raised border, serous exudate, and a crusted surface.

    b. **Regional lymphadenopathy** may be present.

3. **Differential diagnoses** include herpes simplex virus-type 1 (HSV-1) infection, chancroid, lymphogranuloma venereum (LGV), traumatic ulcer, furuncle, and carcinoma.

4. **Evaluation.** The clinical diagnosis can be confirmed by **darkfield microscopic examination** or **serologic testing** [e.g., the Venereal Disease Research Laboratory (VDRL) test for screening and the fluorescent treponemal antibody-absorbed (FTA-ABS) test for confirmation].

5. **Therapy.** Primary syphilis can be treated with any of the following antibiotic regimens:
    a. **Benzathine penicillin G** (one dose of 2.4 million U administered intramuscularly)
    b. **Doxycycline** (100 mg twice daily for 2 weeks administered orally)
    c. **Tetracycline** or **erythromycin** (500 mg four times daily for 2 weeks administered orally)
    d. **Ceftriaxone** (250 mg for 10 days administered intramuscularly)

6. **Disposition.** The patient should follow up with a physician in 1 month for serologic confirmation of cure.

B **Genital herpes**

1. **Cause.** Genital herpes is caused primarily by **herpes simplex virus-type 2 (HSV-2).**

2. **Clinical features**
    a. **Lesion.** Genital herpes is characterized by **painful, recurrent, ulcerated lesions** on the genitalia, perineum, thigh, sacrum, buttocks, anus, or rectum. The lesions begin as erythematous papules that develop into groups of vesicles in a herpetiform arrangement. These vesicles become pustules, which erode to form ulcerations with a moist or crusted appearance.
    b. **Lymphadenopathy.** The lesions are usually accompanied by **tender inguinal** or **femoral lymphadenopathy** that is usually **unilateral.**

3. **Differential diagnoses** include syphilis, chancroid, and gonococcal erosions.

4. **Evaluation**
    a. **Tzanck smear.** A Tzanck smear is positive in 75% of cases.
    b. **Viral culture** confirms the diagnosis in 1–10 days.
    c. **Serologic evaluation** can detect the presence of antibodies to HSV-1 or HSV-2.

5. **Therapy** is indicated for patients with severe disease and for immunocompromised patients. Sexual contacts should be notified and treated as well.
    a. In most patients, **acyclovir** is administered orally to treat outbreaks and prevent recurrence.
        (1) Acyclovir (400 mg three times daily) is administered for 10 days to treat the first outbreak.
        (2) For recurrent episodes, patients begin treatment with acyclovir (400 mg three times daily for 5 days) at the beginning of the prodrome or within 2 days of the onset.
        (3) Acyclovir, 400 mg three times daily, is administered to prevent recurrence of disease.
    b. In HIV-infected patients, **acyclovir** or **foscarnet** may be administered intravenously to treat genital herpes.

6. **Disposition.** Patients who are being treated with acyclovir should schedule follow-up appointments with their primary care physicians. Patients should be advised to avoid sexual contact when ulcerations are present.

C **Chancroid**

1. **Causes.** Chancroid is caused by *Haemophilus ducreyi* infection and is endemic in tropical and subtropical Third World countries.

2. **Clinical features**

a. **Lesion.** The characteristic lesion is a tender papule with an erythematous border that evolves from a pustule to an erosion and, eventually, to an ulcer with a friable base, granulation tissue, and exudate. Lesions are typically found on the genitalia, breasts, fingers, thighs, or oral mucosa.

b. **Lymphadenopathy.** Chancroid is characterized by a **suppurative regional lymphadenopathy (bubo).**

3. **Differential diagnoses** include genital herpes, syphilis, LGV, and traumatic lesions.

4. **Evaluation.** Scrapings from the ulcer base or pus from a bubo will reveal clusters or parallel chains of Gram-negative rods. Culture of *H. ducreyi* is difficult, and no serologic tests are available.

5. **Therapy.** Appropriate antibiotic regimens include the following:
    a. **Erythromycin,** 500 mg orally four times daily for 7 days
    b. **Ceftriaxone,** one 250-mg intramuscular dose
    c. **Azithromycin,** one 1.0-g dose administered orally
    d. **Amoxicillin,** 500 mg, **plus clavulanic acid,** 125 mg, orally three times daily for 7 days
    e. **Ciprofloxacin,** 500 mg orally twice daily for 3 days

6. **Disposition.** Patients should be treated as outpatients. A follow-up appointment 1 week later with a primary care physician should be scheduled.

D **LGV**

1. **Cause.** LGV is caused by **C. trachomatis, immunotypes** L^1, L^2, and L^3, and is endemic in East and West Africa, India, South America, and the Caribbean.

2. **Clinical features.** LGV is characterized by painless genital lesions and a suppurative, diffuse, painful lymphadenopathy.
    a. **Primary stage.** Any of the following types of lesions may be present on the genitalia or in the vagina or urethra during the primary stage: papules, shallow erosions, ulcers, or a herpetiform arrangement of lesions with a lymphangial nodule (bubonulus) that may rupture, causing deforming scars.
    b. **Secondary stage**
        (1) **Inguinal syndrome.** The inguinal syndrome is characterized by **unilateral buboes** (one third of which rupture) and the **groove sign** (i.e., the depression made by Poupart's ligament that separates inflamed femoral and inguinal nodes).
        (2) **Anogenitorectal syndrome** is characterized by proctocolitis that leads to perirectal abscesses, ischiorectal and rectovaginal fistulas, anal fistulas, and rectal strictures.

3. **Differential diagnoses** include genital herpes, primary syphilis, and chancroid.

4. **Evaluation**
    a. **Serologic studies.** *C. trachomatis* can be identified using a **complement-fixation test.**
    b. **Histologic identification** of *C. trachomatis* in a biopsy sample is also possible.
    c. **Culture** on tissue-culture cell lines is positive in approximately 30% of cases.

5. **Therapy.** The following regimens are appropriate for the treatment of LGV:
    a. **Doxycycline,** 100 mg orally, twice daily for 21 days
    b. **Erythromycin** or **sulfisoxazole,** 500 mg orally, four times daily for 21 days

6. **Disposition.** The patient should be reevaluated at the end of the antibiotic course.

E **Condylomata acuminatum (genital warts)**

1. **Cause.** Genital warts are sexually and nonsexually transmitted by skin-to-skin contact. The pathogen is **human papilloma virus (HPV).**
    a. Types 6 and 11 are the most common "low-risk" oncogenic types of HPV.
    b. Types 16, 18, 31, and 33 are the major causes of dysplasia and carcinoma of the cervix, vulva, penis, and anus.

2. **Clinical features**
   a. **Lesions** develop from papules to filiform, sessile, or cauliflower-like masses, usually located in clusters on the genitalia, perineum, urethra, anus, rectum, or perioral or perianal regions. The lesions are painless.
   b. **Lymphadenopathy.** No significant lymphadenopathy is associated with condylomata acuminatum.
3. **Differential diagnoses** include molluscum contagiosum, folliculitis, skin tags, and cancer.
4. **Evaluation.** Diagnosis is confirmed by biopsy, but is suggested by whitening of the lesions when 5% acetic acid is applied for 5 minutes.
5. **Therapy.** Methods of wart removal include:
   a. Cryosurgery with **liquid nitrogen**
   b. Topical application of **podophyllin** (10%–25%) in compound tincture of benzoin or **trichloroacetic acid** (80%–90%)
   c. **Electrodesiccation, electrocautery,** or **laser surgery**
6. **Disposition.** The patient should be warned that the lesions are highly contagious and advised to follow up with a primary care physician for long-term treatment.

F **Molluscum contagiosum**

1. **Causes.** Molluscum contagiosum is a sexually and nonsexually transmitted disease caused by **poxvirus.**
2. **Clinical features.** The lesions are painless, well-defined, umbilicated, pearly white papules (1–10 mm in diameter) on the neck, trunk, genitalia, or eyelids.
   a. HIV-positive patients are more likely to have multiple lesions.
   b. The lesions may be pruritic if they are secondarily infected.
3. **Differential diagnoses** include **keratoacanthoma** and **basal cell carcinoma.**
4. **Evaluation.** Microscopic examination of a **Giemsa-stained central core biopsy specimen** reveals "molluscum bodies." If sexual abuse is suspected, serotyping may be performed.
5. **Therapy.** Spontaneous remission occurs in the majority of cases. Curettage, topical application of liquid nitrogen, or electrocautery may be employed if spontaneous remission does not occur.
6. **Disposition.** The patient should be discharged if there are no risk factors for HIV and the patient desires no further treatment.

G **Pediculosis pubis (phthiriasis, pubic lice, crabs)**

1. **Causes.** The pathogenic organism is the pubic louse, *Phthirus pubis.* Transmission is through close physical contact.
2. **Clinical features**
   a. **Lesions.** The lice appear to be brown specks, 1–2 mm in diameter. The eggs (nits) appear to be white specks attached to the hair. The area is pruritic.
   b. **Lymphadenopathy.** Secondary infection of excoriations may be associated with regional lymphadenopathy.
3. **Differential diagnoses** include eczema, tinea, and folliculitis.
4. **Evaluation.** Diagnosis is based on clinical assessment.
5. **Therapy**
   a. **Permethrin (1%) rinse** or **0.5% malathion** is applied topically.
      (1) Shaving hair in the affected area may help.
      (2) Treatment of contacts is mandatory.
   b. **Antibiotics** may be indicated for infected excoriations.

6. **Disposition.** Patients should be reevaluated in 1 week if symptoms persist because retreatment may be necessary.

VI MALE UROGENITAL PROBLEMS

A **Disorders affecting the penis**

1. **Phimosis,** the inability to retract the foreskin proximally over the glans, rarely brings patients to the ED.
   a. **Cause.** Phimosis may occur secondary to chronic infection or as a consequence of poor hygiene.
   b. **Clinical features.** Patients may present with poor hygiene, painful erections, or urinary retention. If infection (balanoposthitis) is present, prepuce tenderness with associated erythema, edema, and purulent drainage may be seen.
   c. **Therapy.** Consultation with a urologist is advisable. Phimosis is usually treated surgically (e.g., by making an operative dorsal slit or circumcising the patient).

2. **Paraphimosis** results when the foreskin is retracted proximal to the coronal sulcus of the glans and cannot be reduced distally.
   a. **Clinical features.** The retracted foreskin becomes edematous leading to edema of the glans. Eventually, necrosis of the glans occurs when the venous congestion progresses to arterial compromise.
   b. **Therapy.** Applying pressure to the glans for 5 minutes may reduce the tissue edema, allowing reduction of the foreskin. If applying pressure is unsuccessful, making a dorsal slit following local infiltration with 1% lidocaine will allow for decompression of the glans and foreskin reduction.

3. **Balanoposthitis** is inflammation of the glans (balanitis) and of the foreskin (posthitis).
   a. **Cause.** If the condition is recurrent, diabetes mellitus should be excluded as the cause.
   b. **Clinical features.** The foreskin and glans appear erythematous and are tender. A malodorous, purulent exudate is present.
   c. **Therapy** entails practicing local hygiene with soap and water and applying a topical antifungal cream. If bacterial infection is present, a broad-spectrum antibiotic should be prescribed.

4. **Penile fracture** is disruption of the tunica albuginea of the penis.
   a. **Clinical features.** The patient usually describes experiencing a sudden, acute pain in the penis during sexual intercourse that is accompanied by a "cracking" sound. The penis is swollen and tender to palpation.
   b. **Evaluation.** A retrograde urethrogram using 15–20 mL of water-soluble contrast material should be obtained to rule out urethral injury.
   c. **Therapy.** Immediate urologic consultation should be obtained for penile hematoma evacuation and repair of the tunica albuginea.

5. **Constriction**
   a. **Causes**
      (1) **Constrictive penile bands** are used to prolong erections. Progressive edema may develop, preventing easy removal.
      (2) **Human hair** may accidentally encircle the coronal sulcus in circumcised young boys.
   b. **Clinical features.** Constriction may lead to local tissue damage, urethral injury, and venous and arterial blood supply interruption with eventual tissue necrosis.
   c. **Evaluation.** A retrograde urethrogram should be obtained if urethral injury is suspected.
   d. **Therapy.** Local anesthesia with 1% lidocaine without epinephrine may be required to remove the offending object. Metal cutters or a ring removal saw may be needed to remove metal constricting bands. Urologic consultation is required with evidence of tissue necrosis or urethral injury.

6. **Zipper entrapment.** Local anesthesia is all that is usually required to allow the zipper to be unzipped. Intravenous conscious sedation (e.g., with midazolam 0.1 mg/kg to a maximum dose of 2 mg) may be beneficial in children.

7. **Urethral foreign bodies.** Patients of all ages may have various objects placed into the urethra. The placement of foreign objects in the urethra may be related to curiosity or sexual experimentation, but an abusive situation should also be considered.
   a. **Clinical features.** Patients may present with penile pain associated with dysuria and hematuria.
   b. **Evaluation**
      (1) **Physical examination.** A physical examination, including a **rectal examination,** should be carried out.
      (2) **Laboratory studies. Urinalysis** and **urine culture** should be performed.
      (3) **Radiographs.** Views of the **penis** and **KUB** views should be obtained.
   c. **Therapy.** Immediate urologic referral for foreign body removal is required, followed by retrograde urethrography or endoscopy.

8. **Urethral stricture**
   a. **Causes.** Urethral stricture occurs secondary to **trauma** (including instrumentation) and **sexually transmitted infections** (e.g., gonococcal and chlamydial infections).
   b. **Clinical features.** Patients may present with urinary retention, difficulty initiating the urinary stream, voiding in small amounts, and a sensation of incomplete voiding.
   c. **Differential diagnoses** include BPH, prostate cancer, foreign body obstruction, and bladder stones.
   d. **Evaluation**
      (1) **Retrograde urethrography** or **urethrocystoscopy** should be performed by a urologist to determine the cause of the stricture.
      (2) **Laboratory studies. Urinalysis** and **urine culture** may identify the cause.
   e. **Therapy.** If the patient is unable to void or has significant urinary retention (as evidenced by a postvoid residual of more than 300 mL of urine), he or she must be catheterized. Consultation with a urologist prior to discharge is required.

9. **Priapism** is a painful, prolonged penile erection without accompanying sexual desire.
   a. **Causes**
      (1) **Medications** (e.g., trazodone, phenothiazine)
      (2) **Spinal cord injury**
      (3) **Hematologic disorders** (e.g., sickle cell disease, leukemia)
      (4) **Iatrogenic causes** (e.g., papaverine injection for impotence)
      (5) **Idiopathic causes**
   b. **Clinical features.** Patients present with a history of a painful erection that has lasted for several hours. The corpus cavernosum is firm and tender to palpation. The glans and corpus spongiosum are soft and uninvolved.
   c. **Evaluation**
      (1) **Patient history.** A complete history is necessary to identify the possible etiology.
      (2) **Laboratory studies.** A **CBC** and **sickle cell preparation** should be obtained.
   d. **Therapy.** Consultation with a urologist is necessary.
      (1) **Acute therapy** entails the subcutaneous administration of **terbutaline** (0.25–0.5 mg) every 4–6 hours.
      (2) **Definitive therapy**
         (a) **Identifiable causes** should be treated accordingly. For example, iatrogenic causes respond to corpus cavernosum blood aspiration followed by the intracorporeal injection of an α-adrenergic agent.
         (b) **Surgical treatment. Shunting** between the corpus cavernosum and the glans or corpus spongiosum or dorsal vein may be required.

B **Disorders affecting the testicles and epididymis**

1. **Testicular torsion** occurs most commonly during the second decade of life.

a. **Cause.** Testicular torsion occurs when the tunica vaginalis envelops the testis and attaches above the epididymis, rather than attaching at the posterior aspect of the testis. The anatomic defect (referred to as "bell-clapper deformity") is bilateral and allows the testicle to rotate within the tunica vaginalis.

b. **Clinical features**

(1) **Symptoms.** The patient reports the acute onset of **severe testicular pain** that **may radiate to the abdomen. Nausea** and **vomiting** are common.

(2) **Physical examination findings**

(a) The involved testicle is high-riding, may be positioned horizontally, and is markedly tender to palpation. The overlying scrotum is erythematous and edematous.

(b) Elevation of the scrotum to the symphysis does not relieve the pain (i.e., Prehn's sign is absent). The cremasteric reflex is often absent as well.

c. **Differential diagnoses** include acute epididymitis, orchitis, appendicitis, testicular or epididymal appendix torsion, hernia, tumor, and hydrocele.

d. **Evaluation**

(1) **Laboratory studies.** A **CBC** may reveal leukocytosis. Pyuria is absent on **urinalysis.**

(2) **Radionuclide scanning** with **technetium-99m pertechnetate** is the test of choice but may not be readily available.

(3) **Doppler ultrasound** examination is rapid and should be arranged as soon as possible.

e. **Therapy.** A urologist should be consulted immediately. **Manual** or **surgical detorsion** must occur within 4–6 hours; treatment should not be delayed to await ancillary test results.

(1) **Sedation and analgesia.** Sedation, provided by the intravenous administration of midazolam (2 mg), and analgesia, provided by the intravenous administration of meperidine (50–75 mg) and promethazine hydrochloride (25–50 mg) or fentanyl (1–4 μg/kg), is necessary. Spermatic cord blocks, accomplished by the administration of 10 mL of 1% lidocaine high in the scrotum, may prove beneficial, although the use of a spermatic cord block eliminates the endpoint of pain relief with detorsion.

(2) **Reduction.** Initial attempts at reduction should be toward the ipsilateral thigh because the torsion usually occurs toward the midline (i.e., the patient's left testicle should be rotated clockwise and the patient's right testicle counterclockwise as the physician faces the patient).

(3) **Bilateral orchiopexy** is necessary to prevent recurrence.

2. **Testicular** or **epididymal appendage torsion** occurs most commonly in prepubescent boys.

a. **Clinical features.** The patient complains of the **sudden onset of pain** near the location of the appendage (e.g., at the head of the epididymis or the superior pole of the testicle). A **"blue dot" sign** is seen as the engorged, cyanotic appendage approaches the overlying scrotal skin.

b. **Differential diagnoses** include testicular torsion, epididymitis, orchitis, and testicular trauma.

c. **Evaluation.** Often the diagnosis is clear following physical examination. Doppler ultrasound may be helpful. If the diagnosis is still uncertain, urologic surgical exploration may be required.

d. **Therapy.** Symptomatic relief is provided with oral analgesics. Some urologists may consider excision.

e. **Disposition.** Following discharge from the ED, patients should see a urologist or primary care physician within 1 week.

3. **Acute epididymitis**

a. **Causes**

(1) **Sexually transmitted epididymitis** is often associated with urethritis. The most common causative organisms include *C. trachomatis* and *N. gonorrhoeae.*

(2) **Non–sexually transmitted epididymitis** is often associated with prostatitis or UTI. The most common causative organisms are *E. coli, Pseudomonas,* and *Klebsiella.*

b. **Clinical features**
  (1) **Symptoms.** Patients report the gradual onset of **scrotal pain** that becomes progressively more severe. The pain may radiate along the spermatic cord. **Urinary symptoms** are often present.
  (2) **Physical examination findings**
    (a) **Epididymal swelling** and **tenderness** may prevent the examiner from distinguishing the testes from the epididymis.
    (b) **Fever** and **urethral discharge** may be observed.
    (c) **Prehn's sign** is present.
c. **Differential diagnoses** include testicular tumor, testicular torsion, testicular appendix torsion, testicular trauma, and orchitis.
d. **Evaluation**
  (1) **Physical examination.** Prostate palpation (not massage) should be performed to rule out prostatitis.
  (2) **Laboratory studies**
    (a) **Urinalysis** may reveal pyuria.
    (b) **Urine culture** may identify the organism in cases of non–sexually transmitted infection.
    (c) **Urethral swab.** A urethral swab for *C. trachomatis* and *N. gonorrhoeae* should be performed.
  (3) **Doppler ultrasound** is of limited usefulness in differentiating epididymitis from testicular torsion.
e. **Therapy**
  (1) **Antibiotic therapy**
    (a) **Sexually transmitted epididymitis** is treated with **doxycycline** (100 mg by mouth twice daily for 10 days) and **ceftriaxone** (one 250-mg dose administered intramuscularly). Treatment of sexual partners is required.
    (b) Non–sexually transmitted epididymitis is treated with **trimethoprim–sulfamethoxazole** (160/800 mg), one tablet by mouth twice daily, or **ciprofloxacin** (500 mg by mouth twice daily for 10–14 days).
  (2) **Pain relief. NSAIDs** or **narcotics** (e.g., acetaminophen with codeine) can be prescribed to relieve pain.
  (3) **Supportive care.** Bed rest for 2 days is advisable, and physical activity and heavy lifting should be minimized. Patients may be advised to wear an athletic supporter.
f. **Disposition.** Outpatient therapy is usually sufficient, but admission may be required for an ill-appearing patient with severe pain and swelling, leukocytosis, and an elevated temperature.

4. **Orchitis**
  a. **Causes.** Orchitis is usually associated with a systemic infection, particularly mumps, and occurs only in postpubertal patients.
  b. **Clinical features.** Mumps orchitis occurs 3–4 days after the development of parotitis and is bilateral in up to 10% of cases. Physical examination reveals a tender, swollen testicle.
  c. **Differential diagnoses** include epididymitis, testicular torsion, testicular trauma, and testicular tumor.
  d. **Evaluation. Urinalysis** is usually normal. A **CBC** reveals a leukocytosis.
  e. **Therapy** entails bed rest, local application of heat, oral analgesics, and antipyretics as needed. Patients may be advised to wear an athletic supporter.

5. **Testicular masses**
  a. **Clinical features.** Only 10% of patients present with acute pain as a result of hemorrhage or infarction. Another 10% may present with complaints related to malignant disease.
  b. **Evaluation.** Any patient with a painless testicular swelling or mass must be referred to a urologist for evaluation. Misdiagnoses are not uncommon and include epididymitis, hydrocele, spermatocele, and orchitis.

C **Disorders affecting the scrotum** Idiopathic synergistic necrotizing fasciitis (**Fournier's gangrene**) is a rapidly spreading infection of the scrotum that progresses to gangrene. Patients with diabetes and immunocompromised patients are most often affected.

1. **Causes.** The infection is polymicrobial; causative organisms originate from the integument, urethra, or rectum. Commonly isolated organisms include:
   a. Hemolytic streptococci and *Clostridium*
   b. *E. coli*
   c. *Bacteroides*

2. **Clinical features.** Early in the course of the disease, a simple cellulitis or abscess may be misdiagnosed.

3. **Therapy.** Patients should be admitted to the hospital. Consultation with a urologist is necessary.
   a. **Broad-spectrum intravenous antibiotic coverage** should be initiated.
   b. **Wide surgical debridement** is required.
   c. **Hyperbaric oxygen** should be considered.

D **Disorders affecting the prostate** include **acute prostatitis, chronic prostatitis, nonbacterial prostatitis** (Table 5–4), and **prostatodynia.**

1. **Acute prostatitis**
   a. **Causes.** The most commonly infecting organisms are *E. coli* (80% of cases), *Pseudomonas, Klebsiella, Proteus,* and *Enterococcus.*
   b. **Clinical features**
      (1) **Symptoms.** Patients present with an acute **febrile illness** characterized by chills, myalgias, arthralgias, and low back, perineal, or rectal pain. **Urinary frequency, urgency, nocturia, dysuria,** and varying degrees of **urinary retention** may exist.
      (2) **Physical examination findings.** Rectal examination reveals a prostate that is painful, swollen, firm, and warm to touch.
   c. **Differential diagnoses** include cystitis, pyelonephritis, diverticulitis, and perirectal abscess.
   d. **Evaluation**
      (1) **CBC.** A CBC may reveal leukocytosis.
      (2) **Urine culture** usually identifies the offending organism.
      (3) **Prostate secretion analysis and culture.** Prostate massage should not be performed because of the risk of bacteremia.
   e. **Therapy.** Most patients with prostatitis may be managed as outpatients with appropriate antibiotic therapy and supportive measures. Patients who are febrile and present with urinary retention may require hospitalization and intravenous antibiotics.

TABLE 5–4 **Comparison of Findings in Acute, Chronic, and Nonbacterial Prostatitis**

	Acute Prostatitis	**Chronic Prostatitis**	**Nonbacterial Prostatitis**
Constitutional symptoms	Severe	Mild	Mild
Urinary symptoms	Severe	Mild	Mild
Rectal examination findings	Painful, swollen, firm, warm prostate gland	Normal or boggy prostate gland	Normal
Expressed prostate fluid analysis	Not performed	>10 WBCs per high-power field	>10 WBCs per high-power field
Expressed prostate fluid culture	Not performed	Positive	Negative
Urine culture	Positive	Positive	Negative
Complete blood count (CBC)	Leukocytosis	Usually normal	Normal

WBCs = white blood cells.

(1) **Supportive measures** include hydration, antipyretics, analgesics, and stool softeners.

(2) **Outpatient antibiotic therapy** must be continued for a minimum of 2 weeks.

  (a) **First-line agents.** Fluoroquinolones are prescribed until culture and sensitivity testing results are known. Appropriate regimens might include oral **ciprofloxacin** (500 mg twice daily) or **ofloxacin** (200–300 mg twice daily).

  (b) Depending on the results of sensitivity testing, the following drugs may be administered:

    (i) **Trimethoprim–sulfamethoxazole** (160/800 mg), twice daily

    (ii) **Tetracycline** (250–500 mg), four times daily

    (iii) **Doxycycline** (100 mg), twice daily

    (iv) **Erythromycin** (500 mg), four times daily

(3) **Inpatient antibiotic therapy. Ciprofloxacin** (400 mg intravenously every 12 hours) or **gentamicin** (1 mg/kg every 8 hours) **plus ampicillin** (2 g every 6 hours) is continued for 1 week, followed by oral antibiotics.

2. Chronic prostatitis

  a. Causes. The most commonly infecting organisms are *E. coli, Pseudomonas, Proteus, Enterobacter, Staphylococcus,* and *Streptococcus.*

  b. Clinical features

  (1) **Signs and symptoms.** Fever and chills are uncommon, except with acute exacerbations. **Urinary symptoms** of frequency, urgency, nocturia, and dysuria may be present and are associated with **low back, perineal,** or **suprapubic pain.**

  (2) **Physical examination findings.** Rectal examination may reveal a normal or boggy prostate gland.

  c. Evaluation

  (1) **CBC.** Typically, the CBC is normal.

  (2) **Urine culture.** The offending organism can usually be cultured from the urine.

  (3) **Prostate secretion analysis and culture.** Generally, more than 10 WBCs per high-power field and a large number of macrophages are noted. Culture usually identifies the responsible organism.

  d. Therapy. Supportive measures and antibiotic choices are similar to those for acute prostatitis, although the antibiotics must be continued for up to 12 weeks.

3. Nonbacterial prostatitis

  a. Cause. Nonbacterial prostatitis may be caused by *Mycoplasma, Chlamydia,* or *Ureaplasma.*

  b. Clinical features. The presenting signs and symptoms are similar to those of chronic prostatitis.

  c. Evaluation

  (1) **Urine cultures** are negative.

  (2) **Prostate secretion analysis and culture.** Analysis reveals more than 10 WBCs per high-power field, but culture is negative.

  (3) **CBC** results are normal.

  d. Therapy. A clinical trial of antibiotics may be tried for a minimum of 4 weeks. Commonly used agents include **erythromycin** (500 mg by mouth four times daily) and **doxycycline** (100 mg by mouth twice daily for 14 days).

4. Prostatodynia

  a. Cause. The cause is unknown.

  b. Clinical features are similar to those of chronic noninfectious prostatitis.

  c. Evaluation

  (1) **Urine cultures** are negative.

  (2) **Prostate secretion analysis** reveals fewer than 10 WBCs per high-power field, and cultures are negative.

  d. Therapy. α-Adrenergic blocking agents may provide relief.

Study Questions

Directions: *Each of the numbered items or incomplete statements in this section is followed by answers or by completions of the statement. Select the ONE lettered answer or completion that is BEST in each case.*

1. What is the most common cause of intrinsic acute renal failure?
   - A Congestive heart failure (CHF)
   - B Urethral stricture
   - C Ischemia
   - D Benign prostatic hypertrophy (BPH)
   - E Dehydration

2. What is the most common cause of urinary retention in men?
   - A Prostate cancer
   - B Urethral stricture
   - C Nephrolithiasis
   - D Neurogenic bladder
   - E Benign prostatic hypertrophy (BPH)

3. Which one of the following is the most likely value for the fractional excretion of sodium (FENa) in a patient with intrinsic acute renal failure?
   - A Greater than 2.0
   - B 1.0–2.0
   - C 0.5–1.0
   - D Less than 1.0

4. Which antibiotic regimen is appropriate for the treatment of a urinary tract infection (UTI) in a patient in the third trimester of pregnancy?
   - A Trimethoprim–sulfamethoxazole, 160/800 mg orally, once daily for 7 days
   - B Nitrofurantoin, 50–100 mg orally, four times daily for 7–10 days
   - C Ciprofloxacin, 250 mg orally, twice daily for 3 days
   - D Norfloxacin, 400 mg orally, twice daily for 3 days
   - E Ofloxacin, 200 mg orally, twice daily for 7 days

5. What is the test of choice for diagnosing testicular torsion?
   - A Doppler ultrasound
   - B Angiography
   - C Radionuclide scanning with technetium-99m pertechnetate
   - D Magnetic resonance imaging (MRI)
   - E Plain radiograph

6. Which disease process may predispose patients to the formation of urinary stones?
   - A Diabetes mellitus
   - B Irritable bowel syndrome
   - C Osteoarthritis
   - D Dermatomyositis
   - E Inflammatory bowel disease

7. A 23-year-old man presents to the emergency department (ED) complaining of scrotal pain. The pain began 4 days ago and has gradually worsened. The patient now feels hot and his scrotum is too tender to allow for an adequate examination. What is the most likely diagnosis?

- A Testicular torsion
- B Hydrocele
- C Epididymitis
- D Urethritis
- E Spermatocele

8. What is the initial therapy in the management of a patient diagnosed with Fournier's gangrene?

- A Intravenous antibiotics
- B Surgical debridement
- C Oral analgesics
- D Hyperbaric oxygen
- E Retrograde urethrography

9. A 25-year-old man presents to the emergency department (ED) because of a painless, ulcerated lesion on the shaft of his penis. His left inguinal lymph nodes are enlarged and painful; occasionally, a yellowish fluid drains from them. Which of the following is the most likely diagnosis?

- A Herpes
- B Genital warts
- C Syphilis
- D Molluscum contagiosum
- E Lymphogranuloma venereum (LGV)

Answers and Explanations

1. The answer is C Acute tubular necrosis (ATN) secondary to ischemia is the most common cause of intrinsic acute renal failure (i.e., renal failure as a result of direct injury to the renal parenchyma). Other causes include glomerulonephritis, acute interstitial nephritis, poststreptococcal nephritis, rhabdomyolysis, hypertension, and diabetes. Dehydration can be a prerenal cause of acute renal failure. Urethral stricture and BPH are causes of obstructive urinary retention.

2. The answer is E Urinary retention may have an obstructive, neurologic, or pharmacologic cause. In men, obstruction as a result of BPH is the most common cause of urinary retention. All patients with acute urinary retention require catheterization.

3. The answer is A Intrinsic acute renal failure is characterized by the inability of the kidney to concentrate urine (i.e., to reabsorb sodium). Therefore, the FENa, which is equal to the urine sodium:serum sodium ratio divided by the urine creatinine:serum creatinine ratio multiplied by 100, is greater than 2, because the concentration of sodium in the urine is higher than that found in the serum.

4. The answer is B Nitrofurantoin, amoxicillin, or cefpodoxime is indicated for the treatment of a UTI in a pregnant woman. Fluoroquinolones (e.g., ciprofloxacin, norfloxacin, ofloxacin) are contraindicated in pregnancy and any sulfa-containing drug (e.g., trimethoprim–sulfamethoxazole) is contraindicated during the third trimester.

5. The answer is C Radionuclide scanning with technetium-99m pertechnetate is the test of choice for diagnosing testicular torsion. Doppler ultrasound is a quick test, but has a high false-negative rate. When clinically suspected, intravenous pain medications or conscious sedation followed by manual detorsion should be attempted immediately. Consultation with a urologist, surgical exploration, and bilateral orchiopexy are mandatory with suspected torsion. In order to ensure a high salvage rate, treatment should be initiated before ancillary test results are available.

6. The answer is E Patients with inflammatory bowel disease are predisposed to the development of urinary calculi. Other clinical conditions that may predispose to stone formation are gout, hyperparathyroidism, hyperuricemia, and immobilization. Some drugs, such as diuretics, may also increase a patient's risk of forming stones.

7. The answer is C This patient most likely has acute epididymitis. The patient does not complain of penile discharge or dysuria, making urethritis less likely. Spermatocele and hydrocele are generally not associated with testicular tenderness. Testicular torsion tends to produce a more acute clinical picture [the patient probably would have presented to the ED within 6 hours of the onset of pain] and is not commonly associated with fever.

8. The answer is A Fournier's gangrene, or idiopathic synergistic necrotizing fasciitis, is a rapidly spreading infection of the scrotum that is treated with intravenous antibiotics, followed by surgical debridement. Hyperbaric oxygen may also be a useful therapeutic modality, but is less urgent than the administration of antibiotics or surgical debridement.

9. The answer is E LGV is a sexually transmitted disease that manifests as a painless lesion accompanied by painful buboes. Buboes are suppurative, enlarged lymph nodes that may drain purulent fluid. The actual lesion may form a nodule that then ruptures, leaving a scar. Genital warts are raised cauliflower-like structures that do not usually cause lymphadenopathy with drainage.

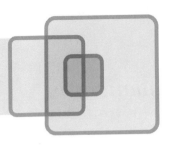

chapter 6

Infectious Disease Emergencies

DAVID E. WILLIAMS · RODNEY BERGER

I   **SEPSIS**

A **Discussion**   Sepsis should be considered a clinical syndrome.

1. **Etiology.** Although most cases of sepsis are caused by Gram-negative or Gram-positive bacteria, mycobacteria, rickettsiae, fungi, viruses, and protozoa have also been implicated.

2. **Pathogenesis.** The pathogenesis of sepsis is complex, is only partially understood, and usually involves many organ systems.
   a. A **focal infection** results in invasion of the bloodstream by the organism or proliferation of the organism at the site of infection. Actual microbial invasion of the bloodstream is not necessary for the development of sepsis, which is caused by the release of large quantities of **endotoxins, exotoxins,** and **other substances into the tissues and the bloodstream.**
   b. The release of these toxins induces the release of **endogenous mediators** by activated host cells. Depending on the timing and the quantity of their release, these endogenous mediators may either help or hinder the host response.
      (1) **Tumor necrosis factor (TNF),** described by some as a proinflammatory substance, shifts the immune system into an overresponsive phase, causing a reaction analogous in some respects to anaphylaxis.
      (2) **Platelet activating factor** is associated with systemic activation of the coagulation system, leading to disorders of homeostasis. Simultaneous systemic clotting and bleeding resulting from the deposition of fibrin in small blood vessels cause **disseminated intravascular coagulation (DIC),** microvascular thrombosis leads to **organ failure,** and **consumption coagulopathy** occurs.
      (3) **Myocardial depressant substance** is also released.

3. **Predisposing factors** include, but are not limited to, the following:
   a. **Extremes of age**
   b. **Iatrogenic procedures** (e.g., indwelling catheters, surgical or invasive diagnostic procedures)
   c. **Medical conditions** (e.g., cirrhosis, burns, multiple trauma, diabetes mellitus, cancer, complicated pregnancy or delivery)
   d. **Social factors** (e.g., alcoholism, substance abuse, intravenous drug abuse)
   e. **Immunosuppression** (e.g., neutropenia, complement deficiencies, hypo- or agammaglobulinemia, splenectomy, HIV infection)
   f. **Malnutrition**

B **Clinical features** vary considerably depending on whether the patient is in the early, intermediate, or late phase of the syndrome.

1. **General symptoms and physical examination findings**
   a. **Systemic findings** may include fever, chills, rigors, or hypothermia.
   b. **Neuromuscular findings** may include myalgias and arthralgias.
   c. **Neurologic findings** may include altered mental status.

d. **Cardiopulmonary findings** may include tachycardia, arrhythmias, hypotension, hypertension, a widened pulse pressure, or tachypnea. A primary tachypnea, directly related to sepsis and associated with acute hyperventilation and primary respiratory alkalosis, is thought to be caused by endotoxins, kallikreins, bradykinin, prostaglandins, and/or complement activation.

e. **Dermatologic findings.** Dermal lesions that should increase clinical suspicion of sepsis include petechiae, embolic lesions, and ecthyma gangrenosum.

2. **Site-specific symptoms and physical examination findings**

a. **Skin.** Findings that might be indicative of the initial focal source include erythema, a localized increase in temperature, lymphadenitis, induration, fluctuation, and pus. [In an immunosuppressed or neutropenic patient, a localized area of painful erythema may well indicate an initial focal source, even in the absence of localized warmth and swelling and irrespective of the absolute white blood cell (WBC) count.]

b. **Heart or lungs.** Findings may include a cough, sputum, dyspnea, chest pain, cyanosis, rales, or edema.

c. **Urinary tract.** Findings may include urinary urgency, frequency, dysuria, tenesmus, flank pain, oliguria, or anuria.

d. **Gastrointestinal tract.** Findings may include abdominal pain, nausea, vomiting, diarrhea, constipation, or jaundice. When the initial focus of infection is difficult to discern ("primary bacteremia"), one must strongly consider the probability of infection originating in the gastrointestinal tract (especially in patients on chemotherapy).

e. **Central nervous system (CNS).** Findings may include an altered sensorium, headache, stiff neck, focal neurologic signs, photophobia, retinal hemorrhages, cotton wool spots, conjunctival petechiae, endophthalmitis, or panophthalmitis.

C **Differential diagnoses** include the following:

1. **Viral diseases** (e.g., influenza, dengue fever, coxsackie B virus infection)

2. **Spirochetal diseases** (e.g., syphilitic Jarisch-Herxheimer reaction, leptospirosis, relapsing fever caused by *Borrelia* infection)

3. **Rickettsial diseases** (e.g., Rocky Mountain spotted fever, endemic typhus)

4. **Protozoal diseases** (e.g., *Toxoplasma gondii* infection, *Trypanosoma cruzi* infection, *Pneumocystis carinii* infection, *Plasmodium falciparum* infection)

5. **Endocrine diseases** (e.g., adrenal insufficiency, thyroid storm)

6. **Nonseptic causes of shock** (e.g., cardiogenic shock, hypovolemic shock, neurogenic shock, pulmonary embolism, cardiac tamponade, anaphylaxis, dissecting aortic aneurysm)

7. **Collagen vascular diseases**

8. **Vasculitides**

9. **Thrombocytic thrombocytopenic purpura/hemolytic–uremic syndrome**

D **Evaluation**   There is no single reliable laboratory test for the diagnosis of sepsis. Although the **history** and **physical examination** form the basis of the presumptive diagnosis, the following additional testing is still considered essential.

1. **Laboratory studies**

a. **Blood cultures** and **site-specific cultures** [e.g., sputum, urine, cerebrospinal fluid (CSF)] should be obtained prior to initiating empiric antibiotic therapy.

b. **Gram staining** of site-specific samples is indicated.

c. **Serologic studies** (e.g., counterimmune electrophoresis, latex agglutination) are useful when infection with pneumococcus, *Haemophilus influenzae*, meningococcus, or group B streptococcus is suspected.

    d. Complete blood count. Findings compatible with a diagnosis of sepsis include leukocytosis, eosinopenia, anemia, leukopenia, and thrombocytopenia.

    e. Urinalysis. Proteinuria is a finding that supports a diagnosis of sepsis.

    f. Coagulation profile. Findings that would support a diagnosis of sepsis include a prolonged prothrombin time (PT) and thrombocytopenia.

    g. Arterial blood gas (ABG) profile. Findings in a patient with sepsis could include hypoxemia and lactic acidosis.

    h. Serum biochemical profile. Supportive findings would include hypoferremia, hyper- or hypoglycemia, hypocalcemia, hyperbilirubinemia, and azotemia.

2. Imaging studies. Site-specific **radiographs, ultrasonograms, computed tomography (CT) scans,** or **magnetic resonance imaging (MRI) scans** may be appropriate.

3. Other studies. Evaluation of site-specific samples obtained by **biopsy** or **aspiration** may be helpful.

E Therapy

1. Supportive measures

    a. Mechanical ventilation is necessary for patients with respiratory insufficiency.

    b. Volume replacement is necessary for hypotensive patients. **Pressor agents** may also be required.

        (1) Norepinephrine is rarely, if ever, indicated. (It has an intense peripheral vasoconstricting activity, causes ischemic tissue necrosis in the case of extravasation, compromises the perfusion of vital organs, and increases myocardial irritability.)

        (2) Dopamine should be administered only after aggressive volume replacement and after the central venous and pulmonary artery wedge pressures have increased to the upper limits of normal. (If this agent is used in the presence of reduced intravascular fluid volume, the vasodilatation secondary to the β-adrenergic stimulation can cause a paradoxic decline in blood pressure and decreased tissue perfusion because of the sudden drop in effective intravascular volume.)

    c. Transfusion

        (1) Whole blood transfusion is indicated if the patient is anemic and hypotensive with a low central venous pressure and pulmonary artery wedge pressure.

        (2) Plasma fraction transfusion is indicated if the patient is not anemic, but has a low blood pressure, central venous pressure, and pulmonary artery wedge pressure.

        (3) Fresh frozen plasma transfusion is necessary for patients with depleted levels of coagulation factors.

        (4) Platelet transfusions are indicated when the patient has thrombocytopenia.

        (5) Cryoprecipitate transfusions are indicated for patients with hypofibrinogenemia.

        (6) Granulocyte transfusions (initially used in neutropenic patients) have fallen into disuse because of:

           (a) The high complication rate associated with WBC transfusions

           (b) The high incidence of pulmonary complications

           (c) The significant incidence of related viral infections

           (d) The results of a recent, large, well-documented, and randomized study showing no significant difference in recovery rates or survival, even in the subset of patients without evidence of bone marrow recovery

    d. Correction of metabolic abnormalities. Acidemia, hypoxia, hyper- or hypoglycemia, electrolyte imbalances, and nutritional deficiencies must be corrected.

    e. Supportive pharmacologic therapy

        (1) Corticosteroids are indicated only in the presence of hypoadrenalism.

        (2) Heparin has been shown in numerous studies to be capable of temporarily terminating DIC. It is considered the drug of choice for patients with coexistent deep venous thrombophlebitis.

(3) **Diuretics** are indicated only when volume expansion is not adequate to maintain urine output, even in the presence of central venous and pulmonary artery wedge pressures in the upper limits of normal.

(4) **Recombinant colony-stimulating factors** are currently being evaluated in clinical trial studies and have replaced granulocyte transfusions.

(5) **Naloxone,** an antagonist of opiates and β endorphins, has been shown in one small human study to produce a 45% increase in systolic blood pressure lasting 45 minutes, but in another small study, the drug failed to demonstrate any benefit when administered to patients with septic shock caused by a Gram-negative organism.

(6) **Other drugs.** Phenothiazines, antihistamines, indomethacin, ibuprofen, glucagon, α-adrenergic blocking agents, vasodilators, cyclooxygenase inhibitors, pentoxifylline, antiserums, immunoglobulin M (IgM) monoclonal antibodies, anticytokines, and other newer agents are currently under study.

2. **Specific measures**
   a. **Surgery.** Septic foci must be removed or drained.
   b. **Antibiotic therapy.** All patients with septic shock should receive empiric antibiotic therapy as soon as possible. Once the source of the infection has been identified, the spectrum of antibiotic coverage may be narrowed, and once the culture and sensitivity results are available, it may be possible to narrow the spectrum of coverage even further.
      (1) **Selecting empiric antibiotics.** Knowledge of preexisting immune dysfunction can be useful for targeting antibiotics for initial empiric therapy (Table 6–1). Empiric therapy should be effective against Gram-positive and Gram-negative bacteria, and given intravenously in the maximum doses allowed.
      (2) **Specific drug combinations** are summarized in Table 6–2.

F **Disposition**   Clinically unstable patients must be treated in the intensive care unit (ICU). Chemistries and CBCs should be monitored closely in all patients.

G **Prevention**

1. **Gamma-globulin** should be administered to hypo- or agammaglobulinemic patients.
2. **Pneumococcal vaccination** and **vaccination against *H. influenzae*** are indicated for geriatric patients and patients with certain chronic diseases.

II ACQUIRED IMMUNE DEFICIENCY SYNDROME (AIDS)

A **Discussion**

1. **Etiology.** AIDS is caused by HIV, a cytopathic retrovirus. Transmission of HIV can occur via semen, vaginal secretions, blood or blood products, or transplacental transmission in utero. HIV

TABLE 6–1   Organisms Commonly Associated with Infections in Patients with Immune Dysfunction

Immune Dysfunction	Potential Causes	Commonly Associated Microbes
Granulocytopenia	Myelosuppressive therapy, irradiation	Gram-negative bacilli (e.g., *Pseudomonas aeruginosa*, staphylococci)
Cellular immune dysfunction	Congenital defects, Hodgkin's disease, AIDS, antineoplastic therapy (e.g., for lymphoma), immunosuppressive therapy (e.g., to prevent transplant rejection)	*Mycobacterium,* fungi, *Listeria, Pneumocystis carinii,* herpesviruses
Humoral immune dysfunction	Splenectomy, untreated multiple myeloma	*Streptococcus pneumoniae, Haemophilus influenzae*

TABLE 6–2   Drug Regimens Used in the Empiric Treatment of Sepsis

Patient Profile	Regimen
Adult without an obvious source of infection	Basic regimen: Third-generation cephalosporin OR an antipseudomonal β-lactamase–susceptible penicillin + an antipseudomonal aminoglycoside OR imipenem
Adult with a high probability of having a Gram-positive infection (e.g., intravenous drug abuser, patient with toxic shock syndrome, patient with infection secondary to an indwelling vascular catheter)	Basic regimen + nafcillin or vancomycin[†]
Adult with a high probability of having an anaerobic infection (e.g., intra-abdominal or biliary tract infection, female genital tract infection, necrotizing cellulitis, aspiration pneumonia, dental infection, soft tissue infection)	Basic regimen + metronidazole or clindamycin
Adult suspected of having a *Legionella* infection	Basic regimen + erythromycin
Neonate	Ampicillin or ticarcillin with clavulanic acid + an aminoglycoside[†]
Infant (1–3 months)	Ampicillin + ceftriaxone or cefotaxime
Child older than 3 months	Ceftriaxone OR cefotaxime
Nonneutropenic patient with a nosocomial infection	Third-generation cephalosporin + metronidazole OR ticarcillin, ampicillin, or piperacillin with the corresponding β-lactamase inhibitor + an aminoglycoside[†] OR imipenem +/− an aminoglycoside[†]
Neutropenic patient with a nosocomial infection	Third-generation cephalosporin + metronidazole + an aminoglycoside[†] OR ticarcillin, ampicillin, or piperacillin with the corresponding β-lactamase inhibitor + an aminoglycoside[†] OR imipenem + an aminoglycoside[†]
Patient with thermal injuries to >20% of the body surface area	Ceftriaxone + an aminoglycoside[†] OR an antipseudomonal penicillin + an aminoglycoside + vancomycin[†]
Pregnant woman	β Lactam or erythromycin; gentamicin is also considered appropriate under these circumstances[*]

[*]Amikacin should be used when gentamicin resistance is known or suspected.
[†]Peak and trough levels for aminoglycosides and vancomycin must be monitored.

has been isolated from saliva, urine, CSF, brain tissue, tears, breast milk, alveolar fluid, synovial fluid, and amniotic fluid. Transmission has not been documented via casual contact.

2. **Pathogenesis.** HIV selectively attacks cells involved in immune function, primarily the CD4 (helper T) cells. As a result, profound defects in the host's immune system develop, leading to a variety of opportunistic infections and neoplasms. HIV infection progresses through four stages:

   a. **Acute illness associated with seroconversion.** Within a few weeks of HIV infection, patients may present with malaise, fever, rash, arthralgias, lymphadenopathy, and weight loss secondary to the acute, initial, primary infection. This phase is self-limited.

   b. **Asymptomatic stage.** An asymptomatic period that may last 10 years or more follows. During this phase, the patient's CD4 count is normal (greater than 800/mm^3) and he or she is fully immunocompetent. The virus is actively replicating, but the host's immune response is still capable of keeping the virus in check.

   c. **Early symptomatic AIDS.** Eventually, however, the pendulum swings in favor of the virus, and the CD4 count gradually declines as the infection wins over the host's defenses. When the

CD4 count falls to around 500/mm³, the patient becomes more susceptible to opportunistic infections.

d. **Late symptomatic AIDS.** As the CD4 count falls below 100/mm³, the immune system is severely compromised and all types of life-threatening opportunistic infections [e.g., toxoplasmosis, coccidioidomycosis, cytomegalovirus (CMV) infection, *Mycobacterium avium-intracellulare* (MAI) infection] and neoplasms (e.g., Hodgkin's disease, non-Hodgkin's lymphoma) are likely to occur.

B **Clinical features** The spectrum of disease caused by HIV infection is immense. Because of the complexity of HIV infection, the role of emergency department (ED) personnel is to diagnose and treat those complications that arise in HIV infection that may lead to acute morbidity and mortality.

a. **Symptomatic HIV infection.** Fever, malaise, weight loss, and night sweats in the absence of any opportunistic disease in a previously asymptomatic HIV-positive patient mark the transition toward symptomatic disease. Once these symptoms appear, systemic infection and malignancy must be ruled out.

b. **Cutaneous manifestations.** Skin disorders secondary to HIV are commonly encountered in the ED.

(1) **Kaposi's sarcoma** is one of the most common manifestations of AIDS, second only to *P. carinii pneumonia* (PCP).

(2) **Xerosis (dry skin)** and **pruritus** are common.

(3) **Bullous impetigo, ecthyma,** or **folliculitis** may be seen with *Staphylococcus aureus* infection.

(4) **Ulcerations** and **macerations** may be seen with *Pseudomonas aeruginosa* infection.

(5) **Herpes simplex, herpes zoster, syphilis,** and **scabies** are all commonly seen.

(6) **Molluscum contagiosum, intertriginous infections** (often caused by candidiasis or *Trichophyton* infection), **seborrheic dermatitis, condylomata acuminata** [caused by human papilloma virus (HPV)], **psoriasis, atopic dermatitis,** and **alopecia** are also commonly seen.

c. **Neurologic manifestations.** CNS disease occurs in 75%–90% of patients with AIDS, and 10%–20% of AIDS patients initially present with CNS symptoms. The most common symptoms are seizures and altered mental status.

(1) **Toxoplasmosis** is the most common cause of focal encephalitis in patients with AIDS. Symptoms include fever, headache, focal neurologic symptoms, altered mental status, or seizures.

(2) **AIDS dementia complex** is a progressive dementia, with symptoms of impaired short-term memory and confusion. It is caused by the direct effect of HIV on the brain cells, and occurs in over one third of patients with AIDS.

(3) **Cryptococcal CNS infection** may be seen in up to 10% of AIDS patients and may cause either focal cerebral lesions or diffuse meningoencephalitis. Symptoms may include headache, light-headedness, depression, seizures, or cranial nerve palsies.

(4) **Tuberculous meningitis** and **HSV encephalitis** are also common.

d. **Psychiatric manifestations**

(1) **Depression** is common among AIDS patients and may initially manifest as a primary complaint or a suicide attempt.

(2) **AIDS psychosis** is poorly understood, and the patient may present with hallucinations, delusions, or other abnormal behavioral changes.

e. **Ophthalmologic manifestations.** CMV retinitis occurs in 10%–15% of patients and accounts for the majority of retinitis among AIDS patients. It may be asymptomatic or patients may present with photophobia, scotoma, redness, pain, or diminished visual acuity. CMV retinitis is characterized by **cotton wool spots,** fluffy white retinal lesions that are often perivascular.

f. **Pulmonary manifestations.** Lung infections are one of the most common reasons HIV-positive patients present to the ED. The most common pulmonary disorders in HIV-positive patients include PCP, *Mycobacterium tuberculosis* infection, CMV infection, *Cryptococcus neoformans* infection, *Histoplasma capsulatum* infection, and neoplasms. PCP is the most common opportunistic infection among AIDS patients—over 80% will acquire PCP at some time during their illness.

   (1) Nonproductive cough and the presence of a diffuse infiltrative process on chest radiography suggest PCP, CMV infection, or Kaposi's sarcoma.

   (2) Hilar adenopathy with a diffuse pulmonary infiltrate may be associated with *C. neoformans* infection, histoplasmosis, *M. tuberculosis* infection, or neoplasia.

g. **Gastrointestinal manifestations.** Approximately 50% of patients will present with gastrointestinal complaints at some time during their illness. The most common presenting symptoms include abdominal pain, bleeding, and diarrhea. Esophagitis may present as dysphagia or odynophagia. Common causes of gastrointestinal complications include *Candida* infection, Kaposi's sarcoma, MAI infection, herpes simplex virus-type 1 (HSV-1) or herpes simplex virus-type 2 (HSV-2) infection, CMV infection, *Campylobacter jejuni* infection, *Shigella* infection, salmonellosis, giardiasis, cryptosporidiosis, *Entamoeba histolytica* infection, and *Isospora* infection.

C **Differential diagnoses**   The list of differential diagnoses for HIV and all of its manifestations is lengthy because virtually any disease process can mimic an illness associated with HIV infection. A patient should be screened for HIV infection when there is prolonged illness without a ready explanation.

D **Evaluation**

1. **Confirmation of HIV infection.** A person suspected of being infected by HIV should be serologically tested using **enzyme-linked immunosorbent assay (ELISA)** or **Western blot assays** to confirm the presence of the virus. These tests are usually not performed in the ED because of issues of confidentiality, counseling, and follow-up. If the patient's presenting complaint necessitates admission, then the testing should be performed as an inpatient. Otherwise, the patient should be given appropriate referrals for outpatient testing.

2. **Evaluation of presenting symptoms.** Additional tests depend on the symptoms at the time of presentation to the ED.

   a. **Systemic symptoms**

      (1) **History and physical examination.** A complete history should be obtained and a thorough physical examination should be performed.

      (2) **Laboratory studies.** A CBC, serum biochemical profile, blood and urine cultures, urinalysis, liver function tests, chest radiographs, and serologic test results for syphilis, *Toxoplasma*, and *Coccidioides* should be obtained.

   b. **Neurologic symptoms.** For an HIV-infected patient presenting with headache, focal neurologic changes, or altered mental status, a CBC and serum biochemistry profile should be obtained, as well as a CT scan (with and without contrast). A lumbar puncture should be performed to obtain samples for serology to exclude toxoplasmosis, CMV infection, *Cryptococcus* infection, HSV infection, tuberculosis, and lymphoma.

   c. **Pulmonary symptoms.** The work-up for any pulmonary complaint should include the following:

      (1) Chest radiograph

      (2) ABG analysis

      (3) Sputum culture, Gram stain, and acid-fast stain

      (4) Blood cultures

   d. **Gastrointestinal symptoms**

(1) Diarrhea is the most common gastrointestinal complaint. ED evaluation may include microscopic examination of a stool sample for leukocytes, acid-fast staining of a stool sample, and examination for ova and parasites, as well as bacterial culture of stool and blood.

(2) Esophagitis. Endoscopy, fungal stains, viral cultures, or biopsy may be necessary to establish the diagnosis. An air-contrast barium swallow may be necessary to confirm a diagnosis of *Candida* esophagitis.

E **Therapy**   The role of the ED physician is rarely to treat directly the underlying HIV infection, because the internist or infectious disease specialist is better able to follow the patient and monitor the efficacy and side effects of the drugs involved over a long-term basis. Instead, the ED physician's focus should be the acute presentations of the common opportunistic infections and how to treat them in order to avoid unnecessary morbidity.

1. **Primary disease.** Zidovudine (AZT) and its related analogs, dideoxycytidine (ddC) and dideoxyinosine (ddI), protease inhibitors, and CD4 receptor blockers have formed the mainstay of direct treatment for HIV infection over the past 10 years. The ED physician should be aware that AZT prophylaxis is usually initiated when the patient's CD4 count drops below 500/mm^3. Therefore, a medication history that includes trimethoprim–sulfamethoxazole or AZT can provide clues to the patient's CD4 count and can help guide the ED physician in deciding if an HIV-positive individual should be considered immunocompromised at that time.

2. **Complications of HIV infection**
   a. **Cutaneous complications.** Most skin disorders can be treated by referral to a dermatologist for work-up and treatment on an outpatient basis.
      (1) Xerosis can be treated with emollients; **pruritus** may respond to oatmeal baths or antihistamines.
      (2) *S. aureus* **infection,** *P. aeruginosa* **infection, herpes zoster, syphilis,** and **scabies** can all be treated with standard therapies.
      (3) HSV lesions can be treated with **acyclovir** (200 mg orally five times daily for 10 days or, for extensive disease, 30 mg/kg/day intravenously).
      (4) Kaposi's sarcoma is generally not associated with significant morbidity or mortality. Chemotherapy (e.g., with vincristine, vinblastine, or doxorubicin) or radiation therapy is warranted only for extensive, painful, or cosmetically disfiguring lesions.
      (5) Molluscum contagiosum. Cryotherapy or curettage can be used to remove the small, flesh-colored papules of molluscum contagiosum.
      (6) Intertriginous infections (e.g., such as can occur with *Candida* or *Trichophyton* infection) can be treated with **topical imidazole creams** (e.g., clotrimazole, miconazole, ketoconazole).
      (7) Seborrheic dermatitis is treated with **topical steroids.**
      (8) HPV infections are treated for cosmesis with cryotherapy, topical therapy, or laser therapy.
   b. **Neurologic complications**
      (1) Toxoplasmosis is treated with oral **sulfadiazine** (100 mg/kg/day) and **pyrimethamine** (25–50 mg/kg/day) with **folic acid** to reduce the incidence of hematologic toxicity. Short courses of **steroids** may be employed, and chronic suppressive therapy is needed after acute treatment.
      (2) Cryptococcosis. Treatment for cryptococcal infection includes **amphotericin** (0.4–0.6 mg/kg/day intravenously), with or without **flucytosine** (75–100 mg/kg/day). Sixty percent of patients respond to this therapy. Initial therapy should continue for 6 weeks, and chronic suppressive therapy is often indicated.
      (3) Other infections (e.g., bacterial meningitis, brain abscess, CMV infection, HSV encephalitis, neurosyphilis) should be treated according to the standard therapies in place for each disease process.

c. **Psychiatric complications.** Hospitalization should be instituted when necessary for patients with depression, acute delirium, or incapacitating dementia.

d. **Ophthalmologic complications.** No specific therapy is indicated for cotton wool spots. CMV retinitis is treated with **ganciclovir** (5 mg/kg twice daily) for 2 weeks, followed by long-term maintenance therapy. All patients with eye complaints should be referred to an ophthalmologist for further evaluation.

e. **Pulmonary complications**
   (1) **PCP.** Relapses are common—65% of patients will have a reinfection within 18 months.
      (a) **Trimethoprim** (20 mg/kg/day) and **sulfamethoxazole** (100 mg/kg/day) should be administered either orally or intravenously for 2–3 weeks.
      (b) **Pentamidine** (4 mg/kg/day) may be used as an effective alternate therapy.
      (c) **Oral steroid therapy** should be instituted for those patients with an arterial oxygen tension (PaO$_2$) less than 70 mm Hg, or an alveolar–arterial (A-a) gradient greater than 35. The usual regimen consists of **prednisone,** 80 mg/day for 5 days, followed by 40 mg/day for 5 days, and then 20 mg/day for 11 days.
   (2) *M. tuberculosis* **infection** is treated with a triple drug regimen of **isoniazid, rifampin,** and **ethambutol.** This regimen may be supplemented with **pyrazinamide** and **streptomycin.**

f. **Gastrointestinal complications**
   (1) **Diarrhea.** Dehydration should be corrected. Antibiotic therapy should be initiated when appropriate.
   (2) **Oral candidiasis** is treated with **clotrimazole troches** five times daily until clear, or oral **ketoconazole** or **fluconazole.**
   (3) **Other oral lesions** (e.g., HSV infection, Kaposi's sarcoma) are common and can usually be managed on an outpatient basis with symptomatic therapy.

F **Disposition** should be based on the ability to rule out any life-threatening complications of HIV infection.

1. **Discharge.** Many HIV-infected patients with fever may be managed as outpatients if the source of the fever does not dictate admission, appropriate laboratory studies have been initiated, the patient is able to function adequately at home (i.e., he or she is able to ambulate and maintain adequate oral intake), and appropriate medical follow-up can be arranged.

2. **Admission**
   a. Patients with a CD4 count below 500/mm^3 and an unknown source of fever are usually admitted for further observation and evaluation.
   b. If a life-threatening illness cannot be ruled out, or the patient is debilitated beyond the point where he or she can be cared for adequately at home, then the patient should be admitted for further treatment and evaluation.

III CENTRAL NERVOUS SYSTEM INFECTIONS

A Meningitis

1. **Discussion.** Meningitis is inflammation of the membranes of the brain and the spinal cord. The mortality rate ranges from 10%–50%.
   a. **Etiology.** Infectious meningitis may be caused by bacteria, viruses, fungi, or parasites.
   b. **Pathogenesis.** Meningitis is usually caused by hematogenous bacterial seeding of the subarachnoid space, but direct inoculation via a dural defect (e.g., after trauma or neurosurgery) or direct spread of organisms from parameningeal infections (e.g., sinusitis or otitis media) can also occur.
   c. **Clinical syndromes**
      (1) **Acute meningitis.** Onset of symptoms occurs within 24 hours and patients have a rapidly progressive downhill course (the treated mortality rate is 50%). Most likely pathogens are

Streptococcus pneumoniae and *Neisseria meningitides,* or *H. influenzae* in the nonimmunized pediatric population.

(2) **Subacute meningitis** presents in 1–7 days and is usually caused by viruses or fungi.

(3) **Chronic meningitis.** Symptoms persist for longer than 1 week and the disease follows a prolonged, indolent course. Causes include some viral meningitides as well as *M. tuberculosis, Treponema pallidum, Cryptococcus,* and other fungi.

2. **Clinical features**

a. **Bacterial meningitis.** The classic presentation of acute bacterial meningitis is fever, headache, photophobia, nuchal rigidity, lethargy, malaise, altered sensorium, seizures, vomiting, and chills. Complications include hyponatremia, hydrocephalus, and cerebrovascular accident.

b. **Fungal meningitis** often has a more subacute course than bacterial meningitis, with the same range of symptoms but often to such a mild degree that the diagnosis may not be considered.

c. **Tuberculous meningitis** often has a protracted course and a vague, nonspecific presentation of fever, weight loss, night sweats, and malaise, with or without headache and meningismus.

d. **Viral meningitis.** The presentation can range from acute to protracted with nonspecific findings.

3. **Differential diagnoses** include encephalitis, brain abscess, neoplasm, trauma, subdural hematoma, subarachnoid hemorrhage, systemic lupus erythematosus (SLE), sarcoidosis, rheumatoid arthritis, toxic encephalopathy, metabolic encephalopathy, multiple sclerosis, and granulomatous angiitis.

4. **Evaluation**

a. **CSF analysis** for cell count and differential, Gram staining, counterimmunoelectrophoresis (CIE), and culture are the diagnostic procedures of choice. Increased intracranial pressure (ICP) is a relative contraindication to performing a lumbar puncture, but a CSF sample can still be obtained in the presence of increased ICP by using a small-bore (25-gauge) needle, keeping the stylet partially within the needle during puncture to control CSF flow, and collecting only enough fluid (about 1 mL) to perform Gram staining and culture.

(1) **Cell count and differential**

(a) **Bacterial meningitis.** An increase in the leukocyte count to greater than 5 cells/mm³, a CSF:serum glucose ratio of less than 0.5 in normoglycemic subjects, and a CSF protein level greater than 45 mg/dL are all indicators of a bacterial infection.

(b) **Viral meningitis.** A marked lymphocytosis is evident on the differential, but this finding is not diagnostic for viral meningitis because 6%–13% of all bacterial meningitides are also characterized by a marked lymphocytosis.

(2) **Staining.** A Gram stain can rapidly detect the presence and type of bacterial organism, and an India ink preparation can identify cryptococcal meningitis in 33% of patients.

(3) **CIE** detects specific bacterial antigens. If the procedure is performed simultaneously on blood, urine, and CSF, its diagnostic accuracy approaches 100%. It is 90% accurate for detecting cryptococcal disease.

b. **CT scan.** If there are any signs of focal neurologic deficits or altered mental status, a head CT scan should be obtained prior to a lumbar puncture, to rule out mass lesions or other evidence of increased ICP.

5. **Therapy**

a. **Antibiotics.** Patients with an acute presentation should receive antibiotics within 30 minutes of presentation. Studies have shown that early antibiotic therapy will not significantly affect CSF analysis results or CSF cultures drawn within 6 hours of antibiotic administration, but failure to promptly administer antibiotics may dramatically affect patient morbidity and mortality.

(1) In the absence of knowledge of the offending organism, empiric therapy could be initiated with a **penicillin** or a **third-generation cephalosporin** (current practice favors ceftriaxone or cefotaxime). Dosages are as follows:

(a) **Penicillin** (for adults, 12 million U/day intravenously in six to eight divided doses)

(b) **Ampicillin** (2 g intravenously every 12 hours)

(c) **Ceftriaxone** (2 g intravenously every 12 hours for adults; 50–75 mg/kg/day every 12–24 hours for children)

(d) **Cefotaxime** (2 g intravenously every 4–6 hours for adults; 200 mg/kg/day every 8 hours for children)

(2) If infection with *Staphylococcus* or a Gram-negative bacillus is a concern (e.g., in a patient with a history of recent neurosurgery, head trauma, or a CSF shunt), then **vancomycin** (25 mg/kg administered as an intravenous bolus) plus **ceftazidime** (2 g intravenously every 8 hours for adults; 90–150 mg/kg every 8 hours for children) should be used.

(3) If the host is immunocompromised and infection with *Listeria monocytogenes, N. meningitidis,* or aerobic Gram-negative bacilli is a concern, then **vancomycin, ceftazidime,** and **ampicillin** should be used.

b. **Steroids.** The use of steroids in the pediatric population is controversial, but many authors favor steroid use to decrease inflammation and possibly decrease the incidence of long-term sequelae (e.g., hearing loss associated with bacterial meningitis caused by *S. pneumoniae* or *H. influenzae*). Current guidelines are to administer **dexamethasone** (0.15 mg/kg intravenously) at the time of antibiotic administration.

6. **Disposition.** All patients with suspected meningitis should be admitted to the hospital for further evaluation.

a. If the results of CSF analysis are normal but the patient still shows clinical signs of infection, a repeat lumbar puncture should be performed in 8–12 hours and antibiotics should be initiated empirically before the second lumbar puncture is performed.

b. The diagnosis of aseptic or viral meningitis should be made only after hospital admission and the appropriate CSF cultures have proven negative for other forms of meningitis.

B **Encephalitis**

1. **Discussion.** Encephalitis is an infection of the cerebrum, cerebellum, and brain stem. Two thousand cases of encephalitis are reported in the United States annually. Encephalitis may be caused by a number of organisms, including HSV and arboviruses (e.g., Eastern equine encephalitis virus, Western equine encephalitis virus, St. Louis encephalitis virus, California encephalitis virus), *Mycoplasma, Toxoplasma, Coccidioides, Cryptococcus, T. pallidum, Borrelia burgdorferi, Naegleria,* and *Mycobacterium.*

2. **Clinical features** are very similar to those of meningitis. An altered level of consciousness ranging from lethargy and irritability to frank obtundation and coma is common. Seizures and gait ataxia also occur.

3. **Differential diagnoses** include meningitis, brain abscess, neoplasm, trauma, subdural hematoma, subarachnoid hemorrhage, SLE, toxic encephalopathy, and metabolic encephalopathy.

4. **Evaluation.** CSF analysis and a head CT scan form the cornerstone of diagnosis. The diagnosis of encephalitis is usually made by first ruling out the presence of meningitis using Gram staining, antibody titers, India ink preparations, and CSF cultures.

a. **CSF analysis.** A CSF sample obtained via a lumbar puncture usually shows a normal glucose level, an elevated protein level, and marked pleocytosis in patients with encephalitis, but these signs are nonspecific. When HSV or *Naegleria* is the causative organism, an elevated CSF red blood cell (RBC) count is common. Specific CSF and blood serum titers for specific encephalitides (e.g., *Toxoplasmosis*) are available and useful for identifying the causative agent.

b. **Brain biopsy** used to be performed routinely to rule out HSV as a cause, but the procedure has fallen out of favor because of the morbidity associated with it.

5. **Therapy.** Because differentiating encephalitis from meningitis is very difficult, presumptive therapy should be initiated for bacterial meningitis even before the initiation of the work-up. Treatment is generally supportive. HSV can be treated with acyclovir.

6. **Disposition.** All patients suspected of having encephalitis should be admitted to the hospital for further evaluation and treatment.

C Brain abscess

1. **Discussion**
   a. **Incidence.** Brain abscesses are rare. The greatest incidence is seen in patients between the ages of 20 and 40 years; men are affected twice as often as women.
   b. **Pathogenesis**
      (1) Abscesses usually occur secondary to a focus of infection outside the CNS.
         (a) Brain abscesses arise from the middle ear, mastoid, and paranasal sinuses 40% of the time.
         (b) Hematogenous spread of bacteria from remote sites causes 30% of infections.
         (c) Twenty percent of brain abscesses have no clear cause.
      (2) Inflammation of the cerebrum progresses to abscess formation, and finally encapsulation. Three major complications can cause sudden deterioration: uncal or tonsillar herniation, spontaneous hemorrhage, and rupture of the abscess into the ventricular or subarachnoid space. Patients presenting with signs of brain herniation have a mortality rate greater than 50%.
   c. **Risk factors** for brain abscess include AIDS, immunosuppression, and intravenous drug abuse.

2. **Clinical features.** The clinical presentation may mimic that of a brain tumor, but the presentation of an abscess usually evolves more rapidly (e.g., within days to weeks). The classic presentation is one of headache, recent seizure, low-grade fever, and a focal neurologic deficit.
   a. **Headache** is the most common symptom; it is present in 70%–90% of affected patients.
   b. **Focal neurologic deficits** are found in 75% of patients.
   c. **Seizures** are found in 30% of patients; **fever** in 50% of patients.

3. **Differential diagnoses** include a tumor, encephalitis or meningitis, cerebrovascular accident, subarachnoid hemorrhage, migraine, and an extradural abscess.

4. **Evaluation.** A **head CT scan** is the procedure of choice, with and without contrast. Laboratory values are rarely helpful, although the WBC count is elevated in 30% of patients.

5. **Therapy.** Definitive care entails surgical intervention and antibiotic therapy.
   a. **Supportive therapy.** If there are signs of increased ICP, the physician may need to elevate the bed 30°, intubate and hyperventilate the patient, and institute dexamethasone therapy (10–12 g intravenously every 6 hours for adults; 0.6 mg/kg every 6 hours for children).
   b. **Antibiotic therapy.** Drugs should be selected using susceptibility testing as a basis (Table 6–3), and therapy should be continued for 4–6 weeks.

6. **Disposition.** Patients with brain abscesses require hospital admission and immediate neurosurgical consultation.

D Rabies

1. **Discussion**
   a. **Etiology.** Rabies is caused by an RNA-carrying reovirus and is transmitted by infectious saliva. In developing countries, dogs are the primary reservoir; in the United States, skunks (60%), bats (15%), raccoons (10%), and cows (4%) predominate.
   b. **Pathogenesis.** The rabies virus spreads across the motor endplates along the peripheral nervous system to the spinal cord and then to the CNS, where it replicates. Incubation periods average 35–64 days.

2. **Clinical features**
   a. Initial symptoms are nonspecific: fever, malaise, headache, nausea, sore throat, cough, and pain and paresthesias at the inoculation site.

TABLE 6–3 Antibiotic Therapy for Brain Abscess

Type of Infection	Drug	Regimen	
		ADULT DOSAGE	PEDIATRIC DOSAGE
Staphylococcus aureus or coagulase-negative staphylococci	Nafcillin	2 g intravenously every 4–6 hours	50 mg/kg/day intravenously every 4 hours
	Vancomycin (for MRSA)	1 g intravenously every 12 hours	15 mg/kg/day intravenously every 4–6 hours
Streptococcus	Penicillin G	2–4 million U intravenously every 4 hours	250,000 U/kg/day intravenously every 4 hours
Enteric Gram-negative bacilli or *Pseudomonas*	Piperacillin	4 g intravenously every 4–6 hours + an aminoglycoside	. . .
Mixed anaerobic/aerobic	Ticarcillin + clavulanic acid	3.1 g intravenously every 6 hours	200–300 mg/kg/day intravenously every 4–6 hours
	Ampicillin + sulbactam	3 g intravenously every 6 hours	. . .
	Piperacillin + tazobactam	3.375 g intravenously every 6 hours	. . .

MRSA = methicillin-resistant *Staphylococcus aureus*.

    b. After 1–4 days, altered mental status, opisthotonos, painful visible spasms, and motor paresis occur. In 20% of patients, an ascending, symmetric, flaccid areflexia paralysis similar to that seen in Landry's syndrome and Guillain-Barré syndrome may occur.

    c. Hypersensitivity to secondary stimuli and hydrophobia occur in the later stages. Death usually occurs within 4–7 days in untreated patients; coma, convulsions, and apnea occur immediately prior to death.

3. Differential diagnoses include encephalitis, polio, tetanus, meningitis, brain abscess, septic cavernous virus thrombosis, cholinergic poisoning, Landry's syndrome, and Guillain-Barré syndrome.

4. Evaluation. The diagnosis of rabies in animals and humans is made by **analysis of biopsied brain tissue.** Histologic examination will reveal Negri bodies; fluorescent antibody testing can also be performed.

5. Therapy

    a. Postexposure immunoprophylaxis should be instituted as soon as possible. Both of the following therapies are safe for pregnant women.

        (1) Rabies immune globulin (RIG) is administered as follows: 20 IU/kg daily, with half the dose infiltrated locally at the exposure site and the other half administered intramuscularly.

        (2) Human diploid cell vaccine (HDCV) is given in five 1-mL doses on days 0, 3, 7, 14, and 28.

    b. Prompt cleansing and debridement of the wound and **tetanus prophylaxis** should also be initiated.

6. Disposition. Any patient suspected of having rabies should be admitted to the ICU for supportive management.

7. Prevention. Preexposure rabies prophylaxis should be considered for people involved in wildlife trapping or rabies vaccine production, animal handlers, and travelers to underdeveloped countries.

E **Tetanus**

    1. Discussion

a. **Etiology.** Tetanus is an acute, frequently fatal illness that results from infection of a wound with *Clostridium tetani,* an anaerobic, Gram-positive rod that can exist in either a vegetative or sporulated form.

b. **Pathogenesis.** The spores are resistant to destruction and can survive in the soil for years. Once a spore is introduced into a wound, any factor that lowers the oxidation-reduction potential, such as crushed, devitalized tissue, can favor the transformation of *C. tetani* from its sporulated form to its toxin-producing vegetative form.

   (1) The incubation period is 24 hours to 1 month. The shorter the incubation period is, the more severe the disease is.

   (2) *C. tetani* produces an exotoxin, **tetanospasmin,** which is transported to the CNS by retrograde axonal transport and via the bloodstream. Tetanospasmin acts on the motor endplates of the skeletal muscles and on the spinal cord, brain, and sympathetic nervous system to prevent transmission at inhibitory interneurons in the CNS.

c. **Incidence.** In the United States, approximately 60 cases of tetanus are reported each year, with an overall fatality rate of 21%. Most of these cases occur in individuals older than 50 years who are inadequately immunized.

2. **Clinical features** include muscular rigidity, violent muscular contractions, and autonomic dysfunction. Clinical tetanus has four forms.

   a. **Local tetanus** is persistent rigidity of the muscles in close proximity to the site of injury.

   b. **Generalized tetanus** begins as pain and stiffness in the jaw muscles and progresses to involve muscular contractions and rigidity of the whole body.

   c. **Cephalic tetanus** follows injuries to the head, involves cranial nerve dysfunction, and has a particularly poor prognosis.

   d. **Neonatal tetanus** is an important cause of infant mortality in developing countries and carries an extremely high mortality rate.

3. **Differential diagnoses** include strychnine poisoning, neuroleptic malignant syndrome, meningitis, encephalitis, hypocalcemia tetany, rabies, and temporomandibular joint (TMJ) disease.

4. **Evaluation.** The diagnosis is purely clinical.

5. **Therapy**

   a. **Treatment of complications.** Respiratory compromise may require immediate neuromuscular blockade and orotracheal intubation.

   b. **Minimizing the spread of toxin**

      (1) **Wound debridement.** All wounds into which spores were potentially introduced must be identified and débrided. A wound may not be identified in up to 20% of patients.

      (2) **Tetanus immune globulin (TIG)** is administered as a single intramuscular dose of 3000–5000 U to neutralize circulating toxin. Although TIG does not ameliorate the patient's symptoms, studies have shown that it does significantly decrease mortality.

      (3) **Penicillin G** (10 million U intravenously every 24 hours) or **erythromycin** (2 g/day intravenously) are the drugs of choice to eradicate the organism.

   c. **Treatment of autonomic dysfunction.** Autonomic dysfunction can be successfully treated with **labetalol** (0.25–1 mg/min continuous intravenous infusion), **magnesium sulfate** (a loading dose of 70 mg/kg intravenously followed by infusion of 1–4 mg/hour to maintain a serum level of 2.5–4 mm/L), and **morphine sulfate** (5–30 mg intravenously every 2–8 hours) or **clonidine** (300 μg every 8 hours per nasogastric tube).

   d. **Immunization.** Patients who recover from tetanus must undergo active immunization because the disease does not confer immunity. **Tetanus toxoid** (0.5 mL) should be administered at 1 and 6 weeks and at 6 months after injury.

6. **Disposition.** All patients suspected of having tetanus must be admitted to the ICU for further treatment and evaluation.

IV **SEXUALLY TRANSMITTED DISEASES (OTHER THAN AIDS)**

A **Gonorrhea**

1. **Discussion**
   a. **Etiology.** Gonorrhea is caused by *Neisseria gonorrhoeae.*
   b. **Pathogenesis.** The organism attaches to the surface of epithelial cells, especially in the urethra, genital tract, rectum, and throat.
   c. **Incidence.** Gonorrhea is the most frequently reported communicable disease in the United States (over 1 million cases reported annually). The highest incidence is in men between the ages of 20 and 24 years.

2. **Clinical features**
   a. **Local disease**
      (1) **Acute urethritis** is the most common presentation in heterosexual men. Symptoms begin within 1–14 days of exposure and consist of dysuria and penile discharge. Three to ten percent of men with gonorrhea may be asymptomatic.
      (2) **Cervicitis.** Primary gonorrhea in women is **usually asymptomatic,** and when symptoms do occur, they are usually mild and nonspecific. Up to 20% of women with primary gonorrhea develop **pelvic inflammatory disease (PID),** and 33%–81% of women with PID have gonorrhea.
      (3) **Pharyngeal gonorrhea** is **usually asymptomatic.** The pharynx is colonized in 3%–7% of heterosexual men, 5%–20% of women, 10%–25% of homosexual men, and 39%–96% of pregnant women.
      (4) **Anorectal gonorrhea** is common in both heterosexual women and homosexual men, and is **often asymptomatic.** When symptoms occur, they are usually **mild pruritus** and **rectal discomfort.**
   b. **Disseminated gonorrhea** may complicate the disease course in 1%–3% of patients with localized disease and is manifested most commonly as an **acute arthritis** or **dermatitis syndrome.**

3. **Differential diagnoses**
   a. **Gonococcal urethritis** must be differentiated from nongonococcal urethritis caused by *Chlamydia trachomatis.*
   b. **Disseminated gonorrhea.** *N. meningitidis* infection, acute rheumatic fever, and Reiter's syndrome must be ruled out. Differential diagnoses for skin lesions include syphilis, HIV infection, and condyloma acuminata.

4. **Evaluation.** Gram stain and culture of discharges are the cornerstone of diagnosis. All patients evaluated for gonorrhea should also have blood drawn for syphilis serology.

5. **Therapy.** For uncomplicated cervicitis or urethritis, **ceftriaxone** (250 mg intramuscularly) and **doxycycline** (100 mg orally twice daily for 14 days, to cure possible concomitant *Chlamydia* infection) are the standard therapy.
   a. **Cefixime** (400 mg orally in a single dose), **ciprofloxacin** (500 mg orally in a single dose), or **ofloxacin** (400 mg orally as a single dose) are all approved alternatives to ceftriaxone.
   b. **Erythromycin** (500 mg orally four times daily for 7 days) can replace doxycycline in pregnant patients or those allergic to tetracyclines.

6. **Disposition**
   a. Uncomplicated gonorrhea is managed on an outpatient basis. All sexual contacts must be identified and treated, and HIV testing should be considered by the patient with his or her primary physician at a later date.
   b. Patients with disseminated gonorrhea require hospitalization.

B **Syphilis**

1. **Discussion**

   a. Etiology. Syphilis is caused by *T. pallidum.*
   b. Incidence. There are 29,000 new cases of syphilis each year. This figure represents probably only 10% of actual cases.

2. **Clinical features**
   a. Primary syphilis. After an average incubation period of approximately 3 weeks, a smooth, painless ulcer called a **chancre** appears at the site of primary inoculation. The chancre heals without treatment in approximately 3–6 weeks; at about the same time, a painless uni- or bilateral regional **adenopathy** develops.
   b. Secondary syphilis represents disseminated disease and occurs in all patients with untreated primary infection. The lesions of secondary syphilis are **papulosquamous lesions** that occur over the entire trunk, extremities, penis, and buttocks. **Fever** and **weight loss** occur in 70% of patients.
   c. Tertiary syphilis occurs at least 10 years after the primary infection in at least 30%–35% of untreated patients. The two most important manifestations of tertiary syphilis are **cardiovascular syphilis,** causing thoracic aneurysms, and **neurosyphilis,** causing meningitis, stroke, seizures, dementia, general weakness, and posterior column dysfunction.

3. **Differential diagnoses** include chancroid, HSV-1 infection, lymphogranuloma venereum (LGV), tinea, sarcoid, lichen planus, seborrhea dermatitis, molluscum contagiosum, traumatic ulcer, furuncle, and carcinoma.

4. **Evaluation.** The clinical diagnosis can be confirmed by **darkfield microscopic examination** or **serologic testing** (see Chapter 5 V A 4).

5. **Therapy**
   a. The standard treatment for **primary, secondary,** and **early tertiary syphilis** is **benzathine penicillin G** (2.4 million U administered intramuscularly as a single dose). **Ceftriaxone, ciprofloxacin, ofloxacin,** and **cefixime** can also be used in the same doses used to treat gonorrhea.
   b. For **late tertiary syphilis** or **neurosyphilis, benzathine penicillin G** (2.4 million U, three doses administered intramuscularly 1 week apart) is used. **Doxycycline** (100 mg orally twice daily for 14 days) can be given to patients who are allergic to penicillin.

6. **Disposition**
   a. Primary and secondary syphilis can be treated on an outpatient basis.
   b. Patients with neurosyphilis or major cardiovascular manifestations require admission for intravenous therapy.

C Chlamydia

1. **Discussion**
   a. Etiology. Chlamydia is caused by *C. trachomatis,* an obligate intracellular bacterium.
   b. Pathogenesis. The incubation period is typically 1–3 weeks and symptoms, if present, can range from mild burning or irritation to those of peritonitis.

2. **Clinical features.** Chlamydia infections present a wide range of clinical manifestations.
   a. In **men,** infection causes **urethritis, epididymitis,** and **proctitis.**
   b. In **women, urethritis, cervicitis,** and **PID** are common.
   c. LGV. Chlamydia can cause painless, shallow ulcerations or nodular lesions with lymphadenopathy. These lesions, along with the associated lymph nodes and sinus tracts, can become fluctuant and are accompanied by constitutional symptoms of fever, chills, headache, and malaise.
   d. The incidence of **asymptomatic infection** is high, from 3%–20%.

3. **Differential diagnoses** include gonorrhea and urinary tract infection (UTI).

4. **Evaluation.** Although the organism can be cultured, the yield is relatively low. **ELISA** is currently the most accurate means of diagnosis.

5. **Therapy. Doxycycline** (100 mg orally twice daily by mouth) has been the standard therapy, but **azithromycin** (1 g orally in a single dose) appears to be as effective.

6. **Disposition.** Once treated, patients can be discharged with strict instructions to have their partners checked and to follow up for culture results.

D **Chancroid** is discussed in Chapter 5 V C.

E **Trichomoniasis**

1. **Discussion.** Trichomoniasis is caused by the protozoan *Trichomonas vaginalis.* It is contracted through contact with genital secretions.

2. **Clinical features.** After an incubation period of 4–20 days, women develop vaginitis characterized by a **copious, foamy, yellow discharge with a foul odor.** Men are usually asymptomatic.

3. **Differential diagnoses** include *Gardnerella* vaginitis, candidiasis, gonorrhea, syphilis, and HSV infection.

4. **Evaluation.** Diagnosis is by microscopic identification of the motile, flagellated parasites on a wet-mount slide.

5. **Therapy. Metronidazole** (250 mg orally three times daily for 7 days or 2 g orally as a single dose) is recommended. In pregnant women, a 7-day course of **1% clotrimazole vaginal cream** is used.

F **Herpes**

1. **Discussion.** Herpes is the most common ulcerative sexually acquired lesion in the United States.
   a. **Etiology.** There are two clinically indistinguishable forms of the virus, HSV-1 and HSV-2. Although HSV-2 more commonly causes lesions in the genital area and HSV-1 more commonly causes lesions on the face, the two forms can exist (together or separately) anywhere on the body.
   b. **Pathogenesis.** Infants may acquire the infection while passing through the birth canal, leading to meningitis and ophthalmic involvement. The incubation period is 2–21 days.

2. **Clinical features.** HSV causes recurrent, painful, vesicular ulcerations, most commonly on the cervix and vulva in women and the glans and prepuce in men. The initial episode may last several weeks and be accompanied by a flu-like illness, but subsequent recurrences are usually shorter in duration and less intense than the initial episode.

3. **Differential diagnoses** include chancroid, LGV, and syphilis.

4. **Evaluation.** Diagnosis is usually made by history and physical appearance of the lesions and confirmed by culture of the serous fluid from the lesions.

5. **Therapy.** There is currently no cure.
   a. Initial episodes may be treated with **acyclovir** (200 mg five times daily for 7 days), which usually decreases the duration and the intensity of the episode.
   b. Treatment of recurrent episodes is usually not very effective unless initiated early in the presentation of the episode. Early initiation of therapy may shorten the course of the illness by 1–2 days. Suppressive acyclovir therapy has been used with some success for those patients who have multiple recurrent episodes, although the episodes usually return once suppressive therapy is discontinued.

6. **Disposition.** Herpes is treated on an outpatient basis.

V   **UPPER RESPIRATORY TRACT INFECTIONS**

A **Streptococcal pharyngitis**

1. **Discussion.** Pharyngitis (infection of the pharynx and tonsils) is commonly caused by viruses and bacteria. **Group A β-hemolytic streptococci** are clearly the most important causative

agents, accounting for half of all pharyngeal infections in patients between the ages of 5 and 15 years.

2. **Clinical features.** Although no set of symptoms is classic for streptococcal pharyngitis, the sudden onset of a fever and sore throat with enlargement of the cervical lymph nodes and red, swollen tonsils and palate are common. The presence of a scarlatiniform rash in the presence of pharyngitis practically identifies a group A β-hemolytic streptococcus as the causative agent. Headache, vomiting, abdominal pain, meningismus, and torticollis can occur as well.

3. **Differential diagnoses** include viral illnesses, diphtheria (*Corynebacterium diphtheriae* infection), *N. gonorrhoeae* infection, and Epstein-Barr virus infection.
    a. **Pharyngeal diphtheria** is characterized by tissue necrosis and the creation of a **pseudomembrane** over the tonsils, soft palate, uvula, or pharyngeal wall that can lead to airway obstruction (see V B).
    b. **Pharyngeal gonorrhea.** *N. gonorrhoeae* causes a mild or asymptomatic pharyngitis seen in some sexually active adults and victims of child abuse [see IV A 2 a (3)].
    c. **Infectious mononucleosis.** Epstein-Barr virus usually causes asymptomatic infections early in childhood and adolescence, but has been associated with isolated tonsillopharyngitis characterized by malaise, fatigue, and sore throat. There is an increase in the number of atypical lymphocytes on peripheral blood smear and the heterophil antibody is present in over 90% of patients older than 5 years. Infectious mononucleosis is generally a benign, self-limited, somewhat prolonged illness.

4. **Evaluation**
    a. **Throat culture** is the mainstay of diagnosis.
    b. **Serology.** Rapid streptococcal antigen detection techniques that involve extraction of group A carbohydrate antigen from a throat swab and combination of the antigen with a latex agglutination, conglutination, or ELISA take 10–30 minutes to perform and have sensitivities of 50%–90% and specificities of 98%–100% when compared with throat culture (the gold standard).

5. **Therapy.** The objectives of management are to prevent rheumatic fever and suppurative complications, and to hasten recovery.
    a. **Antibiotic therapy**
        (1) A single dose of intramuscular **penicillin G benzathine** (600,000–1.2 million U for an average-sized adult) is very effective.
        (2) Oral **penicillin V** (250 mg four times daily for 10 days) is equally effective.
        (3) **First-** and **second-generation cephalosporins** and **erythromycin** are popular alternatives for patients who are allergic to penicillin.
    b. **Symptomatic therapy** includes acetaminophen, over-the-counter throat sprays and lozenges, and warm fluids.
    c. **Tonsillectomy.** Indications for tonsillectomy remain controversial, though some authors feel that children with many recurrent episodes of tonsillitis (more than seven in 1 year) may benefit from surgical management.

6. **Disposition.** Pharyngitis is managed primarily on an outpatient basis.

B **Diphtheria** is an acute infectious disease characterized by the formation of a fibrinous pseudomembrane on the respiratory mucosa. Cutaneous diphtheria lesions are also common.

1. **Discussion**
    a. **Etiology.** Diphtheria is caused by *C. diphtheriae.*
    b. **Pathogenesis**
        (1) Transmission is via the secretions of infected individuals or carriers, or via contaminated fomites.

(2) Following a short incubation period (1–4 days), the bacillus begins to destroy a layer of superficial epithelium, forming an exudate that coagulates to form a grayish pseudomembrane containing bacteria, fibrin, leukocytes, and necrotic epithelial cells.

(3) The multiplying microbes produce an exotoxin that is lethal to host cells. Damage to the myocardium, nervous tissue, and renal tissue occurs following hematogenous transport of the exotoxin. Complications that can occur if treatment is not prompt include:

  (a) Myocarditis (days 10–14), congestive heart failure (CHF), and arrhythmias
  (b) Peripheral nerve palsies (weeks 3–6), bilateral flaccid weakness or paralysis, decreased deep tendon reflexes, ptosis, strabismus, and the inability to accommodate

  c. **Predisposing factors.** Crowded habitats and low socioeconomic status predispose to the spread of diphtheria. The most significant risk factor, however, is inadequate immunization.

2. **Clinical features**
   a. **Symptoms.** Patients complain of a sore throat, dysphagia, and a low-grade fever accompanied by nausea, vomiting, chills, and a headache. The patient's breathing may be labored as a result of upper airway edema or sudden detachment of the pseudomembrane, leading to sudden respiratory obstruction.
   b. **Physical examination findings** include tachycardia and the pseudomembrane. Attempts to remove the pseudomembrane usually result in bleeding.

3. **Differential diagnoses** include streptococcal pharyngitis, viral pharyngitis, gonococcal pharyngitis, oral syphilis, Vincent's angina, epiglottitis, and (in the late stages of disease) Guillain-Barré syndrome.

4. **Evaluation.** The diagnosis is largely based on the clinical appearance of the membrane.
   a. **Culture.** If antibiotic therapy has not been initiated, growth on Loeffler's agar will reveal an aerobic, motile organism in 8–12 hours.
   b. **Gram staining** of the membrane may show Gram-positive, club-shaped rods.

5. **Therapy.** Spontaneous reversal occurs slowly over many weeks, but prompt treatment is essential to avoid complications. Recovery is slow, and too rapid a return to even "normal" levels of physical activity may worsen toxin-induced myocarditis.
   a. **Diphtheria antitoxin** is derived from horse serum (therefore, sensitivity testing is recommended) and administered intramuscularly to neutralize the toxin. Antitoxin neutralizes only that toxin that is not yet bound to cells and should be administered immediately, without waiting for culture results. The dosage of the antitoxin is based on the patient's clinical presentation, not on age or weight.
   b. **Antibacterial therapy.** Penicillin G eliminates the carrier state but has not been shown to alter the course, complications, or outcome of diphtheria. Erythromycin, ampicillin, clindamycin, and rifampin may also be useful.
   c. **Supportive therapy**
      (1) If oxygenation is impaired or obstruction appears imminent secondary to dislodgement of the membrane, tracheostomy is preferred over endotracheal intubation.
      (2) Nutritional status, hydration status, and electrolyte balance should be addressed as necessary.
      (3) Neurologic and cardiovascular status should be monitored continuously and carefully.

6. **Disposition.** Patients require immediate admission to the ICU.

7. **Prevention**
   a. Contacts of patients with negative cultures and no symptoms should maintain adequate immunization status.
   b. Asymptomatic carriers (those with positive cultures but no symptoms) should be treated with a full course of antibiotics and isolation at home.
   c. Symptomatic carriers should be treated with antibiotics and antitoxin.

C **Epiglottitis**

1. **Discussion.** Inflammatory disorders of the laryngeal region may be either supraglottic (i.e., affecting the supraglottis or epiglottis) or infraglottic (i.e., affecting the larynx or trachea). The disease entity known as epiglottitis would be more appropriately called supraglottitis in that the pathologic changes involve not only the epiglottis, but also the aryepiglottic folds and the false vocal cords.

   a. **Etiology.** Epiglottitis can result from:
      (1) **Chemical damage** (e.g., aspiration of gasoline)
      (2) **Mechanical injury** (e.g., trauma, burns)
      (3) **Sarcoidosis** (causes chronic epiglottitis)
      (4) **Infection**
         (a) **Viruses** (e.g., parainfluenza virus, adenovirus, respiratory syncytial virus, herpes virus)
         (b) **Bacteria** (e.g., *H. influenzae,* group A β-hemolytic streptococci, *S. pneumoniae, Haemophilus parainfluenzae, Klebsiella pneumoniae, Fusobacterium necrophorum, Pasteurella multocida*)
         (c) **Fungi** (e.g., *Aspergillus, Candida*)

   b. **Pathogenesis.** Resistance to flow within a cylinder is proportional to the length of the cylinder divided by the cylinder's radius to the fourth power. Therefore, a decrease in the radius of only 2 mm will produce a 16-fold increase in the resistance to airflow! The pathogenesis of airway obstruction at this level includes:
      (1) Mucosal edema
      (2) Inspissation of secretions
      (3) Aspiration of secretions
      (4) Laryngospasm of the inflamed hyperesthetic larynx

2. **Clinical features.** Epiglottitis is characterized by a sudden, fulminant course.
   a. **Patient history.** Usually, there is no history of a prodromal upper respiratory tract infection. (This is in contrast to what is normally observed in patients with croup.)
   b. **Symptoms** include a disproportionately sore throat, fever, a muffled voice (versus the hoarseness seen in croup; see Chapter 15 III), minimal coughing (versus the bark-like cough seen in croup), dysphagia, and respiratory distress.
   c. **Physical examination findings** include:
      (1) Drooling, dyspnea, tachypnea, inspiratory stridor (softer and less prominent than that seen with croup), and use of the accessory respiratory muscles
      (2) Cervical adenopathy
      (3) Tripod position (patient leans forward, supporting him- or herself with both hands, and hyperextends his or her neck)
      (4) Toxic or septic appearance

3. **Differential diagnoses** include croup, sepsis, aspirated foreign body, peritonsillar or retropharyngeal abscess, diphtheria, lingual tonsillitis, angioedema, pharyngitis, drug allergy, inhalation or ingestion of toxic substances, acute thyroiditis, and epiglottic hematoma.

4. **Evaluation.** Examination of the pharynx and administration of sedatives should be avoided when evaluating a patient with suspected epiglottitis. No patient in respiratory distress or with any indications of potential airway compromise should ever be transferred to another institution.
   a. **Laryngoscopy** can be used to view the pharynx and larynx in adults.
      (1) **Indications.** Oral instrumentation (e.g., indirect laryngoscopy) is indicated in the following circumstances:
         (a) Patients in whom epiglottitis is only suspected and with mild to moderate signs and symptoms
         (b) Patients without any indicators of potential airway compromise

(2) Extreme caution should be employed. The procedure should be performed only in EDs with immediately accessible complete resuscitation equipment by a physician experienced in laryngoscopy.

   b. **Radiography.** A portable lateral neck radiograph is adequate for the diagnosis of epiglottitis and is much safer than allowing the patient to leave the ED. Most radiographic studies are inconclusive and should not be performed until experts on airway intervention are on-site. However, soft tissue lateral neck radiographs may demonstrate enlargement of the epiglottis (greater than 8 mm) and aryepiglottic folds (greater than 7 mm) and/or ballooning of the hypopharynx with air.

5. **Therapy**
   a. **Intubation** (in a controlled setting, ideally in the operating room, by an anesthesiologist, oto-laryngologist, or pediatric surgeon) is necessary.
      (1) Venipuncture, injections, ABG analysis, the use of oxygen masks, and the taking of radiographs should be avoided until the patient is successfully intubated.
      (2) Blind nasal or orotracheal intubation should never be attempted.
   b. **Administration of a helium–oxygen mixture** (e.g., Heliox 80:20 or 70:30) has been recommended as a temporizing measure in the acute phase while preparing for definitive treatment. The density of helium is less than that of nitrogen and therefore decreases airflow resistance and turbulence through narrowed conduits. **Administration of racemic epinephrine is contraindicated.**
   c. **Antibiotic therapy** should be initiated immediately after blood and epiglottic cultures are taken and successful intubation has occurred.
      (1) The antibiotic of choice is **cefotaxime** (50 mg/kg every 8 hours) or **ceftriaxone** (50 mg/kg/day administered intravenously in four equal doses).
      (2) As an alternative, **ampicillin** (200 mg/kg/day administered intravenously in four equal doses) together with **chloramphenicol** (100 mg/kg/day administered intravenously in four equal doses) can be used until the results of cultures and sensitivities are available. Drug levels should be monitored.
   d. **Surgical intervention.** Bedside cricothyrotomy or tracheostomy may be necessary. Transtracheal needle jet ventilation in children younger than 8 years old may be done as a temporizing measure until the tracheostomy can be performed in the operating room.

6. **Disposition.** Laryngoscopy should be repeated prior to extubation, which is usually accomplished in 24–48 hours with appropriate treatment. ICU monitoring is indicated for 24 hours following extubation.

7. **Prevention**
   a. **Rifampin prophylaxis** (20 mg/kg/day once daily for 4 days, maximum 600 mg/day) is indicated for all family members and household and day-care contacts.
   b. **Vaccination against** *H. influenzae* is an excellent prophylactic measure but obviously is not 100% effective.

D Laryngitis

1. **Discussion.** Laryngitis in the adult is usually synonymous with hoarseness.
   a. **Etiology**
      (1) **Acute laryngitis.** Causes of acute laryngitis include:
         (a) **Trauma** (e.g., laryngeal hematoma, edema secondary to exposure to heated gasses or liquids, dislocation or disruption of an arytenoid)
         (b) **Infection**
            (i) **Viruses** (e.g., adenoviruses, coronaviruses, parainfluenza viruses, respiratory syncytial viruses)

        (ii) Bacteria (e.g., *Staphylococcus, H. influenzae, C. diphtheriae,* mycobacteria)

        (iii) Fungi

    (2) Chronic laryngitis

      (a) Intralaryngeal causes include benign laryngeal disease (e.g., benign polyps, vocal fatigue) and malignant laryngeal disease.

      (b) Extralaryngeal causes

        (i) Perilaryngeal causes include infiltrating thyroid carcinoma, lymphoma, and deep neck infection.

        (ii) Remote causes include recurrent entrapment from lung cancer and stroke.

        (iii) Systemic causes include neuromuscular disorders, rheumatoid disorders, and infiltrative processes.

2. Clinical features. Hoarseness is the most common manifestation of laryngeal disease regardless of its cause.

  a. Symptoms include dysphagia, odynophagia, and hoarseness. If the hoarseness presents as a part of the self-limited coryza syndrome (the most common form of adult laryngitis), it usually develops 2–4 days into the illness and lasts from 1–3 weeks.

  b. Physical examination findings may include stridor; aspiration; a gray pseudomembrane attached to the posterior pharynx; lesions on the nose, pharynx, larynx, skin, penis, vagina, or bladder; peripheral neuritis or cranial nerve dysfunction; and signs of myocarditis (e.g., heart failure, dysrhythmias).

3. Differential diagnoses

  a. Epiglottitis. Laryngitis must be differentiated immediately from epiglottitis.

    (1) Clinically, findings such as the tripod position, drooling, reluctance to speak, extreme apprehension, stridor, and retractions clearly indicate impending airway obstruction.

    (2) Radiographic findings may help (see V D 4 b).

  b. Diphtheria must also be considered, especially in nonimmunized, not currently immunized, immunocompromised, and immunosuppressed patients. This point is crucial because the treatment of diphtheria is completely different and the need for treatment is urgent.

  c. Aspiration

4. Evaluation

  a. Laboratory studies are generally not helpful diagnostically but may be useful for baseline and follow-up. Diphtheria may be an exception (see V B 4).

  b. Radiography. Radiographic findings in patients with epiglottitis may include a swollen epiglottis ("thumbprint") and a nonuniform hypopharynx that is distended proximal to the point of obstruction. In contrast:

    (1) In mild laryngitis, the radiograph may appear normal.

    (2) In a more severe case of laryngitis, the radiograph may show a normal epiglottis, possibly a distended hypopharynx, and a narrowed subglottic airway.

5. Therapy

  a. Coryza syndrome. Treatment is symptomatic and includes voice rest.

  b. *Staphylococcus* or *H. influenzae* infection. Treatment with a third-generation cephalosporin is effective.

6. Disposition

  a. Discharge. Most patients are discharged for follow-up with their family physician. Patients with hoarseness persisting more than 4–6 weeks should be referred to an otorhinolaryngologist for further evaluation.

  b. Admission. Patients with a clinical presentation suggestive of impending airway obstruction are admitted to the hospital and treated as described for epiglottitis.

VI SKIN AND SOFT TISSUE INFECTIONS

A **Staphylococcal scalded skin syndrome (SSSS)** is an acute, widespread, erythematous process characterized by peeling of the epidermis. Neonates, infants, young children, and immunosuppressed patients are most often affected.

1. **Discussion**
   a. **Etiology.** SSSS is caused by group II coagulase-positive *S. aureus*, phage type 71.
   b. **Pathogenesis**
      (1) **Transmission** is usually via direct contact or through inhalation.
         (a) Epidemics often occur in nurseries or day-care centers.
         (b) In children and immunosuppressed adults, the disease is sporadic.
      (2) The bacteria produce an **epidermolytic toxin** that separates the superficial part of the epidermis from the granular cell layer. The toxin then enters the circulation and causes a rash similar to that of scarlet fever. Loss of the protective skin barrier then exposes the patient to sepsis and fluid and electrolyte imbalance.

2. **Clinical features**
   a. In neonates and infants, the syndrome usually begins as a localized crusted (impetigo-like) infection at the umbilical stump or in the diaper area. In children, it usually starts as a superficially crusted lesion around the nose or ear.
   b. Within 24 hours, tender scarlet areas appear around the crusted lesions. The areas become painful and rapidly progress to large, flaccid blisters that break easily, producing erosions. The epidermis peels off easily in large sheets, leaving moist, glistening surfaces and progressing rapidly (within 36–72 hours) to widespread desquamation of the skin. Minor pressure produces skin separation (Nikolsky sign). Systemic symptoms, including fever, chills, and malaise, ensue.

3. **Differential diagnoses**
   a. **Toxic epidermal necrosis (TEN;** see Chapter 11 X A). A rapid and accurate differential diagnosis between SSSS and TEN is essential because the approach to treatment is completely different.
      (1) SSSS occurs in infants, children, and immunocompromised patients and begins with a staphylococcal infection (which may not have been noted initially).
      (2) TEN usually occurs in older patients and is usually associated with an adverse reaction to a medication. TEN usually has an acute onset and is symmetric.
   b. **Drug hypersensitivity rashes, viral exanthems,** and **the rash of scarlet fever** are usually acute, symmetrical, associated with systemic signs, and nonpainful.
   c. **Toxic shock syndrome (TSS)** presents with a diffuse sunburn-like erythroderma, followed several days later with desquamation of the skin and epidermal sloughing (especially of the palms and soles). The clinical course of the dermatologic lesions readily differentiates the two disease entities, but at a single point in time the two may be difficult to differentiate.
   d. **Thermal burns, genetic bullous diseases, pemphigus vulgaris,** and **bullous pemphigoid** are also characterized by bullae, erosions, and easily loosened epidermis and must be differentiated from SSSS.

4. **Evaluation**
   a. **Cultures** should be taken from the skin, nasopharynx, and blood.
   b. **Skin biopsy** can be used to define the level of epidermal cleavage, allowing SSSS to be differentiated from TEN. Biopsy in SSSS shows cleavage and blister formation within the outermost layer of the epidermis (i.e., the granular cell layer), whereas biopsy in TEN shows subepidermal blister formation (i.e., at the level of the basal cell).

5. **Therapy.** Because the epidermal cleavage is superficial, the stratum corneum is quickly replaced and rapid healing occurs within 5–7 days of appropriate treatment.

    a. **Antibiotic therapy.** Treatment with **systemic penicillinase-resistant antistaphylococcal antibiotics** (e.g., **nafcillin,** 50–100 mg/kg/day) should be initiated immediately on the basis of the clinical diagnosis.

    b. **Supportive therapy**

       (1) If the disease is widespread and the lesions are weeping, the skin should be treated as for burns. **Hydrolyzed polymer gel dressings** are useful and reduce the number of dressing changes.

       (2) **Intravenous fluids** should be administered to combat dehydration.

    c. Corticosteroids are contraindicated, and topical therapy and patient handling must be minimized.

B **TSS** is a severe illness characterized by a high fever of sudden onset associated with vomiting, diarrhea, myalgias, and a rash. Hypotension rapidly progressing to shock follows. Although most commonly associated in the public mind with the use of superabsorbent tampons, women who do not use tampons and men have also been affected.

1. **Discussion**

    a. **Etiology.** Although endotoxins have recently been implicated, the most consistent finding and presumed etiology are an **exotoxin [toxic shock syndrome toxin-1 (TSST-1)]** produced by a strain of phage group I *S. aureus.*

    b. **Pathogenesis.** The organism has been isolated from mucosal surfaces (e.g., the nasopharynx, trachea, vagina) and the skin, empyemas, abscesses, and wounds. It is thought that the exotoxin enters the blood through breaks in the mucosa or the peritoneal cavity. TSS has been seen in postoperative patients; typically, the wound associated with this disease is characteristically very benign in appearance.

2. **Clinical features** include the sudden onset of fever (102°F–105°F), headache, intermittent confusion, lethargy, and an absence of focal neurologic findings. Patients may have a sore throat and nonpurulent conjunctivitis. Vomiting and profuse watery diarrhea are also noted. The characteristic rash is a diffuse sunburn-like erythroderma, which between days 3 and 7 desquamates, leading to epidermal sloughing that is readily noticed on the palms and soles. Hypotension is associated with peripheral and pulmonary edema in the absence of an elevated central venous pressure.

3. **Differential diagnoses** include SSSS, TEN, streptococcal toxic shock–like syndrome, Kawasaki syndrome, meningococcemia, scarlet fever, and viral exanthems.

4. **Evaluation**

    a. **Laboratory studies**

       (1) **CBC.** A CBC will reveal a mild nonhemolytic anemia, a moderate leukocytosis with a predominance of bands, and an early thrombocytopenia followed later by a thrombocytosis.

       (2) **Coagulation tests.** Mild prolongation of the PT and PTT is observed (although clinically apparent bleeding is not).

       (3) **Serum biochemistry.** The blood urea nitrogen (BUN) and creatinine levels are elevated in the presence of oliguria.

       (4) **Liver function tests.** Liver enzyme levels are elevated.

    b. **Culture.** All probable and possible sources of infection should be cultured and Gram stained. *S. aureus* can be cultured from a wound or the vagina in 90% of patients. Rarely, a positive culture for *S. aureus* can be obtained from the blood.

    c. **Serology.** Serum antibodies to TSST-1 are not detectable, but serology performed on an *S. aureus* isolate may be positive.

    d. **Skin biopsy** shows subepidermic cleavage (as in TEN).

5. **Therapy.** Foreign objects (e.g., tampons, diaphragms, sponges) must be removed immediately, and hypotension or shock should be treated with fluids and electrolytes. Treatment with a **β lactamase–resistant penicillin** or **cephalosporin** should be initiated immediately.

6. **Disposition.** Patients must be admitted to the ICU immediately. The mortality rate is 10%–15%.

C **Streptococcal toxic shock–like syndrome** is a life-threatening infectious syndrome characterized by fever, rash, rapidly progressive and destructive soft tissue infection, and hypotension. In the lay press, after the death of the famous puppeteer Jim Henson, this disease became known as the "flesh-eating disease."

1. **Discussion**
   a. **Etiology.** Streptococcal toxic shock–like syndrome is caused by *Streptococcus pyogenes*, a group A β-hemolytic streptococcus.
   b. **Pathogenesis.** Bacteremia is the pathogenic mechanism of the ensuing shock.

2. **Clinical features.** Streptococcal toxic shock–like syndrome presents in a fashion very similar to TSS, except that the source of the soft tissue infection is exceedingly obvious.

3. **Differential diagnoses** include TSS, SSSS, and TEN.

4. **Evaluation.** Diagnosis is based on the clinical presentation and the dermatologic findings. Site and blood cultures will grow *S. pyogenes.*

5. **Therapy.** Antibacterial therapy must be effective against both *S. aureus* and *S. pyogenes,* because until the culture results are available, the diagnosis cannot be made with absolute certainty on clinical grounds alone.

6. **Disposition.** All patients must be admitted to the ICU. In nonimmunocompromised patients, the mortality rate is 30%; in immunocompromised patients, the mortality rate is 60% within 24 hours.

D **Cellulitis** is a diffuse, spreading, acute inflammatory process affecting solid tissues and characterized by hyperemia, leukocytic infiltration, and edema without cellular necrosis or suppuration.

1. **Discussion**
   a. **Etiology.** *S. pyogenes* is the most common cause. Other less common causes include other serologic groups of β-hemolytic streptococci (B, C, and G), *S. aureus, P. multocida* (from cat or dog bites), *Aeromonas hydrophila* (from fresh water), *Vibrio vulnificus* (from warm salt water), and aerobic Gram-negative bacilli (in patients with granulocytopenia, diabetic foot ulcers, or severe tissue ischemia).
   b. **Pathogenesis.** The diffuse spread of infection occurs because streptokinase, DNase, and hyaluronidase (enzymes produced by *S. pyogenes*) degrade cellular components that would otherwise contain and localize the inflammatory process.
   c. **Predisposing factors** include skin trauma or ulceration, preexisting infections (e.g., tinea pedis), scars (especially from saphenous vein removal), immunocompromise, and edema.

2. **Clinical features.** The major findings are local erythema and tenderness, often with lymphangitis and lymphadenopathy.
   a. The skin is hot, red, and edematous and the borders of the lesions are usually indistinct. Peau d'orange and petechiae are frequently observed. Vesicles and bullae may develop and rupture. Occasionally, necrosis of the involved skin is noted. Rarely, there are large areas of ecchymosis.
   b. Systemic manifestations may include fever, chills, and tachycardia.

3. **Differential diagnoses** include erysipelas (spreading infection of the skin and mucous membranes that is usually observed on the face). The rash of **erysipelas** differs from that of cellulitis in that the raised margins are sharply demarcated.

4. **Evaluation.** The diagnosis depends mainly on the clinical findings.
   a. **Laboratory studies.** Leukocytosis is common.
   b. **Culture.** Culturing of the etiologic organism is difficult, even with aspiration or biopsy of the involved area, unless pus has formed or the wound is open. (One must also consider that a positive culture may be detecting a secondary pathogen.) Blood cultures are only occasionally positive.
   c. **Serology.** Serologic tests (e.g., measurement of anti-DNase B) confirm a streptococcal cause, but should not be necessary.

5. **Therapy**
   a. **Supportive therapy**
      (1) The affected area should be elevated and immobilized to help reduce the edema.
      (2) Cool, wet dressings should be applied to relieve local discomfort.
   b. **Antibacterial therapy**
      (1) **Streptococcal cellulitis.** Penicillin is the drug of choice. Alternatives are erythromycin, clindamycin, or macrolides. Neutropenic patients should be started empirically on gentamicin and mezlocillin.
      (2) **Staphylococcal cellulitis.** Dicloxacillin is the drug of choice. Vancomycin, cephalosporins, sulpha, or macrolides should be considered if the infection is caused by a resistant strain (MRSA).
      (3) *P. multocida* **cellulitis.** Penicillin is the drug of choice.
      (4) *A. hydrophila* **cellulitis.** An aminoglycoside should be used.
      (5) *V. vulnificus* **cellulitis.** Tetracycline is the drug of choice.
      (6) **Recurrent cellulitis.** If the recurrent cellulitis affects a lower extremity, treatment for tinea pedis should be undertaken to eliminate a source of infection. If antifungal medication fails, or tinea is not present, recurrent cellulitis can be prevented by monthly administration of benzathine penicillin G, oral penicillin, or erythromycin.

6. **Complications** are rare but could be serious and include:
   a. Severe necrotizing subcutaneous infection
   b. Necrotizing fasciitis
   c. Bacteremia with or without metastatic foci
   d. Chronic lymphatic obstruction
   e. Chronic edema or elephantiasis
   f. Osteomyelitis underlying the infection or hematogenous spread.

E **Lymphangitis** is an acute inflammation of the subcutaneous lymphatic channels.

1. **Discussion**
   a. **Etiology.** *S. pyogenes* is the most common causative agent.
   b. **Pathogenesis.** The microbes usually enter the lymphatic channels from a wound or abrasion, or from a preexisting infection (e.g., a cellulitis).

2. **Clinical features.** Red, warm, tender streaks extend proximally from a peripheral lesion toward regional lymph nodes, which may eventually also become enlarged and tender. Systemic manifestations (e.g., fever, chills, headache) may actually precede any obvious signs of cutaneous infection.

3. **Differential diagnoses** include erythema marginatum (rheumatic fever), cutaneous larva migrans, and erythema chronicum migrans (Lyme disease).

4. **Evaluation.** Diagnosis is clinical. Leukocytosis is usually noted.

5. **Therapy.** Most patients respond readily to appropriate antibiotic therapy (e.g., penicillin for streptococcal infections, cephalosporin for staphylococcal infections). In addition, rest, elevation, and moist head will improve healing.

VII BONE INFECTIONS (OSTEOMYELITIS)

A **Discussion**   Osteomyelitis is microbial invasion and destruction of bone. The elderly, intravenous drug abusers, patients with sickle cell disease, and immunocompromised patients are at the most risk.

1. **Etiology**
   a. *S. aureus* is the most common cause of osteomyelitis in adults.
   b. *P. aeruginosa* and *Serratia marcescens* are more frequently implicated in intravenous drug abusers.
   c. *Salmonella* infection is associated with osteomyelitis in patients with sickle cell disease.

2. **Pathogenesis.** Infection can occur by hematogenous spread, by direct extension, from a retropharyngeal abscess, or by direct contamination.

B **Clinical features** Typical findings are fever and bone pain, but these symptoms occur in only approximately 50% of patients. Localized tenderness over the affected area of the bone or joint that is not relieved by rest is another major sign.

C **Differential diagnoses** include malignancy, degenerative joint disease, and trauma.

D **Evaluation**

1. **Laboratory studies.** An elevated erythrocyte sedimentation rate (ESR) is the most significant finding. The WBC count is also commonly elevated.

2. **Culture.** Blood cultures are positive in approximately 50%–60% of patients.

3. **Imaging studies**
   a. **Plain radiographs** do not usually show the classic findings of lytic lesions, periosteal elevation, and cortical irregularity or destruction until 7–14 days after the onset of symptoms.
   b. **CT scans** and **MRIs** are more sensitive than radiographs. MRI is the best imaging technique, with a sensitivity of 96%, a specificity of 92%, and an accuracy of 94%. **Bone scan** may be used to help localize bone involvement but it is not specific to infection, as cancer and fractures may also show up.

4. **Bone biopsy or aspiration** is necessary to make the diagnosis if blood cultures are negative.

E **Therapy** The current regimen is 4–6 weeks of parenteral antibiotic therapy followed by a prolonged course of oral antibiotics. Because a wide variety of organisms can cause osteomyelitis, proper identification of the causative organism by blood cultures or bone biopsy is essential.

F **Disposition** All patients must be admitted to the hospital for administration of antibiotics and immobilization. An orthopedic or neurosurgical evaluation should always be sought.

VIII   OTHER INFECTIONS

A **Parasitic infections**

1. **Discussion.** The incidence of parasitic disease is increasing in the United States due to immigration from other countries, increased travel, and an increase in immunosuppression caused by HIV.

2. **Clinical entities**
   a. **Ascariasis** is caused by *Ascaris lumbricoides.* The larvae hatch from ingested eggs and migrate through the bloodstream to the lungs, causing **fever, cough, dyspnea, hemoptysis,** and **eosinophilia.**
   b. **Pinworm infection** is caused by *Enterobius vermicularis.* The eggs hatch in the cecum, appendix, ileum, and ascending colon. The gravid female migrates to the anus (usually at night), where it causes an intense pruritus (**pruritus ani**).
   c. **Hookworm infection** is caused by *Necator americanus,* which is prevalent in southern climates. Infection is associated with human waste used as fertilizer and the lack of shoes and latrines. Because each worm feeds on 0.03–0.2 mL of blood per day, chronic infection leads to **chronic anemia,** especially in children. Patients may present with a **cough, low-grade fever, abdominal pain, diarrhea, weakness, weight loss, guaiac-positive stools,** and **eosinophilia.**
   d. **Threadworm infection** is caused by *Strongyloides stercoralis,* which infests the mucosa of the small intestine. The parasite invades the body by penetrating the skin, leading to **pruritus** and an **erythematous rash (cutaneous larval migrans).** As the worms migrate through the lungs to the gastrointestinal tract, they also cause **cough, dyspnea,** and **pneumonia.** After they reach

the intestine, they produce **abdominal pain** and **bloody mucoid diarrhea.** Fatalities have occurred in elderly and immunocompromised patients.

e. **Whipworm infection** is caused by *Trichuris trichiura,* a parasite most often found in rural communities in the United States. Children may become infected when playing in soil contaminated by ova. The adult worm resides in the cecum, causing **anorexia, insomnia, abdominal pain, fever, flatulence, diarrhea, weight loss, pruritus, eosinophilia,** and **microcytic hypochromic anemia.** *Trichuris* infestation can result in **colitis** and **rectal prolapse** in children.

f. **Trichinellosis** is caused by *Trichinella.* Transmission is by the ingestion of infected pork, beef, or walrus meat. Symptoms depend on the number of worms ingested, the number of larvae produced, and the site of invasion, though the primary lesions are in striated muscle; clinical manifestations include **acute myocarditis, nonsuppurative meningitis, bronchopneumonia,** or **catarrhal enteritis.** Patients may present with nausea and vomiting, diarrhea, fever, urticaria, periorbital edema (which is pathognomonic), splinter hemorrhages, myalgia, muscle spasms, a stiff neck, headache, and psychiatric disorders.

g. **Schistosomiasis** is caused by *Schistosoma.* The parasite penetrates the skin, creating a maculopapular rash, and the adult parasites then reside in the venous system.

  (1) **Acute disease (Katayama fever)** is severe but rarely seen; **lymphadenopathy** and **hepatosplenomegaly** are characteristic.

  (2) **Chronic disease.** More typically, patients present in the chronic state with granulomas in the liver (leading to portal hypertension) and bladder (leading to obstructive hydroureter). Patients may present with **diarrhea, abdominal pain, melena, hepatosplenomegaly, hematemesis, ascites,** and **liver failure.** With *S. haematobium* infection, **dysuria** and **hematuria** may be found.

h. **Tapeworm infections** are caused by *Taenia solium* (**pork tapeworm**), *Taenia saginata* (**beef tapeworm**), and *Diphyllobothrium latum* (**fish tapeworm**).

  (1) **Pork tapeworm** is indigenous to Central America and the Middle East. *T. solium* larvae may encyst in the subcutaneous tissues, eye, brain, and heart, causing **seizures, myocarditis, periorbital edema,** and sometimes morbidity.

  (2) **Beef tapeworm** is more common. Adult worms live in the small intestine. Infected patients can present with **nausea, vomiting, headache, abdominal pain, pruritus, constipation, diarrhea,** and **intestinal obstruction,** or they may be **asymptomatic.**

  (3) **Fish tapeworm.** Consumption of raw or undercooked fish (e.g., sushi; sashimi; pickled, salted, or smoked fish) is the most common method of transmission to humans. The parasite resides in the intestine and absorbs vitamin B_{12}, causing a **pernicious anemia.**

i. **Amebiasis** is caused by *E. histolytica.* The amoebae inhabit the cecum and large intestine, causing ulcers and diffuse inflammation that generally mimic ulcerative colitis. Fifty percent of infected patients are **asymptomatic;** the remaining 50% may experience **nausea, vomiting, anorexia, diarrhea, fever, abdominal pain,** and **leukocytosis.** Rarely, amebiasis can develop in the liver and produce an abscess.

j. **Giardiasis** is caused by *Giardia lamblia* and is the most common parasitic intestinal infection in the United States. Cysts are ingested in fecally contaminated water or are passed by hand-to-mouth transmission; once ingested, the parasite inhabits the host's duodenum and upper jejunum. Symptoms include **explosive, foul-smelling diarrhea, flatus, abdominal distention, fatigue, fever, weight loss,** and **malaise.**

k. **Trypanosomiasis** is caused by *Trypanosoma* species.

  (1) *T. cruzi,* the American variety, causes **Chagas' disease.** The acute phase of illness can last 2–3 months and consists of **fever, headache, anorexia, conjunctivitis,** and **myocarditis.** Infants can develop **meningoencephalitis,** and heart involvement can lead to **CHF** and **ventricular aneurysms.** The organism can attack the myenteric plexus of the gastrointestinal tract, resulting in **megacolon.**

      (2) *T. brucei rhodesiense* and *T. brucei gambiense,* the African varieties, cause **sleeping sickness.**

  3. Differential diagnoses include bacterial or viral infection, collagen vascular disease, and neoplasia.

  4. Evaluation is mainly by **fecal analysis** and **serology.**

    a. Ascariasis is diagnosed by finding eggs of the adult worm in the stool sample. Serologic tests (e.g., bentonite flocculation, ELISA, indirect hemagglutination) may also be useful.

    b. Pinworm infection is diagnosed by finding eggs or worms on a cellophane tape swab of the anus. Accuracy is improved by examination and testing in the early morning.

    c. Hookworm infection is diagnosed by finding ova in the stool sample.

    d. Threadworm infection is diagnosed by finding ova in a stool sample or a duodenal aspirate.

    e. Whipworm infection is diagnosed by finding ova in the stool sample.

    f. Trichinellosis is characterized by leukocytosis, eosinophilia, elevated serum creatine phosphokinase levels, and nonspecific electrocardiogram (ECG) charges. The diagnosis can be confirmed with a latex agglutination skin test and a complement fixation or bentonite flocculation test [available from the Centers for Disease Control (CDC)]. ELISA is very sensitive and specific after the third week, and biopsy of tender muscle may be helpful after the fourth week of infection.

    g. Schistosomiasis is diagnosed by observing eggs in the feces or on rectal biopsy.

    h. Tapeworm infection, amebiasis, and **giardiasis** are diagnosed by ova and parasite stool examination and ELISA.

    i. Chagas' disease is characterized by anemia, leukocytosis, an elevated ESR, and ECG changes (PR- and R-wave changes, heart block, arrhythmias). During the acute phase, ELISA tests are helpful and trypomastigotes can be seen on a peripheral smear. In the chronic phase, the diagnosis is made with a complement fixation test or biopsy of the liver, spleen, or bone marrow.

  5. Therapy

    a. Ascariasis, pinworms, and **hookworms** are treated with **mebendazole** or **pyrantel pamoate.**

    b. Whipworms and **trichinellosis** are treated with **mebendazole.**

    c. Threadworms are treated with **thiabendazole.**

    d. Schistosomiasis and **tapeworms** are treated with **praziquantel.**

    e. Amebiasis is treated with **metronidazole** followed by **iodoquinol.**

    f. Giardiasis can be treated with **quinacrine** or **metronidazole.**

    g. Chagas' disease is treated with **nifurtimox.**

  6. Disposition. Most parasitic infections are treated on an outpatient basis, although complications such as dehydration secondary to gastritis or myocardial involvement may require inpatient therapy for supportive care.

B **Tick-borne disease**

  1. Lyme disease

    a. Discussion. Lyme disease, caused by the spirochete **B. burgdorferi,** is the most frequently transmitted tick-borne disease. It is prevalent in 33 of the 50 states, with the highest incidence in the Northeast. The majority of cases occur in the late spring and late summer.

    b. Clinical features. Lyme disease has three stages.

      (1) Stage I is characterized by **erythema chronicum migrans** (an annular lesion) and **flu-like symptoms** of fever, chills, headache, malaise, and weakness. Symptoms appear 3–32 days after the tick bite.

      (2) Stage II begins 4 weeks later. Ten percent of untreated patients develop **neurologic disorders** (e.g., headache, meningoencephalitis, facial nerve palsy, radiculoneuropathy) and **cardiac disease** [e.g., first-, second-, or third-degree atrioventricular (AV) block].

      (3) Stage III occurs in 60% of patients with untreated Lyme disease several weeks or years after infection. Patients develop **migratory polyoligoarthritis** that most often involves the knee, shoulder, and elbow.

   c. Differential diagnoses include viral syndromes, connective tissue disease, Guillain-Barré syndrome, and rheumatoid arthritis.

   d. Evaluation. Diagnosis is best made by careful history and physical examination.

      (1) Laboratory studies. The ESR is usually elevated and the lymphocyte count slightly decreased.

      (2) Serology. Both immunosorbent and immunofluorescent assays are accurate in identifying antibodies to *B. burgdorferi,* but these studies are usually negative during the early stages of the disease; patients may not show a specific rise in antibody titers until stage II or stage III.

   e. Treatment

      (1) Tick removal. If the patient presents with stage I symptoms, a careful search for the tick should ensue. The tick is best removed by grasping the head with forceps and gently pulling it away from the skin.

      (2) Antibacterial therapy

         (a) Adults and nonpregnant women. Treatment is with **doxycycline** (100 mg orally twice daily for 10–21 days).

         (b) Children, allergic patients, and pregnant women. Amoxicillin (40 mg/kg/day three times daily), **penicillin,** or **erythromycin** (30–50 mg/kg/day five times daily for children) can be used.

         (c) Patients with stage II disease. For patients with severe neurologic or cardiac symptoms, **ceftriaxone** (1 g intravenously every 12 hours for 10–14 days) is recommended.

   f. Disposition. Lyme disease can usually be treated on an outpatient basis, regardless of the stage of disease.

2. Rocky Mountain spotted fever

   a. Discussion. Rocky Mountain spotted fever, caused by ***Rickettsia rickettsii,*** is the second most common tick-borne disease. Rocky Mountain spotted fever occurs primarily in the northwest United States, but has also been reported in the southern and eastern states.

      (1) Incidence. There are 500–1000 cases annually. Peak incidence occurs from late spring to early fall.

      (2) Pathogenesis. The bacteria invade small blood vessels throughout the body, leading to vascular damage and a vasculitis secondary to an immunologic response that produces rash, fever, edema, DIC, encephalitis, myocardial necrosis, pulmonary interstitial disease, and adult respiratory distress syndrome (ARDS). The disease can progress to shock and death.

   b. Clinical features. Rocky Mountain spotted fever has a wide clinical spectrum. The triad of fever, headache, and rash is seen in 55%–65% of patients.

      (1) Initial symptoms are fever, followed by an erythematous, maculopapular, blotchy rash that ultimately becomes petechial. The rash is present in 75%–80% of patients, begins at the flexor surfaces of the wrists and ankles, and spreads centripetally.

      (2) Other symptoms are vomiting (66% of patients), myalgia (85% of patients), cough (33% of patients), and signs of meningoencephalitic involvement (25% of patients).

   c. Evaluation. The diagnosis of Rocky Mountain spotted fever is difficult. In addition to the physical examination and history, **immunofluorescent antibody staining** can be performed on a skin biopsy specimen obtained from an area of rash. This test is 100% specific and 70% sensitive. The only other recommended scientific test is the **fluorescent antibody test,** but this test is most often negative in the early phases of the illness. A titer greater than 1:64 or a fourfold rise is diagnostic.

   d. Therapy for Rocky Mountain spotted fever is **tetracycline** (10–70 mg/kg given intravenously in one dose for 10 days for adults and children older than 8 years) or **chloramphenicol** (80 mg/kg given intravenously in one dose for children younger than 8 years).

   e. Disposition. Patients usually require admission.

3. **Tick paralysis**
   a. **Discussion.** Tick paralysis is a relatively uncommon tick-borne disease resulting in an ascending paralysis.
      (1) **Incidence.** Incidence is highest in late spring to late summer and is higher in girls than in boys. The mortality rate in untreated cases may exceed 12%.
      (2) **Pathogenesis.** Tick paralysis is believed to be caused by a venom secreted from the female tick salivary glands during feeding—most probably a neurotoxin that produces a block of the peripheral motor nerve endplate, resulting in a failure of acetylcholine release at the neuromuscular junction.
   b. **Clinical features.** Symptoms of tick paralysis develop within 4–7 days and consist of **restlessness** and **paresthesias of the hands or feet.** Within 1–2 days, the presenting symptoms are followed by a **symmetric, ascending, flaccid paralysis** accompanied by **loss of deep tendon reflexes.** Death can result from respiratory paralysis.
   c. **Evaluation.** Tick paralysis is diagnosed by symptoms and discovery of the tick.
   d. **Therapy.** Tick paralysis is treated by tick removal.
   e. **Disposition.** Admission to the hospital may be required if the patient's symptoms are severe.

4. **Relapsing fever**
   a. **Discussion.** Relapsing fever is an uncommon acute recurrent febrile illness caused by a spirochete of the *Borrelia* species. It is isolated to the western and southwestern United States, with peak incidence in the summer months.
   b. **Clinical features.** After an incubation period of 5–9 days, individuals with **relapsing fever** may experience a febrile episode lasting 3 days, followed by an afebrile period and a return of fever. The fever is accompanied by **chills, malaise, vomiting, headache,** and **myalgias.** Splenomegaly (40% of patients), hepatomegaly (20% of patients), and neurologic involvement (10% of patients) may also be noted.
   c. **Evaluation.** There are no helpful serologic tests for relapsing fever, but peripheral blood smears show spirochetes in up to 70% of patients. Clinical presentation usually points to the diagnosis.
   d. **Therapy.** Relapsing fever is treated with **tetracycline** (500 mg orally four times daily for 10 days) or **erythromycin** (250 mg orally four times daily for 10 days).
   e. **Disposition.** Admission to the hospital may be required if the patient's symptoms are severe.

5. **Q fever** is caused by *Coxiella burnetii* and presents as a flu-like illness characterized by fever, myalgias, headache, and cough. Q fever is diagnosed by complement fixing antibody titers and clinical presentation. The flu-like syndrome resolves spontaneously in 2–4 weeks, but treatment is with tetracycline. Hospital admission may be required in the presence of severe symptoms.

6. **Tularemia**
   a. **Discussion.** Tularemia is caused by the bacterium *Francisella tularensis.* Although it was originally thought that tularemia was spread by rabbits and rabbit meat, it is now recognized that ticks are the most frequent vector. Peak incidence occurs in the summer months; most cases occur in the southern and Midwestern states.
   b. **Clinical features.** Tularemia has two major presentations.
      (1) **Ulceroglandular tularemia** is the most common (occurring in approximately 50% of patients) and presents as lymphadenopathy, fever, and reddened nodules that indurate and then ulcerate.
      (2) **Typhoidal tularemia** presents with fever, chills, debility, abdominal pain, diarrhea, anorexia, and weight loss.
   c. **Evaluation.** Tularemia is diagnosed on the basis of history and physical examination findings. Acute specific agglutination titers greater than 1:160 are diagnostic.

    d. Therapy. Tularemia is treated with **streptomycin** (30–40 mg/kg given in one dose for 4–7 days). **Tetracycline** (50–60 mg/kg given in four divided doses daily for 14 days) is an alternative for patients who are sensitive to streptomycin.

    e. Disposition. Hospital admission is usually required.

7. Babesiosis

    a. Discussion. Babesiosis is caused by ***Babesia,*** an intraerythrocytic protozoal parasite that causes a malaria-like syndrome. The distribution is similar to that of Lyme disease; in fact, the two entities have been seen concurrently in the same patient. Babesiosis was originally reported in only splenectomized individuals, but since 1969 there has been an increased incidence in all patients.

    b. Clinical features. Babesiosis has a broad range of clinical presentations, from a brief febrile illness to severe disease characterized by hemolytic anemia, hemoglobinuria, and death.

        (1) Fever, malaise, anorexia, and fatigue are almost universally present. Headache and mild to moderate hemolytic anemia are also commonly seen.

        (2) The physical examination is usually nonspecific, although splenomegaly is seen in 40% of patients.

    c. Evaluation. Thick and thin Giemsa-stained blood smears will usually show intraerythrocytic organisms. A presumptive diagnosis can also be made by using indirect immunofluorescent staining for antibody if the titers are greater than 1:256.

    d. Therapy

        (1) Antibacterial therapy. Babesiosis can be treated with **clindamycin** (600 mg orally twice daily for adults; 20–30 mg/kg/day every 6 hours for children) and **quinine** (650 mg orally twice daily for adults; 25 mg/kg/day every 8 hours for children) for 14 days.

        (2) Exchange transfusion has been effective in severe cases.

    e. Disposition. Hospital admission is indicated for patients with severe disease.

8. Colorado tick fever

    a. Discussion. Colorado tick fever is caused by an orbivirus of the family Reoviridae. Only 200 cases are reported annually.

    b. Clinical features. Patients develop the sudden onset of fever, headache, lethargy, myalgias, and anorexia within 3–6 days of exposure.

    c. Evaluation is by the clinical presentation and history.

    d. Therapy. Colorado tick fever is a self-limited disease. Patients usually recover in 3 weeks and treatment is supportive.

    e. Disposition. Patients with severe symptoms may require hospital admission.

Study Questions

Directions: *Each of the numbered items or incomplete statements in this section is followed by answers or by completions of the statement. Select the ONE lettered answer or completion that is BEST in each case.*

1. Which one of the following treatments is appropriate for a 25-year-old man who was bitten by a dog while vacationing in Mexico City? (The dog was unprovoked, and the patient's last tetanus shot was 2 years ago.)
   - (A) Wound cleansing and debridement, 20 IU/kg rabies immune globulin (RIG; half of the dose at the bite site, and half intramuscularly), and the first of five doses of human diploid cell vaccine (HDCV)
   - (B) Wound cleansing and debridement, 10 IU/kg RIG intramuscularly, and the first of five doses of HDCV
   - (C) Wound cleansing and debridement, 20 IU/kg RIG (half of the dose at the bite site, the other half intramuscularly), the first of five doses of HDCV, and 0.5 mL tetanus toxoid administered intramuscularly
   - (D) Wound cleansing and debridement and the first of five doses of HDCV

2. A woman presents with a painless ulcer measuring 3 mm on her vulva, and has associated tender abdominal and inguinal lymphadenopathy. The woman also complains of mild lower abdominal discomfort and a clear vaginal discharge. What is the most likely diagnosis?
   - (A) Condyloma lata
   - (B) Herpes simplex virus (HSV) infection
   - (C) Lymphogranuloma venereum (LGV)
   - (D) Chancroid
   - (E) Granuloma inguinale

3. An 8-year-old boy in Oklahoma is brought to the emergency department (ED) over the Fourth of July weekend because of fever, chills, malaise, arthralgias, and a headache. Physical examination reveals a maculopapular rash that is most prominent on his wrists and ankles. What is the most likely diagnosis?
   - (A) Meningitis
   - (B) Lyme disease
   - (C) Rabies
   - (D) Rocky Mountain spotted fever
   - (E) Babesiosis

4. A 20-year-old woman complains of progressive weakness in her lower extremities but denies having any other symptoms. Physical examination reveals an afebrile patient with absent deep tendon reflexes. What is the most likely diagnosis?
   - (A) Rabies
   - (B) Tetanus
   - (C) Relapsing fever
   - (D) Tick paralysis
   - (E) Lyme disease

5. Which common parasite can cause rectal prolapse in children?
   - (A) *Ascaris lumbricoides*
   - (B) *Enterobius vermicularis*
   - (C) *Trichuris trichiura*
   - (D) *Trichinella*
   - (E) *Taenia solium*

6. A pregnant woman who has been vacationing at Martha's Vineyard presents to the emergency department (ED) complaining of photophobia and a mild frontal headache. On further evaluation, she is found to have third-degree atrioventricular (AV) block. What is the appropriate treatment for this patient at this time?

- (A) Doxycycline (100 mg orally twice daily for 14 days) and discharge
- (B) Amoxicillin (500 mg orally three times daily for 14 days) and discharge
- (C) Chloramphenicol (50 mg/kg/day intravenously) and admission
- (D) Ceftriaxone (1 g intravenously every 12 hours), temporary pacemaker placement, and admission
- (E) Tetracycline (500 mg intravenously every 6 hours), temporary pacemaker placement, and admission

7. Which of the following drugs or fluids is not considered useful in the treatment of septic shock?

- (A) Isoproterenol
- (B) Normal saline
- (C) Lactated Ringer's solution
- (D) Dopamine
- (E) Norepinephrine

Answers and Explanations

1. The answer is A In a patient who has been bitten by an unfamiliar dog, especially one in a developing country, possible rabies exposure should be assumed. The correct treatment is 20 IU/kg of RIG, half of the dose administered at the bite site and half administered intramuscularly, plus the first of five vaccinations with HDCV. HDCV will be administered again on days 3, 7, 14, and 28. Prompt cleansing and debridement of the wound are also indicated. Because the patient has had a tetanus booster within the last 5 years, a second booster is not necessary at this time.

2. The answer is C LGV is characterized by painless, ulcerated lesions associated with lymphadenopathy. Caused by *Chlamydia trachomatis,* LGV can also be associated with the classic presentation for pelvic inflammatory disease (PID). The lesions of chancroid, while ulcerative, are usually painful. Granuloma inguinale presents with painless lesions that can develop into extensive ulcerative lesions, but this infection is very rare in the United States. HSV infection causes multiple, vesicular, painful lesions. Condyloma lata are flat, wart-like, painless lesions seen most often in patients with secondary syphilis.

3. The answer is D The 8-year-old boy most likely has Rocky Mountain spotted fever. Although meningitis can have a very similar clinical picture, the fact that the rash began on the boy's wrists and ankles, in addition to where the boy lives (Oklahoma) and the time of year (July), make Rocky Mountain spotted fever a more likely diagnosis. Stage I Lyme disease can present with flu-like symptoms, but its characteristic rash is a single, "bull's-eye"–type lesion (erythema chronicum migrans). Neither rabies nor babesiosis is associated with a rash.

4. The answer is D Only tick paralysis always presents with a clinical picture that can be identical to that of Guillain-Barré syndrome (i.e., a symmetric, ascending, flaccid paralysis accompanied by loss of the deep tendon reflexes). Removal of the tick is curative. Rabies can also cause a Guillain-Barré–like syndrome in 20% of affected patients, but usually other symptoms of fever, malaise, altered mental status, and muscle spasms predominate. Usually, muscle spasms and autonomic disturbances, but not paralysis, are seen in patients with tetanus. Neither Lyme disease nor relapsing fever is characterized by paralysis.

5. The answer is C *Trichuris trichiura* (whipworm) is acquired by children playing in contaminated soil. The adult worm resides in the colon. Heavy worm burdens in children can result in colitis or rectal prolapse.

6. The answer is D This patient has stage II Lyme disease and is showing both neurologic symptoms of meningoencephalitis and cardiac symptoms of complete heart block. The patient should be started on ceftriaxone and needs a thorough work-up, including a lumbar puncture to exclude other forms of meningitis and temporary pacemaker placement to counteract the heart block. Because she is pregnant, tetracycline and doxycycline are not acceptable. Chloramphenicol is not recommended for the treatment of Lyme disease.

7. The answer is E Norepinephrine's intense peripheral vasoconstricting activity, myocardial hyperexcitatory activity, vital organ hypoperfusion tendencies, and extravasation-related ischemic tissue necrosis make its use in the treatment of sepsis rarely, if ever, indicated. Volume replacement (with normal saline or lactated Ringer's solution) is necessary for hypotensive patients. Isoproterenol and dopamine should be administered only after aggressive volume replacement and after the central venous and pulmonary artery wedge pressures have increased to the upper limits of normal.

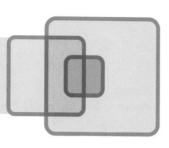

chapter 7

Metabolic Emergencies

WILLIAM GOSSMAN

I · SODIUM IMBALANCE

A · Hyponatremia

1. **Discussion**
   a. **Definition.** Hyponatremia is defined as a serum sodium level that is less than 135 mEq/L.
      (1) **True hyponatremia** is usually characterized by a serum sodium concentration less than 125 mEq/L and a serum osmolality less than 250 mOsm/kg.
      (2) **Pseudohyponatremia** occurs secondary to severe hyperglycemia, hyperproteinemia, or hyperlipidemia. The serum sodium level is decreased but the total body sodium level is unchanged.
   b. **Causes**
      (1) **Hypovolemic hyponatremia**
         (a) **Extrarenal losses.** In patients with hypovolemic hyponatremia as a result of extrarenal sodium loss, the urinary sodium level is less than 20 mEq/L. **Sweating, vomiting, diarrhea,** and **third-space sequestration** (e.g., as a result of burns, peritonitis, or pancreatitis) are common sources of extrarenal sodium loss.
         (b) **Renal losses.** In patients with hypovolemic hyponatremia as a result of renal sodium loss, the urinary sodium level is greater than 20 mEq/L. **Loop** or **osmotic diuretics, Addison's disease, ketonuria,** and **renal tubular acidosis** are sources of renal sodium loss.
      (2) **Euvolemic hyponatremia** occurs due to an increase in total body water; the total body sodium level is normal. **Hypothyroidism** and the **syndrome of inappropriate antidiuretic hormone (SIADH)** are causes of euvolemic hyponatremia. SIADH is associated with tumors, central nervous system (CNS) disease, pulmonary disease, hypopituitarism, medications, idiopathic causes, and a reset osmostat.
      (3) **Hypervolemic hyponatremia** occurs with **renal failure, cirrhosis, congestive heart failure (CHF),** and **nephrotic syndrome.**
2. **Clinical features.** The influx of water into brain cells may lead to apathy, agitation, headaches, altered consciousness, seizures, coma, weakness, nausea, anorexia, and vomiting.
3. **Differential diagnoses** include **pseudohyponatremia,** which can be caused by diabetic ketoacidosis and a hyperosmolar state (leading to hyperglycemia), multiple myeloma (leading to hyperproteinemia), or hypertriglyceridemia (leading to hyperlipidemia).
4. **Evaluation**
   a. **Laboratory studies** should include a serum electrolyte panel (i.e., sodium, potassium, chloride, and bicarbonate); serum glucose, blood urea nitrogen (BUN), and creatinine levels; and urinalysis (to determine the urine sodium level and osmolality).
   b. **Electrocardiography.** An electrocardiogram (ECG) should be obtained.

5. Therapy

a. **Fluid restriction** or **replacement**

(1) **Hypervolemic** and **euvolemic hyponatremia** usually result from hemodilution; **fluid restriction** is the initial treatment in stable, asymptomatic patients. Inhibition of water reabsorption caused by SIADH can be treated on an inpatient basis using demeclocycline (600–1200 mg/day) or furosemide.

(2) **Hypovolemic hyponatremia** can usually be treated with **isotonic saline.**

b. **Sodium replacement.** Sodium deficits can be calculated as follows:

$$Na^+ \text{ deficit (mEq)} = 0.6 \times (\text{wt kg}) \times (140 - \text{serum } Na^+)$$

(1) If the hyponatremia is acute, is severe (i.e., the serum sodium level is less than 120 mEq/L), and results in CNS symptoms, administration of **3% (hypertonic) saline solution** at 25–60 mL/hour is indicated.

(a) The serum sodium concentration should not increase at a rate that exceeds 2 mEq/hour.

(b) Hypertonic saline should be discontinued when sodium levels increase to 120 mEq/L or when the patient shows significant clinical improvement.

(2) In patients with chronic severe hyponatremia, the rate of serum sodium correction should not exceed 0.5 mEq/L/hour (12 mEq/L/day). Correcting the sodium deficiency too quickly could cause central pontine myelinolysis. If the hyponatremia is severe (i.e., serum sodium levels less than 120 mEq/L) and develops rapidly with CNS manifestations, 3% saline should be administered at a rate of 25–100 mL/hour.

6. Disposition

a. **Admission** is required for symptomatic patients, patients who have a serum sodium concentration below 125 mEq/L (with or without symptoms), patients who require intravenous or pharmacologic correction of the sodium imbalance, and patients who have significant comorbid factors (e.g., diabetes, advanced age, sepsis).

b. **Discharge.** If the patient is being discharged, the case should be discussed with a primary care physician and a follow-up appointment should take place within 48–72 hours.

B **Hypernatremia**

1. Discussion

a. **Definition.** Clinically significant effects occur at serum sodium levels greater than 155 mEq/L.

b. **Causes**

(1) **Reduced water intake** can be caused by a **defective thirst mechanism, unconsciousness,** an **inability to drink,** or a **lack of access to water.**

(2) **Increased water loss** can be caused by **vomiting, diarrhea, sweating, fever, hyperventilation, diabetes insipidus, osmotic diuresis, thyrotoxicosis,** and **severe burns.**

(3) **Increased sodium intake** or **renal salt retention** is due to **hypertonic saline ingestion** or **infusion, sodium bicarbonate administration, hyperaldosteronism, Cushing's disease,** and **congenital adrenal hyperplasia.**

2. Clinical features

a. **Symptoms** can include confusion, weakness, muscle irritability, tremulousness, seizures, and coma. Hypocalcemia, which is frequently seen in patients with hypernatremia, may contribute to the neurologic symptoms.

b. **Physical examination findings** may include flat neck veins, orthostatic hypotension, tachycardia, poor skin turgor, dry mucous membranes, tonic spasms, and respiratory paralysis.

3. Evaluation

   a. **Laboratory studies** should include a complete blood count (CBC); serum electrolyte panel; serum glucose, BUN, and creatinine levels; and urinalysis (to determine the urine sodium level and osmolality).
   b. **Electrocardiography.** An ECG should be obtained.
4. **Therapy**
   a. **Fluid replacement.** The amount of water needed to correct hypernatremia can be estimated as follows:

$$\text{Water deficit (L)} = 0.6 \times (\text{usual body wt in kg})$$
$$\times (\text{measured Na}^+ \text{ concentration} - \text{desired Na}^+ \text{ concentration})$$
$$/ \text{ measured Na}^+ \text{ concentration}$$

   (1) When dehydration is severe, normal saline or lactated Ringer's solution should be administered to improve blood pressure and tissue perfusion.
   (2) Once perfusion is reestablished, 0.45% saline is administered to maintain a urine output of 0.5 mL/kg/hour.
   b. **Sodium reduction.** The rate of sodium reduction should not exceed 10–15 mEq/L/day. The goal is to reach a normal serum sodium value in 48–72 hours.
6. **Disposition**
   a. **Admission.** Symptomatic patients, patients who have a serum sodium concentration greater than 160 mEq/L (with or without symptoms), patients who require intravenous or pharmacologic correction of the sodium imbalance, and patients who have significant comorbid factors require admission.
   b. **Discharge.** Before discharging a patient, the case should be discussed with a primary care physician and arrangements should be made for appropriate follow-up.

II   POTASSIUM IMBALANCE

A Hypokalemia

1. **Discussion**
   a. **Definition.** Hypokalemia, the most common electrolyte abnormality, is defined as a serum potassium level that is less than 3.5 mEq/L.
   b. **Causes**
      (1) **Extrarenal causes** include **inadequate dietary intake, diarrhea, vomiting,** and **redistribution** (e.g., as a result of insulin administration, epinephrine infusion, or acute alkalemia).
      (2) **Renal causes**
         (a) **Drug-induced** renal losses are caused by **loop diuretics, penicillin, aminoglycosides,** and **amphotericin B.**
         (b) **Hormone-induced** renal losses can occur as a result of **primary adrenal adenomas, adrenal hyperplasia, ectopic adrenocorticotropic hormone (ACTH) syndrome, renin-secreting tumors, renal artery stenosis,** and **malignant hypertension.**
         (c) **Renal tubular acidosis, Bartter's syndrome,** or **chronic magnesium depletion** can also lead to hypokalemia.
2. **Clinical features**
   a. **Symptoms** include weakness, paresthesias, and polyuria.
   b. **Physical examination findings** include areflexia, orthostatic hypotension, ileus, paralysis, and arrhythmias.
3. **Evaluation**
   a. **Laboratory studies** should include a serum electrolyte panel; serum BUN, creatinine, creatinine phosphokinase, phosphate, magnesium, and glucose levels; and urinalysis.

(1) **Serum evaluation** may show elevated creatinine phosphokinase levels.

(2) **Urinalysis.** The urine specimen may be dipstick-positive for red blood cells (RBCs). Formal urinalysis may reveal myoglobin, consistent with rhabdomyolysis.

b. **Electrocardiography.** ECG findings include T-wave flattening or inversion, U waves, ST-segment depression, premature ventricular contractions (PVCs), and a wide QRS complex.

4. **Therapy**
   a. **Potassium replacement**
   (1) If the serum potassium level is greater than 2.5 mEq/L and there are no ECG abnormalities, 40–80 mEq of **potassium chloride** should be administered per day until the imbalance is corrected, with no more than 40 mEq given as a single dose.
   (2) Severe hypokalemia (i.e., a serum potassium level less than 2.5 mEq/L) is treated by infusing 10 mEq of potassium chloride per hour in 50–100 mL of 5% dextrose in water or normal saline by intravenous piggyback for 3–4 hours.
      (a) No more than 40 mEq of potassium should ever be put in a single liter of intravenous fluid and no more than 10 mEq should be given per hour.
      (b) Continuous cardiac monitoring is required.
   b. **Magnesium replacement** with 2 g of magnesium sulfate in 50 mL of 5% dextrose in water administered over 20 minutes may be necessary.
   c. **Phosphate replacement.** If the serum phosphate level is low, **potassium phosphate** may be used instead of potassium chloride. The recommended daily dose is 2.5 mg/kg.

5. **Disposition**
   a. **Admission**
   (1) Patients with serum potassium concentrations of less than 2.5 mEq/L require admission to the hospital.
   (2) Patients with malignant cardiac dysrhythmias, digitalis toxicity, profound weakness with impending respiratory failure, rhabdomyolysis, hepatic encephalopathy, or a serum potassium level of less than 2.0 mEq/L require admission to the intensive care unit (ICU).
   b. **Discharge.** Patients with mild hypokalemia (serum potassium concentration = 2.5–3.5 mEq/L) can usually be managed as outpatients with gradual oral potassium repletion, provided they do not have ECG abnormalities, profound muscular weakness, ileus, or other serious effects. Patients who are discharged on oral supplementation should have a follow-up appointment within 48–72 hours.

B **Hyperkalemia**

1. **Discussion**
   a. **Definition.** Hyperkalemia is defined as a serum potassium level that exceeds 5.5 mEq/L.
   b. **Causes**
   (1) **Extrarenal causes** of hyperkalemia include **insulin deficiency, acidemia, hyperosmolality, β blocker** administration, oral or intravenous **potassium supplements, penicillin potassium salts, massive blood transfusion, crush injuries, burns, mesenteric** or **muscular infarction,** and **tumor lysis syndrome.**
   (2) **Renal causes.** Hyperkalemia is most commonly encountered in patients with **chronic renal insufficiency. Acute renal failure, hypoaldosteronism,** and **drugs** [e.g., nonsteroidal anti-inflammatory drugs (NSAIDs), cyclosporine, heparin, angiotensin-converting enzyme (ACE) inhibitors, potassium-sparing diuretics] can also cause hyperkalemia.
   (3) **Laboratory error** is the most common cause of hyperkalemia.

2. **Clinical features**
   a. **Symptoms** may include weakness, paresthesias, and confusion.
   b. **Physical examination findings** may include paralysis, areflexia, ileus, respiratory insufficiency, or cardiac arrest.

3. **Differential diagnoses** include **pseudohyperkalemia,** which can occur as a result of hemolysis, extreme leukocytosis, acidosis, thrombocytosis, or cold agglutinins. Laboratory error may also lead to a misdiagnosis of hyperkalemia.

4. **Evaluation**

   a. **Laboratory studies** include a serum electrolyte panel and serum BUN, creatinine, glucose, and magnesium levels. If the potassium level is extremely high or if the sample was hemolyzed, it may be advisable to check another blood sample.

   b. **Electrocardiography.** The patient should be placed on a continuous cardiac monitor, and an ECG should be obtained. Early ECG findings include peaked T waves and a shortened QT interval. Later, widened QRS complexes, prolonged PR intervals, low-amplitude P waves, and elevation or depression of the ST segment are seen. Advanced changes include absent P waves, marked QRS complex widening, and tall T waves, resulting in a sine wave pattern, ventricular fibrillation, and asystole (Figure 7–1).

5. **Therapy**

   a. **Acute therapy.** There are several approaches to acutely lowering potassium levels.

      (1) **Calcium chloride (CaCl),** 5 mL of a 10% solution (13.6 mEq/10 mL) or 10 mL of a 10% **calcium gluconate** solution (4.6 mEq/10 mL), is administered over 2 minutes and repeated in 5–10 minutes if necessary. This approach, which works by stabilizing cell membranes without altering potassium levels, is the most rapid way of lowering potassium. CaCl should ideally be infused through a central line as it causes severe skin injury if accidentally infiltrated from peripheral IV lines.

      (2) **Sodium bicarbonate** [44 mEq (1 ampule) administered intravenously over 5 minutes and repeated 10–15 minutes later if necessary] causes an intracellular influx of potassium. Onset of action occurs in approximately 15 minutes.

      (3) **Regular insulin** (10–20 U administered via an intravenous push) with **10% dextrose** (500 mL in water) administered over 1 hour, or 10 U of insulin administered via an intravenous push with 1 ampule (25 g) of 50% glucose administered over 5 minutes will lower potassium by causing an intracellular shift. Effects occur 30–60 minutes after administration.

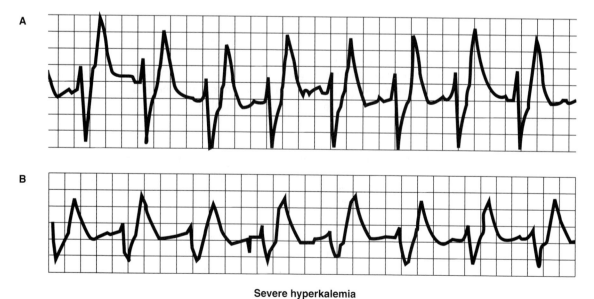

Severe hyperkalemia

FIGURE 7–1 **(A)** Typical electrocardiogram (ECG) in a patient with early hyperkalemia. Notice the peaked T waves. **(B)** Typical ECG in a patient with severe hyperkalemia. Notice the absent P waves, widening of the QRS complex, and tall T waves.

(4) Furosemide, bumetanide, and **acetazolamide** all increase potassium excretion.

(5) Sodium polystyrene sulfonate (Kayexalate) (15–30 g administered orally every 2–4 hours, or 50 g in 200 mL as a retention enema every 2–6 hours) causes a sodium–potassium exchange in the colon.

(6) Dialysis should be considered for patients with severe hyperkalemia who have failed to respond to pharmacologic attempts at lowering the potassium level, and for patients with acute or chronic renal failure.

b. **Maintenance of potassium balance.** Potassium balance is maintained by:

(1) Diuretics and **fludrocortisone**

(2) Cation-exchange resins, such as sodium polystyrene sulfonate

(3) Aldosterone, either as **desoxycorticosterone acetate** (15–20 mg/day intramuscularly) or **fludrocortisone acetate** (0.2–0.6 mg/day orally)

6. **Disposition**

a. **Admission.** When ECG abnormalities or clinical manifestations of hyperkalemia are present, admission to the ICU with continuous cardiac monitoring is required.

b. **Discharge.** Patients with mild serum potassium elevations in the absence of clinical and ECG abnormalities can be discharged, provided any identifiable predisposing factors have been corrected. Patients should have a follow-up evaluation within 48–72 hours.

III CALCIUM IMBALANCE

A Hypocalcemia

1. **Discussion**

a. **Definition.** Hypocalcemia is defined as an ionized calcium level below 2.0 mEq/L or a total serum level below 8.5 mg/dL.

b. **Causes** of hypocalcemia include **shock, sepsis, renal failure, pancreatitis, hypomagnesemia, alkalosis, decreased serum albumin, hypoparathyroidism** (idiopathic or as a result of irradiation or surgery), **pseudohypoparathyroidism, osteoblastic metastasis, malabsorption,** and **excess phosphates.** Medications that cause hypocalcemia include **cimetidine, phosphate laxatives, phenytoin, phenobarbital, gentamicin, heparin, theophylline, loop diuretics,** and **glucocorticosteroids.**

2. **Clinical features**

a. **Symptoms** can include circumoral and distal extremity paresthesias, irritability, weakness, fatigue, muscle cramps, and seizures.

b. **Physical examination findings** often include hyperreflexia, carpopedal spasm, tetany, laryngospasm, Trousseau's sign (carpopedal spasm after arterial occlusion of the arm for 3 minutes), and Chvostek's sign (contraction of the facial muscles after percussion over the facial nerve).

3. **Evaluation**

a. **Laboratory studies** should include serum albumin, calcium, magnesium, phosphate, BUN, and creatinine levels; liver studies; amylase and lipase levels; ionized calcium levels; a serum electrolyte panel; and a CBC.

b. **Electrocardiography.** ECG findings may include a prolonged QT interval, sinus bradycardia, complete heart block, ventricular arrhythmias, and ventricular fibrillation.

c. **Radiology.** When hypocalcemia occurs in the context of osteomalacia, radiographic findings can include craniotabes, frontal skull bossing, rachitic rosary ribs, a widened rib cage (Harrison's groove), bowed legs, demineralization, and thinning of the cortical bone.

4. **Therapy**

a. Patients with **acutely symptomatic hypocalcemia** should be treated with 10 mL of **10% calcium gluconate** infused intravenously over 10–15 minutes, followed by a maintenance infusion of 1–2 mg/kg/hour over 6–12 hours. Calcium must be given cautiously to patients receiving digitalis because calcium can worsen digoxin toxicity or cause sudden death.

b. For **asymptomatic** patients, oral therapy with elemental calcium (with or without vitamin D) may be all that is required. The rapid intravenous administration of calcium to asymptomatic patients with mild to moderate hypocalcemia is contraindicated because doing so can cause severe cardiovascular, neuromuscular, or renal complications.

5. **Disposition**

a. **Admission.** Patients with symptomatic hypocalcemia who require intravenous replacement therapy must be admitted to the hospital. These patients should be placed on continuous cardiac monitoring, and serial serum calcium levels should be obtained.

b. **Discharge.** Asymptomatic patients may be discharged with appropriate follow-up.

B Hypercalcemia

1. **Discussion**

a. **Definition.** Hypercalcemia is defined as a total calcium level exceeding 10.5 mg/dL or an ionized calcium level exceeding 2.7 mEq/L.

b. **Causes**

(1) **Endocrine causes** of hypercalcemia include **primary hyperparathyroidism, hyperthyroidism, pheochromocytoma, adrenal insufficiency,** and **acromegaly.**

(2) **Malignancies** that present with hypercalcemia include **squamous cell carcinoma of the lung, breast cancer, kidney cancer, myeloma,** and **leukemia.**

(3) **Granulomatous disorders** that can cause hypercalcemia include **sarcoid, tuberculosis, histoplasmosis,** and **coccidioidomycosis.**

(4) **Medications.** Excessive **vitamin D or A intake, thiazides, lithium,** and **hormonal therapy for breast cancer** can cause hypercalcemia.

(5) **Miscellaneous causes** include **immobilization, Paget's disease, dehydration, excess calcium ingestion,** and **milk-alkali syndrome.**

2. **Clinical features**

a. **Signs and symptoms** can include weakness, depression, confusion, lethargy, personality changes, nausea, vomiting, anorexia, constipation, headache, and abdominal pain.

b. **Physical examination findings** often include dehydration, decreased motor strength, decreased mental status, ataxia, hyporeflexia, fractures, hypertension, weight loss, renal insufficiency, and cardiac arrest.

3. **Evaluation**

a. **Laboratory studies** should include ionized calcium levels; serum calcium, protein, phosphate, magnesium, BUN, creatinine, glucose, amylase, and lipase levels; a serum electrolyte panel; and a CBC.

b. **Electrocardiography.** ECG abnormalities include shortening of the QT interval, widening of T waves, bradyarrhythmias, bundle branch blocks, and second-degree and complete heart block.

4. **Therapy.** Treatment is required for symptomatic patients with calcium levels greater than 12 mg/dL who are unable to maintain a good fluid intake or have abnormal renal function.

a. **Fluid replacement.** Because patients with hypercalcemia are usually dehydrated, the initial and safest treatment is restoration of volume with large amounts of saline (5–10 L of normal saline in the first 24 hours).

b. **Pharmacologic therapy**

(1) **Furosemide** (1–3 mg/kg) can be administered intravenously to enhance urinary output and increase renal excretion of calcium.

(2) **Mithramycin** (15–25 mg/kg in 5% dextrose administered intravenously over 3 hours), a cytotoxic agent that also decreases the serum calcium level, may be useful in patients with metastatic bone disease.

(3) **Calcitonin** (2–4 IU/kg intramuscularly every 12 hours) diminishes calcium levels, usually within 12 hours. Calcitonin is useful for the initial treatment of hypercalcemia, but generally not for long-term management.

(4) **Hydrocortisone** (3 mg/kg/day) can be administered intravenously in divided doses every 6 hours. Hydrocortisone inhibits bone resorption and gastrointestinal absorption of calcium.

c. **Dialysis** should be considered for patients with severe symptoms and for patients with cardiac or renal disease.

5. **Disposition.** Patients with a calcium level greater than 12 mg/dL, symptoms, or abnormal renal function require admission for continuous cardiac monitoring and serial calcium levels.

IV MAGNESIUM IMBALANCE

A Hypomagnesemia

1. **Discussion.** Clinically important hypomagnesemia occurs when the serum magnesium concentration falls below 1.0 mEq/L.

2. **Clinical features**
   a. **Symptoms.** Complaints include malaise, diffuse weakness, anorexia, nausea, vomiting, and seizures.
   b. **Physical examination findings.** The clinical features mimic those of hypocalcemia, with nervous system complaints dominating the clinical picture. Findings may include Chvostek's sign, Trousseau's sign, tremors, twitching, clonus, increased deep tendon reflexes, carpopedal spasm, frank tetany, delirium, movement disorders, and dysarthria.

3. **Evaluation**
   a. **Laboratory studies** include serum magnesium, calcium, BUN, creatinine, and glucose levels and a serum electrolyte panel. Because only approximately 1% of the total body magnesium is sampled with a serum laboratory test, **patients with symptomatic hypomagnesemia may have normal or only minimally decreased serum magnesium levels.**
   b. **Electrocardiography.** ECG findings include atrial and ventricular tachyarrhythmias, torsades de pointes, and a prolonged QT interval. Arrhythmias caused by hypomagnesemia may not respond to the usual antiarrhythmic therapy, but they may respond well to intravenous magnesium. Magnesium (2 g) should be administered rapidly over 2 minutes via an intravenous line to patients in pulseless ventricular tachycardia suspected of being hypomagnesemic (e.g., a patient with myocardial infarction who is taking diuretics).
   c. **Ancillary tests** (e.g., radiographs) may be required to diagnose the underlying cause.

4. **Therapy**
   a. **Mild hypomagnesemia** is treated with oral supplementation. **Magnesium hydroxide** (200–600 mg, four times daily) is usually used.
   b. **Severe hypomagnesemia,** characterized by marked neurologic manifestations or malignant ventricular arrhythmias, is treated with 2–4 g of **magnesium sulfate** administered in 100–200 mL of 5% dextrose in water over 20 minutes. Additional treatment should be directed toward correcting the underlying cause of the hypomagnesemia.

5. **Disposition.** Indications for admission include a serum magnesium level below 1 mEq/L, severe central neurologic manifestations, cardiac arrhythmias, and severe underlying disorders.

B Hypermagnesemia

1. **Discussion**
   a. **Definition.** Hypermagnesemia is defined as a serum magnesium level greater than 2.5 mEq/L.
   b. **Causes.** Because the kidney is efficient in excreting excess magnesium, hypermagnesemia is uncommon except in the presence of **renal failure** or an **iatrogenic cause.** Other causes of

hypermagnesemia include **rhabdomyolysis, tumor lysis, burns, tissue trauma, diabetic ketoacidosis, hypothyroidism, cathartic abuse, antacids, eclampsia treatment,** and **adrenal insufficiency.**

2. **Clinical features**
   a. **Symptoms.** Common but nonspecific findings include nausea, vomiting, lethargy, mental confusion, and coma.
   b. **Physical examination findings** become apparent when the magnesium level exceeds 4 mEq/L and include depression of the deep tendon reflexes, marked muscle weakness, bulbar paralysis, and respiratory insufficiency.

3. **Evaluation**
   a. **Laboratory studies** include serum calcium, ionized calcium, BUN, and creatinine levels and a serum electrolyte panel.
   b. **Electrocardiography.** Dysrhythmias and cardiac arrest can occur at serum magnesium levels exceeding 8 mEq/L, but the ECG manifestations of hypermagnesemia are variable and nonspecific.

4. **Therapy**
   a. **Exogenous sources of magnesium should be removed.**
   b. **Pharmacologic therapy**
      (1) **Calcium gluconate** or **calcium chloride.** Because calcium transiently reverses the effects of hypermagnesemia by acting as a direct antagonist, 10 mL of 10% calcium gluconate or calcium chloride solution can be given intravenously in symptomatic patients.
      (2) **Furosemide.** In patients with normal renal function, brisk diuresis with intravenous normal saline and furosemide will enhance urinary magnesium excretion.
   c. **Dialysis.** In patients with very high magnesium levels or in patients with renal failure, emergency peritoneal dialysis or hemodialysis may be required.

5. **Disposition.** Patients with magnesium levels above 8 mEq/L require admission to a monitored bed and should be considered for early dialysis. For patients with lower magnesium levels, admission depends on the underlying cause, the patient's hemodynamic status, and the presence of any comorbid factors (e.g., renal failure, cancer, psychiatric problems).

V   ACID–BASE IMBALANCE

A Normal physiology   Acid–base balance refers to the maintenance of blood hydrogen ion concentration. The negative logarithm of this concentration, pH, is usually closely maintained between 7.35 and 7.45. Three homeostatic mechanisms maintain this balance:

1. **Buffer systems.** Soluble buffers mediate an immediate response to changes in pH. Carbonic acid, phosphoric acid, hemoglobin, and plasma proteins account for one third of the body's buffering capacity. Intracellular tissue proteins are responsible for the remaining two thirds.

2. **Respiratory mechanisms.** Through a respiratory response, changes in alveolar ventilation can promptly cause hydrogen ions to be excreted or retained by changing the concentration of components of the carbonic acid buffer system.

3. **Renal mechanisms** mediate a slow response to change in the total body hydrogen ion load by causing net excretion or production of hydrogen ions.

B Respiratory acidosis

1. **Discussion**
   a. **Definition.** Respiratory acidosis is characterized by a blood carbon dioxide tension (P_{CO_2}) greater than 40 mm Hg and a decreased blood pH. It is associated with inadequate elimination of carbon dioxide by the lungs.

       (1) **Acute respiratory acidosis** is characterized by acute carbon dioxide retention leading to an increased P_{CO_2} but a minimal change in plasma bicarbonate concentration. For each 10-mm Hg increase in P_{CO_2}, the plasma bicarbonate level increases 1 mEq/L and the blood pH decreases by 0.08.

       (2) **Chronic respiratory acidosis** becomes apparent after 2–5 days. Renal compensation (i.e., increased hydrogen ion secretion and bicarbonate production in the distal nephron) is seen. For every 10-mm Hg increase in P_{CO_2}, the plasma bicarbonate level increases 3–4 mEq/L and the blood pH decreases by 0.03.

    b. Causes of respiratory acidosis include all disorders that reduce pulmonary function and carbon dioxide clearance:

       (1) CNS lesions

       (2) Sedative therapy and overdose

       (3) Neuromuscular disorders (e.g., kyphoscoliosis, scleroderma, flail chest, rib fractures)

       (4) Pleural disease

       (5) Obstructive airway disease [e.g., asthma, chronic obstructive pulmonary disease (COPD)]

2. Clinical features. Respiratory acidosis may lead to symptoms of generalized CNS depression, reduced cardiac output, and pulmonary hypertension.

3. Evaluation

    a. Laboratory studies should include an arterial blood gas (ABG) report; a serum electrolyte panel; and BUN, creatinine, and glucose levels. It might also be useful to obtain urine drug screen results and a serum ethanol level.

    b. Electrocardiography and **radiography** may be useful.

    c. Ancillary tests (e.g., muscle biopsy) should take place outside of the ED.

4. Therapy

    a. Correction of the underlying cause should be attempted. For example, in the case of drug-induced hypoventilation, vigorous attempts should be made to clear the offending agent from the body.

    b. Assisted ventilation. A P_{CO_2} of more than 60 mm Hg may be an indication for assisted ventilation if CNS or pulmonary muscular depression is severe. Care must be taken not to normalize the P_{CO_2} in patients with chronic respiratory disturbances. Because renal compensatory mechanisms have already normalized the blood pH in these patients, rapid correction of the respiratory parameters can lead to a dangerous elevation of the blood pH.

C Respiratory alkalosis

1. Discussion

    a. Definition. Respiratory alkalosis is characterized by a decreased P_{CO_2} and an increased pH. It is associated with excessive elimination of carbon dioxide by the lungs.

       (1) **Acute respiratory alkalosis.** For each 10-mm Hg decrease in P_{CO_2}, the plasma bicarbonate level decreases by 2 mEq/L and the blood pH increases by 0.08. The serum chloride level also increases.

       (2) **Chronic respiratory alkalosis.** For each 10-mm Hg decrease in P_{CO_2}, the plasma bicarbonate level decreases by 5–6 mEq/L and the blood pH increases by 0.02. The serum chloride level also increases.

    b. Causes

       (1) **Anxiety** is the most common cause of respiratory alkalosis.

       (2) **Hypoxia** results in an increased respiratory rate and, thus, respiratory alkalosis.

       (3) **Primary pulmonary disorders** (e.g., pneumonia, asthma, pulmonary fibrosis, pulmonary embolism) lead to stimulation of the ventilatory rate, resulting in a low P_{CO_2}.

       (4) **Salicylate toxicity** initially causes overstimulation of the respiratory center, resulting in respiratory alkalosis.

(5) **CNS disorders** (e.g., cerebrovascular accident, tumor, infection, trauma) may be associated with inappropriate stimulation of ventilation.

(6) **Pregnancy** and **progesterone therapy** cause an increase in respiratory rate, thereby decreasing the P_{CO_2}.

(7) **Early Gram-negative septicemia** results in a respiratory alkalosis by an unknown mechanism.

2. **Clinical features.** Acute alkalemia results in a generalized feeling of anxiety, severe obtundation, a tetany-like syndrome, and depressed cardiac function at a blood pH exceeding 7.73.

3. **Evaluation.** The ordering of tests should be directed toward finding the underlying cause. Some basic tests include an ABG, a CBC, a serum electrolyte panel, serum BUN and creatinine levels, a urine pregnancy test, liver studies, a salicylate level, a blood culture, and a chest radiograph.

4. **Therapy.** The primary goal of therapy is to correct the underlying cause. Most cases of respiratory alkalosis require no direct treatment.

D Metabolic acidosis

1. **Discussion.** Metabolic acidosis is defined by a decreased blood pH and a decreased plasma bicarbonate concentration (less than 24 mEq/L).

2. **Causes.** Metabolic acidosis is caused by the loss of bicarbonate or the accumulation of an acid other than carbonic acid (e.g., lactic acid). The causes of metabolic acidosis can be divided into those associated with a normal anion gap and those associated with an elevated anion gap. The gap represents anions that are present in the serum but are not routinely measured. The anion gap is calculated from the electrolyte values: anion gap $= ([Na^+] + [K^+]) - ([HCO_3^-] + [Cl^-])$. The normal range is 10–12 mEq/L.

   a. **Anion gap metabolic acidosis.** The causes of an anion gap metabolic acidosis can be remembered using the mnemonic, "A MUDPILE CAT" (Figure 7–2). The following are broad categories of disorders associated with anion gap metabolic acidosis:

   (1) **Lactic acidosis** results from decreased oxygen delivery to tissues and is caused by conditions such as sepsis and shock. Lactic acidosis is the most common cause of anion gap metabolic acidosis.

Alcohol

Methanol

Uremia

Diabetic ketoacidosis

Paraldehyde

Iron and **I**soniazid

Lactic acidosis

Ethylene glycol

Carbon monoxide

Aspirin

Toluene

FIGURE 7–2 Mnemonic for remembering the causes of anion gap metabolic acidosis.

   (2) **Ketoacidosis** is a condition characterized by increased ketone body formation that occurs as a complication of diabetes mellitus, prolonged starvation, and prolonged alcohol abuse.

   (3) **Renal failure** leads to an increased anion gap due to the accumulation of various organic and inorganic anions associated with a reduced glomerular filtration rate (GFR).

   (4) **Chemicals.** A variety of chemical substances (e.g., salicylates, methanol, ethylene glycol, paraldehyde, iron, isoniazid) can result in the accumulation of organic acids. An anion gap greater than 35 mEq/L is usually caused by ethylene glycol, methanol, or lactic acidosis.

  b. **Nonanion gap metabolic acidosis** is caused by:

   (1) **Conditions that lead to the renal loss of bicarbonate** (e.g., proximal tubular acidosis, distal tubular acidosis, acetazolamide therapy leading to carbonic anhydrase inhibition)

   (2) **Conditions that lead to the gastrointestinal loss of bicarbonate** (e.g., diarrhea, pancreatic fistula, ureterosigmoidostomy)

   (3) **Administration of hydrochloric acid, ammonium chloride, arginine hydrochloride,** or **oral calcium chloride**

3. **Clinical features.** The clinical features of metabolic acidosis are usually related to the underlying disorder. pH levels below 7.2 lead to decreased cardiac output, resistance to catecholamines, hypotension, and Kussmaul's respiration (i.e., a rapid, regular, and deep respiratory rate).

4. **Evaluation**

  a. **Laboratory studies** should include an ABG; a CBC; a serum electrolyte panel; serum creatinine, BUN, and glucose levels; and urinalysis.

   (1) The calculated osmolarity, which is used to calculate the osmolar gap, can be calculated as follows:

$$\text{Calculated osmolority (mOsm/L)} = 2\,(\text{Na}) + (\text{glucose}/18) + (\text{BUN}/2.8)$$

    The osmolar gap (i.e., the difference between the measured osmolality and the calculated osmolarity) can aid in diagnosing the cause of an anion gap acidosis. Normally, the osmolar gap is 275–285 mOsm/L. Different substances increase the osmolar gap to varying degrees (Table 7–1).

   (2) Laboratory data may provide other clues as to the cause of the anion gap metabolic acidosis. For example:

    (a) Hyperglycemia and glucosuria are characteristic of diabetic ketoacidosis, while the blood glucose level is lower and glucosuria is mild or absent in alcoholic ketoacidosis.

    (b) Serum lactic acid levels are elevated in lactic acidosis, although the differential for an elevated serum lactic acid level is broad.

    (c) Calcium oxalate or hippurate crystals may be evident in the urine of patients with anion gap metabolic acidosis as a result of ethylene glycol intoxication.

  b. **Ancillary tests** may be necessary to determine the specific cause of the metabolic acidosis.

TABLE 7–1 Effect of Various Chemicals on the Osmolar Gap in Anion Gap Metabolic Acidosis

Substance	Amount Needed to Increase the Serum Osmolarity 1 mOsm/L (in mg/dL)	Increase in mOsm/L as a Result of Each mg/dL of Substance
Methanol	2.6	0.38
Ethanol	4.3	0.23
Ethylene glycol	5.0	0.20
Acetone	5.5	0.18
Isopropyl alcohol	5.9	0.17
Salicylate	14.0	0.07

5. **Therapy.** Metabolic acidosis may be treated with **sodium bicarbonate** when the blood pH is less than 7.2.

   a. The following equation is used to calculate the required amount of bicarbonate:

   $$\text{Bicarbonate deficit (mEq)} = (24 - HCO_3^-)(0.4)(\text{wt kg})$$

   b. Complications of bicarbonate administration include hypernatremia, paradoxic cerebrospinal fluid (CSF) acidosis, hypokalemia, hyperosmolality, and the induction of dysrhythmias.

E Metabolic alkalosis

1. **Discussion**

   a. **Definition.** Metabolic alkalosis is characterized by an increased pH and an increased plasma bicarbonate concentration.

   b. **Causes.** Increased bicarbonate results from either increased endogenous production with reduced renal excretion or exogenous administration of bicarbonate or another alkali.

      (1) **Vomiting** or **nasogastric suction** causes a loss of gastric hydrochloric acid that leads to an increase in plasma bicarbonate. The decreased extracellular volume due to vomiting plus the chloride deficits reduce the GFR and increase the rate of bicarbonate and sodium reabsorption, helping to maintain the alkalosis.

      (2) **Diuretics** that increase sodium chloride loss lead to hydrogen ion loss, resulting in decreased bicarbonate production. Volume depletion by the sodium deficit reduces the GFR, stimulates proximal tubular reabsorption of bicarbonate, and maintains the metabolic alkalosis.

      (3) **Conditions characterized by excessive mineralocorticoid action** (e.g., Cushing's disease, hyperaldosteronism, Bartter's syndrome) stimulate hydrogen ion secretion, thereby raising the plasma bicarbonate level. Potassium depletion by a similar mechanism is also noted.

      (4) **Administration of alkali,** either as sodium bicarbonate or as organic ions (e.g., lactate, citrate, acetate), results in an increased plasma bicarbonate level.

      (5) **Rapid correction of hypercapnia** in patients with a chronic state of respiratory acidosis leads to a transient state of hyperbicarbonatemia and an elevated pH.

2. **Clinical features.** Signs and symptoms of metabolic alkalosis are usually dominated by the underlying disease state.

3. **Evaluation**

   a. **Laboratory tests** should include an ABG report, a serum electrolyte panel, and serum glucose, BUN, and creatinine levels.

   b. **Ancillary tests** may be necessary to identify the underlying cause of the metabolic alkalosis.

4. **Therapy.** The primary goal of therapy is to correct the underlying cause. Frequently, volume expansion with sodium chloride–containing solutions is required.

Study Questions

Directions: Each of the numbered items or incomplete statements in this section is followed by answers or by completions of the statement. Select the ONE lettered answer or completion that is BEST in each case.

1. A 69-year-old woman complains of weakness. The results of laboratory studies are as follows: serum sodium, 122 mEq/L; serum potassium, 4.5 mEq/L; serum chloride, 110 mEq/L; plasma bicarbonate, 24 mEq/L. The serum sodium level is noted to be chronic. What treatment is required?

   A Administer 3% saline at a rate of 100 mL/hour
   B Administer normal saline at a rate that does not exceed 0.5 mEq/L/hour
   C Administer demeclocycline (600–1200 mg/day)
   D Administer furosemide
   E Admit the patient for observation

2. Which of the following agents most rapidly counteracts the cardiac effects of severe hyperkalemia?

   A Calcium gluconate
   B Furosemide
   C Insulin–dextrose
   D Sodium bicarbonate
   E Cation exchange resin

3. An abnormally low serum level of which one of the following electrolytes results in prolongation of the QT interval?

   A Chloride
   B Sodium
   C Calcium
   D Potassium
   E Phosphate

4. What is the most common cause of a high anion gap metabolic acidosis?

   A Ketoacidosis
   B Lactic acidosis
   C Persistent diarrhea
   D Pancreatic fistula
   E Anxiety

5. Pseudohyponatremia occurs secondary to which disorder?

   A Central nervous system (CNS) disease
   B Addison's disease
   C Renal tubular acidosis
   D Hyperglycemia
   E Hypopituitarism

6. A 55-year-old man with a history of lung cancer with metastasis to the pelvis presents with weakness, depression, confusion, and abdominal pain. The serum calcium level is noted to be 13 mg/dL. After initiating infusion of normal saline in the emergency department (ED), what is the next intervention?

   A Administration of mithramycin (15–25 mg/kg in 5% dextrose) intravenously over 3 hours
   B No additional treatment is required

C Administration of calcitonin (2–4 IU/kg) intramuscularly every 12 hours

D Administration of a cation-exchange resin

E Intravenous infusion of insulin–glucose

7. A 20-year-old pregnant woman receiving magnesium sulfate intravenously in the emergency department (ED) as a treatment for preterm labor begins to complain of nausea and weakness. On physical examination, her deep tendon reflexes are depressed. What should be done for this patient?

A Peritoneal dialysis should be performed

B Furosemide should be administered

C Magnesium sulfate infusion should be terminated

D No treatment is required

E Calcitonin (2–4 IU/kg every 12 hours) should be administered

8. In acute respiratory acidosis, for each 10-mm Hg increase in carbon dioxide tension (P_{CO_2}), the pH decreases by

A 0.08

B 0.03

C 0.02

D 2

E 5

9. In hypomagnesemia, clinical features mimic those of

A hyponatremia

B hypercalcemia

C hyperkalemia

D hypocalcemia

E hypokalemia

10. Consider the following values: pH, 7.25; carbon dioxide tension (P_{CO_2}), 40 mm Hg; oxygen tension (P_{O_2}), 92 mm Hg; plasma bicarbonate, 14 mEq/L. With which type of acid–base disturbance are they most consistent?

A Respiratory alkalosis

B Respiratory acidosis

C Metabolic acidosis

D Metabolic alkalosis

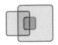

Answers and Explanations

1. The answer is B In a stable patient with a chronically low sodium level, normal saline should be administered at a rate that does not exceed 0.5 mEq/L/hour (12 mEq/L/day). Correcting the sodium deficiency too quickly could cause central pontine myelinolysis. Patients with acute, severe hyponatremia accompanied by central nervous system (CNS) symptoms should be administered 3% saline (25–60 mL/hour). Demeclocycline and furosemide are used to treat hyponatremia caused by the syndrome of inappropriate antidiuretic hormone (SIADH).

2. The answer is A The most rapid way to counteract the cardiac effects of hyperkalemia is by calcium gluconate or calcium chloride infusion. Calcium stabilizes cell membranes without altering potassium levels. Bicarbonate causes an intracellular influx of potassium and takes 15 minutes to work. An insulin–glucose infusion also shifts potassium into cells; the onset of action occurs in 30–60 minutes. Definitive therapy involves eliminating potassium by stimulating renal excretion (e.g., by administering cation exchange resins or performing dialysis).

3. The answer is C Hypocalcemia causes prolongation of the QT interval and may cause ventricular arrhythmias, but more commonly results in sinus bradycardia or complete heart block. QT-interval prolongation is also seen with hyperphosphatemia (not hypophosphatemia). Hypokalemia causes flattening of the T waves and a prominent U wave, which may look like QT-interval prolongation on the electrocardiogram (ECG), but really is not. Hyponatremia and hypochloremia do not alter the ECG significantly.

4. The answer is B Lactic acidosis, which results from decreased oxygen delivery to the tissues, is the most common cause of a high anion gap acidosis. Lactic acidosis is caused by conditions like sepsis and shock. Ketone body formation as a result of diabetes mellitus or prolonged starvation leads to anion gap metabolic acidosis, but is not the most common cause. Pancreatic fistulas and persistent diarrhea cause a nonanion gap metabolic acidosis. Anxiety accompanied by an increase in respiratory rate is the most common cause of respiratory alkalosis.

5. The answer is D Pseudohyponatremia is defined as a decrease in serum sodium concentration that is not accompanied by a decrease in the plasma osmolality. Pseudohyponatremia is seen with severe hyperglycemia, hyperproteinemia, and hyperlipidemia. Addison's disease and renal tubular acidosis cause renal loss of sodium with a resultant decrease in serum osmolality. Hypopituitarism and CNS disease can cause the syndrome of inappropriate antidiuretic hormone (SIADH).

6. The answer is A This patient requires treatment for hypercalcemia because he is symptomatic and has a serum calcium level greater than 12 mg/dL. Once the patient's fluid status has been corrected, mithramycin is the treatment of choice for this patient because of his metastatic bone disease. Calcitonin may be started but it requires more than 12 hours to work and does not have any cytotoxic properties. Cation-exchange resins and an insulin–glucose drip are used to treat hyperkalemia, not hypercalcemia.

7. The answer is C The initial treatment for this patient would be to stop the magnesium infusion and place the patient under observation. Peritoneal dialysis is reserved for patients in renal failure or with very high magnesium levels. Furosemide along with forced saline diuresis will enhance renal excretion of magnesium, but is reserved for more severe cases of hypermagnesemia. Calcitonin is used for hypercalcemia, not hypermagnesemia.

8. The answer is A In acute respiratory acidosis, the pH decreases by 0.08 and the bicarbonate level increases by 1 mEq/L for every 10-mm Hg increase in P_{CO_2}. In chronic respiratory acidosis, the pH decreases by 0.03 for every 10-mm Hg rise in the P_{CO_2}. Chronic respiratory alkalosis leads to a bicarbonate decrease of 5–6 mEq/L and a pH increase of 0.02 for each 10-mm Hg decrease in P_{CO_2}.

9. The answer is D Hypomagnesemia and hypocalcemia are both associated with hyperreflexia, tetany, seizures, Trousseau's sign, and Chvostek's sign. There are no specific physical findings associated with hyponatremia. Hyperkalemia and hypokalemia lead to areflexia, ileus, paralysis, and orthostatic hypotension. Hypercalcemia is associated with ataxia, hyporeflexia, dehydration, and hypertension.

10. The answer is C Metabolic acidosis is characterized by a decreased (acidic) blood pH and a decreased plasma bicarbonate concentration (i.e., less than 24 mEq/L). In this patient, the pH is in the acidic range (7.25), the P_{CO_2} and P_{O_2} are normal, and the plasma bicarbonate concentration is abnormally low (14 mEq/L). These findings are indicative of a primary metabolic acidosis.

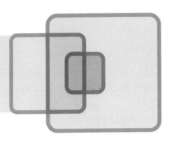

chapter **8**

Endocrine Emergencies

LESLIE S. ZUN

I   **HYPOGLYCEMIA**

A **Discussion**

1. **Definition.** Hypoglycemia is generally considered to be present when the serum glucose level is **less than 50 mg/dL.**

2. **Etiology.** Glucose homeostasis is the result of a complex interaction between insulin (secreted by the pancreas), counterregulatory hormones (e.g., glucagon, catecholamine, glucocorticoids), and growth hormone (GH). Traditionally, hypoglycemia is classified as either postprandial (reactive) or fasting.

   a. **Spontaneous hypoglycemia**

      (1) **Postprandial (reactive) hypoglycemia** is characterized by declining glucose levels after a glucose load.

      (2) **Alimentary hypoglycemia** occurs in patients who have recently undergone gastrointestinal surgery.

      (3) **Prediabetic glucose intolerance.** Hypoglycemia may be an early manifestation of non–insulin-dependent diabetes mellitus.

      (4) **Functional (idiopathic) hypoglycemia.** Hypoglycemia occurs between the fed and fasting state.

      (5) **Fasting hypoglycemia** occurs in patients with significant underlying pathologic conditions.

      (6) **Endogenous insulin excess** may result from **insulinomas** (nonmalignant pancreatic tumors) or **extrapancreatic neoplasms.**

      (7) **Regulatory hormone deficiencies.** Acquired or congenital deficiencies of glucagon, glucocorticoids, or GH can lead to hypoglycemia.

      (8) **Organ failure.** Impaired liver or kidney function can lead to hypoglycemia.

      (9) **Systemic disease.** Shock, sepsis, and starvation can cause hypoglycemia.

   b. **Induced hypoglycemia**

      (1) **Insulin-induced hypoglycemia,** seen in patients with diabetes, is the most common cause of hypoglycemia seen in the emergency department (ED).

      (2) **Factitious hypoglycemia** may be seen in psychiatric patients (e.g., as a result of the ingestion of oral hypoglycemic agents by a patient with Münchhausen syndrome).

      (3) **Chemical-induced.** Alcohol-induced hypoglycemia is found in malnourished, alcoholic patients. Other chemicals and medications can also induce hypoglycemia.

3. **Risk factors.** Young children and elderly patients are at high risk for the development of hypoglycemia.

B **Clinical features** are caused by the direct effects of hypoglycemia on the central nervous system (CNS), as well as its indirect effects on the sympathetic nervous system. Patients may be asymptomatic, or they may present with a wide variety of symptoms.

1. **Nonspecific systemic symptoms** include sweating, palpitations, hypertension, peripheral vasodilation, hyperventilation, tachycardia, dyspnea, pallor, and tremulousness.

2. **Neurologic symptoms** include paresthesia, neurologic deficit, diplopia, clonus, and transient hemiplegia.

3. **Psychiatric manifestations** include impairment of memory, change of personality, combative behavior, fatigue, headache, insomnia, nightmares, visual problems, catatonia, convulsions, and general sluggishness.

C **Differential diagnoses**   Hypoglycemia may masquerade as neurologic, psychiatric, or cardiovascular disease. Stroke, diabetic ketoacidosis, nonketotic hyperosmolar coma, alcohol intoxication, alcohol withdrawal, and other causes of coma must all be ruled out.

D **Evaluation**   Bedside glucose testing is a reliable test for ruling out hypoglycemia. Repeat laboratory measurements are required to confirm the diagnosis in patients who do not respond to glucose administration or who experience the recurrence of symptoms after treatment.

E **Therapy**

1. Prehospital providers commonly administer one ampule (25 g) of **50% dextrose** intravenously. Alcoholic patients should receive **thiamine** (100 mg administered intravenously) prior to receiving dextrose to prevent Wernicke-Korsakoff syndrome (see VIII). If intravenous access is unavailable, **glucagon** (0.5–2.0 mg) is administered intramuscularly or subcutaneously. The glucagon dose can be repeated twice.

2. A **meal high in complex carbohydrates** should be provided following initial treatment. If the patient is unable to swallow, an intravenous infusion of 5% dextrose in water should be initiated.

F **Disposition**

1. **Admission** is indicated for patients who have taken an oral hypoglycemic agent or long-acting insulin. Patients in whom no obvious cause for the hypoglycemia can be identified and patients with persistent neurologic deficits or cardiac complications (e.g., coronary or cerebrovascular insufficiency) should also be admitted.

2. **Discharge.** Patients whose symptoms are rapidly reversed without complications and in whom a clear cause for the hypoglycemia has been identified may go home. Patients with diabetes who experience a hypoglycemic episode should be taught how to adjust their insulin dose, food intake, or both based on their level of physical activity.

II   **DIABETIC KETOACIDOSIS**

A **Discussion**

1. **Definition.** Diabetic ketoacidosis (DKA) is a disorder found in insulin-dependent patients that is characterized by **hyperglycemia, ketonemia,** and **acidosis.**

2. **Etiology.** Diabetic ketoacidosis is caused by a relative or absolute deficiency of insulin and increased levels of stress hormones (e.g., catecholamines, cortisol, GH). Insulin deficiency leads to lipolysis, which in turn leads to the production of ketone bodies, resulting in an acidosis.

3. **Precipitating factors** include lack of insulin, infection, injuries, emotional stress, alcohol use, myocardial infarction (MI), and cerebrovascular accident.

B **Clinical features**

1. **Symptoms** include nausea, vomiting, abdominal pain, polyuria and polydipsia, and altered mental status.

2. **Physical examination findings**
   a. **Kussmaul's respirations** (i.e., rapid, shallow breathing) may be noted, and the breath often smells like **acetone.**

b. **Dehydration** may be reflected by **hypotension, reflex tachycardia, dry skin,** and **dry mucous membranes.**

C **Differential diagnoses** Hypoglycemia, nonketotic hyperosmolar coma, isopropyl alcohol ingestion, alcoholic ketoacidosis, lactic acidosis, uremia, toxin ingestion, and starvation ketosis must be ruled out.

D **Evaluation**

1. **Laboratory studies**
   a. A provisional diagnosis can be obtained via **arterial blood gas (ABG)** and **bedside glucose determinations.**
      (1) **Hyperglycemia** (defined as a serum glucose level of at least 300 mg/dL) will be evident.
      (2) **Metabolic acidosis** is demonstrated by a serum bicarbonate concentration of less than 15 mEq/L and a pH of less than 7.3.
   b. A **serum biochemical profile** [including **electrolytes, blood urea nitrogen (BUN),** and **creatinine levels**], **urinalysis,** and **ketone levels** confirm the diagnosis.
      (1) **Ketonemia** results from β-hydroxybutyrate and acetoacetate. Qualitative tests (e.g., the nitroprusside test) detect acetoacetate, but not β-hydroxybutyrate.
      (2) **Electrolyte derangements** may be present, depending on the patient's hydration status.
   c. **Other studies,** such as a complete blood count (CBC), a chest radiograph, or an electrocardiogram (ECG), may be indicated to identify precipitating causes.

E **Therapy**

1. **Normal saline** should be administered at an initial rate of 1 L/hour for the first 2–3 hours. The average fluid deficit is 5–10 L. Clinical response and urine output are the best indicators of fluid status. Be careful to correct fluid deficits over several hours as rapid fluid administration may result in cerebral edema, especially in children.

2. **Insulin** is usually administered intravenously using a low-dose technique (i.e., 5–10 U/hour) until the ketonemia and acidosis have resolved.

3. **Potassium** (20 mEq/L) should be added to the intravenous fluids early in therapy to correct the profound potassium deficiency associated with diabetic ketoacidosis. During the first day of treatment, the patient usually requires 100–200 mEq of potassium. Potassium levels must be closely monitored throughout therapy.

4. **Phosphate.** It is unclear whether phosphate replacement is necessary. Phosphate is given either orally or intravenously if the patient's serum phosphate level decreases to below 1.0 mg/dL.

F **Disposition** Most patients with diabetic ketoacidosis need to be admitted, often to an intensive care unit (ICU). In patients with mild diabetic ketoacidosis, the ketoacidosis may resolve in the ED. These patients should be placed under observation until any underlying precipitating causes can be ruled out.

III NONKETOTIC HYPEROSMOLAR COMA

A **Discussion**

1. **Definition.** Nonketotic hyperosmolar coma is a syndrome characterized by severe hyperglycemia, hyperosmolarity, and dehydration. Nonketotic hyperosmolar coma is less common than diabetic ketoacidosis and commonly occurs as an early manifestation of non–insulin-dependent diabetes. Occasionally, both nonketotic hyperosmolar coma and diabetic ketoacidosis are seen in the same patient.

2. **Etiology**
   a. **Diabetic patients** who have been subjected to a stressor (e.g., infection, stroke, gastrointestinal bleeding, pancreatitis) or who are taking thiazide diuretics, corticosteroids, phenytoin, cimetidine, propranolol, or calcium channel blockers may develop nonketotic hyperosmolar coma.

   b. Nondiabetic patients. Situations that cause severe dehydration or excessive glucose load (e.g., burns, heat stroke, peritoneal dialysis, hemodialysis, the ingestion of enormous amounts of sugar-containing foods) may cause this disorder in nondiabetic patients.

3. **Pathogenesis.** Nonketotic hyperosmolar coma and diabetic ketoacidosis represent different ends of a spectrum of lipid mobilization. Nonketotic hyperosmolar coma is precipitated by stress that increases glucose levels over days or weeks. The presence of a small amount of insulin is thought to suppress ketogenesis. Significant osmotic diureses lead to severe dehydration and altered mental status.

B **Clinical features**

1. **Patient history.** Most patients are elderly with either non–insulin-dependent diabetes (67% of patients) or insulin-dependent diabetes (33% of patients).

2. **Symptoms.** Patients develop polydipsia and polyuria initially, followed by alterations in mental status. The disorder may go unrecognized until stupor and coma develop. The severity of the altered mental status depends on the glucose level.

3. **Physical examination findings.** Principal findings include dehydration, fever, hypotension, tachycardia, and variable respiratory patterns. A variety of neurologic signs, such as tremors, fasciculations, hemisensory deficits, and hemiparesis, may occur.

C **Differential diagnoses**   Any disorder that can cause altered mental status (e.g., hepatic failure, uremia, sepsis, stroke, drug ingestion, lactic acidosis) must be considered.

D **Evaluation**

1. **Glucose, ketones,** and calculated and measured **serum osmolarity values** are essential.
   a. The **glucose level** is typically 1000 mg/dL or more.
   b. Although **ketones** may be present in small amounts, there is usually an absence of ketonemia and ketonuria.
   c. The **serum osmolarity** is greater than 350 mOsm/kg.

2. **Serum electrolyte, BUN,** and **creatinine levels; urinalysis;** and **ABG determinations** are indicated.
   a. Serum **sodium** ranges from 120–160 mEq/L and **potassium** depletion is usually severe.
   b. The **BUN** is usually elevated; the **BUN:creatinine ratio** usually exceeds 30:1.

3. **Other studies.** It is important to search for the underlying cause. A chest radiograph, ECG, computed tomography (CT) head scan, lumbar puncture, or cultures may be appropriate.

E **Therapy**

1. **Fluid resuscitation.** The average fluid deficit is 8–12 L; therefore, administration of half-normal saline (or normal saline for hypotensive patients) is indicated. One half of the patient's fluid deficit should be administered in the first 12 hours, and the remainder administered over the next 24 hours.

2. **Potassium** should be replaced early in the course of therapy. Usually, an infusion at a rate of 10–20 mEq/L for the first 24–36 hours is initiated if the patient's fluid status is such that he or she is able to produce urine.

3. **Insulin** is administered by continuous infusion (0.1 U/kg/hour) or intramuscular injection. The insulin should be stopped when the blood glucose level reaches 300 mg/dL.

4. **Glucose** is indicated if the glucose level is below 250 mg/dL.

5. **Phosphate.** Administration of phosphate is controversial.

6. **Low-dose heparin** may be used to prevent arterial and venous thrombosis.

F **Disposition**   Nonketotic hyperosmolar coma is associated with a high mortality rate. Patients are very ill and should be admitted to an intensive care service. Until the patient has been stabilized and other etiologies ruled out, transfer to other institutions is not advised.

IV **ALCOHOLIC KETOACIDOSIS**

A **Discussion**

1. **Definition.** Alcoholic ketoacidosis is usually seen in alcoholic patients who are forced to abruptly cease drinking alcohol after a drinking binge, but it may also be seen in first-time drinkers. These patients do not have diabetes mellitus. Alcoholic ketoacidosis is characterized by an anion gap acidosis and a high ketone level.

2. **Pathogenesis.** The pathogenesis is uncertain. It is related to low insulin levels, reduction of available nicotinamide adenine dinucleotide (NAD), and increased ketone formation.

B **Clinical features**

1. **Patient history.** The patient has recently stopped or limited alcohol consumption because of abdominal pain, nausea, and vomiting, not from a desire to stop drinking.

2. **Symptoms**
   a. **Diffuse abdominal pain** is typically present. Abdominal pain may be caused by alcohol-related diseases (e.g., pancreatitis, gastritis, hepatitis), or it may be caused by disorders unrelated to alcoholism (e.g., sepsis, pneumonia, pyelonephritis).
   b. **Symptoms of alcohol withdrawal** or **delirium tremens** may be noted.

3. **Physical examination findings**
   a. **Hydration status.** Dehydration occurs secondary to vomiting, diaphoresis, and decreased oral intake. The patient is acutely ill with **hypotension** and **tachycardia.**
   b. **Vital signs. Kussmaul's respirations** may be present, and the **temperature may be elevated** or normal.
   c. **Mental status** varies from **normal to comatose.**
   d. **Stigmata of alcoholism** (e.g., spider angiomata) may be noted.

C **Differential diagnoses** Any disorder that causes an anion gap acidosis must be ruled out. The most significant disorders to consider are diabetic ketoacidosis, hyperemesis gravidarum, starvation, cyanide poisoning, and isopropyl alcohol intoxication.

D **Evaluation**

1. **Serum biochemical profile** and an **ABG determination** will establish the presence of an anion gap acidosis. Although most patients have an acidic blood pH, a few patients may have normal or alkalotic pH values. A mixed disorder may also be found (e.g., metabolic ketoacidosis may occur from vomiting and respiratory alkalosis may occur from fever, sepsis, or alcohol withdrawal).

2. **Ketone studies.** β-Hydroxybutyric acid is the predominant ketone formed in alcoholic ketoacidosis. Because the nitroprusside test detects acetoacetate but not β-hydroxybutyrate, this test is of limited usefulness in patients with alcoholic ketoacidosis. As the patient undergoes treatment, acetoacetate levels increase, suggesting a fictitious worsening of the ketoacidosis.

3. **Bedside glucose determination.** The blood glucose level may be low, normal, or minimally elevated. Most patients have normal to increased glucose levels.

E **Therapy** The reversal of ketoacidosis can take 12–18 hours.

1. **Saline solutions containing glucose** and **thiamine** are administered to treat dehydration. Glucose appears to improve the clinical response. Magnesium and vitamin supplements should be given if poor oral intake is suspected.

2. **Insulin.** Administration of insulin is not indicated unless the patient has concomitant diabetes mellitus.

3. **Bicarbonate.** Administration of bicarbonate is controversial. Many authors would recommend administering a small amount of bicarbonate if the blood pH falls below 7.1, especially if myocardial disease, cardiac dysfunction, or arrhythmias are present.

F **Disposition**

1. **Admission.** Patients who cannot tolerate oral fluids or who have a significant metabolic acidosis should be admitted. Underlying or precipitating illnesses and abdominal pain must be evaluated prior to discharge. Patients usually respond to therapy in 12–24 hours and may be discharged at that time.

2. **Discharge.** If the patient responds well to therapy in the ED, he or she may be discharged. Close follow-up and referral for alcoholism treatment are essential.

V **LACTIC ACIDOSIS**

A **Discussion**

1. **Etiology**
   a. D-**Lactic acidosis** is associated with shortened bowel syndrome and is caused by bacterial fermentation. Treatment is neomycin or vancomycin.
   b. **Type A lactic acidosis** is caused by tissue hypoxia and is associated with a high mortality rate. The hypoxia may be related to hemorrhage or hypovolemic, cardiogenic, or septic shock.
   c. **Type B lactic acidosis** is not associated with tissue hypoxia. This type of acidosis may occur abruptly or over a few hours. The mechanism predisposing a patient to type B lactic acidosis is not well understood.
      (1) **Type B_1 lactic acidosis** is found in patients with diabetes, liver disease, sepsis, seizures, renal disease, and neoplasia.
      (2) **Type B_2 lactic acidosis** is associated with drugs, toxins, and chemicals. Ethanol is most commonly associated with this type of lactic acidosis; phenformin, fructose, and salicylate ingestion are also associated with type B_2 lactic acidosis.
      (3) **Type B_3 lactic acidosis** is associated with inborn errors of metabolism and is rare. Type I glycogen storage diseases and hepatic fructose biphosphate deficiency also cause type B_3 acidosis.

2. **Pathogenesis.** Lactic acidosis is caused by a buildup of lactic acid, which produces an anion gap acidosis.
   a. Lactate is a by-product of glycolysis. Lactate dehydrogenase (LDH) catalyzes the following reaction:

   $$Pyruvate + NADH + H^+ \rightarrow Lactate + NAD$$

      (1) Nicotinamide adenine dinucleotide (NADH) is reoxidized to NAD along the electron transport chain. This process is halted during anoxia, leading to the accumulation of lactate under the conditions of shock or tissue hypoxia.
      (2) The lactate-neutral ratio of lactate to pyruvate is 10:1. Alterations in this ratio create a high anion metabolic acidosis.
   b. The acidosis develops because the rate of production of lactate is greater than the rate of lactate utilization by the liver and kidneys.

B **Clinical features** are nonspecific. The onset of illness is usually abrupt. The patient appears ill, and hypoventilation or Kussmaul's respiration may be observed. Alterations in mental status range from lethargy to coma. Vomiting and abdominal pain may be present.

C **Differential diagnoses** include those disorders that produce an anion gap acidosis (e.g., diabetic ketoacidosis, alcoholic ketoacidosis, renal failure, salicylate toxicity, methanol toxicity, ethylene glycol toxicity, paraldehyde toxicity, cyanide poisoning).

D **Evaluation**

1. ABG determinations; serum electrolyte, glucose, BUN, and creatinine levels; liver function studies; and a drug screen are necessary to make the diagnosis.

2. Measurement of lactate levels is indicative but not diagnostic of lactic acidosis. The normal lactate level (0.5–1.5 mEq/L) is increased to 5–6 mEq/L or more in patients with lactic acidosis. However, clinically insignificant factors that can increase the lactate level include exercise; hyperventilation; infusion of glucose, saline, and bicarbonate; and injections of insulin or epinephrine.

E **Therapy**

1. If it can be identified, the underlying cause of the lactic acidosis should be treated.

2. **Adequate ventilation** and **volume replacement** are essential. Vasopressors are not indicated because they may actually decrease tissue perfusion.

3. **Diuresis** is encouraged with adequate fluids and loop diuretics; the urine output should be 300–500 mL/hour. Oliguric patients may require hemodialysis with administration of bicarbonate.

4. **Sodium bicarbonate** is considered when the pH falls below 7.2.
   a. The dose of bicarbonate is calculated as discussed in Chapter 7 V D 4.
   b. The bicarbonate may be given as a push or as an infusion of 3–4 ampules of bicarbonate in 1 L of 5% dextrose in water.

5. **Other approaches.** Many other treatment modalities (e.g., insulin, thiamine, dichloroacetate) have been attempted, but none has been effective.

F **Disposition**   Patients with lactic acidosis are seriously ill and usually need to be admitted to the ICU.

VI   THYROID DISORDERS

A **Thyroid storm**

1. **Discussion**
   a. **Definition.** Thyroid storm is a rare, life-threatening manifestation of hyperthyroidism that affects 1%–27% of hyperthyroid patients.
   b. **Patient profile.** It is not possible to predict which hyperthyroid patients will develop thyroid storm. Patients commonly have hyperthyroidism for up to 2 years prior to the onset of thyroid storm, and most have antecedent Graves' disease. Patients with hyperthyroidism who are undiagnosed or untreated are at risk for thyroid storm.
   c. **Etiology.** Thyroid storm is thought to be caused by changes in thyroid production or secretion, alteration of the body's response to thyroid hormone, and adrenergic hyperactivity.
   d. **Precipitating factors.** There are many nonspecific stressors that can precipitate a thyroid storm. Infection, pulmonary emboli, nonketotic hyperosmolar coma, diabetic ketoacidosis, surgery, burns, emotional stress, and trauma can cause thyroid storm. Iodine[131] therapy, thyroid hormone ingestion, premature withdrawal of antithyroid therapy, and contrast radiographic material can also precipitate storm.

2. **Clinical features**
   a. **Thyroid storm** is difficult to diagnose because the manifestations are protean. The clues to diagnosis include a history of hyperthyroidism, ocular signs of Graves' disease, a widened pulse pressure, and a palpable goiter.
      (1) **Systemic manifestations.** Heat intolerance and fever are commonly present. The pulse rate ranges from 120–200 beats/min but is out of proportion to the fever. Sweating is profuse and leads to dehydration.
      (2) **Cardiovascular manifestations** include increased systolic blood pressure, an elevated pulse pressure, a systolic flow murmur, sinus tachycardia, and atrial fibrillation. Cardiac arrhythmia, congestive heart failure (CHF), and pulmonary edema are also found.
      (3) **CNS manifestations** are common and vary from agitation and restlessness to psychosis and mental confusion to obtundation and coma. Proximal muscle weakness and myopathy may also be seen.

      (4) **Gastrointestinal disturbances** are variable, and weight loss is common. Nausea, vomiting, anorexia, abdominal pain, and hepatic dysfunction with jaundice may occur.

    b. **Apathetic thyrotoxicosis** is a rare form of thyroid storm found in patients in their seventh decade or older. In patients with apathetic thyrotoxicosis, the usual hyperkinetic manifestations of thyroid storm are absent. Patients present with lethargy, slow mentation, placid apathetic facies, goiter blepharoptosis, and proximal muscle weakness. Atrial fibrillation and CHF may obscure the underlying thyrotoxicosis.

3. **Differential diagnoses.** Conditions that cause hypermetabolic states (e.g., cocaine intoxication, sympathomimetic excess, pheochromocytoma) should be considered in the differential diagnosis.

4. **Evaluation**

    a. **Thyroid function tests.** An elevated free thyroxine (T_4) level and a suppressed, unmeasurable thyroid-stimulating hormone (TSH) level confirm the diagnosis. In the rare condition of triiodothyronine (T_3) thyrotoxicosis, elevated T_3 levels are found in the presence of normal T_4 and TSH levels.

    b. **Other laboratory tests** that are frequently obtained include a serum electrolyte panel, cortisol levels, calcium levels, glucose levels, a CBC, and liver function tests.

        (1) Elevated glucose and calcium levels are a common finding.

        (2) Normochromic, normocytic anemia, depressed cholesterol levels, and elevations in liver enzyme activity are fairly common.

5. **Therapy.** The underlying causes or precipitating events need to be evaluated and treated. No precipitating event is found in up to 50% of cases.

    a. **General supportive measures** include:

        (1) Intravenous fluids to replace losses

        (2) Supplemental oxygen to compensate for increased consumption

        (3) Acetaminophen and cooling blankets to reduce fever

        (4) Digitalis and diuretics to treat CHF

        (5) Antiarrhythmics (except atropine) to treat cardiac arrhythmias

        (6) Hydrocortisone (300 mg daily administered intravenously), thought to increase survival by an unknown mechanism

    b. **Minimization of thyroid hormone synthesis and release**

        (1) **Propylthiouracil** (**PTU**, 900–1200 mg) or **methimazole** (90–120 mg) can be administered orally or via a nasogastric tube to inhibit thyroid hormone synthesis.

        (2) **Iodine** [in the form of **strong iodine solution** (1 mL three times daily), **potassium iodine** (10 drops of a solution containing 1 g/mL every 4–6 hours), or **sodium iodine** (1 g every 8–12 hours by slow intravenous infusion)] will prevent thyroid hormone release. Iodine preparations should be **administered 1 hour after the administration of PTU or methimazole** to prevent the synthesis of new hormone. Potassium-sparing diuretics and potassium-containing drugs should be used with caution in patients receiving potassium iodine because they can increase potassium load.

    c. **Symptomatic treatment.** Administering **propranolol** (1 mg/min up to 10 mg) blocks the peripheral thyroid effects. Propranolol also blocks the peripheral conversion of T_4 and T_3. Pregnant patients and patients with reactive airway disease, diabetes mellitus, or CHF should not receive propranolol. Reserpine and guanethidine are alternatives to propranolol.

6. **Disposition.** Patients diagnosed as having thyroid storm must be admitted to the ICU.

B Hypothyroidism and myxedema coma

1. **Discussion**

    a. **Hypothyroidism** is a slow, progressive disorder usually caused by subtotal thyroidectomy or radioactive iodine treatment. The prevalence of hypothyroidism varies from 0.1%–1%, and increases with age. Hypothyroidism is more prevalent in women.

(1) **Primary hypothyroidism** is failure of the thyroid gland to respond to TSH. It may be caused by therapy for Graves' disease, subtotal thyroidectomy, autoimmune thyroiditis, iodine deficiency, or antithyroid drugs, or it may be congenital.

(2) **Secondary hypothyroidism** is caused by failure of the anterior pituitary gland to release TSH. Causes include pituitary tumors, postpartum hemorrhage, and infiltrative disorders.

b. **Myxedema coma** is a rare but life-threatening expression of hypothyroidism. It is most common during the winter months in elderly women with long-standing hypothyroidism. There are many precipitating factors, including infection, cardiovascular events, hemorrhage, and trauma. The mortality rate is as high as 50%, even with treatment.

2. **Clinical features**
   a. **Hypothyroidism**
      (1) **Symptoms.** Patients present with fatigue, weakness, cold intolerance, constipation, weight gain, muscle cramps, diminished hearing, and mental disturbances. The voice may deepen. Neurologic manifestations include paresthesia, ataxia, delusions, hallucinations, and psychosis.
      (2) **Physical examination findings.** The skin feels dry and waxy, and nonpitting edema is present. Bradycardia, mild hypertension, and cardiac enlargement are also found.
   b. **Myxedema coma.** Patients present with the symptoms of hypothyroidism and are comatose.
      (1) **Vital signs.** Eighty percent of myxedema coma patients are hypothermic.
      (2) **Pulmonary signs.** Patients have respiratory distress characterized by hypoventilation, hypercapnia, and hypoxia.
      (3) **Cardiovascular manifestations** include cardiomegaly, ventricular arrhythmias, hypotension, and bradycardia.
      (4) **Neuropsychiatric manifestations** include seizures, ataxia, tremors, slow mentation, delusions, and psychosis.
      (5) **Gastrointestinal and renal manifestations.** Patients frequently present with or have symptoms of megacolon, urinary retention, and abdominal distention.

3. **Differential diagnoses.** The differential diagnoses for myxedema coma include:
   a. **All causes of coma** (e.g., hypothermia, respiratory failure, electrolyte imbalance, hypoglycemia, stroke, drug overdose)
   b. **Chronic renal failure**
   c. **Nephrotic syndrome**

4. **Evaluation.** The diagnosis of myxedema coma is made on the basis of signs and symptoms of coma in a patient with hypothyroidism.
   a. Thyroid function tests and serum TSH levels can usually confirm the diagnosis, although results are not usually available in the ED.
   b. Laboratory studies and radiologic evaluation should be tailored to the presenting complaint.
      (1) Patients may need a CBC, blood cultures, liver function tests, cholesterol levels, a serum electrolyte panel, renal function tests, ABG determinations, and/or serum calcium levels.
         (a) Classic findings include hyponatremia, hypochloremia, hypoxia, and hypercapnia. Elevated serum creatinine kinase, aspartate aminotransferase (AST), and lactate dehydrogenase (LDH) are found.
         (b) Variable potassium, calcium, and glucose levels are found.
      (2) A chest radiograph and ECG are usually necessary. A CT head scan and obstructive gastrointestinal series may also be necessary. The chest radiograph demonstrates an enlarged cardiac silhouette, and the ECG usually shows bradycardia, T-wave inversion, prolongation of the PR interval, and low voltage.

5. **Therapy.** Administration of medications, even in a normal dose, should be performed with caution.
   a. **General supportive measures**
      (1) Oxygen and ventilatory support

(2) Correction of hypothermia

(3) Correction of electrolyte and glucose abnormalities

(4) Administration of vasopressors

(5) Administration of antibiotics if the possibility of infection exists

(6) Administration of hydrocortisone (300 mg/day) to ensure an adequate cortisol level

    b. Specific therapy is the administration of **intravenous thyroxine** (400–500 mg infused slowly, followed by 50–100 mg daily). **Triiodothyronine** could be given instead at a dose of 25–50 mg intravenously.

6. Disposition. All patients with myxedema coma need to be admitted to an ICU. Patients with uncomplicated hypothyroidism can be treated at home.

VII ADRENAL INSUFFICIENCY AND ADRENAL CRISIS

A Discussion

1. Normal physiology

    a. The **adrenal medulla** secretes **catecholamines.**

    b. The **adrenal cortex** secretes **cortisol, aldosterone,** and **androgens.** Androgen production is significant in women but not in men.

        (1) Cortisol is a potent hormone affecting glucose metabolism and water distribution. It also influences the pressor effects of catecholamines.

        (2) Aldosterone increases sodium reabsorption and potassium excretion.

2. Adrenal insufficiency is a chronic disorder characterized by a lack of cortisol and aldosterone.

    a. Primary adrenal insufficiency results from the failure of the adrenal gland to produce cortical hormones. Primary insufficiency is uncommon and is most frequently caused by idiopathic autoimmune adrenalitis.

    b. Secondary adrenal insufficiency results from failure of the pituitary gland to secrete adrenocorticotropic hormone (ACTH). Secondary insufficiency is frequently caused by steroid suppression of the hypothalamic-pituitary-adrenal axis.

3. Adrenal crisis is a medical emergency that can affect patients with chronic adrenal insufficiency who experience an acute stressful event (e.g., surgery, trauma, infection).

B Clinical features

1. Patients present with nonspecific complaints of weakness, fatigue, lethargy, anorexia, nausea, vomiting, abdominal pain, diarrhea, dizziness, and weight loss. Dehydration, hypotension, postural orthostasis, tachycardia, decreased heart size, lowered cardiac output, and decreased urine output are seen. The skin is cold and dry with increased brownish pigmentation over the exposed areas of the body. Mentation may be slowed but coma is unlikely.

2. In patients with secondary adrenal insufficiency, signs and symptoms of hypothalamic or pituitary disease (e.g., loss of sexual performance, menstrual irregularities, headache, galactorrhea, visual disturbances, features of acromegaly, and signs of hypothyroidism) may be noted as well.

C Differential diagnoses

1. The signs and symptoms of **adrenal insufficiency** are nonspecific and similar to those caused by many **viral illnesses.**

2. In patients with **adrenal crisis,** any illness that causes cardiovascular compromise (e.g., **acute MI, sepsis, pulmonary embolism, heart failure, hypovolemia**) should be considered.

D Evaluation

1. Laboratory studies

   a. **Serum biochemical profile and ABG determination.** Findings include mild to moderate hyponatremia, mild hypokalemia, hypoglycemia, hypercalcemia, moderate increases in BUN levels, and a mild metabolic acidosis.
   b. **CBC.** Findings include lymphocytosis and mild eosinophilia.
   c. **ACTH test.** This test can be used to differentiate primary from secondary causes of adrenal insufficiency. Baseline ACTH and cortisol levels should be drawn. Thirty minutes following the intravenous administration of 250 mg ACTH, a cortisol level is obtained. The administration of ACTH may be therapeutic as well as diagnostic. Dexamethasone will not interfere with this test.

2. **Electrocardiography.** An ECG shows flattened T waves, a prolonged QT interval, low voltage, prolongation of the PR or QRS intervals, ST-segment depression, and signs of hyperkalemia.

3. **Radiography.** A chest radiograph demonstrates a small, narrow heart. An abdominal radiograph may show calcification of the adrenal glands.

E **Therapy**

1. **General supportive measures.** Fluids and vasopressors are administered to counteract dehydration and shock. Cardiac monitoring and determination of the central venous pressure can be used to monitor the response. It may be necessary to administer as many as 2–3 L of fluid over the first 8 hours.

2. **Therapy for adrenal crisis.** Patients suspected of having adrenal crisis should be treated before the confirmatory laboratory studies are returned.
   a. **Hydrocortisone.** An intravenous push of 100 mg should be given, and 100 mg should be added to the intravenous bottle.
   b. **Fludrocortisone** (0.05–0.1 mg) daily may be needed if hypotension and volume depletion persist.

F **Disposition**   All patients with adrenal crisis must be admitted to the ICU.

VIII   WERNICKE-KORSAKOFF SYNDROME

A **Discussion**

1. **Definition.** Wernicke-Korsakoff syndrome is a potentially fatal neurologic disorder, found in alcoholics with poor nutritional status, that is caused by chronic vitamin B_1 deficiency.

2. **Pathogenesis.** Alcoholism interferes with the gastrointestinal absorption of vitamin B_1 and impairs conversion of vitamin B_1 to its active metabolite. In many patients, concomitant liver disease impairs storage of vitamin B_1.
   a. The administration of glucose to an alcoholic patient with an inadequate supply of thiamine may precipitate this disorder.
   b. Some patients with Wernicke-Korsakoff syndrome have a genetic defect in transketolase that is only manifested when there is a thiamine deficiency.

B **Clinical features**   The classic triad of findings is abnormal mental status, ophthalmoplegia, and gait ataxia. Patients are disoriented and unable to identify familiar objects. Patients may also have hypothermia, hypotension, coma, and circulatory collapse.

C **Differential diagnoses** include any process that causes altered mental status (e.g., alcohol intoxication and withdrawal, trauma, and metabolic, infectious, or toxic disorders).

D **Evaluation**   The diagnosis is usually made clinically. If the diagnosis is in question, additional testing is needed. Laboratory evaluation and CT head scanning may be appropriate. The diagnosis of thiamine deficiency can be confirmed by enzymatic analysis, but patients need to be treated immediately.

E **Therapy**   With prompt therapy, the ophthalmoplegia usually resolves within hours and the coma resolves in hours to days, but the memory deficit may never resolve.

1. **Thiamine** (100 mg) administered intravenously is the treatment of choice. Thiamine (50–100 mg intravenously) is continued daily until the patient has achieved proper oral nutritional status.
   a. It is essential that thiamine be given prior to the administration of glucose.
   b. The administration of thiamine is standard protocol for patients with altered mental status and for those who are alcoholic and malnourished.

2. **Magnesium.** Hypomagnesemia must also be corrected.

F **Disposition**   Patients with Wernicke-Korsakoff syndrome must be admitted to the hospital. This syndrome is associated with a 15%–20% mortality rate.

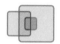

Study Questions

Directions: Each of the numbered items or incomplete statements in this section is followed by answers or by completions of the statement. Select the ONE lettered answer or completion that is BEST in each case.

1. What is the mortality rate associated with Wernicke-Korsakoff syndrome?
   - A 0%–5%
   - B 5%–10%
   - C 10%–15%
   - D 15%–20%
   - E 20%–25%

2. A 75-year-old woman is brought to the emergency department (ED). She has signs and symptoms of congestive heart failure (CHF), and atrial fibrillation is detected on the electrocardiograph (ECG). What other symptom may also be observed?
   - A Blepharoptosis
   - B Exophthalmos
   - C Stare
   - D Lid lag

3. What is the correct sequence of agents in the treatment of thyroid storm?
   - A Propranolol, propylthiouracil (PTU), iodine
   - B Iodine, PTU, propranolol
   - C PTU, iodine, propranolol
   - D PTU, propranolol, iodine

4. How should insulin be administered to patients with nonketotic hyperosmolar coma?
   - A Bolus
   - B Bolus plus infusion
   - C Continuous infusion
   - D No insulin should be administered

5. A 50-year-old man is brought to the emergency department (ED) following a drinking binge that has lasted for 3 days. Acute abdominal pain has caused the patient to temporarily stop consuming alcohol. The patient is found to have alcoholic ketoacidosis. What is the usual treatment?
   - A Administration of fluids and bicarbonate
   - B Administration of fluids, glucose, and thiamine
   - C Administration of fluids, glucose, thiamine, and bicarbonate
   - D Administration of fluids

6. What laboratory test assists in making the diagnosis of lactic acidosis?
   - A Serum electrolyte panel
   - B Serum lactate level
   - C Serum ketone level
   - D Serum glucose level

7. A 70-kg, 25-year-old man is brought to the emergency department (ED) and a diagnosis of diabetic ketoacidosis is made. Administration of intravenous fluids is indicated. How much fluid should be given in the first 2 hours of therapy?

- A 500 mL
- B 1000 mL
- C 2000 mL
- D 10 mL/kg
- E 20 mL/kg

8. Which one of the following is NOT commonly a precipitant of nonketotic hyperosmolar coma?

- A Hydrochlorothiazide
- B Cimetidine
- C Heat stroke
- D Aspirin

Answers and Explanations

1. The answer is D Wernicke-Korsakoff syndrome is associated with a mortality rate of 15%–20%. The ophthalmoplegia and coma usually resolve, but the memory deficit may persist.

2. The answer is A This elderly woman most likely has apathetic thyrotoxicosis, a rare form of thyroid storm found in patients older than 60 years. These patients often have CHF and atrial fibrillation. Blepharoptosis (i.e., drooping of the upper eyelid) is commonly found in these patients. The other ocular symptoms of Graves' disease that are usually seen in patients with thyroid storm (e.g., stare, exophthalmos, lid lag) are not usually found in patients with apathetic thyrotoxicosis.

3. The answer is C In patients with thyroid storm, the synthesis of new hormone must first be prevented, followed by the retardation of thyroid hormone release. PTU is administered first to inhibit thyroid hormone synthesis. Iodine is administered 1 hour later to prevent the release of thyroid hormone. Propranolol is used to block thyrotoxic symptoms and is administered last.

4. The answer is C Insulin is administered as a continuous infusion (0.1 U/kg/hour) to patients with nonketotic hyperosmolar coma. Insulin is not usually indicated in patients with alcoholic ketoacidosis, because these patients do not usually have diabetes.

5. The answer is B Administration of saline (normal or half-normal) with glucose is the mainstay of treatment for alcoholic ketoacidosis. Thiamine administration is indicated prior to administration of the glucose to prevent Wernicke-Korsakoff syndrome. Insulin is not used to treat this disorder. The administration of bicarbonate is controversial; it may be indicated in patients with a blood pH below 7.1 who are experiencing cardiac dysfunction or arrhythmias.

6. The answer is A The diagnosis of lactic acidosis is made by finding an anion gap acidosis in the context of a process that can cause an accumulation of lactate. Elevated lactate levels can be found in lactic acidosis as well as in many conditions not associated with acidosis. Lactic acidosis is not characterized by ketonemia.

7. The answer is C Patients with diabetic ketoacidosis are significantly dehydrated and often have a fluid deficit of 5–10 L. Generally, 2–3 L of fluid are administered during the first hour of therapy.

8. The answer is D Many agents and procedures can precipitate nonketotic hyperosmolar coma. Often, these precipitating factors are factors that can induce hyperglycemia or glucose loads. Aspirin therapy is not a precipitating factor for nonketotic hyperosmolar coma. Thiazide diuretics (e.g., hydrochlorothiazide) and cimetidine can induce nonketotic hyperosmolar coma in patients with diabetes. Conditions that cause severe dehydration, such as heat stroke, can cause nonketotic hyperosmolar coma in nondiabetic patients.

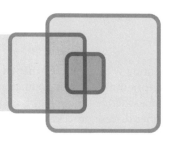

chapter **9**

Neurologic Emergencies

LESLIE S. CARROLL · NICHOLAS LORENZO

I ALTERED MENTAL STATUS AND COMA

A **Discussion**

1. **Pathogenesis.** Coma or a change in mental status implies bilateral cortical disease or suppression of the reticular activating system.

2. **Causes.** The potential causes of altered mental status and coma are innumerable. The mnemonic **"AEIOU TIPS"** is an organized way of remembering the various potential causes of altered mental status and coma.

   a. **A** stands for **alcohol** (and **drugs** and **toxins**). Pharmacologic agents alter mental status through bilateral cortical suppression.

   b. **E** stands for **endocrine** and **environmental** causes.
      (1) **Endocrine causes** include **hyperammonemia** (e.g., secondary to liver disease), **electrolyte abnormalities** (e.g., hyponatremia), and **hypo-** and **hyperthyroidism.**
      (2) **Environmental causes** include **hypo-** and **hyperthermia.**

   c. **I** designates **insulin poisoning** and **impaired glucose utilization.**
      (1) **Hypoglycemia** is the most common cause of altered mental status seen in the emergency department (ED). Hypoglycemia may occur in any patient but is more commonly seen in patients with diabetes, alcoholics, neonates, patients with toxic ingestions, patients with poor nutrition states, and patients with pancreatic tumors or retroperitoneal sarcomas. Hypoglycemia may also occur secondary to infection, metabolic derangements, insulin poisoning, and oral hypoglycemic dosing.
      (2) **Hyperglycemia** leading to diabetic ketoacidosis may cause altered mental status.

   d. **O** signifies **oxygen deprivation** and **opiate poisoning.**
      (1) **Oxygen deprivation (hypoxemia)** has multiple causes (e.g., pneumonia, cerebral hypoperfusion secondary to shock or cardiac arrhythmias, pulmonary embolism, bronchospasm).
      (2) **Opiate poisoning** depresses central respiratory centers, leading to acute hypoxia.

   e. **U** signifies **uremia.** Coma may occur secondary to rapid changes in the blood urea nitrogen (BUN) level.

   f. **T** stands for **trauma.** Hypoperfusion and cerebral trauma may induce a change in mental status.

   g. **I** signifies **infection.** Both systemic and neurologic infection (e.g., meningitis, encephalitis) may induce a change in mental status.

   h. **P** designates **psychiatric causes** and **porphyria.** Attributing a change in mental status to a psychiatric cause is a diagnosis of exclusion.

   i. **S** stands for **space-occupying lesions,** which induce an altered state of consciousness or coma by involving the bilateral cortical hemispheres or suppressing the reticular activating system.
      (1) Bilateral cortical disease is generally secondary to metabolic or toxic causes.
      (2) Space-occupying lesions induce coma by increasing pressure on the reticular activating system, not by causing local neuronal destruction.

B **Evaluation**   The patient presenting with an altered mental status requires a thorough physical examination, appropriate laboratory and diagnostic evaluation, and immediate treatment. The goal of the ED physician is to determine whether the etiology is metabolic or toxic in nature (as opposed to a structural defect). The former disease process is managed medically, whereas the latter is a potential surgical emergency.

1. **Stabilization**
   a. **ABCs and vital signs.** The airway, breathing, and circulatory status of the patient must be evaluated initially, and a full set of vital signs is essential.
   b. **Intravenous access, cardiac monitoring,** and **supplemental oxygen** should be established.
   c. **Oxygen and glucose levels** should be evaluated using **pulse oximetry** and an **accucheck.**
      (1) **Hypoxemia** is corrected by administering **supplemental oxygen. Naloxone** should be administered intravenously in an adult to reverse opiate-induced respiratory depression. There are no case reports of adverse effects secondary to naloxone dosing; however, the patient may experience an acute opiate withdrawal syndrome.
      (2) **Hypoglycemia** is rapidly corrected by administering glucose. **Thiamine** should be administered prior to administering **glucose** in an adult to avoid precipitating Wernicke's encephalopathy.

2. **Physical examination.** A thorough physical examination is essential.
   a. **General examination.** The patient should be undressed and the entire body examined. Clues to the cause of the altered mental status may include evidence of trauma, needle marks, perspiration, skin discoloration (e.g., jaundice), odors (e.g., alcohol, acetone), and rashes.
   b. **Head, ears, eyes, nose, and throat (HEENT)**
      (1) **Head.** The head should be inspected for evidence of trauma. **Bilateral periorbital ecchymosis ("raccoon's eyes")** or **ecchymosis around the mastoid area (Battle's sign)** suggests a basilar skull fracture.
      (2) **Eyes**
         (a) **Pupils.** Pupillary size and reactivity should be assessed.
            (i) **Miosis** results from multiple causes, which can be remembered using the mnemonic **"COPS²":**
               Clonidine and imidazoles
               Opiates
               Phenothiazines (especially Thorazine)
               Sedative-hypnotic agents
               Cholinergics (e.g., pilocarpine, physostigmine)
               Organophosphates and carbamates
               Pontine hemorrhage
               Sleep
            (ii) **Mydriasis** may result from anticholinergic agents or sympathomimetic agents. A fixed and dilated pupil suggests uncal herniation of the temporal lobe on the ipsilateral side with resultant compression of cranial nerve III. However, in an alert patient, a fixed and dilated pupil may be secondary to therapy with a cycloplegic agent or aneurysmal compression of cranial nerve III.
         (b) **Fundi.** The fundi should be inspected to rule out increased intracranial pressure (ICP).
      (3) **Ears.** The tympanic membranes should be inspected to rule out blood behind the membrane, which would indicate a basilar skull fracture.
      (4) **Nose.** The nares are inspected to rule out a cerebrospinal fluid (CSF) leak.
      (5) **Throat.** The pharynx should be inspected and a gag reflex elicited. An absent gag reflex predisposes a patient to aspiration and may be an indication for intubation.
   c. **Neck.** Palpation of the cervical spine in a comatose patient is unnecessary. A cervical injury should be assumed and the neck immobilized. If the history and physical examination are not consistent with a traumatic injury, then the neck should be evaluated for signs of meningismus.

d. **Heart.** The heart should be examined for arrhythmias, murmurs (suggesting endocarditis), and rubs (suggesting uremic pericarditis). Blood pressure must be serially evaluated to rule out hypo- or hypertension.

e. **Lungs.** The respiratory rate and pattern must be evaluated.

   (1) **Hypoventilation** may occur secondary to metabolic abnormalities or toxicity. An acute opiate overdose may present as a depressed level of consciousness and a decreased respiratory rate.

   (2) **Hyperventilation** may be seen in numerous disease states (e.g., metabolic acidosis, salicylate poisoning, hypoxia, hypercarbia).

   (3) **Cheyne-Stokes respiration** is a crescendo–decrescendo pattern of breathing that implies bilateral hemispheric dysfunction with an intact brain stem. This type of breathing accompanies metabolic disorders and may be the first sign of transtentorial herniation.

   (4) **Apneustic breathing** is characterized by a prolonged pause after inspiration (similar to breath holding) and is seen in patients with pontine infarction.

   (5) **Ataxic breathing** is irregular breathing without a pattern; this type of breathing is preterminal.

f. **Abdomen and rectum.** A thorough abdominal examination, including a rectal examination, may aid in the diagnosis of an altered state of consciousness.

   (1) The abdomen should be inspected for signs of trauma. **Cullen's sign (periumbilical ecchymosis)** and **Grey Turner's sign (flank ecchymosis)** suggest retroperitoneal hemorrhage.

   (2) **Organomegaly** (e.g., hepatomegaly, splenomegaly, distended bladder), **ascites, bruits, masses, heme-positive stools,** and the presence or absence of **bowel sounds** may aid in determining the cause of the altered mental status. For example, a patient with an altered mental status who has no bowel sounds and a distended bladder may have ingested an anticholinergic medication. A patient with hepatomegaly and ascites may be suffering from hepatic encephalopathy.

3. **Neurologic examination.** The neurologic examination evaluates mental status, cranial nerve involvement, motor responses, cerebellar integrity, and reflexes.

   a. **Glasgow coma scale** (Table 9–1). The Glasgow coma scale uses a point score (from 3–15) to categorize eye, verbal, and motor responses according to the severity of impairment.

      (1) Any patient who can move a body part on command is demonstrating high-level motor system functioning.

      (2) Movement of limbs in response to a noxious stimulus implies motor system involvement, at least at the diencephalic level.

      (3) **Decorticate posturing** (i.e., hyperextension of the legs and flexion of the elbows, drawing the hands toward the center of the body) suggests lesions of the internal capsule or upper midbrain that interfere with the corticospinal pathways.

      (4) **Decerebrate posturing** is hyperextension of the arms and legs. This type of posturing is seen in severe disease in which only the lower brain stem is intact.

      (5) Total paralysis in a comatose patient implies that no brain stem functioning is occurring and is extremely grave.

   b. **Mental status exam.** The mental status exam primarily addresses the patient's orientation to person, place, and time. The ability to respond to voiced commands is then tested. If the patient does not respond to verbal stimuli, then response to noxious stimuli should be attempted.

   c. **Cranial nerve assessment** is described in Table 9–2.

   d. **Muscle strength assessment.** If the patient is able to follow simple commands, then the motor strength in major muscle groups should be documented on a point scale of 0–5 (Table 9–3).

   e. **Sensory examination.** Responses to light touch, pain, proprioception, and a sensory level (in patients with spinal injuries) should be evaluated. Figure 9–1 shows the sensory dermatomes.

TABLE 9–1   Glasgow Coma Scale

Category	Response	Score
Eyes	Open spontaneously	4
	Open in response to verbal command	3
	Open in response to pain	2
	No response	1
Best verbal response	Oriented and conversant	5
	Disoriented but conversant	4
	Inappropriate words	3
	Incomprehensible sounds	2
	No response	1
Best motor response	Obeys commands	6
	Responds to painful stimulus	5
	Withdraws from painful stimulus	4
	Decorticate posturing	3
	Decerebrate posturing	2
	No response	1
Total score		3–15

   f. **Reflexes** should be assessed and graded on a scale from 0–4: 0 = no response, 1 = hypoactive, 2 = normal, 3 = brisk but not pathologic, and 4 = abnormally brisk with or without clonus. Reflexes tested include the biceps (C5–6), triceps (C7–8), brachioradialis (C5–6), quadriceps (L3–4), ankle (S1–2), and Babinski (pathologic extension of the toes on lateral stroking of the plantar surface of the foot).

   g. **Cerebellar function** is assessed by gait, finger-to-nose testing, and heel-to-shin testing.

TABLE 9–2   Cranial Nerve Examination

Cranial Nerve		Function	Assessment
I	Olfactory	Smell	Ask patient to identify odors
II	Optic	Vision	Ask patient to read or count fingers
III	Oculomotor	Eye movement, pupillary constriction, and pupillary accommodation	Test eye movement, pupillary constriction, and pupillary accommodation
IV	Trochlear	Eye movement	Test eye movement; have patient follow object
V	Trigeminal	Facial sensation, masseter muscle innervation	Test facial sensation; have patient bite while palpating masseter muscle
VI	Abducens	Abducts eye	Ask patient to look to the side
VII	Facial	Facial movement, taste (anterior two thirds of tongue)	Ask patient to wrinkle forehead and close eyes
VIII	Vestibulocochlear	Hearing and balance	Test hearing and balance
IX	Glossopharyngeal	Taste (posterior one third of tongue), gag reflex, salivation	Test patient's gag reflex with a tongue depressor
X	Vagus	Lifts palate	Ask patient to say "ah" and observe symmetric elevation of the palate with the uvula midline
XI	Accessory	Innervates sternocleidomastoid and trapezius muscles	Ask patient to shrug shoulders and move head from side to side
XII	Hypoglossal	Innervates tongue	Ask patient to move tongue from side to side

TABLE 9–3   Evaluation of Muscle Strength

Grade	Equivalent Patient Ability
0/5	No detectable contraction
1/5	Palpable contraction, trace movement
2/5	Able to move when gravity is eliminated
3/5	Able to move fully against gravity but not resistance
4/5	Able to oppose gravity and resistance
5/5	Normal

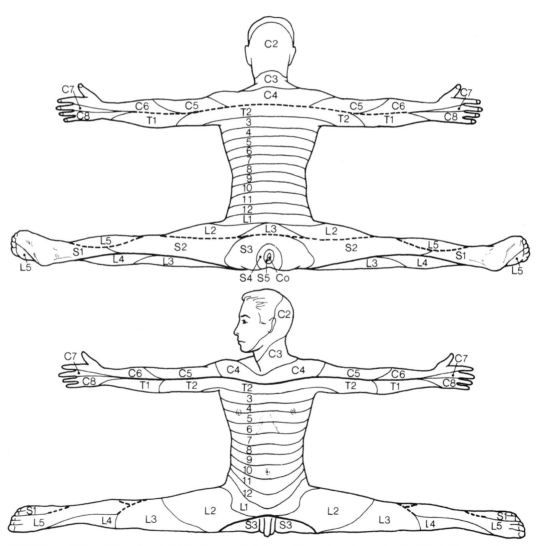

FIGURE 9–1   Pattern of dermatomal distributions and their innervation by the spinal roots. (Reprinted with permission from Haymaker W, Woodhall B. *Peripheral Nerve Injuries.* 2nd Ed. Philadelphia: WB Saunders, 1953:19.)

4. **Laboratory studies**
   a. **Complete blood count (CBC).** A CBC should be performed to detect abnormalities (e.g., anemia, leukemia) or to confirm suspicions of an infective process.
   b. **Electrolyte status.** The discovery of electrolyte disturbances (e.g., hypo- or hypernatremia), a rapid change in BUN level, or detection of an osmolar gap (typical in patients with toxic alcohol ingestions) may aid in diagnosis.
   c. **Arterial blood gas (ABG) analysis.** All patients with an altered mental status should undergo ABG analysis to determine the acid–base status and to detect hypoxia and hypercarbia.
   d. **Urine drug screen.** A urine drug screen may reveal the cause of the change in mental status.
   e. **Specific levels** (e.g., ammonia, calcium, thyroid hormone, salicylate, lithium, phenobarbital, carbamazepine, phenytoin, valproic acid, digoxin) may be ordered, depending on the patient's history and examination findings.
   f. **CSF analysis.** A lumbar puncture may be necessary to rule out meningitis or encephalitis.

5. **Diagnostic studies**
   a. **Electrocardiogram (ECG).** An ECG should be obtained to rule out a myocardial infarction, which may decrease cardiac output enough to elicit cerebral hypoperfusion. Brady- or tachyarrhythmias may also lead to cerebral hypoperfusion and a change in mental status.
   b. **Computed tomography (CT) scan.** A brain CT scan may help to rule out mass lesions.
   c. **Cervical spine series.** A patient with a change in mental status may have suffered trauma; a cervical spine series should be performed to rule out injury.
   d. **Electroencephalogram (EEG).** An EEG is an inpatient procedure designed to assess potential seizure activity and cortical functioning.

C **Disposition** of the patient with an altered level of consciousness depends entirely on the diagnosis. For example, a patient presenting with hypoglycemia secondary to inappropriate insulin dosing may be observed and subsequently discharged, a trauma patient with an acute intracranial bleed requires neurosurgical consultation, and a patient suffering acute salicylate poisoning may require urgent dialysis.

II   HEADACHE

A **Migraine**

1. **Discussion.** Migraine headaches are generally recurrent attacks that vary widely in intensity, duration, and frequency.
   a. **Onset.** They usually begin in adolescence or early adult life, although onset may occur in childhood. The development and persistence of migraines in later life are most unusual.
   b. **Predisposing factors.** Women are afflicted three times more often than men. There is a definite relationship to the menstrual cycle, with more attacks occurring during menses. During pregnancy, most women are symptom-free during the third trimester.
   c. **Pathophysiology**
      (1) **Vascular hypothesis.** According to this theory, put forth by Graham and Wolff in 1938, the aura is secondary to vasoconstriction, and the headache is secondary to subsequent vasodilatation.
      (2) **Neuronal hypothesis.** In 1944, Leao described a slowly spreading wave of cortical activity ("spreading depression") as being responsible for migraine headache.
      (3) **Neurovascular hypothesis.** Presently, an integrated theory of migraine headache has developed. A patient with a low threshold for migraine headache responds to excessive afferent input or an endogenous stimulus (e.g., stress) by developing a headache. The cortex and hypothalamus act on brain-stem nuclei to induce changes in the cerebral vasculature. Stimulation of the locus ceruleus results in cerebral vasoconstriction, initiating the aura. The vasoconstriction is followed by a neurogenic sterile inflammatory reaction

around the trigeminal axons, leading to extracranial vessel dilation. Trigeminal nerve input is carried to the brain and is perceived as painful.

2. **Clinical features.** Migraines are usually unilateral, throbbing, and associated with anorexia, nausea, and vomiting.

   a. Classic migraine occurs in only 12% of patients with migraine and is often familial.

     (1) The prodromal phase is sharply defined, with the aura beginning up to 1 hour prior to the start of head pain. Contralateral manifestations include scotomas, fortification spectra, visual field defects, and transient amblyopia. Occasionally, the prodromal symptoms are motor or sensory.

     (2) The aura is followed by a unilateral throbbing headache associated with nausea, vomiting, photophobia, and sonophobia.

   b. Common migraine is the most common migraine syndrome, occurring in over 80% of migraine patients.

     (1) The prodromal symptoms are not sharply defined and may consist of mood disturbances, fatigue, nausea, and vomiting. Visual disturbances are not present. The prodromal phase may precede the headache by hours or days.

     (2) The headache is unilateral, throbbing, and associated with photophobia, sonophobia, anorexia, nausea, vomiting, and general malaise.

   c. Complicated migraine occurs when the neurologic symptoms persist beyond the headache phase of a classic migraine. These patients often present with disorders of speech including dysarthria, aphasia, dyslexia, and dysgraphia. Permanent sequelae may result from major or minor strokes secondary to ischemic or hemorrhagic infarcts.

   d. Basilar artery migraine primarily affects young, menstruating women.

     (1) The prodromal symptoms are typically visual and include visual scintillations and visual loss throughout both visual fields. The visual disturbances are quickly followed by vertigo, ataxia, dysarthria, or tinnitus and peripheral paresthesias. Loss of consciousness may occur.

     (2) The prodrome lasts from a few minutes to up to an hour and is followed by a severe throbbing occipital headache and vomiting.

   e. Ophthalmic and hemiplegic migraines are rare; young adults are usually affected. The neurologic deficits of both headaches rarely persist after the attack.

     (1) Ophthalmic migraine. In ophthalmic migraine, the headache is ipsilateral to an ocular nerve palsy. A third nerve palsy combined with pupillary dilatation is common. The migraine cannot be differentiated from an intracranial aneurysm compressing cranial nerve III in the region of the carotid or at the junction of the internal carotid and the posterior communicating artery. This headache is a diagnosis of exclusion; a normal cerebral angiogram may be required to make this diagnosis.

     (2) Hemiplegic migraine is characterized by neurologic deficits that range from mild hemiparesis to full hemiplegia associated with a contralateral headache. Hemiplegic migraine is also a diagnosis of exclusion.

3. **Differential diagnoses.** There are numerous causes of headache. Some of the more common causes include temporomandibular joint (TMJ) syndrome, head injury, anemia, uremia, toxic effects from drugs or fumes, dental disease, Paget's disease, sinusitis, refractive error, hypertension, hypoxia, temporal arteritis, and tumors.

4. **Therapy**

   a. Acute therapy

     (1) Sumatriptan is a serotonin agonist that induces vasoconstriction. Sumatriptan is administered subcutaneously in 6-mg dosages, 1 hour apart. No more than 12 mg should be administered in a 24-hour period. Contraindications to sumatriptan include ischemic heart disease, hypertension, headache with neurologic symptoms, concurrent ergotamine administration, and intravenous drug use. Several other triptan (e.g., naratriptan, zolmitriptan) medications, all of which have similar mechanisms of action, are also available for use. It is important to note that these headache patients may respond to one triptan but not another. Thus, multiple trials of the different triptans are appropriate before declaring the patient "triptan unresponsive."

    (2) **Ergotamines** are potent vasoconstrictors. Contraindications are similar to those for sumatriptan.

        (a) **Oral or sublingual ergotamines** are administered in 2-mg dosages at 30-minute intervals, to a total dose of 6 mg.

        (b) **Dihydroergotamine (DHE)** is administered intramuscularly or intravenously in 1-mg dosages at 1-hour intervals, to a maximum dose of 6 mg in 1 week.

    (3) **Antiemetics** (e.g., metoclopramide, prochlorperazine, domperidone, cyclizine) are often used successfully as first-line treatment for migraine; often, the headache will resolve with this treatment alone. If the headache persists, then either sumatriptan or DHE may be given (in the absence of contraindications).

    (4) **Analgesics** and **nonsteroidal anti-inflammatory drugs (NSAIDs)** are also part of the treatment armamentarium. Narcotic analgesics are sporadically used but are usually avoided because of the potential for addiction and respiratory depression.

  b. **Prophylactic treatment.** ED physicians generally do not prescribe prophylactic treatment for migraines; however, the ED physician should be familiar with these medications because the patient may be taking them at the time he or she presents to the ED. Prophylactic agents include β-adrenergic blocking agents, ergotamine preparations, methysergide, cyproheptadine, monoamine oxidase (MAO) inhibitors, NSAIDs, tricyclic antidepressants, and calcium channel blockers.

B Cluster headache (histamine headache, migrainous neuralgia)

1. **Discussion.** Cluster headaches occur several times daily for weeks or months and are followed by long periods of pain-free intervals. The headaches are more common in the spring and fall.

  a. **Incidence.** Cluster headaches occur in 2%–9% of patients who complain of headaches.

  b. **Predisposing factors.** Men are affected four to five times more frequently than women. Cluster headaches are often precipitated by ingestion of alcohol, use of nitroglycerin- or histamine-containing products, stress, changes in climate, and allergens.

2. **Clinical features.** Cluster headaches are characterized by unilateral excruciating facial pain that is often accompanied by ipsilateral nasal congestion, lacrimation, and conjunctival injection. Horner's syndrome (i.e., ptosis, miosis, and anhidrosis) may be seen; the ptosis and miosis are ipsilateral.

3. **Therapy. One hundred percent oxygen** (8–10 L/min for 10–15 minutes) has been found to be helpful in treating cluster headaches. **Ergotamines, triptans** (e.g., sumatriptan, naratriptan), and **analgesics** are also used.

C Post–lumbar puncture headache

1. **Discussion.** Five to thirty percent of patients who undergo lumbar puncture develop a headache within hours or a few days of the procedure. The headache is thought to be secondary to low CSF pressure and a continuous CSF leak.

2. **Clinical features.** Patients present with a bilateral pulsatile headache associated with nausea and vomiting that is exacerbated by sitting upright and relieved by supination.

3. **Therapy**

  a. Mildly symptomatic patients should receive **antiemetics, intravenous fluids,** and **analgesics.**

  b. Patients with persistent symptoms may require a trial of intravenous **caffeine sodium benzoate** to increase the CSF pressure via cerebral vasoconstriction. Caffeine is administered as a 500-mg bolus over 15 minutes, and then as a continuous drip of 500 mg over 2–3 hours.

Caffeine administration is generally reserved for younger patients and is contraindicated in patients with coronary artery disease or hypertension, patients taking theophylline, patients with a history of arrhythmias, and patients at risk for a vasospastic event.

c. Severely symptomatic patients may require a **"blood patch"** (i.e., autologous transfer of blood to the epidural space at the site of the previous lumbar puncture). This procedure is thought to stop leakage of CSF, thus restoring cerebral pressure. Consultation with an anesthesiologist is necessary when considering this treatment, as the anesthesiologist may perform this simple procedure and discharge the patient home if improved.

4. **Disposition.** Most patients with post–lumbar puncture headaches are discharged. Patients with complicating features require admission.

D **Hypertensive headaches** are rare and overly diagnosed in the ED. An acute hypertensive headache requires a diastolic blood pressure elevation of approximately 25% or a sustained diastolic blood pressure greater than 130 mm Hg. Patients present with hypertension and a throbbing occipital headache. Treatment with antihypertensive agents relieves the headache and most patients can be discharged. Patients with hypertensive urgency or crisis require admission (see Chapter 2 VI).

E **Pseudotumor cerebri (benign intracranial hypertension)** occurs in young, obese females with irregular menses or amenorrhea. The patient presents with a severe headache, nausea, vomiting, and visual complaints. Papilledema is evident on physical examination. A CT scan will demonstrate signs of increased ICP without mass effect; the ventricles are slit-like. Lumbar puncture reveals CSF pressures greater than 250 mm Hg. Therapy consists of repeated lumbar punctures to relieve pressure. Steroids may also be administered. Most patients are discharged, but patients with severe symptoms that fail to resolve with lumbar puncture require admission.

F **Temporal arteritis**

1. **Discussion.** Temporal arteritis is a vasculitis of the temporal artery. The disease occurs in elderly patients (the average age at the time of onset is 70 years). Left untreated, temporal arteritis may result in bilateral blindness.

2. **Clinical features.** Patients present with unilateral, excruciating, burning pain over the affected artery. The disease is often associated with polymyalgia rheumatica (PMR) and may present with systemic involvement including fever, polymyalgia, malaise, weight loss, and anorexia. Patients complain of decreased visual acuity. Physical examination reveals a tender, inflamed temporal artery. An afferent pupillary defect may be present.

3. **Evaluation.** Diagnosis is made by history, physical examination, and the demonstration of an erythrocyte sedimentation rate (ESR) greater than 50 mm/hour. Definitive diagnosis is established through arterial biopsy.

4. **Therapy** consists of the administration of high-dose steroids.

5. **Disposition.** Patients should be admitted to the hospital for the administration of systemic steroids and close observation. Consultation with a rheumatologist is necessary.

G **Trigeminal neuralgia** affects older patients, especially women. The pain is secondary to trigeminal nerve hyperactivity. Clinically, patients present with unilateral facial pain (most commonly in the V2 distribution, although the V1 and V3 distributions may be affected). The pain is generally brief, intermittent, and described as "electric." The pain is triggered by eating, talking, or touching the face. Physical examination is unremarkable, and there are no neurologic deficits. Carbamazepine is the outpatient treatment of choice.

H **Other causes of headache**

1. **Subarachnoid hemorrhage (SAH)**

a. **Discussion**

    (1) **Etiology.** SAH most commonly results from rupture of an **intracranial aneurysm.** The second most common cause is rupture of an **arteriovenous malformation.** Twenty-five percent of patients with a ruptured aneurysm will die the same day. Of the patients who survive, most are left with severe neurologic deficits. SAH is found in 1% of all ED patients with a headache. Always maintain a low index of suspicion.

    (2) **Pathophysiology.** Saccular aneurysms occur most commonly at the bifurcations of the large arteries and subsequently rupture into the subarachnoid space.

b. **Clinical features**

    (1) **Headache.** Patients complain of the sudden onset of a headache that they may describe as "the worst headache of my life." The headache may be nonlocalized or may be localized to the occipital area and neck.

    (2) **Loss of consciousness** occurs in 45% of patients secondary to decreased cerebral perfusion.

    (3) **Vomiting** occurs secondary to increased ICP.

    (4) **Focal neurologic deficits.** Most commonly, SAH is not associated with focal neurologic deficits. However, the presence of a focal neurologic deficit may aid in localization of the aneurysm. For example, an aneurysm at the junction of the posterior communicating artery and the internal carotid artery may result in a third nerve palsy associated with pupillary dilatation, loss of light reflex, and retro-orbital pain.

    (5) **Meningismus** may be evident on physical examination secondary to irritation of the meninges.

c. **Evaluation**

    (1) **CT scan.** An unenhanced brain CT scan will detect an SAH in approximately 95% of affected patients within the first 24 hours. However, the sensitivity of CT for detecting SAH drops significantly if the SAH occurred more than 36–48 hours prior to the scan.

    (2) **Lumbar puncture.** If the CT scan is unrevealing, then a lumbar puncture must be performed to rule out SAH.

    (3) **Cerebral angiography** will localize the site of aneurysm or rupture prior to neurosurgical intervention.

    (4) **ECG.** The ECG will frequently show ST-segment changes consistent with an ischemic process. Other abnormalities may include a widened QRS complex, an increased QT interval, and inverted T waves. Deeply inverted T waves are suggestive of an intracerebral hemorrhage (ICH; see III A 1 b 1).

d. **Therapy.** Urgent neurosurgical consultation is required. Supportive measures include hyperventilation (to control cerebral edema) and nimodipine (to reduce vasospasm, which can lead to the development of ischemic stroke).

e. **Disposition.** Following neurosurgical correction of the bleed, patients are monitored in the intensive care unit (ICU).

2. **Primary central nervous system (CNS) tumors**

a. **Discussion.** The principal primary tumors affecting the brain include **astrocytomas (glioblastoma multiforme** is the most devastating), **oligodendrogliomas, meningiomas, schwannomas,** and **lymphomas.**

b. **Clinical features**

    (1) **Headache** is insidious in onset. The pain is most severe on awakening. A new or unfamiliar headache should increase suspicion of a brain tumor.

    (2) **Signs of increased ICP** (e.g., nausea, vomiting) may be present.

    (3) **Focal neurologic signs** and **seizures** may occur.

c. **Evaluation.** Imaging studies [e.g., an enhanced CT scan or magnetic resonance imaging (MRI)] aid in diagnosis.

d. **Therapy. Neurosurgery, radiation therapy,** and **chemotherapy** are often necessary. **Corticosteroid therapy** may be beneficial.

e. **Disposition.** Outpatient work-up is often acceptable; however, patients with a change in mental status or focal deficits need inpatient evaluation.

3. **Infections,** such as **meningitis, brain abscess,** and **sinusitis** (see Chapter 6 III A, C, and V A, respectively) can present with headache.

4. **Subdural** and **epidural hematomas** are discussed in Chapter 17 III B 2–3.

5. **Acute angle closure glaucoma** is discussed in Chapter 12.

III   CEREBROVASCULAR ACCIDENT

A Stroke

1. **Discussion.** Stroke is the primary cause of disability in the United States and the third leading cause of death after heart disease and cancer. Economically, this disease is devastating in terms of hospital costs, removal of patients from the work force, and rehabilitation expenses. Emotionally, the patient and family suffer immensely.

   a. **Ischemic strokes**

      (1) **Thrombotic strokes**

         (a) **Atherosclerotic disease** predisposes patients to thrombotic strokes and is responsible for the majority of all strokes. The atherosclerotic vessel is hyperplastic and contains fibrous deposits that cause plaque formation in the subintimal area. Plaque formation leads to vessel narrowing and platelet adhesion, eventually leading to occlusion and infarction.

         (b) **Vasculitis, polycythemia, hypercoagulable states,** and **dissection** can also cause thrombotic stroke.

      (2) **Embolic strokes** occur when a thrombus is released from a proximal site and lodges in a distal vessel, occluding the blood supply. The most common sources of emboli are the heart and major vessels (i.e., the carotid and vertebral arteries).

         (a) **Cardiac sources of emboli** include mural thrombi (secondary to myocardial infarction and arrhythmias, especially atrial fibrillation), valvular heart disease with resultant thrombus formation, ventricular septal defects with thrombus formation, and cardiac tumors.

         (b) **Rare causes of emboli** include septic emboli secondary to endocarditis, fat emboli secondary to long bone fractures, and particulate emboli seen in intravenous drug abusers.

      (3) **Hypoperfusion strokes** generally result from decreased cardiac output. The areas of the brain most susceptible to hypoperfusion injury are the "watershed" areas, located at the periphery of the major vessels. Ischemic hypoperfusion strokes do not present with a discrete syndrome because a diverse population of neurons is affected.

   b. **Hemorrhagic strokes** may be intracerebral or subarachnoid.

      (1) **ICH.** In an ICH, bleeding occurs directly into the cerebral parenchyma.

         (a) **Etiology.** The majority of ICHs are associated with **chronic hypertension.**

         (b) **Pathophysiology.** Small intracerebral vessels are damaged by long-standing hypertension and eventually rupture and bleed. Hypertensive bleeds most commonly occur in the putamen and internal capsule, thalamus, pons, and cerebellum. The hemorrhage enlarges, leading to compression of local neurons. Increased ICP may lead to neuronal dysfunction in adjacent brain tissue. A large hematoma may gain access to the ventricular system and displace midline structures, leading to coma and death.

      (2) **SAH** is discussed in II H 1.

2. **Clinical features.** Only the clinical features of the major syndromes are discussed here. The easiest method of approaching stroke is to think about the vascular distribution of the brain (Figure 9–2).

   a. **Middle cerebral artery.** Patients present with contralateral hemiplegia, hemianesthesia, and homonymous hemianopsia (blindness affecting either the right or left half of the visual fields

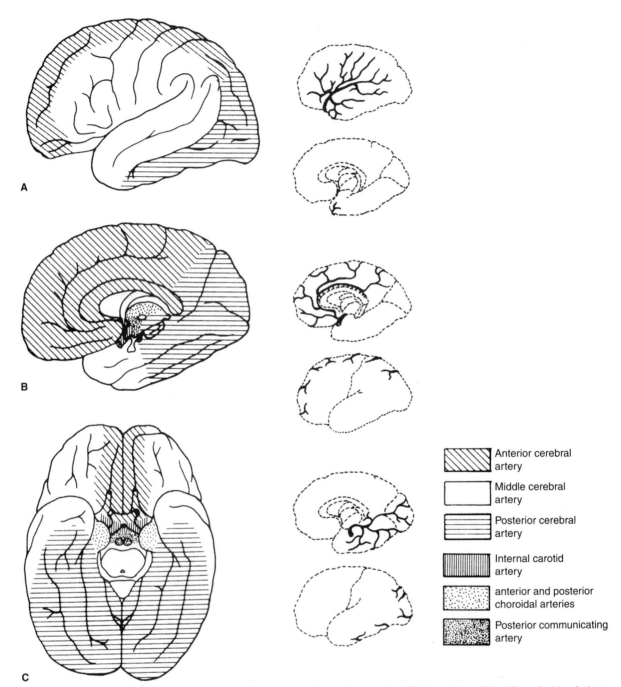

FIGURE 9–2 Surface distribution of the anterior, middle, and posterior cerebral arteries. **(A)** Lateral view of the left cerebral hemisphere. **(B)** Medial view of the left cerebral hemisphere. **(C)** Ventral view of the cerebrum. The figures to the right show the branches of the arteries. (Reprinted with permission from DeMyer. *NMS Neuroanatomy.* 2nd Ed. Baltimore: Williams & Wilkins, 1997:403.)

of both eyes). Aphasia occurs when the hemisphere dominant for language is affected. Patients may display conjugate eye deviation toward the side of the lesion (away from the deficit).

    b. Anterior cerebral artery. Patients display contralateral paralysis and sensory loss of the lower extremity, urinary incontinence, infantile reflexes such as suck and grasp, and slowness in mentation with perseveration.

c. Internal carotid artery. A patient with a stroke localized to the internal carotid artery shows signs of middle and anterior cerebral artery stroke because both vessels originate from the internal carotid. The internal carotid also supplies the optic nerve; therefore, monocular blindness may occur. Patients with internal carotid lesions will often have an audible bruit over the carotid. Collateral blood flow from the circle of Willis and between the internal and external carotid systems varies from person to person; therefore, complete occlusion of the internal carotid artery may leave a patient with little deficit, or the patient may be semicomatose secondary to the large area of infarction involved.

d. Posterior cerebral artery. Occlusion of the posterior cerebral artery induces a homonymous hemianopsia secondary to visual cortex infarction. The patient may be unaware of the deficit until formally tested.

e. Vertebrobasilar system (Figure 9–3). To appreciate strokes involving the vertebrobasilar artery system, the blood supply must be reviewed. The vertebral arteries ascend along the anterior surface of the medulla and enter the posterior fossa via the foramen magnum. The two vertebral arteries then merge to form the basilar artery. Branches of the basilar artery supply the pons and the cerebellum. The basilar artery then branches into the two posterior cerebral arteries, which supply the occipital lobes, temporal lobes, the thalamus, and the upper brain stem.

(1) Neurologic deficits involving the vertebrobasilar system are often subtle and include vertigo, diplopia, dysphasia, ataxia, cranial nerve palsies, and bilateral limb weakness. Crossed neurologic deficits (e.g., an ipsilateral cranial nerve deficit coupled with contralateral motor weakness) are the hallmarks of vertebrobasilar stroke.

(2) The **lateral medullary (Wallenberg) syndrome** involves the vertebrobasilar system and affects the brain stem and cerebellum (Figure 9–4).

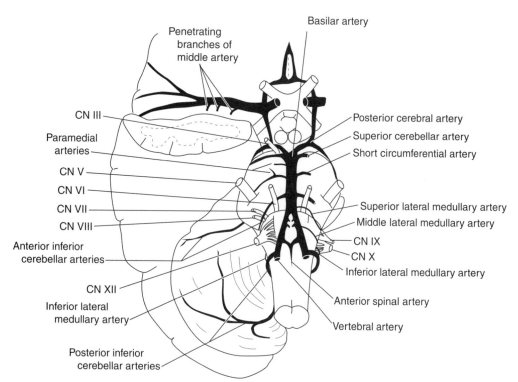

FIGURE 9–3 Vertebrobasilar artery system. *CN* = cranial nerve. (Modified with permission from Mohr JP, Kase CS, Adams RA. Cerebrovascular diseases. In: Petersdorf RG, Adams RD, Braunwald E, et al., eds. *Harrison's Principles of Internal Medicine.* 10th Ed. New York: McGraw-Hill, 1983:2035.)

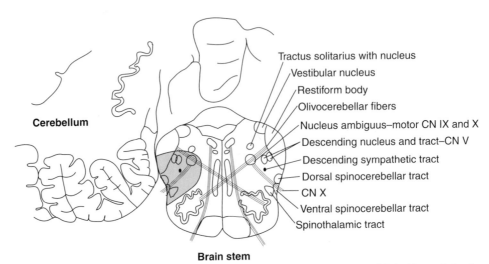

Brain stem

FIGURE 9–4 Lateral medullary (Wallenberg) syndrome (*shaded area*). *CN* = cranial nerve. (Modified with permission from Mohr JP, Kase CS, Adams RA. Cerebrovascular diseases. In: Petersdorf RG, Adams RD, Braunwald E, et al., eds. *Harrison's Principles of Internal Medicine*. 10th Ed. New York: McGraw-Hill, 1983:2037.)

(a) The affected area of the brain stem includes the cranial nerves or nerve tracts that supply cranial nerves V, IV, and X; therefore, the patient experiences hoarseness, dysphasia, and decreased ipsilateral facial sensations.

(b) The vestibular nuclei are affected, leading to nausea, vomiting, and vertigo.

(c) The spinothalamic tract is affected, leading to contralateral loss of pain and heat sensation.

(d) Disruption of the sympathetic tract leads to Horner's syndrome.

(e) Cerebellar dysfunction produces ataxia. Patients experiencing a cerebellar stroke may initially present with the inability to ambulate or a "drop attack," which may be followed by nausea, vomiting, and vertigo. Cranial nerve deficits may also occur.

f. **Small artery disease.** Lacunar infarcts elicit several distinct syndromes and are commonly associated with hypertension. The structures involved include the basal ganglia, internal capsule, thalamus, and brain stem.

(1) Most frequently, a purely motor deficit leading to contralateral motor weakness of the face, arm, and leg results. There is no associated sensory loss. This infarct is localized to the internal capsule or pons.

(2) A pure sensory stroke is secondary to infarction of the ventral posterior nuclei of the thalamus and results in contralateral sensory loss of the face, arm, and leg.

(3) Patients with clumsy hand–dysarthria syndrome present with slurred speech and weakness and ataxia of the upper limb. Lesions of the anterior limb of the internal capsule give rise to this syndrome.

3. **Evaluation**

a. **ABCs.** Airway, breathing, and circulation should be evaluated in all patients who are experiencing a cerebrovascular accident. These patients are potentially critical and should therefore have a safety net of intravenous access, cardiac monitoring, and supplemental oxygen.

b. **Physical examination.** A complete examination should be performed to elucidate clues regarding the cause of the stroke. Major arteries should be auscultated for bruits and arrhythmias and murmurs should be ruled out. The skin should be assessed for signs of peripheral vascular disease, needle marks suggesting intravenous drug abuse, and petechiae or ecchymosis suggesting endocarditis, sepsis, or coagulopathy.

c. Neurologic examination. A complete neurologic examination must be performed.

d. Laboratory studies. A CBC should be performed to rule out anemia or confirm an infective process, electrolytes should be corrected, and baseline coagulation studies should be performed to rule out a coagulopathy and to guide therapy for those patients requiring anticoagulation.

e. Diagnostic studies

(1) A **12-lead ECG** should be used to detect arrhythmias and rule out myocardial infarction.

(2) An **unenhanced CT scan** should be obtained in all patients to rule out ICH. An infarct is treated medically, whereas an intracerebral bleed may need urgent neurosurgical intervention. The CT scan may not detect an ischemic stroke for 6–72 hours after the initial infarct.

(3) **Ancillary tests** generally reserved for inpatients include an echocardiogram to rule out cardiac thrombosis, an angiogram to localize and evaluate the affected vessel, carotid duplex scanning to detect carotid stenosis, and MRI to visualize deficits not seen on the CT scan.

4. Therapy

a. Ischemic stroke

(1) **Management of hypertension.** The management of hypertension during a cerebrovascular accident remains relatively controversial. Only severe hypertension (defined by a systolic blood pressure greater than 220 mm Hg or a diastolic pressure greater than 120 mm Hg) should be treated because a sudden decrease in blood pressure may increase the infarct size. The goal of antihypertensive therapy should be to lower the diastolic pressure to approximately 100 mm Hg. Pharmacologic agents used include nitroprusside, labetalol, hydralazine, and esmolol. All patients should have frequent blood pressure monitoring. Overcorrection of blood pressure may lead to a worse outcome.

(2) **Anticoagulation therapy.** The use of anticoagulation in the ED for a stroke victim should be initiated only in consultation with a neurologist. Immediate heparinization should be considered in those patients with progression of the stroke syndrome in whom an ICH has been ruled out.

(a) An embolic stroke may be treated with anticoagulation; however, anticoagulation is generally withheld for 3–4 days to prevent a hemorrhagic stroke.

(b) Anticoagulation has not proved beneficial in thrombotic strokes.

(3) **Antiplatelet agents** (e.g., **aspirin**). The use of antiplatelet agents is probably not immediately beneficial to the patient; however, a patient with a transient ischemic attack (TIA; see III B) or a small stroke may benefit from chronic treatment with these agents.

(4) **Surgery.** Early neurosurgical consultation is needed for all patients with a cerebellar infarct to determine the need for posterior fossa decompression. Cerebellar swelling can lead to rapid deterioration with herniation.

(5) **Thrombolytic therapy.** Thrombolytic therapy [e.g., with **tissue plasminogen activator (tPA)**] is of limited use during an acute stroke and should be performed with neurologic consultation.

(a) **Eligibility.** Candidates should be older than 18 years and have clinical evidence of an ischemic stroke, and the onset of symptoms must have occurred within the last 3 hours.

(b) **Contraindications** (absolute and relative) include:

(i) Radiologic evidence or high clinical suspicion of ICH

(ii) A history of ICH, neoplasia, arteriovenous malformation, or aneurysm

(iii) Coagulation disorders

(iv) Seizure at the onset of stroke

(v) Severe neurologic deficit

(vi) Evidence on CT scan of stroke (e.g., edema, mass effect, midline shift, effacement of sulci)

(vii) Uncontrolled hypertension (i.e., a systolic blood pressure greater than 185 mm Hg or a diastolic blood pressure greater than 110 mm Hg)

        (viii) A history of surgery, head trauma, or a previous stroke within the previous 3 months

        (ix) Active internal bleeding

        (x) Dementia

        (xi) Age greater than 75 years

    (c) Dosage. In eligible patients, tPA is given at a dose of 0.9 mg/kg intravenously, up to a total dose of 90 mg. No anticoagulants or antiplatelet agents should be administered until 24 hours after the tPA infusion is complete.

  b. Hemorrhagic stroke may require neurosurgical treatment. Supportive measures include actions to decrease the ICP (e.g., hyperventilation, mannitol, diuretics).

5. Disposition. All patients suffering a new stroke should be admitted to the hospital for further work-up, education, and rehabilitation. Patients with large infarcts, an impaired gag reflex, mental status changes, cerebellar strokes, or cerebral hemorrhage should be admitted to the ICU for close monitoring because deterioration of the patient's condition can be devastating.

B TIA

1. Discussion. A TIA is a cerebrovascular accident that resolves within 24 hours. Nearly all thrombotic strokes are preceded by a TIA affecting the same region as the ensuing stroke, although the exact incidence of TIAs progressing to full strokes is unknown. TIAs can result from plaque ulceration or embolism of platelet aggregates from atherosclerotic vessels. Alternatively, embolism from heart valves may result in a TIA. Any hemodynamic insult that results in cerebral hypoperfusion may lead to a TIA.

2. Clinical features. Clinically, TIAs present as a stroke syndrome; however, the symptoms may have resolved at the time of presentation.

3. Evaluation. Work-up in the ED would include a prothrombin time (PT) and partial thromboplastin time (PTT), an ECG, and a CT scan of the head to rule out hemorrhage. Serial examination should follow neurologic symptoms to document progression or resolution.

4. Therapy in the ED entails antiplatelet therapy.

5. Disposition. All patients with new-onset TIAs or increasingly severe TIAs should be hospitalized for further evaluation and treatment. Cerebral circulation and the feasibility of surgery can be evaluated on an inpatient basis using cerebral artery angiography or carotid duplex ultrasonography. Patients with documented vertebrobasilar lesions should be considered potential candidates for anticoagulation.

IV VERTIGO

A Discussion In patients complaining of "dizziness," the primary challenge to the ED physician is to determine what the patient means by that term. Vertigo, the illusion of motion, must be distinguished from light-headedness or near-syncope. Once the diagnosis of vertigo is made, then the task of determining whether the vertigo is of peripheral or central origin remains.

1. Etiology. The end organs of the vestibular system are situated in the bony labyrinths of the inner ear and consist of the semicircular canals and the otolithic apparatus, the utricle and saccule. The neural output of these end organs is conveyed to the vestibular nuclei in the brain stem via cranial nerve VIII. Projections from the vestibular nuclei include cranial nerves III, IV, and VI, the spinal cord, the cerebral cortex, and the cerebellum. Vertigo may occur with disruption of any of these structures.

  a. Peripheral vertigo is caused by dysfunction of structures peripheral to the brain stem.

    (1) Vestibular neuritis is thought to be of viral origin and affects the vestibular nerve. Patients generally present with acute onset of vertigo with associated nausea and vomiting, but no hearing loss. Head positioning worsens the symptoms. History may disclose an upper respiratory tract infection in the weeks preceding the disease. The vertigo may last for days or weeks.

(2) **Labyrinthitis** is characterized by vertigo with associated hearing loss. This disease is presumed to be viral in origin. Bacterial labyrinthitis is extremely rare but may occur secondary to otitis media, mastoiditis, meningitis, or surgery. Labyrinthitis may also occur secondary to trauma as a result of disruption of the otoconia.

(3) **Ménière's disease** classically presents as a triad of hearing loss, tinnitus, and vertigo. The pathophysiology of Ménière's disease is unknown; however, all forms lead to dilation of the endolymphatic systems of the middle ear. The typical patient is older than 50 years and has progressive tinnitus and deafness in the affected ear with acute onset of vertigo. Attacks range from several per week to every few years.

(4) **Benign paroxysmal positional vertigo** occurs when the patient moves his or her head and is the most common cause of vertigo in the elderly. There is no associated hearing loss or tinnitus. The disease is thought to result from calcium carbonate crystal deposition in the inner ear.

(5) **Drug-induced vertigo.** Vertigo may be caused by aminoglycosides, furosemide, NSAIDs (especially indomethacin), cytotoxic agents (e.g., cisplatin), and anticonvulsants (e.g., phenytoin, carbamazepine, ethosuccinate).

b. **Central vertigo** involves disease processes affecting the brain stem or cerebellum.

(1) **Acoustic schwannomas** or **meningiomas** affect cranial nerve VIII. These tumors have the highest incidence in the fifth decade of life. The vertigo, which is of gradual onset, is generally preceded by hearing loss.

(2) **Cerebellar pontine angle tumors** are characterized by vertigo, hearing loss, and nystagmus. Symptoms are gradual in onset. Cranial nerves V, VII, IX, and XII may be affected. Ipsilateral cerebellar abnormalities may also be noted.

(3) **Cerebellar infarction** may cause the sudden onset of vertigo. Cerebellar signs are present along with cranial nerve deficits.

(4) **Cerebellar hemorrhage** is characterized by vertigo and an occipital headache. Gaze is affected secondary to sixth nerve involvement and the patient cannot look toward the side of the lesion. Other cranial nerves are often affected.

(5) **Vertebrobasilar insufficiency** may lead to vertigo. In these patients, cranial nerve function and cerebellar function are disrupted.

B **Clinical features** (Table 9–4)

1. **Peripheral vertigo.** Vertigo of peripheral origin usually is an intense spinning sensation accompanied by nausea and vomiting. The onset is generally acute and the vertigo is aggravated by positional

TABLE 9–4 Peripheral Versus Central Vertigo

	Peripheral Vertigo	Central Vertigo
Onset	Acute	Gradual
Intensity	Moderate to severe	Mild to moderate
Nausea and vomiting	Common	Uncommon
Positionally related	Common	Uncommon
Hearing loss	Common	Uncommon
Neurologic deficits	None	Common
Nystagmus	Fatigable, rotary or horizontal, inhibited by ocular fixation	Nonfatigable, multidirectional, not inhibited by ocular fixation

changes. Tinnitus and hearing loss may accompany the vertigo. The nystagmus is fatigable and inhibited by ocular fixation.

2. **Central vertigo.** Vertigo of central origin is generally less intense and not positionally related. Central vertigo is accompanied by brain stem or cerebellar signs (e.g., cranial nerve dysfunction). Nystagmus is not fatigable and is not inhibited by ocular fixation.

C **Evaluation**

1. **Patient history.** The history is most important in diagnosis.
2. **Physical examination**
   a. **Ears.** The ears should be inspected.
   b. **Eye movements,** with emphasis on nystagmus, are tested. The **Nylen-Bárány maneuver** aids in distinguishing central from peripheral causes of vertigo. From a seated position, the clinician assists the patient in rapidly assuming a supine position with the head lifted 45° from the horizontal and turned to the left 45° from the midline. A positive test, suggesting a peripheral etiology, is defined as either the onset of nystagmus or the production of vertigo. A positive test is then repeated to determine whether the vertigo is less pronounced (i.e., fatigable).
3. **Neurologic examination.** A complete neurologic examination is necessary to determine whether the condition is central or peripheral in origin. For example, any cranial nerve abnormality suggests a central process.
4. **Diagnostic imaging studies.** Cerebral imaging studies are indicated in patients with central vertigo to rule out tumor, hemorrhage, or infarction. In many cases, a CT scan is inadequate for diagnosing a tumor or infarct; thus, the patient may need to undergo MRI.

D **Therapy**

1. **Peripheral vertigo.** Patients suffering from peripheral causes of vertigo benefit from hydration and time. Medications used in the treatment of vertigo include antihistamines, anticholinergics, antiemetics, and benzodiazepines. Most patients require reassurance that their symptoms are benign, and patients must also be advised that their symptoms may be protracted.
2. **Central vertigo.** A patient with central vertigo will need to be seen by a neurologist and, possibly, a neurosurgeon.

E **Disposition**

1. **Peripheral vertigo.** Patients with peripheral vertigo are often discharged after arranging follow-up with an otolaryngologist. Admission is necessary for patients with the potential for self-injury, patients who are experiencing intractable vomiting, and any patient who lives alone.
2. **Central vertigo.** Patients with central vertigo require admission, neurologic or neurosurgical consultation, and additional testing.

V SEIZURES

A **Discussion** Seizures affect approximately 1%–2% of the population. Ten percent of the population will experience at least one seizure in a lifetime.

1. **Definitions**
   a. **Epilepsy** is a clinical condition in which patients are subject to recurrent seizures. The term "epileptic" is reserved for patients with fixed lesions or irreversible causes of seizures.
   b. **Status epilepticus** is defined as continuous seizure activity for more than 30 minutes, or two or more seizures without full recovery between seizures.
2. **Etiology**
   a. **Idiopathic (primary) seizures** have no discernible cause.

    b. Symptomatic (secondary) seizures occur in response to identifiable neurologic pathology. Some of the more common causes of seizures include:

      (1) Structural defects

      (2) Neoplastic disorders

      (3) Vascular disorders (e.g., subdural or epidural hematoma, SAH, arteriovenous malformation, vasculitis)

      (4) Degenerative disorders

      (5) Toxins

        (a) Substance withdrawal (e.g., ethanol, benzodiazepines, barbiturates, clonidine, baclofen)

        (b) Overdose (e.g., theophylline, isoniazid, cyclic antidepressants, anticonvulsants, lithium, sympathomimetics, antihistamines, nicotine, salicylates)

      (6) Metabolic derangements

        (a) Electrolyte imbalance (e.g., hypoglycemia, hyponatremia, hypocalcemia, hypomagnesemia)

        (b) Hypoxia or **anoxic-ischemic injury**

        (c) Uremia, hepatic failure, or **pyridoxine deficiency**

      (7) Infections (e.g., meningitis, encephalitis, brain abscess)

      (8) Eclampsia

      (9) Fever

  3. Classification

    a. Generalized seizures

      (1) Petit mal (absence) seizures

      (2) Grand mal (convulsive) seizures may be **tonic–clonic, clonic, tonic, myoclonic,** or **atonic.**

    b. Partial seizures

      (1) Simple partial seizures may be **motor, somatosensory, autonomic,** or **psychic.**

      (2) Partial seizures with secondary generalization

      (3) Complex partial seizures

    c. Status epilepticus may be **tonic–clonic, absence,** or **focal.**

B Clinical features

1. Generalized seizures are initiated deep within the brain stem and involve both cerebral hemispheres. Consciousness is always lost.

    a. Petit mal seizures, brief periods of loss of consciousness that are not accompanied by motor activity, occur in children 5–10 years of age. The attack ends quickly and the child resumes previous activity. Children with petit mal seizures are often thought to be daydreaming. The attacks may occur frequently, leading to poor academic performance. The frequency of episodes tends to lessen as the child matures.

    b. Grand mal seizures begin with a loss of consciousness.

      (1) Tonic phase. The patient's torso and extremities are extended. The patient may become apneic, lose bowel or bladder control, and vomit.

      (2) Clonic phase. The clonic phase immediately follows; the patient exhibits clonic movements of the torso and extremities. The patient will often inadvertently bite his or her tongue. The attack is generally short-lived, lasting 1–2 minutes.

      (3) Postictal phase. During the postictal period, the patient is flaccid and unconscious. Consciousness then returns gradually; postictal confusion may last for several hours.

2. Partial seizures. Loss of consciousness does not occur.

    a. Simple partial seizures begin in a localized area of the brain and may cause motor, sensory, or psychic symptoms. The occurrence of partial seizures implies a structural brain lesion. Nearby cerebral areas may be affected, leading to localized spread of epileptiform discharges. Thus, a patient may present with twitching of the right thumb that progresses to clonic movements of the entire right extremity and right side of the face. Progression of a partial seizure in this form is termed **"Jacksonian march."**

b. **Secondary generalization of partial seizures** may occur, resulting in loss of consciousness and convulsive motor activity. **Todd's paralysis** is a postictal focal neurologic deficit that can provide a clue as to the seizure focus.

c. **Complex partial seizures (temporal lobe** or **psychomotor seizures)** are initiated in the temporal lobe. Consciousness or mentation is affected. Clinically, patients may experience hallucinations, memory disturbances, visceral symptoms, and/or affective disorders. Patients with temporal lobe epilepsy are often mistakenly referred to a psychiatrist.

C **Evaluation**

1. **Patient history.** An adequate history is essential in all patients presenting with a seizure.
   a. Interviews with bystanders, paramedics, and family members will help to establish that the patient did indeed suffer a seizure.
   b. An attempt should be made to ascertain the cause of the seizure. A history of previous seizures, medical compliance with anticonvulsant medications, coincident illnesses, headaches, head trauma, toxin exposure, toxin withdrawal, pregnancy, or neurologic symptoms may offer a clue.

2. **Physical examination,** including vital signs, may confirm that a seizure actually did occur (e.g., lacerations on the tongue, evidence of bowel or bladder incontinence) and alert the physician to a probable cause (e.g., trauma).

3. **Neurologic examination.** A complete neurologic examination is essential.

4. **Diagnostic imaging studies.** A CT scan with and without contrast is generally performed on a patient with a new-onset seizure to rule out mass lesions. If available, an MRI may be scheduled.

5. **Laboratory studies.** A patient with new-onset seizures must undergo a thorough evaluation to determine a cause. These patients should be monitored and intravenous access obtained. Essential diagnostic studies include pulse oximetry, an accucheck, electrolyte levels (including calcium and magnesium), appropriate cultures if infection is suspected, toxicologic screening, and pregnancy testing. Patients with a normal CT scan presenting with fever, a change in mental status, meningeal signs, or an immunocompromised state should undergo CSF analysis to rule out infection.

D **Therapy** depends on the cause of the seizure and the clinical presentation.

1. **Patients with a seizure history who present to the ED following a seizure** should be questioned in an attempt to discern possible inciting factors.
   a. If the patient recovers from the seizure without any mental or physical abnormalities, then an anticonvulsant drug level should be drawn.
      (1) If the level is found to be low, then the patient may be given a loading dose or started on the appropriate medication.
      (2) If the level is determined to be adequate and it is determined that the patient has experienced a single breakthrough seizure, or if the frequency of breakthrough seizures has increased, then the patient's neurologist should be consulted for continued management.
   b. Should the patient not recover fully from a simple seizure, then the seizure should be considered a new-onset seizure and worked up appropriately.

2. **Patients who are having a seizure** need to be protected from self-harm. The patient should be turned on his or her side to prevent aspiration if vomiting should occur. Side rails should be up and padded. Intravenous administration of anticonvulsant medications is not required for an uncomplicated seizure.

3. **Status epilepticus** is treated aggressively. Stabilization, diagnostic evaluation, and pharmacologic intervention are performed simultaneously.
   a. **Stabilization**
      (1) Airway compromise should be aggressively treated with intubation.

(2) Cardiac monitoring, intravenous access, and supplemental oxygen are instituted. Continuous pulse oximetry and accuchecks are performed throughout the resuscitation. Blood pressure should be closely monitored, and a rectal temperature should be obtained initially and followed. A Foley catheter is inserted to monitor urine output.

b. Diagnostic evaluation

(1) Laboratory studies. Electrolyte levels (including calcium, magnesium, and phosphorus), liver function tests, PT and PTT, ethanol levels, anticonvulsant drug levels, drug levels of potentially convulsant medications, toxicologic screening, pregnancy testing, and creatinine phosphokinase levels (to assess rhabdomyolysis) should be ordered. ABGs are ordered to assess acidemia and hypercarbia.

(2) Diagnostic imaging studies

(a) An **ECG** is obtained to assess for toxicity.

(b) A **brain CT scan** is also performed during the course of treatment; a lumbar puncture should be performed if CT results are unremarkable.

(c) Continuous EEG recordings are performed on paralyzed patients and those in a barbiturate coma.

c. Pharmacologic treatment

(1) Intravenous dextrose is administered to counteract hypoglycemia.

(2) Thiamine (100 mg) and **magnesium sulfate** (2 g) are administered intravenously to alcoholic patients.

(3) First-line agents. Benzodiazepines (e.g., lorazepam, diazepam, midazolam) are first-line agents in the treatment of status epilepticus. Generally, lorazepam in 2-mg increments is administered intravenously (up to a maximum dose of 10 mg).

(4) Co-administration agents. In cases of status epilepticus, benzodiazepines act quickly to control the seizures, but they have a relatively short window of action (30–40 minutes at the most). During this window of opportunity, the patient should be loaded with fosphenytoin (or phenytoin), and if seizures are still not controlled, another intravenous antiseizure medication should be added (e.g., phenobarbital). **Pyridoxine** (6 g, to counteract potential isoniazid poisoning) should also be administered.

(a) Fosphenytoin (or phenytoin) (18 mg/kg, administered at a rate of approximately 50 mg/min). If hypotension occurs, slow the infusion rate but still administer the entire dose.

(b) Phenobarbital (10–20 mg/kg) is administered at a rate of approximately 100 mg/min. The patient should be monitored for hypotension and apnea (with possible intubation).

(5) Pentobarbital anesthesia. If seizures continue in spite of therapy with benzodiazepines, fosphenytoin (phenytoin), and phenobarbital, an anesthesiologist should be consulted for pentobarbital anesthesia. Neurologic consultation must also be obtained for continuous EEG monitoring. Pentobarbital coma is induced by administering a loading dose of 5–15 mg/kg at a rate of 25 mg/min. A maintenance infusion is then initiated at 1–3 mg/kg/hour.

E Disposition   All patients with status epilepticus are admitted to an ICU. Patients with a treatable underlying cause of seizure, patients with uncontrollable seizures, patients with an unclear etiology of the seizure, and patients who may not receive expedient outpatient follow-up should also be admitted to the hospital.

VI   PERIPHERAL NEUROPATHIES

A Chronic neuropathies develop over months to years. Patients presenting to the ED with a history consistent with a chronic neuropathy may be referred to their primary care physicians. Chronic neuropathy has many causes:

1. Diseases (e.g., diabetes, uremia, alcoholism, liver disease, amyloidosis, hypothyroidism, porphyria, lupus, vasculitis, multiple myeloma, polycythemia, sarcoidosis, tuberculosis, scleroderma, hypoglycemia, biliary cirrhosis, acromegaly, malabsorption syndrome, carcinoma, lymphoma, genetic disorders)

2. **Vitamin deficiencies** (e.g., thiamine, pyridoxine, vitamin B_{12}, folic acid, riboflavin, pantothenic acid)

3. **Toxins** (e.g., heavy metals, acrylamide, carbon disulfide, organophosphates, nitrous oxide, hexacarbons, methyl bromide, ethylene oxide, methylbutylketone, pyraminyl, polychlorinated biphenyls)

4. **Drugs** (e.g., amiodarone, colchicine, dapsone, disulfiram, ethambutol, hydralazine, isoniazid, metronidazole, nitrofurantoin, phenytoin, Taxol)

B **Acute neuropathies**

1. **Guillain-Barré syndrome** is an acute inflammatory demyelinating neuropathy.
   a. **Clinical features.** Patients classically present with a prodromal illness, followed in 1–3 weeks by an ascending motor paralysis that peaks in 10–14 days. Diagnosis is based on the history and physical findings consistent with an acute motor neuropathy (e.g., absent reflexes, cranial nerve palsies, autonomic dysfunction).
   b. **Differential diagnoses. Tick paralysis** (see Chapter 6 VIII B 3) has a similar presentation to that of Guillain-Barré syndrome.
   c. **Evaluation.** CSF analysis demonstrates an elevated protein level.
   d. **Therapy** is primarily supportive. Most patients require mechanical ventilation and are admitted to the ICU. Patients with early or severe Guillain-Barré syndrome may benefit from plasmapheresis or intravenous immunoglobulin (IVIG).

2. **Diphtheria,** an acute exudative pharyngeal infection (see Chapter 6 V C), can be complicated by the development of a primarily motor neuropathy days to weeks after the acute illness.
   a. **Clinical features.** Diagnosis rests on an accurate history and physical examination. The eye musculature is most commonly involved, producing ptosis, strabismus, and accommodation difficulties. The pharyngeal musculature may be involved, leading to difficulty in speaking and a change in the quality of the voice. Severe cases may induce proximal muscle weakness that then progresses distally.
   b. **Therapy** is with diphtheria antitoxin; fortunately, immunization has made this disease entity rare.

3. **Botulism** is caused by a preformed toxin elaborated by *Clostridium botulinum.* The toxin acts at the presynaptic terminal to prevent acetylcholine release, leading to paralysis. Sources of infection include improperly prepared food and raw honey.
   a. **Clinical features.** Initial symptoms include nausea, vomiting, and xerostomia. Neurologic findings include cranial nerve palsies (especially affecting the ocular muscles), followed by a descending motor paralysis. Sensation and mental status are not affected.
   b. **Therapy** includes supportive care and, possibly, mechanical ventilation. Decontamination can be attempted with activated charcoal. Botulinum antitoxin may be administered in consultation with an infectious disease specialist.

4. **Bell's palsy** is an idiopathic mononeuritis of cranial nerve VII.
   a. **Clinical features.** The patient presents with paresis of the facial musculature on the affected side. The patient is unable to wrinkle the forehead and close the eye on the affected side. The nasolabial fold is lost, and the mouth sags on the affected side.
   b. **Differential diagnoses** include trauma, otitis media, herpes zoster oticus (Ramsay Hunt syndrome), and tumors.
   c. **Therapy** for idiopathic Bell's palsy consists of patience and the administration of eye lubricants. The use of steroids should be discussed with the otolaryngologist or neurologist who performs the follow-up. Generally, a 2-week steroid taper is utilized.

VII MULTIPLE SCLEROSIS

A **Discussion** Multiple sclerosis is a demyelinating disease that affects the CNS and is characterized by recurrent attacks of focal and multifocal neurologic deficits. The onset of disease occurs during the third and fourth decades of life.

1. **Epidemiology.** Women are affected approximately twice as often as men. Caucasians are affected approximately twice as frequently as non-Caucasians.

2. **Etiology.** The cause of multiple sclerosis is unknown, but the disease is thought to be immune-mediated or infectious in origin. Data supporting these hypotheses are limited. The disease is recognized to be familial; therefore, genetic or environmental factors (or both) may play a role.

3. **Pathogenesis.** The destruction of oligodendrocytes results in myelin sheath destruction. **Plaques** (areas of demyelination in the CNS) are the pathologic hallmark of multiple sclerosis and are most commonly found in periventricular white matter, the brain stem, the optic nerves, and the spinal cord.

B **Clinical features**

1. **Multiple sclerosis.** Patients with multiple sclerosis experience recurrent attacks of neurologic dysfunction with complete to incomplete recovery. Initially, patients generally exhibit the relapsing and remitting form of the disease. This may progress to the relapsing and progressive form of the disease in which patients are left with residual neurologic deficits. The chronic progressive form of the disease is characterized by spinal cord and cerebellar involvement.

   a. **Intranuclear ophthalmoplegia** (Figure 9–5) is a condition in which the medial longitudinal fasciculus (MLF) of the brain stem is ablated. The MLF connects the ipsilateral nucleus of cranial nerve VI with the contralateral nucleus of cranial nerve III.

      (1) A patient with a right MLF lesion will achieve complete abduction of the left eye when asked to look to the left; however, he or she will not be able to move the right eye beyond the midline.

      (2) A patient with bilateral MLF lesions will not be capable of adducting either eye when asked to look to the side. The finding of bilateral ophthalmoplegia is virtually pathognomonic of multiple sclerosis in a young adult. However, multiple sclerosis is a diagnosis of exclusion; space-occupying lesions and vascular abnormalities must be ruled out.

   b. **Optic neuritis** is an inflammatory condition of the optic nerve that occurs as a manifestation of multiple sclerosis in 10%–30% of patients. Patients develop eye pain and visual impairment.

   c. **Transverse myelitis** is an inflammatory disease of the spinal cord resulting in an incomplete to a complete spinal cord syndrome. Spinal cord symptoms generally occur in advanced stages of multiple sclerosis. Transverse myelitis may be associated with mass lesions, postinfectious etiologies, postvaccination syndromes, and vasculitides; therefore, multiple sclerosis is again a diagnosis of exclusion.

   d. **Diplopia** may occur in multiple sclerosis patients secondary to involvement of the cranial nerve pathways involved in extraocular movements. Isolated cranial nerve palsies are rare in multiple sclerosis, but the disorder is included in the differential diagnosis of a young patient presenting with a cranial nerve palsy.

   e. **Ataxia, scanning monotonous speech,** and **intention tremor** are cerebellar manifestations of multiple sclerosis.

   f. **Weakness, hyperreflexia, Babinski's sign,** and **clonus** are upper motor neuron signs resulting from involvement of the corticospinal tracts.

   g. **Decreased vibration** and **position sense** result from posterior column involvement.

   h. **Decreased pain** and **temperature sensations** result from involvement of the spinothalamic tracts (rare).

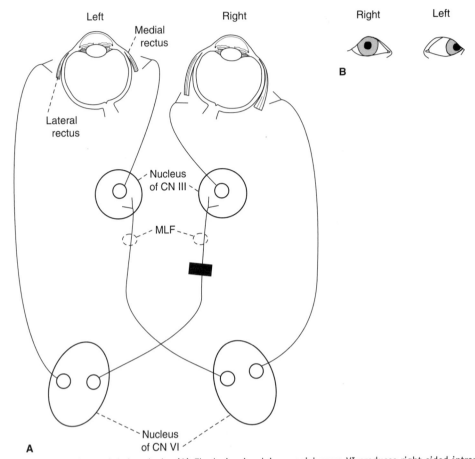

FIGURE 9–5 Intranuclear ophthalmoplegia. **(A)** The lesion involving cranial nerve VI produces right-sided intranuclear ophthalmoplegia **(B)**, in which the patient's attempt to gaze to the left results in complete abduction of the left eye but the inability to move the right eye past the midline. *CN* = cranial nerve; *MLF* = medial longitudinal fasciculus. (Modified with permission from Carpenter MB, Sutin J. *Human Neuroanatomy*. 8th Ed. Baltimore: Williams & Wilkins, 1983:383.)

    i. Urinary retention or **incontinence, constipation,** or **sexual dysfunction** may result from autonomic dysfunction.

    j. Lhermitte's sign is an electric shock–like sensation that occurs in multiple sclerosis patients upon flexion of the neck. This phenomenon occurs secondary to hyperexcitability of demyelinated axons.

  2. Complications. Patients with multiple sclerosis who present to the ED usually present with complications typical of any chronic neurologic debilitating syndrome, such as urinary tract infections (UTIs), decubitus ulcers, aspiration pneumonia, or dehydration. Exacerbations are common secondary to infectious processes and elevated body temperature.

C **Differential diagnoses** Many diseases can cause symptoms similar to those of multiple sclerosis, including amyotrophic lateral sclerosis (ALS), Behçet's disease, brain tumors, CNS infections, neurofibromatosis, pernicious anemia, sarcoidosis, syphilis, syringomyelia, and systemic lupus erythematosus (SLE).

D **Evaluation** Multiple sclerosis is clinically defined as a history of at least two episodes of neurologic deficiency resulting in objective clinical signs of more than one CNS lesion. Although ancillary testing may support the diagnosis of multiple sclerosis, the clinical findings are paramount in the diagnosis.

The diagnosis of multiple sclerosis is generally not made in the ED. Patients suspected of having multiple sclerosis should have all of the potential causes for their symptoms ruled out, and then they should be referred to a neurologist for definitive diagnosis and treatment.

1. **MRI** is the recommended neuroimaging study to support the diagnosis of multiple sclerosis. MRI most commonly detects plaques localized to the periventricular areas. Similar lesions may be detected in the optic nerves, brain stem, and cerebellum.

2. **Evoked response testing** of visual, auditory, and somatosensory afferent pathways may reveal slowed conduction consistent with a demyelination syndrome.

3. **CSF analysis** may disclose oligoclonal banding typical of increased immunoglobulin synthesis.

E **Therapy**   **Intravenous steroids** and other immunosuppressive agents are used in the treatment of acute exacerbations of multiple sclerosis. The treatment of an exacerbation of multiple sclerosis should be handled in consultation with the patient's neurologist.

F **Disposition** depends entirely on the patient's condition upon entering the ED. Patients with multiple sclerosis should be treated like immunosuppressed patients. Any infectious process should be treated aggressively to prevent extension of that process and progression of neurologic dysfunction.

VIII   MUSCLE DISORDERS

A **Myopathies**

1. **Discussion**
   a. Most patients with myopathies present to the ED because of complications of the disease. A patient with a myopathy will eventually not be able to adequately clear secretions and swallow properly; therefore, these patients are susceptible to respiratory tract infections.
   b. The weakness characteristically seen in any myopathy is secondary to **degeneration of muscle fibers.** Initially, the dying fibers are replaced by regeneration. Ultimately, renewal cannot keep pace and progressive fiber loss ensues.

2. **Differential diagnoses.** Myopathies must be differentiated from **neuropathies** and **diseases of neuromuscular transmission** (e.g., myasthenia gravis).
   a. Myopathies generally affect large proximal musculature groups and then progress distally. Neuropathies, on the other hand, usually present with distal symptoms that progress proximally. Diseases of neuromuscular transmission initially affect the extraocular and bulbar musculature.
   b. Neurologic examination of a patient with a myopathy will reveal preservation of sensation and reflexes (as opposed to the findings in a patient with a neuropathy).

3. **Evaluation.** Finding an elevated creatine phosphokinase level, an increased ESR, and leukocytosis may aid in the diagnosis of a myopathy.

4. **Clinical entities**
   a. **Muscular dystrophy.** The muscular dystrophies (Table 9–5) are a group of inherited disorders that lead to muscular degeneration.
      (1) **Duchenne's muscular dystrophy** is an X-linked trait that develops in boys before the age of 5 years, leaving them wheelchair-bound by age 12 years.
      (2) **Fascioscapulohumeral muscular dystrophy** is autosomal dominant, affecting both sexes equally, and beginning in adolescence. The face, shoulder, and pelvic girdle are affected early.
      (3) **Limb–girdle muscular dystrophy** is autosomal dominant and characterized by weakness in the shoulder girdle or the pelvic girdle.
      (4) **Myotonic muscular dystrophy** is an autosomal dominant disease that is characterized by myotonia (i.e., delayed relaxation of muscle after voluntary contraction) as well as weakness.

TABLE 9–5 Muscular Dystrophies

	Duchenne's	Fascioscapulohumeral	Limb–Girdle	Myotonic
Inheritance	X-linked recessive	Autosomal dominant	Autosomal recessive	Autosomal dominant
Sex	Male	Both	Both	Both
Onset	Younger than 5 years	Adolescence	Adolescence	Infancy to adolescence
Initial symptoms	Pelvic girdle	Shoulder girdle	Pelvic girdle or shoulder girdle	Extremities
Progression	Rapid	Slow	Slow	Slow
Serum creatinine phosphokinase	High	Normal	Slightly increased	Normal
Myotonia	Absent	Absent	Absent	Present

    b. Glycogen storage diseases are inherited myopathies in which the muscle enzymes, phosphorylase or phosphofructokinase, are limited, leading to impairment of glycogen breakdown with subsequent intracellular glycogen accumulation and myofilament distortion. The disorder generally affects men in their late teens. After vigorous exercise, the patient complains of muscle pain, stiffness, and weakness. Rhabdomyolysis (see VIII B) may ensue and requires treatment.

    c. Acute periodic paralysis is another inherited disorder that occurs primarily in men during the first two decades of life. The disease may be hypokalemic, hyperkalemic, or normokalemic. History will reveal a period of intense physical exertion, trauma, surgery, or cold weather preceding the attack. Attacks generally last for a few hours and resolve. Laboratory determinations of potassium and creatine phosphokinase should be performed; patients suspected of having the disorder should be referred to a neurologist.

    d. Polymyositis is an inflammatory disorder of skeletal muscle that affects the proximal musculature. **Dermatomyositis** is a form of polymyositis accompanied by a rash that has a predilection for the face and chest and extensor surfaces of the joints.

      (1) Etiology

        (a) Infectious causes of polymyositis include trichinosis, toxoplasmosis, malaria, viral diseases, and Lyme disease.

        (b) Metabolic and endocrine causes of polymyositis include hyper- and hypothyroidism, adrenocortical excess, and hyperparathyroidism.

        (c) Pharmaceutical causes include steroids, aminocaproic acid, clofibrate, colchicine, amiodarone, L-tryptophan, β blockers, chloroquine, D-penicillamine, vincristine, and opiates.

      (2) Predisposing factors. Ten percent of patients diagnosed with polymyositis have an occult malignancy; twenty percent have a connective tissue disorder (e.g., SLE, rheumatoid arthritis, scleroderma). Microscopically, the muscle is infiltrated by lymphocytes, suggesting a cell-mediated autoimmune disorder.

      (3) Therapy is with **steroids.**

B **Rhabdomyolysis** is skeletal muscle injury that leads to the release of myocellular contents into the plasma.

    1. Etiology. Rhabdomyolysis is caused by:

      a. Myopathies

      b. Excessive physical exertion (e.g., seizures)

      c. Muscular ischemia (e.g., compartment syndrome; see Chapter 18 VII A)

      d. Temperature extremes

    e. Direct muscle injury (e.g., burns, trauma)

    f. Toxins (e.g., ethanol, sympathomimetics, seizure-inducing agents)

2. Evaluation. The diagnosis of rhabdomyolysis rests on the laboratory work-up. Serum creatine phosphokinase levels are elevated. Although a urine dipstick will show "large" blood, few or no red blood cells (RBCs) are seen because myoglobin and hemoglobin cross-react on the urine dipstick.

3. Therapy

    a. The primary goal is to halt further muscular destruction. The underlying cause must be treated. Induction of paralysis with a nondepolarizing neuromuscular blocker and subsequent endotracheal intubation may be required to halt muscular activity.

    b. Prevention of complications is also important. The toxic ferrihemate molecule released from myoglobin in patients with rhabdomyolysis produces acute renal tubular necrosis leading to renal failure. Hydration (to the point of a good urine output) and alkalinization of the urine (to prevent the release of ferrihemate from myoglobin) are necessary. A urine pH of greater than 6 and a urine output of 2 mL/kg/hour are desirable.

IX   NEUROLEPTIC MALIGNANT SYNDROME (NMS)

A Discussion   NMS is a clinical syndrome composed of the triad of **hyperthermia, rigidity,** and **altered mental status.**

1. Etiology. NMS occurs secondary to dopamine antagonism, dopamine agonist withdrawal, and dopamine depletion.

    a. Dopamine antagonism

        (1) Therapy with antipsychotic agents (most commonly the depot form of fluphenazine and haloperidol) is the most common cause of NMS.

        (2) Therapy with dopamine antagonists (e.g., metoclopramide) may induce NMS.

        (3) Clozapine therapy has induced NMS. Clozapine was initially suggested as an alternative to neuroleptics in patients who developed NMS because of its low dopamine receptor affinity; however, clozapine has induced NMS.

        (4) Domperidone therapy for gastroparesis has been associated with NMS.

    b. Withdrawal of dopamine agonists (e.g., L-dopa, bromocriptine, amantadine) may precipitate NMS.

    c. Dopamine depletion. Catecholamine-depleting agents (e.g., tetrabenazine) have been implicated in the development of NMS.

2. Incidence. NMS occurs in 0.5%–1.4% of patients taking neuroleptics.

3. Risk factors

    a. A patient restarted on neuroleptics after a prior episode of NMS suffers a recurrence rate of approximately 33%.

    b. Men are affected five times as often as women, and the peak incidence occurs at 20–40 years of age.

    c. Other risk factors include antecedent psychomotor agitation, rate-of-dosage increases, maximum dosages, dehydration, heat, and withdrawal of dopamine agonists.

4. Complications of NMS include rhabdomyolysis with renal failure, metabolic acidosis, dehydration, respiratory failure due to inadequate ventilation, adult respiratory distress syndrome (ARDS), disseminated intravascular coagulation (DIC), hepatitis, and multisystem organ failure.

B Clinical features

1. Fever occurs in 98% of patients. Of these patients, 87% have temperatures greater than 38°C, and 40% have temperatures greater than 40°C.

2. **Altered mental status** occurs in 97% of patients and varies from stupor to coma.

3. **Rigidity** occurs in 97% of patients and may manifest as generalized or "lead pipe" rigidity. Trismus, opisthotonus, myoclonus, and hyperreflexia may occur.

4. **Signs of autonomic instability** are evident in 95% of patients and include sinus tachycardia, hyper- or hypotension, diaphoresis out of proportion to temperature, and tachypnea.

C **Differential diagnoses**

1. **Malignant hyperthermia** can occur 1–2 hours after administration of an anesthetic or paralytic agent. The rigidity associated with NMS is blocked by paralytic agents, whereas that associated with malignant hyperthermia is not. Malignant hyperthermia occurs secondary to abnormal sarcoplasmic reticulum function; therefore, a paralytic agent will not yield any effect.

2. **Serotonin syndrome** results from increased serotoninergic activity. A medication search will differentiate the two syndromes.

3. **Lethal catatonia** occurs in psychiatric patients. This syndrome is not characterized by muscular rigidity.

4. **CNS infections** (e.g., meningitis, encephalitis, sepsis) present with fever and altered mental status, but rigidity is generally not present.

5. **Parkinsonism** may be confused with NMS.

D **Evaluation**

1. **Laboratory studies.** Elevated serum creatine phosphokinase, a sign of rhabdomyolysis, is seen in 95% of patients. Leukocytosis occurs in 98% of patients.

2. **CT** and **lumbar puncture** are negative in 95% of patients.

E **Therapy**   Supportive care is the mainstay of treatment.

1. **ABCs.** Patients with NMS are in critical condition and primary attention to airway, breathing, and circulation should be maintained. Muscular rigidity may affect the thoracic cavity, leading to inadequate respiration.

2. **Cooling measures** should be used to reduce the fever, such as ice packs to the axilla and groin, cooling fan, or a cooling blanket.

3. **Fluid administration** and **alkaline diuresis** are used to treat rhabdomyolysis. Creatine phosphokinase levels and renal function must be monitored.

4. **Pharmacologic therapy**
   a. **Bromocriptine,** a dopamine agonist, is administered orally in dosages of 2.5–7.5 mg every 8 hours.
   b. **Dantrolene** inhibits calcium release from the sarcoplasmic reticulum, thereby preventing muscular contraction. Dantrolene is administered intravenously in 1- to 2-mg/kg increments every 6 hours.
   c. **Nondepolarizing neuromuscular junction blocking agents** may be used to induce paralysis in patients with severe rigidity and hyperthermia. The patient is then intubated.
   d. **Nipride** or **calcium channel blockers** may be used to treat hypertension.

F **Disposition**   Any patient with a tentative diagnosis of NMS is admitted to the ICU for monitoring and therapy.

Study Questions

Directions: *Each of the numbered items or incomplete statements in this section is followed by answers or by completions of the statement. Select the ONE lettered answer or completion that is BEST in each case.*

1. The Glasgow coma scale is used to evaluate a patient who has been brought to the emergency department (ED). The patient opens his eyes only in response to painful stimuli and is making grunting sounds. The patient withdraws from painful stimuli. What is the Glasgow coma scale score for this patient?

- (A) 3
- (B) 6
- (C) 8
- (D) 10
- (E) 12

2. A 70-year-old man comes to the emergency department (ED) because he cannot see out of his right eye and he has a right-sided frontal headache. His erythrocyte sedimentation rate (ESR) is 70 mm/hour. Immediate high-dose steroid therapy is initiated to

- (A) preserve visual acuity in the unaffected eye
- (B) prevent imminent cerebral infarction
- (C) reduce the intracranial pressure (ICP)
- (D) prepare the patient for antibiotic administration
- (E) reduce the inflammatory response caused by the tumor

3. A 60-year-old man presents to the emergency department (ED) because of the sudden onset of nausea, vomiting, and vertigo. Physical examination reveals dysphasia and sagging of the soft palate on the right side. Cerebellar testing reveals right-sided abnormalities with an abnormal heel-to-shin test and past pointing on the right. Motor and sensory examination findings are within normal limits. Where is the lesion most likely located?

- (A) Middle cerebral artery
- (B) Anterior cerebral artery
- (C) Posterior cerebral artery
- (D) Internal carotid artery
- (E) Vertebrobasilar artery

4. A patient with a known seizure disorder presents to the emergency department (ED) because he experienced a seizure the day before. The patient is taking phenytoin. While in the ED, the patient suffers a grand mal seizure. What action should be taken at this time?

- (A) Intravenous access should be established and benzodiazepines administered immediately.
- (B) Pentobarbital anesthesia should be induced, followed by endotracheal intubation.
- (C) The patient should be protected from self-harm.
- (D) A loading dose of phenytoin should be administered intravenously.
- (E) A computed tomography (CT) scan should be performed immediately.

5. A patient with multiple sclerosis is asked to look to her right. She is able to move her right eye normally to the right, but she cannot move her left eye past the midline. This patient may have a lesion of

- (A) the nucleus of cranial nerve VI (left)
- (B) the nucleus of cranial nerve VI (right)
- (C) the nucleus of cranial nerve III (right)

D the nucleus of cranial nerve II (left)

E the medial longitudinal fasciculus (MLF; left)

6. Which of the following does NOT cause pinpoint pupils (miosis)?

A Pontine hemorrhage

B Thorazine

C Clonidine

D Diphenhydramine

E Fentanyl

7. A 65-year-old male arrives by ambulance at the emergency department (ED) with a severe headache after fainting and falling to the ground 30 minutes before. The computed tomography (CT) brain scan is ordered, and it shows an acute finding. Which of the following diagnoses does NOT need urgent neurosurgical consultation and possible surgery?

A Cerebellar infarction

B Subdural hematoma

C Subarachnoid hemorrhage (SAH)

D Embolic stroke

E Epidural hematoma

8. A 58-year-old female presents with severe spinning of the room around her, and she is nauseated and vomiting. Which of the following is NOT typical of peripheral vertigo?

A Acute onset

B Nonfatigable nystagmus

C Absence of neurologic signs

D Nausea and vomiting

E Positive Nylen-Bárány maneuver

Answers and Explanations

1. The answer is C The patient receives 2 points for opening his eyes in response to a painful stimulus, 2 points for incomprehensible sounds, and 4 points for exhibiting flexion-withdrawal (i.e., withdrawing from a painful stimulus), for a total score of 8 on the Glasgow coma scale.

2. The answer is A This patient has temporal arteritis, which, if left untreated, may result in bilateral blindness. The diagnosis is based on the history and the finding of an ESR that is greater than 50 mm/hour. High-dose steroids are initiated to reduce the inflammatory vasculitis, thereby preserving visual acuity in the unaffected eye.

3. The answer is E This patient most likely has lateral medullary (Wallenberg) syndrome, which occurs when a cerebrovascular accident is localized to the vertebrobasilar system. The syndrome results from occlusion of the posterior inferior cerebellar artery; the infarct is localized to the brain stem and cerebellum. The vestibular nuclei are affected, leading to nausea, vomiting, and vertigo. Cerebellar dysfunction produces ataxia. The dysphasia and sagging of the soft palate result from disruption of cranial nerves V, IV, and X. Patients with lesions affecting the middle cerebral artery present with contralateral hemiplegia, hemianesthesia, homonymous hemianopsia, aphasia, and conjugate eye deviation toward the side of the lesion. Patients with lesions affecting the anterior cerebral artery display contralateral paralysis and sensory loss of the lower extremity, urinary incontinence, infantile reflexes, and slowness in mentation with perseveration. Patients with a stroke localized to the internal carotid artery show signs of both middle and anterior cerebral artery stroke.

4. The answer is C This patient is experiencing an uncomplicated seizure. Initially, the patient should be protected from self-harm. If the seizure continues, then intravenous access should be established and benzodiazepines administered. Phenytoin is a second-line agent used for the treatment of status epilepticus. Induction of a barbiturate coma is only indicated for patients experiencing status epilepticus who do not respond to the administration of benzodiazepines or second-line agents. A CT scan would be appropriate if the patient did not have a history of seizures (i.e., to rule out mass lesions).

5. The answer is E Intranuclear ophthalmoplegia occurs when the MLF is ablated. The MLF connects the nucleus of the contralateral cranial nerve VI with the nucleus of the ipsilateral cranial nerve III, resulting in conjugate gaze.

6. The answer is D Diphenhydramine is an anticholinergic agent that induces mydriasis, not miosis. Pontine hemorrhage, phenothiazines (e.g., Thorazine), clonidine, and opiates (e.g., fentanyl) can all cause miosis. An easy way to remember the causes of miosis is to think of the mnemonic "COPS^2."

7. The answer is D Embolic strokes can be treated medically, whereas a cerebellar infarction may lead to swelling and subsequent herniation. Neurosurgical consultation is required to determine the need for posterior fossa decompression. Patients with SAH, subdural hematoma, and epidural hematoma require urgent neurosurgical evaluation and treatment to evacuate blood from the intracranial vault and prevent permanent neurologic damage.

8. The answer is B Peripheral vertigo is acute in onset and associated with nausea and vomiting, hearing loss, absence of neurologic signs, and fatigable nystagmus. If a patient with peripheral vertigo performs the Nylen-Bárány maneuver, unidirectional nystagmus that is fatigable with repeated maneuvers will be induced.

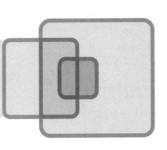

chapter 10

Rheumatologic and Allergic Emergencies

DONNA J. KINSER

I **ANAPHYLAXIS**

A **Discussion**

1. **Anaphylaxis is an acute, life-endangering syndrome** initiated by the precipitous release of substantial amounts of chemical mediators from mast cells and basophils.

a. **Mast cells and basophils** are located in the vicinity of the nerves, lymphatics, and blood vessels of the skin, respiratory tract, gastrointestinal tract, and cardiovascular system. Consequently, these are the sites of the clinical manifestations.

b. **Histamine** is the major preformed chemical mediator. Others are Hageman factor pathway enzymes, proteoglycans, neutrophil chemotactic factor, and eosinophil chemotactic factor. The chemical mediators that are instantly synthesized include the leukotrienes, prostaglandins, and platelet-activating factor (PAF). Other mediators are released secondarily and indirectly, such as serotonin released from platelets by the action of PAF.

2. **Anaphylactic versus anaphylactoid reactions**

a. Anaphylactic reactions involve antibody–antigen interactions mediated by immunoglobulin E (IgE), while anaphylactoid reactions occur via diverse mechanisms that do not involve IgE.

(1) **Anaphylaxis**

(a) In IgE-mediated reactions, there has been prior exposure to the antigen, production of specific IgE by plasma cells, and binding of the IgE to receptor sites on mast cells and basophils. When the antigen is reintroduced, the antigen binds to the antigen-binding fragment (Fab) portion of the specific IgE on the cells. This causes the release of preformed mediators, the synthesis and release of other mediators, and then a series of secondary effects, which culminate in anaphylaxis.

(b) Examples of causes of anaphylaxis include penicillin, foreign proteins (e.g., streptokinase), Hymenoptera venom, foods, preservatives, and antigen skin testing and immunotherapy.

(2) **Anaphylactoid reactions**

(a) Anaphylactoid reactions occur via diverse mechanisms that do not involve IgE. In some cases, the sequence of events involves the direct release of mediators from mast cells and basophils; in other cases, it involves activation of the complement system; and in still other cases, the mechanism is uncertain.

(b) Examples of causes of anaphylactoid reactions include human plasma and blood products, direct histamine releasers (e.g., opiates, curare, dextran, radiocontrast media), and miscellaneous agents and processes, such as exercise, physical factors, nonsteroidal anti-inflammatory drugs (NSAIDs), and mastocytosis.

b. Anaphylactic and anaphylactoid reactions are **clinically indistinguishable** because comparable mediators produce comparable target organ sequelae. The triggering factors and clinical manifestations vary among patients, but may differ little for the individual patient from episode to episode. The **emergency treatment** for anaphylactic and anaphylactoid reactions is directed at the end-organ signs and so **is the same** (although subsequent management may be different, depending on the underlying biochemical mechanism of the triggering factor). For the purpose of this discussion, the term "anaphylaxis" will be used to encompass both IgE and non-IgE reactions.

B **Clinical features** (Table 10–1)

1. Clinical findings prominently involve the skin (urticaria), the upper airways (laryngeal edema, hoarseness, stridor), the lower airways (bronchospasm), the cardiovascular system [hypotension, vasodilation, dysrhythmia, myocardial infarction (MI)], and the gastrointestinal system (abdominal cramps).

2. Symptoms are most likely to occur minutes after exposure to the triggering agent, but may occur in seconds to a few hours. Early or subtle signs and symptoms of anaphylaxis include cutaneous flushing, pruritus, voice change, and sense of impending doom. Usually the later the symptoms occur, the less severe the reaction.

3. Death may occur from respiratory causes (70%) or from cardiovascular causes (25%). Anaphylaxis is fatal in an estimated 0.4 cases per million. Autopsy findings include acute pulmonary hyperinflation, laryngeal edema, visceral congestion, pulmonary edema, intra-alveolar hemorrhage, urticaria/angioedema, and, occasionally, MI.

TABLE 10–1 Possible Clinical Manifestations of Anaphylaxis	
Organ System	**Reaction**
Cutaneous	Diaphoresis
	Flushing
	Pruritus
	Piloerection
	Urticaria
	Angioedema
Head, ears, eyes, nose, and throat	Conjunctivitis
	Rhinorrhea/nasal congestion
	Metallic taste
	Hoarseness
	Stridor
Pulmonary	Tachypnea
	Dyspnea
	Cough
	Wheezing
Cardiovascular	Tachycardia
	Dysrhythmia
	Hypotension
Gastrointestinal	Abdominal cramps
	Nausea and vomiting
	Diarrhea
Neurologic	Altered mental status
	Dizziness
	Seizure

C **Differential diagnoses** The diagnosis of anaphylaxis is generally readily apparent based on history and clinical findings, but may sometimes be confused with overlapping or distinct other problems (Table 10–2). Differential diagnosis involves the following:

1. Judging whether the symptoms and signs represent a simple allergic or pseudoallergic reaction (e.g., asthma exacerbation, urticaria), as opposed to anaphylaxis

2. Considering whether some of the symptoms and signs represent a secondary process (e.g., MI)

3. Determining if a completely different type of problem could be occurring (e.g., drug intoxication, hypovolemic shock)

D **Evaluation** History and physical examination are key for making the diagnosis and for assessing the severity of the reaction in order to plan the management strategy.

1. **Patient history**
   a. **The cause for the anaphylaxis** should be investigated. If the patient, or family member or friend, cannot readily identify the inciting factor, each of the categories of the potential causes needs to be explored (drugs and biologic agents, foods, Hymenoptera venom, and idiopathic and physical factors). **Agents with particular clinical significance** for the emergency practitioner include the following:
      (1) **Penicillin antibiotics** are a leading cause of adverse drug reactions. The overall incidence of adverse reactions to penicillins is estimated to be 2% (range 0.7%–10%). The incidence of anaphylaxis is thought to be 0.015%–0.04% of treatment courses. Approximately 500 deaths per year in the United States are caused by administration of penicillin antibiotics. Virtually all are secondary to the parenteral rather than the oral route.
      (2) **Radiocontrast media,** used for urography, angiography, venography, and enhanced computed tomography (CT), cause anaphylactoid reactions at a rate of 0.22% for ionic (high osmolar) agents. The risk of death has been estimated to be 1 in 10,000 (0.01%). Nonionic (low osmolar) agents cause anaphylactoid reactions at a rate of 0.04%. Although less reactive, nonionic agents have a high cost and have not supplanted ionic agents.
      (3) **Lidocaine and other local anesthetics** rarely cause true allergic reactions, but many patients report "allergy to 'caines' " because a variety of nonallergic reactions are associated with the administration of local anesthesia.
   b. **The route and timing of exposure** should be ascertained. The route may be by injection (e.g., parenteral medications, insect bites), ingestion (accidental or intentional), inhalation, or cutaneous absorption. **The injection route is the most dangerous** because foreign materials are introduced rapidly.
   c. **Additional information** that may have bearing on the assessment and management of the case should be sought (e.g., prior reaction to the same substance and severity of that reaction; underlying medical problems, such as cardiovascular disease or pulmonary disease; current medications, including β blockers, antihistamines, and corticosteroids; and medication allergies).

2. **Laboratory testing** has a subsidiary role.

TABLE 10–2 Differential Diagnoses of Anaphylaxis	
Asthma exacerbation	Hypovolemic shock
Carcinoid syndrome	Mastocytosis
Cerebrovascular accident	Myocardial infarction (MI)
Drug intoxication	Pulmonary embolus
Hereditary angioedema	Seizure disorder
Hyperventilation	Urticarial syndrome
Hypoglycemia	Vasovagal syncope

    a. Immediately available studies may reveal complement abnormalities, hemoconcentration, and leukocytosis. Serum histamine levels may be elevated, but these results are generally not readily available.

    b. Subsequent evaluation, usually done by an allergy specialist, may include testing for specific IgE by prick skin tests or radioallergosorbent blood tests, testing for immune complexes, testing for direct histamine release from mast cells or basophils in vitro, or challenge with the suspected agent (e.g., aspirin) in controlled circumstances.

3. Radiography. A chest radiograph may reveal hyperinflation or atelectasis.

E Therapy

1. Prompt intervention is important. The following protocol should be applied and adapted according to the severity of clinical presentation and response to treatment.

    a. Exposure to antigen must be terminated, and vital signs monitored. Any intravenous infusion of antigen should have been stopped at onset of the reaction and any topical preparations removed. If the agent was recently ingested, gastric lavage should be considered at an appropriate time.

    b. Epinephrine is administered to prevent mediator release, relax laryngeal and bronchial smooth muscle, and support blood pressure.

        (1) Side effects. Epinephrine may cause vomiting, hypertension, tremor, and tachydysrhythmia.

        (2) Possible contraindications include cardiac ischemia, severe hypertension, and pregnancy. When epinephrine is contraindicated, glucagon can be substituted.

        (3) Dosage and administration

            (a) Epinephrine 0.1% (1:1000 preparation). In patients with stable vital signs, epinephrine 0.1% is given subcutaneously or intramuscularly every 15 minutes as required. The dosage is 0.3–0.5 mL for adults and 0.01 mg/kg for children. If the antigen was injected at a peripheral site, absorption may be slowed by proximal application of a tourniquet (which should be loosened every 15 minutes) and local subcutaneous administration of a supplemental dose of 0.1% epinephrine (0.15–0.25 mL for adults; 0.0005 mg/kg for children).

            (b) Epinephrine 0.01% (1:10,000 preparation) is administered intravenously when there is significant airway compromise or shock. For adults, the dosage is 1–3 mL, administered slowly intravenously (or diluted in normal saline to 10 mL and administered via an endotracheal tube). Children receive 0.1 mg/kg by slow intravenous infusion.

    c. Stabilization of airway, breathing, and circulation (ABCs)

        (1) The airway should be observed closely and supported as needed with endotracheal intubation or cricothyrotomy.

        (2) High-flow oxygen should be administered.

        (3) Blood pressure should be supported by placing the patient in a recumbent position or in Trendelenburg's position, by infusing intravenous saline (or colloid), and, if necessary, by administering a pressor such as **dopamine** [400 mg in 500 mL 5% dextrose in water (D5W), at a rate of 2–20 µg/kg/min, titrated, for adults and children] or **norepinephrine** (4 mg in 1000 mL D5W, at a rate of 2–12 µg/min, titrated, for adults).

    d. Treatment of bronchospasm is with β agents primarily and aminophylline secondarily.

        (1) Albuterol 0.5% may be administered via a nebulizer (0.5 mL in 2.5 mL normal saline for adults, 0.1–0.3 mL in 2.5 mL normal saline for children) and may be given continuously if needed, or every 20 minutes. **Nebulized ipratropium bromide** may be used adjunctively.

        (2) Aminophylline is administered intravenously (6 mg/kg over 20 minutes, followed by an infusion at a rate of 0.5–0.9 mg/kg/hour, for children and adults).

    e. **Histamine receptor blockade**

      (1) **Histamine-1 (H_1) receptors** should be blocked with an antihistamine agent such as **diphenhydramine** (1–2 mg/kg intravenously, up to a total dose of 50 mg, initially and every 6–8 hours as needed, for adults and children).

      (2) **Histamine-2 (H_2) receptors.** Blocking of the H_2 receptors with an agent such as **cimetidine** (300 mg administered intravenously initially and every 6 hours as needed, for adults) or **ranitidine** (50 mg administered intravenously initially and every 12 hours as needed, for adults) may also be advantageous.

    f. **Prevention of late-phase reactions.** A **corticosteroid** (e.g., prednisolone, 1–2 mg/kg intravenously every 6 hours until conversion to oral medication) should be administered intravenously in an attempt to abort late-phase reactions.

    g. **Treatment of refractory anaphylaxis.** In the presence of β blockade, anaphylaxis may be particularly refractory to treatment, and **glucagon** (0.05 mg/kg administered as an intravenous bolus, followed by an infusion at a rate of 0.07 mg/kg/hour) may need to be employed. If the patient is not responding to conventional measures, **naloxone** may be tried.

  2. **Late-phase reactions** may occur in the ensuing 6–24 hours. The treatment strategy for a late-phase reaction is the same as that for an initial reaction.

F Disposition

  1. **Discharge.** Patients who present with a mild reaction, respond well to treatment, remain asymptomatic for 4–6 hours, and seem reliable with good support systems may be considered for discharge home.

    a. These patients should be instructed to use oral antihistamines and steroid medication for several days and to return to the emergency department (ED) if there is any change for the worse. They should be advised to avoid the suspected agent or agents and to follow up with their primary care physician.

    b. Patients with conditions such as Hymenoptera-sting anaphylaxis should receive additional advice and care. Additional measures include instructions regarding acquisition of a medical alert bracelet, tag, or card; provision of epinephrine for injection (e.g., Anakit, Epipen) so that early treatment may be self-initiated in the event of another episode of anaphylaxis; and referral to an allergist.

  2. **Admission.** Patients with persistent or recurring airway edema, bronchospasm, hypotension, cardiovascular complications, or altered mental status require hospital admission to an intensive care unit (ICU). Patients who receive treatment for an initially severe anaphylactic reaction but who rapidly become asymptomatic are also usually admitted to the hospital to facilitate treatment in case a late-phase reaction occurs.

G Prevention of anaphylaxis

  1. Allergic reactions should be clearly documented in the medical record.

  2. Inquiries regarding history of allergy should be made before administering a medication, and any worrisome report should be heeded.

  3. When possible, drugs that are highly allergenic should be given orally rather than parenterally. If an injection is given, the patient should be observed for 20–30 minutes.

  4. Desensitization may be feasible and indicated for certain agents such as penicillin, Hymenoptera venom, and aspirin.

  5. Management guidelines for patients who report prior anaphylactic reaction to penicillin antibiotics, radiocontrast media, and local anesthetics are as follows:

    a. **Penicillin.** The potential cross-reactivity among synthetic penicillins, semisynthetic penicillins, carbapenems (e.g., imipenem), and second-generation cephalosporins makes it necessary to avoid this entire family of drugs when selecting an antibiotic regimen for a patient with a history of anaphylaxis to a penicillin antibiotic.

b. Radiocontrast media. When a patient reports a prior reaction to radiocontrast media, one commonly employed clinical option is to select a different test that does not involve the use of radiocontrast media. Another option is to use radiocontrast media, but to diminish the risk by pretreating the patient with antihistamines and corticosteroids. (One recommended protocol is methylprednisolone, 32 mg 12 hours and 2 hours before radiocontrast administration and diphenhydramine, 50 mg orally or intramuscularly 1 hour before radiocontrast administration.)

c. Local anesthetics. The approach to the patient who reports allergy to local anesthesia depends on analysis of the available information. Options may include:

(1) The use of the standard anesthetic when the history supports prior nonallergic reaction to local anesthesia

(2) The use of an agent from a structurally unrelated group when the suspected drug can be identified (Table 10–3)

(3) The use of diphenhydramine 1% for local anesthesia when all local anesthetic agents seem contraindicated

II   URTICARIA AND ANGIOEDEMA

A Discussion   Urticaria and angioedema are associated conditions. Reports indicate 15%–23% of the population of the United States may have had urticaria, and half of the cases are accompanied by angioedema. Occasionally angioedema occurs alone.

1. **Definitions**

   a. **Urticaria** is characterized by pruritic, erythematous, cutaneous elevations that blanch with pressure and clear or migrate within 12–24 hours.

      (1) **Acute urticaria** usually lasts for 2–3 days but may persist for 4–6 weeks. It occurs in younger patients and is more prevalent in those who are atopic. Commonly identified causes include drugs, foods, and infections; however, in over 50% of patients, the cause is not determined.

      (2) **Chronic urticaria** persists for more than 6 weeks. It affects predominantly young adults and is approximately twice as common in women as in men. Occasionally the cause is one of the physical urticarias (see II A 3), but more than 75% of cases are classified as idiopathic. Up to 40% of patients who have chronic urticaria for more than 6 months are still symptomatic to some degree 10 years later.

   b. **Angioedema** is characterized by larger swellings, which originate subcutaneously or submucosally and typically last longer but are less pruritic than the wheals of urticaria.

2. **Pathogenesis** is used to characterize some urticaria/angioedema syndromes.

TABLE 10–3 Local Anesthetic Chemical Groups		
Group I: Esters*	**Group II: Amides†**	**Others‡**
Benzocaine	Bupivacaine	Dibucaine
Procaine	Lidocaine	Dyclonine
Proparacaine	Mepivacaine	Pramoxine
Tetracaine	Prilocaine	

*May cross-react.
†Unlikely to cross-react.
‡For mucous membrane administration.

a. **Immunologic mechanisms**
   (1) **IgE-mediated acute reactions** require prior sensitization to environmental antigens. Examples are foods (e.g., seafood, nuts, eggs), drugs (e.g., penicillins, sulfas, and other antibiotics; streptokinase), Hymenoptera stings (i.e., bees, wasps, hornets, yellow jackets), and inhalants (e.g., pollens, spores). An autoantibody to the IgE receptor has been identified in some cases of chronic urticaria.
   (2) **Complement pathway–mediated reactions** involve C5a and C3a. These reactions are implicated when urticaria occurs in response to infections (e.g., hepatitis, mononucleosis, *Streptococcus*) and in the setting of systemic illness (e.g., connective tissue disorders, thyroid dysfunction, neoplastic disorders).

b. **Nonimmunologic mechanisms**
   (1) Certain agents **may affect mast cells directly,** rather than through interaction with IgE, and thereby cause release of histamine and other preformed mediators. Clinically important agents that may have this effect are opiate derivatives and radiocontrast media.
   (2) Other agents **may affect arachidonic acid metabolism.** Primary examples include aspirin and other NSAIDs.
   (3) Angiotensin-converting enzyme (ACE) inhibitors **may affect the kinin system** to cause angioedema, especially of the face, neck, and upper airway.

3. **Physical urticarias.** The physiologic mechanisms of physical urticarias are not well understood.
   a. Common physical urticarias are **dermatographism,** caused by scratching or stroking the skin, and **cholinergic urticaria,** caused by exercise and sweating.
   b. An uncommon physical urticaria is **cold urticaria** (acquired or familial), which is provoked by exposure to cold temperatures, especially cold water or ice.
   c. Rare physical urticarias are **solar, delayed pressure, aquagenic,** and **localized heat urticarias.** The provocative stimuli are, respectively, light exposure, sustained pressure, water compresses, and hot water.

B **Differential diagnoses**

1. Early maculopapular rashes or local reactions to insect bites may initially resemble urticaria, but over time, urticaria can be diagnosed by its characteristic appearance together with its transient pattern.

2. Distinguishing features of some forms of urticaria that have more serious prognostic significance and special therapeutic implications are as follows:
   a. **Urticarial vasculitis** is characterized by wheals that last more than 24 hours and a biopsy that shows evidence of vascular damage.
   b. **Urticaria pigmentosa** occurs in systemic mastocytosis.
   c. **Hereditary angioedema,** or C1q esterase deficiency, has a predilection for the upper airways. Patients typically have a low level of C4 during and between attacks.

C **Evaluation**

1. **History and physical examination.** Preliminary visual survey usually identifies a patient as having an urticaria/angioedema syndrome. As long as the airway is not compromised and there is not concomitant hypotension or wheezing (which would suggest that the cutaneous findings are actually part of an anaphylactic reaction), evaluation proceeds with detailed history taking in order to establish the cause.
   a. In cases of acute urticaria, history of exposure to agents that may cause an IgE reaction or other type of reaction is sought, plus information that might suggest that this is the first presentation of a systemic illness or physical urticaria.
   b. Patients with chronic urticaria are much less likely to present for emergency care than patients with acute urticaria. Similar questions should be asked in the history.

2. Laboratory studies

a. Laboratory testing in the ED is generally not indicated for acute urticaria and is rarely indicated for chronic urticaria. Of the tests that have immediate turnaround, a complete blood count (CBC) with eosinophil count and erythrocyte sedimentation rate (ESR) might be considered.

b. Clinic evaluation of chronic urticaria may include screening for collagen vascular disease [e.g., ESR, antinuclear antibodies (ANA), rheumatoid factor (RF)], screening for thyroid disease (e.g., thyroid function tests), screening for infections (e.g., stool analysis for ova and parasites if there is eosinophilia; hepatitis panel; Epstein-Barr virus detection), screening for neoplastic disease (e.g., CBC, chest radiograph), and screening for complement pathway disorders (e.g., complement levels). Skin biopsy may be indicated and may possibly challenge testing for physical causes or allergy testing for causative antigens.

D Therapy General measures include avoidance of any identified causative agent and treatment of underlying contributing conditions. In addition:

1. **Antihistamines** are the mainstay of symptomatic management for urticaria and angioedema.

a. The most widely used antihistamines are the traditional H_1-receptor blockers hydroxyzine and diphenhydramine. The newer agents, such as loratadine, have the advantages of being nonsedating and more convenient in terms of dosing, but have the disadvantage of being considerably more expensive.

b. Doxepin is a tricyclic antidepressant drug with marked H_1-receptor antihistaminic activity.

c. Adjunctive treatment with an H_2-receptor antagonist (e.g., cimetidine) may be helpful.

2. **Corticosteroids** (e.g., prednisone, 30 mg orally every morning or 20 mg orally twice daily) are used when antihistamines do not adequately control the signs and symptoms. Because of the potential for adverse long-term side effects, the medication is stopped if ineffective after 1–3 weeks, or is tapered or stopped once symptoms are controlled.

3. **Epinephrine 0.1%** (0.3 mL of 1:1000 preparation subcutaneously) is occasionally necessary for patients with acute, severely symptomatic urticaria or when angioedema may be beginning to compromise the upper airway.

4. **Intubation** may be needed for airway management, especially in patients with a reaction to ACE inhibitors or in patients with hereditary angioedema.

E Disposition

1. **Discharge**

a. Patients with acute urticaria/angioedema may be discharged with prescriptions and instructions to follow up in clinic if medications are ineffective or if the problem persists for more than 6 weeks.

b. Patients with chronic urticaria/angioedema who have not had a diagnostic work-up should be referred to a primary care physician or allergy specialist for evaluation.

2. **Admission.** Only patients with airway compromise need to be admitted to the hospital.

III NECK PAIN

A Discussion

1. **Anatomy**

a. The **musculoskeletal structures of the neck** include the cervical vertebrae, intervertebral disks, supporting muscles, and ligaments.

(1) The **seven cervical vertebrae** are connected by the **anterior** and **posterior longitudinal ligaments.**

(2) Intervertebral disks consist of a shock-absorbing central **nucleus pulposus** surrounded by an **annulus fibrosis.**

(3) Facet joints, one on each side of the spine, connect the vertebral elements posteriorly.

b. Neuroanatomy. The spinal cord is housed in the spinal canal. The individual nerve roots emerge from the spinal canal through the intervertebral neural foramina, located on the right and left sides of the vertebral bodies. There are three main pairs of tracts in the spinal cord:

(1) The **corticospinal tract** provides motor innervation to muscles on the same side.

(2) The **spinothalamic tract,** or **lateral column,** carries superficial pain, deep pain, light touch, and temperature sensation from the opposite side of the body (decussation occurs two dermatome levels above the point of nerve root entry).

(3) The **posterior column** carries proprioception, light touch, and vibration from the same side of the body.

2. Causes of neck pain include:

a. Musculoskeletal disorders

(1) Mechanical disorders

(a) Disk disease. The nucleus pulposus and annulus fibrosis tend to undergo progressive degeneration after the fourth decade of life, decreasing the ability of the intervertebral disk to absorb shocks and stimulating local nerve endings, causing pain that can be perceived along the neck at any level.

(b) Arthritis, and particularly osteoarthritis, may involve the **facet joints** and may also produce pain along the neck at any level.

(c) Muscle spasm or **torticollis** (congenital, spasmodic, drug-induced, hysterical)

(d) Muscle strain or **ligament strain** (acute posterior cervical strain)

(e) Tendinitis (occipital, sternocleidomastoid)

(f) Cervical spondylosis

(g) Thoracic outlet syndrome, which may be confused with cervical disk disease associated with nerve root compression

(h) Skeletal congenital causes, including fused vertebrae, hemivertebrae, instability of the atlantoaxial joint, and spinal stenosis

(2) Medical disorders. Underlying diseases or processes in the bone of the cervical column may cause neck pain and associated symptoms of systemic disease. Specific disorders include:

(a) Inflammatory arthritis (rheumatoid arthritis, juvenile rheumatoid arthritis, ankylosing spondylitis, Reiter's syndrome, psoriatic arthritis, the enteropathic arthritides)

(b) Osteomyelitis (e.g., staphylococcal, tubercular)

(c) Discitis

(d) Abscess

(e) Primary or **metastatic neoplasms** (e.g., multiple myeloma)

(f) Paget's disease

(g) Diffuse idiopathic skeletal hyperostosis

b. Soft tissue disorders. Medical disorders of the soft tissue structures of the neck column, such as the blood vessels, endocrine glands, exocrine glands, respiratory structures, and alimentary structures, can also cause neck pain. The meninges are pain-sensitive, and meningeal irritation may cause symptoms in patients with meningitis or subarachnoid hemorrhage.

(1) Conditions of the soft tissue structures of the neck that can cause neck pain include **thyroiditis, cervical lymphadenitis, pharyngeal infections, sialoadenitis,** and **carotodynia.**

(2) Emergency causes include **meningitis, epidural abscess, carotid dissection,** and **subarachnoid hemorrhage.**

c. Referred pain. The symptom of neck pain may be a referred symptom from a remote somatic or visceral structure that has cervical nerve root innervation based on a common embryologic origin. Pain referred from other sites but perceived in the neck includes pain secondary to tumor or other process in the apex of the lung, and pain secondary to gastrointestinal conditions (e.g., gallbladder disease, pancreatic disease, hiatal hernia, gastric ulcer). Emergency causes include cardiac infarction or ischemia, and thoracic aneurysm.

3. **Pathogenesis**

a. **Neck pain as a result of muscle spasm and ligamentous strain**

(1) **Trauma** may cause muscle spasm or ligamentous strain of the neck. **"Whiplash" (cervical strain syndrome)** describes an injury to muscles and ligaments that have been forcibly extended and flexed.

(2) **"Neck stiffness"** exists as a common disorder in the working population. Sustained position, such as extension of the neck while doing overhead work or flexion of the neck while sitting at a typewriter or computer, causes spasm of the neck muscles and neck pain that may be associated with headache or shoulder-arm-hand pain.

(3) **"Wryneck"** refers to an acutely spasmodic neck, typically asymmetrically so, sometimes noticed after a minor twisting injury or unusual posture of the head. Radiographs, if taken, show straightening of the usual cervical lordosis.

b. **Neck pain as a result of arthritis.** Osteoarthritis, ankylosing spondylitis and the other spondyloarthritides, rheumatoid arthritis, and juvenile rheumatoid arthritis may cause neck pain. Relatively rarely, neck pain is associated with gout and calcium pyrophosphate deposition disease. The pain is usually slowly progressive.

(1) In patients with rheumatoid arthritis, cervical spine disease may progress, placing the patient at risk for neurologic injury.

(2) Atlantoaxial subluxation may be present.

(3) Cord compression may follow minor trauma or be insidious. In patients with spondyloarthropathy, the inflexible cervical spine is susceptible to fracture with minor trauma.

c. **Neck pain as a result of intervertebral disk disease.** Cervical disks, especially the lower cervical disks, may rupture after minor or major trauma. The patient typically presents with the acute onset of pain. In most patients, hyperextension aggravates the pain, and rotation and lateral movements are moderately restricted. There may be bilateral muscle spasm, or occasionally asymmetric muscle spasm. If the cervical disk is large and centrally located, compression of the spinal cord may result. More commonly, however, the disk protrusion impinges on a nerve root and causes radicular symptoms and signs.

d. **Neck pain as a result of cervical spondylosis.** Cervical spondylosis is characterized by degenerative and arthritic changes in the cervical spine that affect nerve roots and the spinal cord. The constellation of pathologic changes includes bone formation in the bony canal (spondylosis), narrowing of the intervertebral disk spaces (by herniation of the nucleus pulposus or by degeneration and desiccation of the disk with aging), formation of osteophytes on the vertebrae, and partial subluxation of one or more vertebrae. Cervical spondylosis is most common at the C5–C6 interspace.

B **Clinical features**

1. **Neurologic signs and symptoms** may result from mechanical or medical musculoskeletal disorders of the neck that involve the nerve roots or spinal cord. The neural foramina and the spinal cord can be encroached upon by a **bulging intervertebral disk** or an **osseous proliferation** from the vertebral body, facet joints, or neural foramina. They may also be encroached upon by masses related to **infection, tumor,** or **bleeding.**

a. **Radicular symptoms and signs.** When the encroachment involves a nerve root, irritation of the dorsal sensory root produces **neuralgic pain,** which is **dermatomal** and **"electric"** in nature, and irritation of the ventral motor root produces **myalgic pain,** which is **sclerotomal** and **"achy"** in nature. Objective signs of nerve root compression are muscle weakness, decreased sensation in a dermatomal distribution, and decreased associated deep tendon reflex.

(1) The first through the seventh cervical nerves exit above the cervical vertebrae of the same number, while the eighth cervical nerve exits below the seventh cervical vertebra. Because

the cervical spinal nerves may consist of separate ventral motor and dorsal sensory bundles at the point of the neural foramina, lesions may present as isolated motor or sensory changes rather than as combined deficits.

(2) Cervical roots 3, 4, and 5 supply innervation to the diaphragm via the phrenic nerves. Innervation in the upper extremity attributable to nerve roots C5–T1 is summarized in Table 10–4. Dermatomes (regions of skin from which afferent fibers converge at a single nerve root) are shown in Chapter 9, Figure 9–1.

b. Spinal cord compression symptoms and signs. When the encroachment involves the spinal cord, patients may present with numb, clumsy hands or spastic paraparesis. The degree of neck pain is variable. When there is extensive spinal cord injury, there can be initial loss of function below the level of the injury, known as spinal shock (see Chapter 17 IV B 3). Specific cord syndromes are discussed in Chapter 17 IV B 2.

2. Systemic signs. Fever or weight loss may be present in patients with infectious, inflammatory, or neoplastic processes.

C **Differential diagnoses**   Although many of the causes of neck pain do not represent an emergency, the **life- or limb-threatening causes of neck pain** must be systematically excluded. These include:

1. Spinal instability resulting from mechanical injury, osteomyelitis, or tumor

2. Cord vulnerability as a result of spinal instability, abscess, hematoma, or tumor

3. Meningitis

4. Subarachnoid hemorrhage

5. MI

6. Thoracic aneurysm

D **Evaluation**   The emergency practitioner typically takes a directed history and performs a focused musculoskeletal examination, a focused neurologic examination, and a general physical examination to develop a preliminary differential diagnosis and plan.

1. Patient history
   a. The time and circumstances of onset, the location, and the quality of the pain should be determined, as well as constancy versus intermittency, and exacerbating or relieving factors.

TABLE 10–4   Innervation of the Upper Extremity

Root	Reflex	Muscles	Action	Sensation
C5	Biceps reflex	Deltoid Biceps	Shoulder abduction Flexion of the supinated forearm	Lateral upper arm
C6	Brachioradialis reflex (biceps reflex)	Extensor carpi radialis, extensor carpi ulnaris Biceps	Wrist extension Flexion of the supinated forearm	Lateral forearm and thumb
C7	Triceps reflex	Flexor carpi radialis, flexor carpi ulnaris Extensor digitorum Triceps	Wrist flexors Finger extension Forearm extension at elbow	Middle finger
C8	None	Flexor digitorum superficialis, flexor digitorum profundus Hand intrinsics	Finger flexion Digit abduction and adduction	Medial forearm and fourth digit
T1	None	Hand intrinsics	Digit abduction and adduction	Median midarm

(1) In cervical spine disorders, stimulation of the simple nerves of the neck can cause pain to be referred to the shoulders and interscapular area. Retro-orbital, temporal, and occipital pain reflects a referral pattern from the areas of the atlas, axis, and C3. Pain with movement of the shoulder is not characteristic of cervical spine disease and suggests the problem is in the shoulder joint or ligaments.

(2) In cervical spine disorders, the degree of pain tends to be affected by various normal movements of the cervical spine.

b. The presence or absence of associated neurologic symptoms or other features needs to be established. Neurologic complaints may reflect nerve root irritation or cord compression; sometimes neck pain is a very minor part of the presentation. Symptoms of dizziness, visual changes, and ataxia may be related to vertebral artery compression by bony spurs encroaching on the vertebral foramina.

c. The past medical history is important, especially in regard to a possible underlying anatomic abnormality, rheumatologic disorder, or immunosuppressive condition. Congenital abnormalities should be considered in children who present with neck pain.

2. Physical examination. In the setting of trauma or suspected neck instability from other causes, prompt and continued immobilization is necessary throughout the evaluation process to minimize the risk of cord injury.

  a. Evaluation of the musculoskeletal structures of the neck

    (1) **Upper body.** The patient's upper body should be inspected for abnormal posture, which may be related to asymmetric muscle spasm or muscle atrophy.

    (2) **Neck.** The neck should be examined with respect to possible bony injury or abnormality. The neck muscles are examined for tenderness or spasm.

    (3) **Range of motion.** If spine instability is not suspected, active range of motion should be tested (i.e., flexion, extension, rotation to the left and right, and lateral bending to the left and right). The shoulders should be examined and range of motion tested.

  b. Evaluation of the soft tissues of the neck

    (1) The soft tissues of the neck should be inspected for swelling or asymmetry, and the midline tracheal position should be verified.

    (2) The patient's neck should be palpated for thyroid abnormalities, lymphadenopathy, enlargements consistent with cysts or other tumors, and areas of induration or fluctuance consistent with abscess. Carotid artery pulsations should be checked.

  c. General physical examination. A general physical examination is performed, paying special attention to the area of concern if a type of referred pain is suspected.

  d. Neurologic examination

    (1) Motor, sensory, and sphincter function should be tested, as well as the reflexes.

    (2) Muscle strength testing in the upper extremities should include the biceps (flexion of the elbow), triceps (extension of the elbow), wrist extensors and flexors, hand and finger flexors, and intrinsic muscles of the hand.

    (3) Sensory testing should include pain and vibration and an attempt to delineate an anatomic deficit.

    (4) Meningeal irritation may be manifested by nuchal rigidity, Kernig sign, and Brudzinski sign.

3. Laboratory and diagnostic imaging studies

  a. If there is **localized spinal tenderness or if the neurologic examination is abnormal,** plain films of the neck should be obtained. If the plain films are suspicious for abnormality or there are neurologic deficits, CT scanning, magnetic resonance imaging (MRI), or myelography should be ordered as indicated and available.

  b. If underlying disease is suspected based on the patient's age, risk factors, or positive review of systems, appropriate and thorough evaluation should be undertaken. In the ED, this may include a CBC, an ESR, radiographs of the cervical spine and chest, a CT scan of the head, an

MRI or CT scan of the neck, and/or cerebrospinal fluid (CSF) analysis for evaluation for meningitis or hemorrhage.

c. If the patient is assessed as having **neurologic deficits associated with the pain,** neurologic or neurosurgical consultation is usually necessary, often before specialized radiographic studies are ordered.

E Therapy

1. **Spasm, strain, or sprain**

   a. Cervical symptoms caused by simple spasm, strain, or sprain are managed with anti-inflammatory medications, ice packs advancing to heat packs, and mobilization as guided by pain control. Improvement should occur within 1–2 weeks.

   b. For patients with more severe pain or spasm, narcotic analgesics or muscle relaxants may also be prescribed. Local injection of an anesthetic agent at key anatomic points may be considered for selected patients. In patients with marked muscle spasm, a soft cervical collar may be appropriate. A hard collar should be used for patients in whom a suspicion of injury remains despite nondiagnostic films.

2. **Disk disease and cervical spondylosis.** Treatment usually includes rest and anti-inflammatory and analgesic medications. Indications for surgical intervention include persistence of symptoms for more than 6 weeks or progressive neurologic deficits from nerve root involvement.

3. **Chronic pain syndromes.** Therapy is best provided according to a therapeutic plan developed by the patient's primary care physician or specialist.

4. **Nonmusculoskeletal causes of neck pain** (e.g., meningitis). Treatment is specific to the problem.

F Disposition

1. **Discharge.** Most patients with musculoskeletal neck pain, including patients with stable cervical disk disease, may be discharged home with arrangements for outpatient follow-up.

2. **Admission.** Patients with rapidly progressive neurologic symptoms or findings consistent with cord compression are emergently evaluated and managed. Patients in whom a serious medical condition (e.g., meningitis, osteomyelitis, abscess, hemorrhage) is suspected require an in-depth work-up and treatment in the hospital.

IV THORACIC AND LUMBAR BACK PAIN

A Discussion

1. **Anatomy**

   a. **Musculoskeletal structures.** The thoracic spine consists of 12 vertebrae and the lumbar spine consists of five vertebrae, with interposed intervertebral disks. The back column is supported by strong ligaments and paraspinous muscles. The posterior aspects of the vertebrae form the spinal canal, neural foramina, and facet or apophyseal joints. The sacrum connects with the iliac bones of the pelvis.

   b. **Neuroanatomy.** The sinuvertebral nerve is the major sensory nerve of the lower back; the pattern of innervation is a complex anastomosis that serves multiple structures and levels, explaining the diffuse and nonspecific nature of pain associated with back disorders of varying causes.

2. **Causes of back pain.** Like neck pain, back pain may be caused by mechanical and medical disorders of the musculoskeletal structures of the spine. The precise cause of back pain can be identified in less than 25% of patients. Herniated disk, spinal stenosis, and compression fracture are identified most often.

   a. **Mechanical causes** of back pain include:

      (1) **Degenerative disk disease**

      (2) **Osteoarthritis** of the facet joints

    (3) **Muscle spasm**

    (4) **Ligament or muscle strain**

    (5) **Intervertebral disk disease**

    (6) **Spinal stenosis**

    (7) **Epidural** or **intradural tumors** in the spinal canal may produce a syndrome similar to that of a ruptured disk.

    (8) **Spondylolysis** and **spondylolisthesis**

    (9) **Spina bifida** (rare)

b. Medical causes of thoracic and lumbar pain include **inflammatory arthritis** (ankylosing spondylitis and the other spondyloarthritides), **infection, neoplasm,** and other underlying diseases and processes (e.g., **spinal osteomyelitis, epidural abscess**).

c. Referred pain. Disorders of the abdominal, retroperitoneal, and pelvic viscera can cause pain that is perceived in the region of the spine. However, back pain is rarely the only symptom, and it is not aggravated by activity or relieved by rest, as is most pain of spinal origin. From an emergency standpoint, it is important to realize that **abdominal aortic aneurysm** and **aortic dissection** may give rise to back pain.

    (1) In general, upper abdominal diseases (peptic ulcer disease, tumors of the stomach, duodenum, and pancreas) are referred to the lower thoracic spine, lower abdominal diseases (colon tumors, colon inflammatory disease) are referred to the lumbar spine, and pelvic diseases (endometriosis; invasive carcinoma of the uterus, cervix, or bladder; uterine malposition; dysmenorrhea; chronic prostatitis; carcinoma of the prostate) are referred to the sacral region.

    (2) Renal pain is perceived in the costovertebral angle.

    (3) Diseases of retroperitoneal structures (e.g., lymphomas, sarcomas) may evoke pain in the adjacent part of the spine. Retroperitoneal bleeding, especially in an anticoagulated patient, can cause back pain.

3. Differential diagnoses

a. Life-threatening causes of back pain, such as abdominal aortic aneurysm or abdominal dissection, must be ruled out.

b. Nonanatomic, nonorganic presentations such as whole leg pain, numbness, and/or weakness are associated with psychological stressors.

4. Clinical findings. Neurologic symptoms may result from mechanical or medical musculoskeletal disorders of the back that involve the nerve roots or spinal cord, such as intervertebral disk protrusion, osseous proliferation, or masses due to infection, tumor, or bleeding.

a. Radicular symptoms and signs are produced when there is nerve root irritation or impingement at the neural foramina. The lumbar and sacral nerve root motor and sensory innervation patterns are summarized in Table 10–5 and Chapter 9, Figure 9–1.

TABLE 10–5 Innervation of the Lower Extremity

Root	Reflex	Muscles	Action	Sensation
L4	Patellar reflex	Anterior tibialis	Dorsiflexion and inversion of foot	Medial regions of lower leg and foot
L5	None	Extensor hallucis longus	Dorsiflexion of great toe	Lateral region of midleg, dorsum of foot
S1	Achilles reflex	Peroneus longus and brevis	Plantar flexion and eversion of foot	Lateral region of foot
S2, S3, S4	Superficial anal reflex	Bladder, foot intrinsics	Toe abduction and adduction	Perianal region

    b. Spinal cord compression symptoms and signs. Specific spinal cord syndromes are discussed in Chapter 17 IV B 2.

      (1) Compression of the spinal cord above T12 results in a constellation of possible **upper motor neuron (UMN)** or **long tract signs:** spasticity, hyperactive deep tendon reflexes, suppressed superficial skin reflexes, positive Babinski sign, acute urinary retention with overflow incontinence, and fecal retention. Acutely, however, these signs may not be apparent because of transient spinal shock producing flaccid paralysis, areflexia, and hypotension.

      (2) Compression in the spinal canal below T12, and specifically below the level of the conus medullaris, results in a constellation of **lower motor neuron (LMN)** or **nerve root signs.** In the **cauda equina syndrome,** flaccid paralysis, areflexia, a negative Babinski sign, and urinary and fecal incontinence due to loss of sphincter tone may be seen.

5. Evaluation. The history and physical examination are key in the initial categorization and management of back pain disorders. Based on clinical complaints and findings, the emergency practitioner classifies the disorder as probably mechanical or probably medical or systemic, with or without associated neurologic involvement.

    a. Patient history

      (1) Possible precipitating factors. In the approach to the patient with back pain, the **patient's age** and the **circumstances of the onset of the pain** are important. There may be **antecedent trauma,** minor to major, or a **history of lifting or strain.** There may be a **history of prior episodes. Occupational history** may be relevant.

      (2) Symptoms

        (a) Characteristics of pain. For the current episode, the acuity, intensity, quality, location, duration, and pattern of the pain should be determined, as well as aggravating and alleviating factors.

        (b) Neurologic symptoms. Information pertaining to possible nerve root irritation, spinal cord compression, or cauda equina syndrome should be elicited. Patients may complain of motor weakness, numbness, paresthesias, or bowel, bladder, or sexual dysfunction.

        (c) Associated symptoms (e.g., fever, weight loss) may be present, or there may be pertinent risk factors for infection, such as chronic steroid use or intravenous drug abuse.

      (3) Past medical history is important in general, and for any prior back pain evaluation and treatment in particular. Medications should be noted.

      (4) Psychosocial issues (e.g., current work status, disability, compensation, litigation) should be discussed because they may influence the assessment, management, and outcome of treatment for back pain.

    b. Physical examination. The back should be examined and a neurologic examination should be performed. The general examination is important to evaluate the patient for a medical disorder as a cause of back pain.

      (1) Examination of the back

        (a) Inspection

          (i) The back should be inspected for **signs of infection and trauma.**

          (ii) Unusual skin markings, which may denote underlying neurologic or bone pathology, should be noted.

          (iii) The **posture** should be analyzed. Are the shoulders and pelvis level? Is midline symmetry present? Does the patient have a gentle lumbar lordotic curve? Listing to one side may be a sign of muscle spasm or accommodation to pain or weakness. The lumbar curve may be straightened by paravertebral muscle spasm.

        (b) Bony palpation of the posterior aspect of the back should be performed. The spinous processes are palpated. Evaluation of the coccyx is accomplished through rectal examination. The sacroiliac joints should be palpated for tenderness.

      (c) Soft tissue palpation of the posterior aspect of the back is also performed.

        (i) The interspinous ligaments connect the adjoining processes, and the supraspinous ligament connects the spinous processes from the seventh cervical vertebra to the sacrum. If either is ruptured, there may be localized pain and a palpable defect between the spinous processes.

        (ii) The paraspinal muscles are palpated for tenderness, spasm, or defects.

        (iii) The sciatic nerve exits the pelvis midway between the greater trochanter and the ischial tuberosity, runs vertically down the midline of the posterior thigh, and divides into the tibial and peroneal nerves. The sciatic nerve is most likely to be palpable with the hip flexed. Tenderness can be caused by a herniated disk or a space-occupying lesion compressing the contributing nerve roots.

      (d) Range-of-motion testing (flexion, extension, lateral bending, and rotation) should be performed to detect restrictions in movement and patterns of exacerbation of pain.

    (2) Selected special tests may be performed.

      (a) Straight leg raising is conducted to reproduce the back or leg pain. The patient may complain of pain in the posterior thigh (hamstring or sciatic), pain all the way down the leg (sciatic), pain in the low back, or pain in the opposite leg. With the leg lowered below the angle producing pain, the foot should be dorsiflexed to stretch the sciatic nerve, which would be expected to reproduce sciatic pain.

      (b) Crossed straight leg raising. In this test, the uninvolved leg is raised. If this produces back and sciatic pain on the opposite side, a herniated disk or comparable condition is suggested, especially in young patients.

      (c) Hoover test. This test gives an estimate of the patient's effort during straight leg raising. The examiner cups one hand under each of the patient's heels. There should be downward pressure from the leg that is not being actively raised.

      (d) Kernig test. This test is designed to stretch the spinal cord and reproduce pain in an effort to determine the origin. While supine, the patient flexes the head onto the chest or attempts to extend the knee after flexing at the hip and the knee. A complaint of pain in the cervical spine, low back, or down the leg is an indication of meningeal irritation, nerve root involvement, or irritation of the dural coverings of the nerve root.

    (3) Neurologic examination of the lower body should be performed, including assessment of motor strength, sensation, reflexes, and sphincter tone.

    (4) Evaluation for extraspinal causes of back and leg pain

      (a) Examination of the abdomen and lower extremities. Pulsatile abdominal masses and bruits, diminished pulses, and color or temperature changes in the distal extremities suggest vascular disease.

      (b) Pelvic examination and **rectal examination** may also be indicated.

c. Diagnostic imaging studies

    (1) Plain films should be obtained for patients older than 50 years, patients with systemic symptoms, patients with an acute injury and localized tenderness, and patients with neurologic deficits.

    (2) Emergent CT, MRI, or myelography is necessary for patients with suspected cord impingement or cauda equina syndrome.

    (3) A CT, an MRI, or a bone scan should be obtained for patients with suspected infectious or malignant conditions.

    (4) Patients with debilitating pain or nerve entrapment neurologic deficits lasting more than 4–6 weeks should also have a CT scan or an MRI.

    (5) Ultrasonography or another imaging study is required when aortic aneurysm is suspected.

d. Laboratory studies should be considered for selected patients. An ESR may be helpful in those with systemic symptoms or with risk factors for inflammatory or infectious diseases. Appropriate arrays of other blood and urine tests specific to the suspected conditions should be conducted for patients being evaluated for medical causes of spinal column disease and for referred pain.

6. **Therapy**
   a. **NSAIDs** or **acetaminophen** is the first line of treatment for most patients with musculoskeletal back pain. Some patients (e.g., those with a compression fracture) require **short-term narcotic analgesics.**
   b. **Short-term muscle relaxants** may benefit patients with muscle spasm.
   c. **Gradual return to tolerated activities** is now believed to be more beneficial than bed rest for most causes of back pain.
   d. **Referrals for unremitting symptoms** are generally most appropriately made by the primary care physician; considerations are for physical therapy, chiropractic care, neurologic evaluation, and orthopedic or neurosurgical intervention.

7. **Disposition**
   a. **Discharge.** Most patients can be discharged home with appropriate medications and instructions for outpatient follow-up.
   b. **Admission** for the purpose of spinal traction is controversial. Admission is necessary for patients with cauda equina syndrome, and for patients with syndromes thought to be infectious or rapidly progressive in terms of neurologic impairment.

B **Specific disorders causing thoracic and lumbar back pain**

1. **Low back strain syndrome.** The most common cause of back pain, low back strain syndrome may be related to muscle spasm and ligamentous strain from a specific traumatic episode or repeated stress. Typically occurring in patients between the ages of 20 and 40 years, the pain may be in the back, buttock, or one or both thighs, and the pain may be accentuated by standing and alleviated by lying. General examination may reveal obesity or leg length discrepancy. The back examination may show the nonspecific signs of muscle spasm and loss of lumbar lordosis, and the neurologic examination is normal.

2. **Herniated intervertebral disk.** Tears in the annulus fibrosus allow the contents of the nucleus pulposus to herniate and compress neural elements. The lower lumbar region (L4, L5, S1) has the most mobility and has the highest incidence of herniated disks; only 1% of all disk herniations are thoracic.
   a. **Patient history.** Patients are typically between the ages of 30 and 50 years. The patient may give a history of acute pain following the sensation of sudden, but minor, pressure on the spine. The pain is often sharp or lancinating in character, and may be associated with nerve root irritation, cord compression, or cauda equina syndrome.
   b. **Signs and symptoms**
      (1) **Sciatic symptoms** are radicular in nature and tend to be exacerbated by maneuvers such as bending, which increase intradiscal pressure. A **positive straight leg raising test** is **75% diagnostically accurate,** and a positive crossed straight leg raising test increases the accuracy.
      (2) **Neurologic symptoms** predict the actual anatomic lesion level approximately 50% of the time, and neurologic signs predict the correct level approximately 75% of the time. In the cauda equina syndrome, a central midline herniation causes paralysis of the sacral roots, leading to bowel and bladder dysfunction and the inability to walk. Prompt recognition and surgical intervention are necessary to minimize permanent bladder and bowel dysfunction.

3. **Spondylolysis and spondylolisthesis.** Spondylolisthesis is forward slippage of one vertebra on another, most often L5 on S1, or L4 on L5. It is secondary to spondylolysis, a separation at the pars interarticularis (a segment near the junction of the pedicle with the lamina). In many cases, spondylolysis seems to be caused by trauma to a congenitally abnormal segment in the pars interarticularis.

    a. **Patient history.** Most often seen in teenagers, spondylolisthesis is associated with backache and is sometimes accompanied by pain that radiates down the legs as a result of stretching of a nerve root or herniation of a disk.

    b. **Physical examination findings.** A palpable "step-off" from one process to another may be an indication of this condition.

4. **Osteoarthritic spinal disease** occurs later in life and may involve any part of the spine; the lumbar area is more often involved than the thoracic area.

    a. The pain is exacerbated by motion and improved with rest; associated complaints include stiffness and limitation of motion. Systemic symptoms are not present.

    b. In osteoarthritis, the severity of the symptoms bears little relation to the radiologic findings. Pain may be present when there are minimal findings on radiographs; conversely, there may be marked spur formation, ridging, and bridging of vertebrae without symptoms.

5. **Ankylosing spondylitis** usually occurs in young adult men. Initial symptoms may be intermittent pain in the middle or low back; occasionally there is radiation of pain to the back of the thighs. Limitation of movement becomes constant and progressive and dominates the clinical picture. Associated musculoskeletal examination findings may be tenderness of the sacroiliac joints, limitation of hip range of motion, and limitation of chest expansion. A similar back pain syndrome may be present in patients with Reiter's syndrome, psoriatic arthritis, and chronic inflammatory bowel disease.

6. **Spinal stenosis** represents a continuum of disease: disk degeneration is followed by posterior facet disease, which then develops into progressive articular facet, laminar, and vertebral encroachment with osteophytic formation and ultimately vertebral fusion.

    a. Initially, patients may have back pain that is related to the disk and facet joint changes. The pain is exacerbated by hyperextension and improved with flexion. When there is involvement of the nerve roots by a disk or bony proliferation, nerve root symptoms and signs are present. The straight leg raising test may be positive.

    b. With advancing age, and particularly in men over the age of 60 years, back symptoms become suggestive of impingement of multiple nerve roots at different levels on both sides of the spinal cord. Once the spinal stenosis stage is reached, patients may have symptoms mimicking those of peripheral vascular insufficiency.

    c. Plain radiographs show degenerative changes in the facet joints and decreased canal diameter on the anterior-posterior (AP) view. A CT scan is better for showing the narrowed canal and the impingement of osteophytes on the intervertebral foramina. Findings of degenerative changes on imaging studies do not correlate well with symptoms.

7. **Vertebral compression fractures** are common, especially in elderly patients, and are usually the result of a flexion injury. The force required to cause the fracture is minimal when there is underlying bone disease (e.g., osteoporosis, multiple myeloma, metastatic cancer).

    a. The thoracic spine is most likely to be affected. In the T2 through T10 area, stable compression fractures with less than 25% anterior wedging tend to occur.

    b. Because of the relative immobility of the thoracic spine (as compared with the lumbar spine), more complicated and unstable fractures tend to occur when the thoracolumbar level of the spine is injured.

    c. Disruption of the posterior ligaments in the lumbar region also produces unstable fractures.

V   MONARTICULAR ARTHRITIS

A **Discussion**   Monarticular arthritis is characterized by **pain** and **inflammation** in an isolated joint. Almost any joint disorder is capable of presenting initially as monarticular arthritis, but usually the practitioner can identify patients who might have an acute inflammatory or infectious condition and appropriately proceed with vigorous evaluation and treatment in the ED.

1. **Septic arthritis** and the **crystal-induced arthropathies** (i.e., **gout, pseudogout**) are the key causes of acute monarticular arthritis that need to be addressed in the ED work-up. Joint infection can coexist with gout or pseudogout: infection in a joint with any microcrystalline deposition process can lead to crystal shedding and subsequent synovitis from both crystals and micro-organisms.

   a. **Septic arthritis** may be **bacterial, tuberculous,** or **fungal** in etiology, and it has the potential for rapid disease progression. Cases are usually classified as those that are caused by *Neisseria gonorrhoeae* (**disseminated gonococcal arthritis**) and those that are caused by all other organisms (**nongonococcal arthritis**).

      (1) **Disseminated gonococcal arthritis.** *N. gonorrhoeae* is the most common cause of bacterial arthritis in urban centers. Disseminated gonococcal arthritis tends to be a disease of young, sexually active, healthy adults. Women, especially pregnant or menstruating women, are affected more often than men.

      (2) **Nongonococcal arthritis**

         (a) **Causes.** *Staphylococcus aureus* is the bacterium most frequently cultured, followed by various species of streptococci. Other causative organisms are *Escherichia coli* and *Pseudomonas aeruginosa* in elderly patients and intravenous drug users, and *Haemophilus influenzae* in young children and, rarely, in adults. When joint infection is present in HIV-positive patients, opportunistic and less common microorganisms, such as *Cryptococcus neoformans* and *Salmonella,* have been identified.

         (b) **Pathogenesis**

            (i) An ongoing illness or problem may allow hematogenous spread of bacteria to a joint. At-risk patients include those with impaired host defense mechanisms, those with indwelling venous catheters, those with chronic arthritis (especially rheumatoid arthritis), and intravenous drug users.

            (ii) Alternatively, micro-organisms may be directly introduced into the joint through a deep penetrating wound (including human bite and animal bite wounds), contiguous osteomyelitis, intra-articular injection or aspiration, arthroscopy, or prosthetic joint surgery.

   b. **Gout.** In this condition, sodium urate crystals precipitate in and around the joints of the extremities when the concentration of urate exceeds its solubility.

      (1) **Patient history.** Gout is more common in men than in women; when it occurs in women, it is most often seen in postmenopausal women. Patients may have a history of food overindulgence, heavy alcohol intake, use of medications (e.g., diuretics), or trauma. Obesity and hypertriglyceridemia are also associated with gout.

      (2) **Phases.** In primary hyperuricemia, the tendency toward acute gout increases with the serum urate level. When the serum urate level exceeds 9 mg/dL, the cumulative incidence of gout reaches 22% in 5 years. In the natural history of gout, the phases include:

         (a) **Asymptomatic hyperuricemia** (serum urate concentration greater than 7 mg/dL)

         (b) **Acute monarticular arthritis with few constitutional symptoms**

         (c) **Arthritis attacks** that are **polyarticular, associated with fever,** and/or **occurring at shorter intervals**

         (d) **Tophi** and **chronic arthritis** with superimposed exacerbations

      (3) **Associated problems** can include renal disease and uric acid nephrolithiasis.

   c. **Pseudogout,** which clinically resembles acute gouty monarthritis, **is a form of calcium pyrophosphate deposition disease (CPPD).** (More chronic forms may resemble osteoarthritis, neuropathic arthropathy, rheumatoid arthritis, and ankylosing spondylitis.) Surveys have shown the radiographic incidence to be as high as 25% in some populations, but many of these patients are asymptomatic.

      (1) **Pathogenesis.** Crystals of CPPD develop in cartilages and other connective tissue. The precise reasons for crystal deposition are not known.

      (2) **Patient history**

(a) CPPD increases in prevalence with age and is somewhat more prevalent in men. It is associated with hyperparathyroidism and hemochromatosis, and CPPD crystalline deposits have been identified in patients with hypothyroidism, urate gout, and Wilson's disease, as well as in kindreds without an identified specific metabolic defect.

(b) An attack of pseudogout may be precipitated by trauma, surgical procedures, or serious medical illness.

2. **Other conditions.** Acute monarticular arthritis may be the atypical presentation of a number of other inflammatory conditions that usually cannot be definitively diagnosed in the ED.

   a. If the patient does not appear ill, the monarticular arthritis may be a presentation of **rheumatoid arthritis** or one of the **seronegative spondyloarthropathies.**

   b. If the patient shows signs of systemic illness, the patient may have **enteropathic arthritis** or **systemic autoimmune disease.**

B **Clinical features**

1. **General**

   a. **Symptoms.** The patient usually describes a short course of increasing pain, redness, swelling, and immobility of a single joint, sometimes associated with fever, skin lesions, or other symptoms and signs related to the specific disease process.

   b. **Physical examination findings.** Examination of the joint usually reveals swelling, warmth, and/or redness that is not present on the contralateral side. Effusion may be present. Special attention should be paid to the patient's temperature, skin, and other joints.

2. **Septic arthritis**

   a. **Disseminated gonococcal infection.** Twenty-five to fifty percent of patients present with a single hot, swollen joint, while the others usually have migratory polyarthralgia or polyarthritis. Fever, dermatitis, and tenosynovitis are the most common findings on the initial examination. The skin lesions are usually small papules located on the trunk or extremities.

   b. **Nongonococcal bacterial arthritis.** Most patients are febrile. Eighty to ninety percent of patients present with monarticular arthritis; the knee is most often affected in adults and the hip is most often affected in children. Other commonly involved sites include the shoulder, wrist, interphalangeal, and elbow joints. Bacterial infection of the sternoclavicular and sacroiliac joints is associated with intravenous drug use.

3. **Gout**

   a. The typical gout attack begins suddenly, often at night, and within a few hours the joint becomes visibly inflamed and exquisitely tender. The skin is often tense and shiny. Swelling is related to synovial effusion and to periarticular edema. Fever, as high as 39.4°C, may occur. The attacks usually subside within a few days to a few weeks, even if untreated. Gout occurring in young adults usually has a more severe course than gout first presenting after middle age.

   b. Gout typically occurs in the lower extremity, and at least half of the initial attacks are confined to the **first metatarsophalangeal (MTP) joint (podagra).** Involvement of other joints of the foot may occur simultaneously or in rapid succession. Acute episodes may also involve tendon sheaths and bursae, especially over the olecranon or patella. In the chronically untreated hyperuricemic patient with recurrent attacks, there is involvement of an increasing number of joints in addition to those of the feet (e.g., the hands, wrists, ankles, knees, elbows). Tophi may be present, but usually not unless the gout has been untreated for approximately 10 years.

4. **Pseudogout**

   a. Pseudogout attacks reach full intensity within 12–36 hours. They generally last up to 10 days, but they may persist for months or occur in clusters. Findings consistent with acute synovitis are noted, and fever (as high as 40.0°C) may occur.

   b. Pseudogout by far most commonly involves the **knee joint.** The other large joints are the next most often affected joints, and the first MTP joint can also be involved. There is a tendency for subsequent attacks to occur in previously involved joints.

C **Differential diagnoses**

1. **Septic arthritis, gout,** and **pseudogout** are the prime diagnostic considerations when a patient presents to the ED with a clinical picture consistent with monarticular arthritis.

2. **Periarticular problems.** Localized periarticular processes (e.g., bursitis, tendinitis, soft tissue infection, bone disease) may cause pain and swelling near a single joint. Bone pain may be caused by Paget's disease or osteomyelitis, or it may be related to hemoglobinopathies, pulmonary hypertrophic osteoarthropathy, or malignancy.

3. **Noninflammatory monarticular arthritis**
   a. **Structural joint problems** may be related to trauma or overuse, internal derangement, loose body, fracture, neuropathic joint, or osteonecrosis.
   b. **Hemarthrosis** is a consideration in patients with bleeding disorders or in those taking anticoagulants.
   c. **Congenital disorders.** Pediatric patients may present with congenital dysplasia of the hip, slipped capital femoral epiphysis, or osteochondritis dissecans.
   d. **Osteoarthritis.** Older patients with osteoarthritis fairly often present with monarthritis of the knee, hip, or other joints.

4. **Underlying inflammatory conditions.** Monarticular arthritis may be part of the pattern of exacerbation and remission of many of the rheumatologic diseases that are usually classified as polyarticular, such as rheumatoid arthritis, psoriatic arthritis, Reiter's syndrome, and systemic lupus erythematosus (SLE). Similarly, enteropathic arthritis is more commonly polyarticular, but monarticular arthritis may be associated with Whipple's disease, intestinal bypass, ulcerative colitis, and regional enteritis.

5. **Rare or less obvious causes of monarticular arthritis.** Hydroxyapatite deposition, crystal-induced arthropathies other than gout and pseudogout, sarcoid, Lyme disease, and myriad other conditions may present as acute monarticular arthritis. Furthermore, when a single joint is persistently inflamed, consideration must be given to the possibilities of indolent infection caused by slow-growing organisms, such as *Mycobacterium tuberculosis, Sporotrichum schenckii,* or *Candida,* and tumors, particularly pigmented villonodular synovitis.

D **Evaluation**

1. **Laboratory studies**
   a. Rapid-turnaround blood tests that may contribute to the diagnosis include a **CBC, ESR,** and **uric acid and calcium levels.** However, a patient with gout may not have hyperuricemia at the time of the acute attack, and most patients with pseudogout do not have hypercalcemia.
   b. If gonococcal arthritis is suspected, **testing for sexually transmitted diseases (STDs)** should be conducted. Genitourinary testing is positive in 80% of patients with disseminated gonococcal infection.
   c. **Blood cultures** are drawn in patients with suspected septic arthritis. In nongonococcal bacterial arthritis, blood cultures are positive approximately 50% of the time, while they are positive less than 20% of the time in patients with disseminated gonococcal infection.

2. **Imaging studies.** Radiographs of the involved joint are usually obtained to rule out fracture and bone disease, and to assess for findings consistent with specific forms of arthritis.
   a. In septic arthritis, routine radiographs generally reveal only joint effusion. A CT scan may be helpful in diagnosing infection of the sternoclavicular or sacroiliac joints.
   b. In early gout, radiographs are expected to be negative, but in chronic gout there may be erosions of bone of 5 mm or more in diameter. Most commonly, erosions are observed in the subchondral areas of the bases or heads of the phalanges and are not associated with the juxta-articular osteopenia seen in rheumatoid arthritis.

   c. In pseudogout, there may be radiographic evidence of calcinosis in cartilage and other structures. Crystal deposition in the knee is recognized as linear or punctate calcification, often localized to the inner two thirds of the meniscus.

3. **Arthrocentesis** is performed to obtain a sample of the joint fluid for study. The joint fluid is analyzed for cell count, glucose and protein levels, viscosity or mucin clot, crystals, and Gram stain characteristics. It is cultured for bacteria (aerobic and anaerobic), acid-fast bacilli, and fungi. Additional special tests may be appropriate in selected cases. Table 10–6 lists findings typical of various conditions.

   a. **Septic arthritis**

     (1) In **disseminated gonococcal arthritis,** *N. gonorrhoeae* is cultured in less than 50% of purulent joints. The mean white blood cell (WBC) count is over 50,000/mm^3.

     (2) In **nongonococcal bacterial arthritis,** the mean synovial fluid WBC count is approximately 100,000/mm^3, but initial counts may be in the same range as inflammatory arthritis. The causative organism is cultured approximately 90% of the time. Low levels of glucose are present in approximately 50% of patients with septic joints, but can also occur in rheumatoid arthritis.

   b. **Gout.** In patients with gout, synovial fluid aspirated early in the clinical course of joint inflammation almost always contains the typical needle-like crystals. The crystals are negatively birefringent using polarized-light microscopy and most commonly are found within polymorphonuclear neutrophils. The WBC count in the synovial fluid is usually approximately 15,000/mm^3, but occasionally is in the range of 70,000/mm^3.

   c. **Pseudogout.** The synovial fluid WBC count is usually less than 15,000/mm^3, although the count may reach 70,000/mm^3 or higher. In pseudogout, the crystals are weakly positively birefringent and rhomboid in shape.

E **Therapy**

1. **Septic arthritis**

   a. **Antibiotics.** The selection of the initial antibiotic is based on the results of the Gram stain and the leading organisms in the differential diagnosis. Table 10–7 contains guidelines regarding empiric therapy.

   b. **Drainage.** Most rheumatologists recommend an initial trial of closed-needle aspiration (arthrocentesis), once or twice daily, in all joints except the hips, which should be managed with open drainage (arthrotomy).

   c. **Immobilization.** A splint or cast is used to immobilize the joint in a position of function. The patient should begin passive range-of-motion exercises as soon as possible.

TABLE 10–6 Synovial Fluid Characteristics

Diagnosis	Appearance	Mucin Clot	WBC/mm^3	Sugar (% of blood level)
Normal	Straw-colored clear	Good	<200	$\cong$ 100
Degenerative joint disease	Slightly turbid	Good	<2000	$\cong$ 100
Traumatic arthritis	Straw-colored bloody, or yellow	Good	$\cong$ 2000	
Rheumatoid arthritis	Turbid	Fair to poor	5000–50,000	<50–75
Spondyloarthropathies	Turbid	Fair to poor	5000–50,000	<50–75
Acute gout, pseudogout	Turbid	Fair to poor	5000–50,000	$\cong$ 90
Septic arthritis	Very turbid or purulent	Poor	50,000–200,000	<50
Tuberculous arthritis	Turbid	Poor	$\cong$ 25,000	<50

WBC = white blood cell.

TABLE 10–7 Suggested Empiric Therapy for Septic Arthritis and Bursitis

Diagnosis	Patient Profile	Likely Causative Organisms	Intravenous Antibiotics
Septic arthritis	Infant (<3 months)	*Staphylococcus aureus* Enterobacteriaceae Group B streptococcus	PRSP + third-generation cephalosporin
	Child (3 months–6 years)	*S. aureus* *Haemophilus influenzae* Streptococci Enterobacteriaceae	PRSP + third-generation cephalosporin
	Adult	*S. aureus* Group A streptococcus Enterobacteriaceae	PRSP + aminoglycoside
	Adult with possible STD contact	Gonococci	Ceftriaxone or cefotaxime
	Prosthetic joint, postoperative, post–intra-articular injection	*S. epidermidis* *S. aureus* Enterobacteriaceae *Pseudomonas* species	Vancomycin + ciprofloxacin
Septic bursitis		*S. aureus*	PRSP (intravenously or orally)

PRSP = penicillinase-resistant synthetic penicillin; STD = sexually transmitted disease.

2. **Crystal-induced arthritis.** When a joint of the lower extremities is involved, a cane or crutches may facilitate limited ambulation.

   a. **Oral NSAIDs** are first-line therapy. **Narcotic analgesics** may be needed adjunctively. All NSAIDs are relatively contraindicated in patients with active ulcer disease because the serious side effects most predominantly involve gastrointestinal bleeding. Low-dose salicylates (less than 3 g/day) should be avoided because they increase hyperuricemia through renal mechanisms.

      (1) **Indomethacin** is the NSAID traditionally used to treat crystal-induced arthritis. The first dose is 75–150 mg, followed by 50 mg every 8 hours. Smaller doses are frequently effective (e.g., 50 mg initially and then 25–50 mg every 8 hours).

      (2) **Other NSAIDs,** such as **ibuprofen** and **naproxen,** are also effective and may have fewer side effects than indomethacin. In adults, **ketorolac** may be administered, 30–60 mg intravenously or intramuscularly, to initiate treatment.

   b. **Colchicine** administration can abort acute gout attacks and may improve the periarthritis associated with sarcoidosis. However, colchicine does not affect the course of rheumatoid arthritis and does not have a predictable effect in pseudogout. The action seems to be related to effects on the polymorpholeukocyte.

      (1) The intravenous dose of colchicine is 2 mg, or 1 mg repeated every 4 hours once or twice. Intravenous administration of colchicine may produce leukopenia in patients with hepatic or renal disease or in those who have been taking colchicine orally.

      (2) The oral dose of colchicine is 0.6 mg every 1–2 hours for up to a maximum of 14 doses. Oral colchicine frequently causes nausea, vomiting, and diarrhea. Significant improvement in signs and symptoms is expected in 12–24 hours, at which point the dosage can be tapered to 0.6 mg two to three times daily.

   c. **Prednisone** may be employed for refractory cases of gout or pseudogout, or when the standard treatment regimens are contraindicated. Glucocorticoids can be administered orally or parenterally. For example, prednisone 60 mg could be given initially and tapered over 7 days. In rare cases, intra-articular glucocorticoids may be considered.

  d. **Allopurinol** or **probenecid** is used to treat hyperuricemia in gout patients after remission of the acute attack.

  e. **Joint aspiration** seems to be therapeutic in patients with pseudogout.

F Disposition

1. **Discharge**

   a. Most patients with straightforward crystal-induced arthritis can be treated as outpatients. Prescriptions are usually written to cover the first week of therapy. Clinic follow-up is important to ensure resolution of the acute episode, and also to address underlying health issues and any recurrent episodes. Possible indications for admission are intractable pain or uncertainty regarding the diagnosis.

   b. When a patient has an acutely inflamed joint but an evaluation not diagnostic and not suspicious for infection, discharge home with cultures pending is acceptable as long as there can be close follow-up. Outpatient work-up, such as serologic tests or special radiographs (to help diagnose noninfectious periarticular causes of acute joint pain and swelling, underlying inflammatory disease, or noninflammatory monarticular arthritis), may be appropriate to initiate from the ED if the institution is set up to do this.

2. **Admission.** Patients who have been diagnosed as having septic arthritis, as well as those suspected of having septic arthritis, should be admitted to the hospital.

VI POLYARTICULAR ARTHRITIS

A Discussion
Polyarticular arthritis is characterized by **pain in multiple joints;** it can be inflammatory or noninflammatory.

1. **Noninflammatory polyarticular arthritis. Osteoarthritis** is the primary disorder in this category. Recognized forms are hereditary osteoarthritis of the hands, hereditary primary generalized osteoarthritis, traumatic osteoarthritis, and osteoarthritis secondary to metabolic disease.

2. **Inflammatory polyarthritis.** Many types of disorders cause inflammatory polyarthritis. They are subdivided according to the location of the arthritis and the number of joints involved: **peripheral polyarticular** (involving five or more joints), **peripheral pauciarticular** (involving two to four joints), and **peripheral with axial involvement** (involving one or both sacroiliac joints and/or the spine).

   a. **Peripheral polyarticular arthritis.** Rheumatoid arthritis is the prototypical inflammatory peripheral polyarthritis. SLE and some forms of viral arthritis, such as that caused by HIV, are also in this group. Psoriatic arthritis occasionally has a polyarticular presentation.

   b. **Peripheral pauciarticular arthritis.** Psoriatic arthritis, Reiter's syndrome, and enteropathic arthritis most frequently present as peripheral pauciarticular disease. Other conditions that are members of this category are rheumatic fever, Behçet's disease, bacterial endocarditis, Lyme disease, sarcoidosis, and polyarticular gout.

   c. **Peripheral polyarthritis with axial involvement** is seen in ankylosing spondylitis. In this condition, the peripheral arthritis may precede the back symptoms, particularly in the juvenile-onset form. A minority of patients with Reiter's syndrome initially presents with polyarthritis and axial involvement, but most develop sacroiliitis or spine disease at some point during the course of the disease. Enteropathic arthritis may present as peripheral arthritis, axial arthritis, or a combination of the two.

B Clinical features
Polyarticular arthritis may present to the ED practitioner as a recurrent symptom in a previously diagnosed disease, as a new symptom in a previously diagnosed disease, or as the first presentation of an as-yet undiagnosed disorder. In patients with inflammatory causes of

polyarthritis, associated inflammatory involvement of other organ systems of the body may also be part of the presentation.

1. **General**
   a. **Patient history**
      (1) For first presentations, in addition to specific joint symptoms and associated symptoms, important aspects of the patient's history include age, gender, acuteness of the illness, anatomic location and symmetry of the arthritis, and relevant exposures.
      (2) For repeat presentations or exacerbations, past medical history is important, including particulars of diagnostic evaluation and treatment.
   b. **Symptoms**
      (1) The patient usually describes onset of pain in multiple joints, with individual joint involvement being simultaneous, additive, or migratory. The patient may describe evidence of inflammation (e.g., redness, warmth, swelling) or evidence of mechanical dysfunction (e.g., joint locking or giving way). In inflammatory arthritis, morning stiffness is a prominent feature.
      (2) There may be nonspecific associated symptoms (e.g., fever, night sweats, weight loss), symptoms suggestive of other musculoskeletal involvement (e.g., back pain), or symptoms suggestive of other organ involvement (e.g., rash, oral or genital lesions, diarrhea, chest pain).

2. **Specific clinical presentations.** Recognition of clinical presentations may assist in determining the diagnosis.
   a. **Osteoarthritis** is the most common cause of polyarthritis.
      (1) **Patient history.** The pathogenesis of osteoarthritis is not well understood, and most cases fall into the category of idiopathic, rather than secondary to other diseases or trauma. Rare in patients younger than 40 years, the incidence of osteoarthritis increases with age.
      (2) **Symptoms** usually develop gradually, but patients may present with the acute development of pain, redness, and swelling.
      (3) **Physical examination findings** include **Heberden's nodes** [i.e., bony enlargements of the distal interphalangeal (DIP) joints] and **Bouchard's nodes** [i.e., bony enlargements of the proximal interphalangeal (PIP) joints]. The next most frequent area of involvement in osteoarthritis is the thumb base, and on examination there may be swelling, tenderness, and crepitus. Other frequently involved sites are the hips, knees, and spine.
   b. **Rheumatoid arthritis,** a systemic chronic inflammatory disorder, is characterized by joint involvement.
      (1) Multiple joints are afflicted at once, usually in the extremities, and usually in a symmetric manner. Associated **extra-articular manifestations** may involve the eyes (e.g., as part of Sjögren's syndrome), the hematologic system (e.g., as part of Felty's syndrome), the lungs, the heart, the blood vessels, and the neuromuscular system.
      (2) The initial presentation of rheumatoid arthritis often is the **symmetric inflammation of the small joints of the hands and feet,** although large joints such as the knees and ankles are sometimes affected first. Monarticular presentation occurs in approximately 15% of patients. In some, systemic manifestations precede overt arthritis.
      (3) **Rheumatoid nodules** (i.e., subcutaneous nodules ranging from a few millimeters to over 20 mm in diameter occurring in areas exposed to pressure) may be found on physical examination in patients with chronic disease. Another finding may be a **Baker's popliteal cyst;** these cysts are lined with synovial membrane, usually communicate with the cavity of the knee joint, and may rupture or dissect.
   c. **Psoriatic arthritis** afflicts 5%–8% of patients with psoriasis. In the asymmetric pauciarticular inflammatory type, the arthritis is typically preceded by psoriasis by many years, and the PIP and DIP joints are most frequently involved. There are also syndromes of symmetric

arthritis and psoriatic spondylitis. Physical examination may reveal sausage-shaped digits (dactylitis), onychodystrophy, and psoriatic skin lesions.

  d. **Enteropathic arthritis** occurs in 10%–20% of patients with ulcerative colitis and Crohn's disease. The arthritis tends to be acute, in association with an initial flare of bowel disease, and does not result in bony destruction. In most patients, the knees, ankles, elbows, and wrists are affected.

  e. **Spondylarthritides.** The spondylarthritides are characterized by involvement of the sacroiliac joints, by peripheral inflammatory arthropathy, by the absence of RF, and by the presence of HLA-B27. Ankylosing spondylitis and Reiter's syndrome fall into this category, as well as the subtypes of psoriatic, juvenile, and inflammatory bowel disease associated with sacroiliitis.

  (1) **Ankylosing spondylitis.** Predominant features are back discomfort and sacroiliitis.

  (a) **Symptoms.** The back pain, which usually first manifests in patients younger than 40, is insidious in onset, persistent, and associated with morning stiffness and improvement with exercise.

  (b) **Physical examination findings**

  (i) **Signs of associated conditions** (e.g., anterior uveitis, aortic valve insufficiency) may be seen.

  (ii) **Local signs.** Patients with ankylosing spondylitis may have **loss of spinal lordosis, muscle spasm,** and **decrease in mobility** in both the anterior and lateral planes of the body.

  (iii) **Peripheral joint involvement** occurs in approximately 25% of cases, especially in the lower limbs, but also in the shoulder and hip. Other musculoskeletal features may be **plantar fasciitis, costochondritis,** and **Achilles tendinitis.**

  (2) **Reiter's syndrome**

  (a) **Patient history.** The syndrome is now recognized as a reactive arthritis, triggered by a specific etiologic agent (e.g., *Shigella, Salmonella, Yersinia, Chlamydia trachomatis, Campylobacter*) in a genetically susceptible host.

  (b) **Signs and symptoms.** The **classic clinical triad** is **urethritis, conjunctivitis,** and **arthritis. Mucocutaneous lesions** may also be present.

  (i) **Arthritis.** In Reiter's syndrome, arthritis is usually asymmetric and additive. It typically involves the joints of the lower extremities, such as the knee, ankle, subtalar, MTP, and toe interphalangeal joints. As in psoriatic arthritis, dactylitis may be a distinguishing feature. Tendinitis and fasciitis are characteristic, especially at the Achilles insertion, at the plantar fascia, and along the axial skeleton.

  (ii) **Mucocutaneous lesions.** The characteristic skin lesions are keratoderma blennorrhagica and lesions of the glans penis (circinate balanitis).

  f. **SLE** is an autoimmune disease with myriad clinical manifestations (see VII B 1). The severity and activity of the disease are highly variable. Almost all patients experience arthralgias and myalgias and most develop intermittent arthritis.

  (1) SLE patients tend to develop fusiform swelling of the joints, diffuse puffiness of the hands and feet, and tenosynovitis. Frequently involved joints are the PIP and metacarpophalangeal (MCP) joints of the hands, the wrists, and the knees, in a symmetric pattern.

  (2) Joint deformities develop in approximately 25% of patients (e.g., a swan-neck deformity or ulnar deviation, as in rheumatoid arthritis).

C   Differential diagnosis

  1. **Inflammatory polyarthritis**

  a. **Rheumatic conditions.** Inflammatory polyarthritis is caused by rheumatic conditions (e.g., rheumatoid arthritis, psoriatic arthropathy, enterohepatic arthropathy, SLE), as well as most variations of juvenile rheumatoid arthritis. It may be a less prominent feature of ankylosing spondylitis, Reiter's syndrome, and the variations of psoriasis, juvenile arthritis, and enteropathic arthritis that involve the spine and sacroiliac joints.

   b. Infection. Inflammatory polyarthritis may occur in conjunction with bacterial infections, such as endocarditis, acute rheumatic fever, brucellosis, and disseminated gonococcal infection. It may also occur in conjunction with viral infections, such as parvovirus 19, rubella, mumps, hepatitis B, and HIV, and in conjunction with the spirochetal infections syphilis and Lyme disease.

   c. Microcrystalline disease. Inflammatory polyarthritis is a possible presentation of microcrystalline disease, such as gout and pseudogout.

2. **Noninflammatory polyarticular arthritis** is generally caused by osteoarthritis. Contributing factors may be heredity, acute or repeated trauma, developmental defects, and metabolic abnormalities including hypothyroidism and the osteoarthritic form of CPPD, as well as hemochromatosis, ochronosis, and acromegaly.

3. **Polyarthralgia** must be distinguished from polyarthritis. Polyarthralgia can occur in serum sickness, drug-induced lupus, and Henoch-Schönlein purpura. It can occur in association with metabolic disorders (e.g., hypothyroidism, hyperthyroidism) or in association with viral infections. Patients with fibromyalgia may be suspected of having polyarthritis or polyarthralgia; however, joint examination is normal and multiple specific tender musculoskeletal sites are present.

4. **Periarticular problems** must also be distinguished from polyarthritis.
   a. Joint pain may be related to trauma or inflammation of the ligaments, tendons, or bursae.
   b. Muscular causes of pain include viral infection, polymyalgia rheumatica (PMR), polymyositis, and dermatomyositis.
   c. Vasculitis and vaso-occlusive disease occasionally present with periarticular pain.
   d. Peripheral neuropathies and compression neuropathies (e.g., carpal tunnel syndrome) may present with periarticular pain.
   e. When axial symptoms are present, nonrheumatologic diseases of the spine (e.g., spinal stenosis, spondylolisthesis) should be considered.
   f. Myeloma, widely metastatic cancers, osteonecrosis, and bone disease associated with sickle cell crises and pulmonary disease may present with bone and joint pain.

D **Evaluation**

1. **Laboratory studies**
   a. Osteoarthritis. No laboratory studies are diagnostic of osteoarthritis, but special laboratory tests may identify one of the causes of metabolic osteoarthritis.
   b. Inflammatory disorders. The inflammatory disorders may be associated with abnormalities of the CBC and ESR. Other tests that may assist in classifying the disorders are RF, ANA, and complement levels; however, the results of these tests are generally not available at the time of the visit to assist in decision making.
      (1) HLA-B27 testing is generally not needed for the diagnosis of ankylosing spondylitis, but may be helpful in classifying one of the variant spondyloarthropathies when radiographs are nondiagnostic.
      (2) Cultures or serologic tests are occasionally helpful in identifying the triggering agent of the reactive arthritis of Reiter's syndrome.
      (3) When an underlying infection (e.g., HIV, gonococcal infection, hepatitis B, Lyme disease, rheumatic fever, endocarditis) is suspected as the basis for polyarthritis, conventional diagnostic testing should be conducted.

2. **Diagnostic imaging studies.** Radiographs of selected involved joints may assist in diagnosis.
   a. Osteoarthritis. Characteristic changes include joint-space narrowing as articular cartilage is lost, subchondral bone sclerosis, subchondral cysts, and marginal osteophytes. Osteophytosis alone may be attributable to aging rather than osteoarthritis. There may be a great dispar-

ity in the severity of the radiographic findings when compared with the severity of the symptoms.

b. **Rheumatoid arthritis.** Characteristic changes include soft tissue swelling, loss of cartilage space, demineralization, erosions, bony ankylosis, subluxations, and subchondral cysts.

c. **Psoriatic arthritis.** Radiographic findings in psoriatic arthritis are similar to those in rheumatoid arthritis, but there may be more involvement of the DIP joints, a "pencil-in-cup" appearance to the proximal and distal terminal phalanx, or an "opera-glass" deformity of one phalanx telescoping into its neighbor. The axial skeleton may show sacroiliitis.

d. **Enteropathic arthritis.** In arthritis associated with gastrointestinal disease, peripheral joint radiographs show soft tissue swelling or effusion without erosion or destruction.

e. **Spondylarthritides**

(1) **Ankylosing spondylitis** is diagnosed by the presence of sacroiliitis, which may be based on the findings of juxta-articular sclerosis, blurring of the joint margin, and narrowing. In more advanced disease of the sacroiliac joint, there may be erosions, joint-space destruction, and total ankylosis. The lumbar spine initially shows squaring of the superior and inferior margins of the vertebral bodies; in some advanced cases, "bamboo spine" is seen. In terms of radiographic differential diagnosis, the spinal changes tend to be similar in the enteroarthropathies, but are more asymmetric and random in spondylitis associated with Reiter's syndrome and psoriatic arthropathy.

(2) **Reiter's syndrome.** Early or mild findings consist of juxta-articular osteoporosis. In more serious disease, marginal erosions and loss of joint space can be seen. As in the other spondyloarthropathies, periostitis occurs. Spurs may occur at the insertion of the plantar fascia.

f. **SLE.** It is rare to find radiographic evidence of cartilage or bone destruction.

3. **Arthrocentesis** and synovial fluid analysis may be performed to determine if the fluid is more consistent with noninflammatory or inflammatory arthritis, and to investigate the possibilities of crystal-induced arthritis and septic arthritis (see Table 10–6).

E Therapy

1. **Osteoarthritis** is treated symptomatically, with NSAIDs or acetaminophen. Narcotics and corticosteroids are rarely indicated. If steroids are used, intra-articular or periarticular injection is preferable to systemic administration, and steroid therapy should be limited to every 4–6 months. Activities and physical therapy should be tailored to the severity of the degenerative process. Orthopedic surgery may be needed in advanced cases.

2. **Acute polyarthritis secondary to rheumatologic conditions** is generally managed with NSAIDs as first-line agents, sometimes supplemented with narcotic analgesics. In more severe cases and flares, systemic corticosteroids are also given. Chronic rheumatoid arthritis is managed with suppressive therapy, such as methotrexate or gold, prescribed in the clinic setting. Ultimately, orthopedic surgery may be necessary. Prolonged administration of a long-acting tetracycline may ameliorate *Chlamydia*-induced Reiter's syndrome.

3. **Acute diseases or underlying conditions causing acute polyarthritis** should be managed according to conventional measures, with symptomatic treatment of the joint pain.

F Disposition

1. **Discharge**

a. Patients with osteoarthritis are managed in the outpatient setting by the primary care physician.

b. Most patients with rheumatologic disorders can be managed as outpatients by the patient's primary care or specialty physician.

c. Patients with psoriasis and underlying conditions such as bowel disease are generally managed according to the severity of the underlying disease rather than the severity of the arthritis.

d. Patients with conditions such as hepatitis B and serum sickness may be managed at home if the diagnosis is clear and the patient is not severely ill.

2. **Admission.** Criteria for admission include:
   a. An unclear diagnosis
   b. Painful and incapacitating arthritis
   c. Severe underlying conditions, such as rheumatic fever or endocarditis

VII CONNECTIVE TISSUE DISORDERS

A Discussion   The cause of relatively few rheumatic diseases is known. Classification is generally based on groupings by one or more common features.

1. **Acquired connective tissue disorders** include SLE, scleroderma, polymyositis and dermatomyositis, mixed connective tissue disease (MCTD), polyarteritis nodosa (PAN), hypersensitivity angiitis, Wegener's granulomatosis, Takayasu's disease, Cogan's syndrome, PMR, and amyloidosis. Some patients who show features of scleroderma, polymyositis, and SLE are considered to have MCTD. The systemic manifestations of the acquired connective tissue disorders are typically complex and often indolent. In some cases they are life-threatening.

2. **Polyarthritides** include rheumatoid arthritis, juvenile rheumatoid arthritis (Still's disease), ankylosing spondylitis, psoriatic arthritis, and Reiter's syndrome [see VI B 2 e (2)].

3. **Other.** Other connective tissue disorders include infectious arthritis, biochemical and endocrine disorders, allergic and reactive disorders, and inherited and congenital disorders.

B Clinical features

1. **SLE** is a **chronic multisystem inflammatory disease** that varies greatly in clinical manifestations, mode of presentation, and clinical course. Most patients are women; presentation often occurs between the ages of 15 and 25 years. Recommended criteria for diagnosis of SLE are presented in Table 10–8.
   a. Joint disorders. SLE patients tend to exhibit **fusiform swelling of the joints, diffuse puffiness of the hands and feet,** and **tenosynovitis.** Frequently involved joints are the PIP and MCP joints of the hands, the wrists, and the knees, in a symmetric pattern. Joint deformities develop in approximately 25% of patients, typically as a swan-neck deformity or ulnar deviation, as in rheumatoid arthritis. A malar rash or other skin rash may be present.
   b. Pleurisy occurs in 50% of patients with SLE during the course of disease, and pleural effusions occur in 30%. These disorders may contribute to significant respiratory compromise. Pulmonary hemorrhage may also occur.
   c. Pericarditis occurs in 30% of SLE patients and is most often seen in elderly patients and during flares. Pericarditis may be asymptomatic, but typically positional chest pain and a pericardial rub are present. Pericardial tamponade and constrictive pericarditis are rare complications.
   d. Myocarditis occurs less frequently than pericarditis.
   e. Central nervous system (CNS) manifestations include **psychoses, seizures,** and **hemiplegias;** these often resolve spontaneously.
   f. Renal failure and **hypertension** may be significant clinical problems. Renal diseases associated with SLE include **nephritis** and **nephrotic syndrome,** which is occasionally complicated by renal vein thrombosis.

2. **Scleroderma (systemic sclerosis)** is characterized by the **deposition of fibrous connective tissue** in the skin and often in many organ systems. Vascular lesions of the skin, lungs, and kidneys may be present.
   a. Cutaneous manifestations. The skin becomes **thickened, atrophic,** and **tight.** Accompanying skin abnormalities that may be present include telangiectasias, calcinosis, and increased melanotic pigmentation.

TABLE 10–8   Criteria for Diagnosis of Systemic Lupus Erythematosus (SLE)*

Criterion	Definition
Malar rash	Fixed erythema, flat or raised, over the malar eminences
Discoid rash	Erythematous raised patches with adherent keratotic scaling and follicular plugging; atrophic scarring may occur
Photosensitivity	Skin rash as a result of unusual reaction to sunlight—documented by patient history or observed by physician
Oral ulcers	Oral and nasopharyngeal ulceration, observed by physician
Arthritis	Nonerosive arthritis involving two or more peripheral joints, characterized by tenderness, swelling, or effusion
Serositis	Pleuritis or pericarditis documented by electrocardiogram or rub **or** Evidence of pericardial effusion
Renal disorder	Proteinuria >0.5 g/day or 3 + **or** Cellular casts
Neurologic disorder	Seizures without other cause **or** Psychosis without other cause
Hematologic disorder	Hemolytic anemia **or** Leukopenia (<4000/mm^3) **or** Lymphopenia (<1500/mm^3) **or** Thrombocytopenia (<100,000/mm^3) in the absence of offending drugs
Immunologic disorder	Positive LE cell preparation **or** Anti-dsDNA **or** Anti-Sm antibodies **or** False-positive test for syphilis
Antinuclear antibodies (ANAs)	An abnormal titer of ANAs by immunofluorescence or an equivalent assay at any point in time in the absence of drugs known to induce ANAs

*If four of these criteria are present at any time during the course of disease, a diagnosis of SLE can be made with 98% specificity and 97% sensitivity.

Reprinted with permission from Tan EM, Cohen AS, Fries JF, et al. The 1982 revised criteria for the classification of systemic lupus erythematosus. *Arthritis Rheum* 1982;25:1271.

   b. **Raynaud's phenomenon** may occur in the extremities; prolonged ischemia may cause pain, ulceration, and gangrene. **CREST syndrome** (**c**alcinosis, **R**aynaud's phenomenon, **e**sophageal hypomotility, **s**clerodactyly, and **t**elangiectasia) is considered a variant of scleroderma.
   c. **Musculoskeletal system manifestations** include **mild inflammatory arthritis, contractures, acral osteolysis** with consequent shortening of the digits, and **myopathy.**

    d. Gastrointestinal system manifestations include **hypomotility of the esophagus** and changes in the small and large intestines.

    e. Pulmonary manifestations may include **pulmonary hypertension** and **interstitial pulmonary fibrosis.** Although pulmonary symptoms are usually chronic, some patients develop acute pulmonary hypertension and rapidly progressive respiratory failure.

    f. Cardiac manifestations, related to cardiac muscle replacement with fibrous tissue, include **arrhythmias, conduction disturbances,** and **congestive heart failure (CHF).** Some patients have pericarditis, which may be accompanied by pericardial tamponade. Some patients with scleroderma have cold-induced vasospastic angina.

    g. Malignant hypertension and **rapidly progressive renal insufficiency** may occur in a subset of patients, typically those with rapidly progressive skin changes.

3. Polymyositis and dermatomyositis. Polymyositis primarily affects skeletal muscle. Dermatomyositis is a variation of polymyositis in which skin eruptions accompany myopathy. Other subdivisions of polymyositis include polymyositis of childhood, polymyositis associated with malignancy, and polymyositis associated with other rheumatic disease. Muscle weakness affects proximal muscles more often than distal muscle groups. The disease is twice as common in women as in men and usually progresses over a period of weeks to months, although expression may be fulminant.

    a. Paralysis of pharyngeal muscles may produce **dysphagia** and **aspiration of ingested materials.**

    b. Respiratory muscle impairment may lead to **respiratory insufficiency** in patients with poorly controlled or chronic disease.

    c. Rhabdomyolysis and **acute renal insufficiency** occasionally develop in patients with florid myositis.

    d. The characteristic **rash of dermatomyositis** is an **erythematous eruption** that occurs over the face, neck, upper chest, and extensor surfaces of joints such as the hands and elbows. Heliotrope erythema or periorbital edema may be present.

4. Temporal arteritis is a granulomatous arteritis of the thoracic aorta and its branches, producing **vasculitis** and **ischemia.** It affects the middle-aged and the elderly.

    a. Signs and symptoms may include headache, tender scalp, visual disturbances, jaw or tongue claudication, and constitutional symptoms. Approximately 25% of patients have the associated condition of polymyalgia rheumatica, in which there is proximal shoulder and hip girdle morning stiffness and aching.

    b. Temporal arteritis may cause blindness before the condition is diagnosed. It may be averted if prodromal symptoms are recognized and treatment initiated.

5. PAN is a **necrotizing vasculitis** of the small and medium-sized muscular arteries. It affects the skin, gastrointestinal tract, and kidneys. Clinical sequelae include nodular, urticarial, or multiform rashes; abdominal angina; hypertension (which can be a significant clinical problem in patients with PAN); and hematuria. Involvement of the coronary arteries may cause cardiac ischemia, regardless of the age of the patient.

6. Kawasaki disease (mucocutaneous lymph node syndrome) is a disease of **young children** and is discussed in detail in Chapter 15 VIII.

C Differential diagnoses

1. Patients who present for the first time with symptoms and signs of a connective tissue disorder may not have a clear clinical diagnosis, and a subset of the various separate syndromes and their variants need to be considered. Nonrheumatologic conditions also enter into the differential diagnosis.

2. When a patient presents with an established connective tissue disorder and worsened or new symptomatology, it becomes necessary to distinguish between an exacerbation of the disease, the development of one of the emergency-associated sequelae, or the occurrence of a concurrent but separate process.

D **Evaluation**

1. **SLE.** Patients may exhibit nonspecific laboratory findings such as anemia, leukopenia, and thrombocytopenia. Urinalysis and coagulation testing may reveal abnormalities. The diagnosis is confirmed through serologic markers. More than 90% of patients with SLE have positive ANA tests, although the test is not entirely specific. Anti-dsDNA antibody levels and low complement levels may reflect disease activity, especially in patients with nephritis. In some patients, the ESR correlates with disease activity.

2. **Scleroderma.** There are no laboratory test abnormalities specific to scleroderma, although there may be abnormalities related to organ involvement. Some seromarkers, such as rheumatoid factor and ANA, may be positive in low titer.

3. **Polymyositis and dermatomyositis.** Muscle enzyme abnormalities are present in polymyositis and dermatomyositis. The presence of one or more muscle enzymes in the blood is necessary to make the diagnosis of polymyositis, and enzymes are valuable for assessing the course of the disease and the response to treatment. Creatinine kinase, transaminases, aldolase, and lactate dehydrogenase (LDH) are the most frequently measured enzymes. Serologic tests are generally not helpful. Characteristic but nonspecific abnormalities may be found on electromyogram.

4. **Temporal arteritis.** In temporal arteritis, the ESR is typically elevated to greater than 50 mm/hour. There may also be anemia and elevations in the liver function tests. The diagnosis is established by temporal artery biopsy.

5. **PAN.** There are no diagnostic serologic tests for PAN. Nonspecific abnormalities that may be present include leukocytosis, anemia of chronic disease, and an elevated ESR. Up to 30% of patients with PAN test positive for hepatitis B surface antigen. Other laboratory findings reflect the particular organ involved. An arteriogram may demonstrate aneurysms in the small and medium-sized arteries of the kidneys and abdominal viscera. Diagnosis can be based on directed biopsy, for example, of the skin or muscle at symptomatic sites.

E **Therapy**

1. **SLE.** Treatment of SLE is not standard because the disease has such a highly variable symptom pattern. Therapy usually involves NSAIDs, antimalarial drugs, corticosteroids, and cytotoxic drugs for patients with more severe or refractory symptoms.
   a. The specific management of pleuritis and pleural effusion may involve anti-inflammatory medication and thoracentesis as indicated. Intubation and ventilatory support may be necessary.
   b. The specific management of pericarditis is usually with NSAIDs; some patients require prednisone.
   c. Glucocorticoids are often given in nephritis and cerebritis, although the degree of benefit is uncertain.

2. **Scleroderma.** Management of scleroderma is mainly directed toward supportive measures and treatment of the involved organ system.
   a. Glucocorticoids are indicated for patients with inflammatory myositis or pericarditis. They are not otherwise indicated in long-term treatment, except perhaps for the prevention of progression of interstitial lung disease.
   b. The hypertension of scleroderma is managed with an ACE inhibitor. Diuretics, which might exacerbate volume contraction, are contraindicated.

3. **Polymyositis and dermatomyositis.** Spontaneous remissions are unusual in polymyositis, so pharmacologic therapy is necessary.
   a. Corticosteroids are the drugs of choice. For example, prednisone may be given in a dose of at least 40 mg/day in divided doses, for up to 4 months or until enzyme levels and clinical manifestations improve. Corticosteroid-resistant patients may respond to cytotoxic drugs.

    b. For acute renal failure due to rhabdomyolysis, the standard treatment modalities apply: administration of normal saline and bicarbonate, and possible administration of furosemide or mannitol in the early phase of renal failure to preserve urine output.

4. Temporal arteritis. Treatment of temporal arteritis should be initiated based on the clinical diagnosis to prevent blindness. Prednisone may be given at a dosage of 60 mg/day.

5. PAN. Treatment is necessary to avoid the otherwise extremely poor prognosis. Prednisone and cyclophosphamide may be given. Patients with concurrent hepatitis B antigenemia may receive vidarabine in combination with plasma exchange with or without glucocorticoids.

6. Kawasaki disease. Treatment is discussed in Chapter 15 VIII E.

F Disposition   It is difficult to make generalizations regarding the disposition of patients with connective tissue diseases because the syndromes are so diverse.

1. Frequently, it is sufficient to initiate the work-up or make a modification in the medication regimen and arrange outpatient follow-up.

2. In unclear or difficult cases, rheumatologic consultation should be obtained.

3. Patients with the manifestations as described in this section or other serious findings should be considered for admission, possibly to the ICU.

Study Questions

Directions: *Each of the numbered items or incomplete statements in this section is followed by answers or by completions of the statement. Select the ONE lettered answer or completion that is BEST in each case.*

1. A 23-year-old secretary taking erythromycin for bronchitis ate cookies that someone had brought into the office. She later learned that the cookies contained walnuts. She had experienced prior urticarial reactions to walnuts, and when she developed hives a few hours later, she presented to the emergency department (ED) requesting medication for severe, widespread pruritus. Which one of the following treatments is most appropriate?

- Ⓐ Ipecac
- Ⓑ Hydroxyzine
- Ⓒ Topical diphenhydramine
- Ⓓ Prednisone
- Ⓔ Epinephrine

2. A patient reports a prior anaphylactic reaction to radiocontrast media. Which one of the following statements regarding this case is correct?

- Ⓐ The risk for the first reaction was 5%–15%, regardless of whether ionic or nonionic radiocontrast media was used.
- Ⓑ The chance of a second reaction would not be substantially reduced by pretreatment with corticosteroids and antihistamines.
- Ⓒ The previous reaction could not have been a vasovagal reaction.
- Ⓓ The recommended alternative for the future is to try to avoid studies involving radiocontrast media entirely.
- Ⓔ Nonionic radiocontrast media is the same price as ionic radiocontrast media.

3. A 38-year-old patient presents with symptoms of L5 nerve root impairment that have been ongoing for 2 weeks. There is no history of trauma or fall. Examination and testing of this patient are likely to reveal which of the following?

- Ⓐ Abnormal findings on plain radiographic films
- Ⓑ Hypesthesia of the entire lower leg on the affected side
- Ⓒ Sensory findings that may include diminished pain on the dorsum of the distal region of the foot
- Ⓓ Motor findings that may include weakness on flexion of the great toe
- Ⓔ Tendon reflexes expected to be diminished at the knee and ankle

4. A 40-year-old male patient presents with knee pain. Joint effusion is aspirated, and synovial fluid shows a white blood cell (WBC) count of 100,000/mm³, weakly positive birefringent rhomboid crystals, and a Gram stain negative for organisms. Which of the following is the appropriate treatment for this patient?

- Ⓐ Reaspirate the joint to drain it completely and then inject Decadron 10 mg intravenously.
- Ⓑ Inject glucocorticoid medication into the joint.
- Ⓒ Prescribe prednisone and indomethacin, and discharge the patient home.
- Ⓓ Admit the patient to the hospital.
- Ⓔ Do not test the serum calcium level as it does not help diagnosis.

5. Which of the paired clinical scenarios and test results is LEAST likely to have clinical significance?

- Ⓐ Young woman with arthritis and rash—positive antinuclear antibody (ANA) test, high titer
- Ⓑ Elderly woman with minimal symptoms—positive ANA test, low titer

C Patient with Raynaud's phenomenon and thickened skin—positive ANA test, low titer

D 60-year-old patient with new headache—elevated erythrocyte sedimentation rate (ESR)

E 42-year-old patient with systemic lupus erythematosus (SLE) and worsening arthritis—elevated ESR

6. Which treatment is LEAST conventional for manifestations of scleroderma?

A General symptom control with glucocorticoids

B Glucocorticoids for pericarditis

C Angiotensin-converting enzyme (ACE) inhibitor for hypertension and renal disease

D Glucocorticoids for myositis

E Nonsteroidal anti-inflammatory drugs (NSAIDs) for pericarditis

7. A 45-year-old male presents with urticaria after ingesting ibuprofen for the first time this year. Which of the following mechanisms or pathways most likely explains his symptoms?

A Arachidonic acid pathway

B Complement pathway

C Direct histamine release

D Immunoglobulin E

E Kinin system

8. A 22-year-old male presents with a history of lower back pain. He admits to being an intravenous drug user. Your evaluation reveals an infection with inflammation of the sacroiliac joint. Which of the following etiologies is most likely?

A *Neisseria gonococcus*

B *Staphylococcus epidermidis*

C *Escherichia coli*

D *Pseudomonas aeruginosa*

E *Staphylococcus aureus*

Answers and Explanations

1. The answer is B In this case, the likely cause of the urticaria was walnut ingestion, based on the prior history of similar reaction, the timing of the development of the hives, and the fact that erythromycin is a rare cause of allergic reaction. First-line treatment for acute urticaria is the oral or parenteral administration of an antihistamine, such as hydroxyzine. Topical medications are generally unsatisfactory for widespread pruritus. Prednisone and epinephrine are not indicated. Ipecac to induce vomiting and rid the gastrointestinal tract of the triggering agent would be unlikely to be helpful hours after the ingestion.

2. The answer is D The ionic type of radiocontrast media is conventionally used because it is less expensive than the nonionic type, and while the estimated risk of reaction to ionic radiocontrast media is higher than that for nonionic radiocontrast media, the risk is still less than 1%. The risk of subsequent reaction to ionic radiocontrast media is approximately 30%, but this risk can be substantially reduced by pretreatment with corticosteroids and antihistamines or by using nonionic media. The decision not to use radiocontrast media at all carries the lowest risk of adverse medication reaction.

3. The answer is C Plain films may be normal or nonspecific in nerve root impingement syndromes. However, because the most likely cause at this level is herniated disk, definitive studies are usually not performed until 4–6 weeks have passed and surgical intervention is being considered. Even the presence of the sensory and motor neurologic findings does not mandate emergency evaluation or hospitalization. However, in some cases intractable pain, debility, or an inconsistent picture may make outpatient management inappropriate. The L4 and S1 levels of the spinal cord supply the nerves for the patellar and ankle reflexes, respectively. The L5 level supplies the posterior tibialis muscle, which provides only a slight, difficult-to-obtain reflex.

4. The answer is D Weakly positive birefringent rhomboid-shaped crystals on polarized microscopy suggest that calcium pyrophosphate deposition disease (CPPD) or pseudogout is ongoing. If the patient has not had the serum calcium level tested previously, it could be checked to rule out hyperparathyroidism as a causative factor. Although the WBC count could be explained by pseudogout alone, it is more consistent with infection. Therefore, the safest approach would be to admit the patient to the hospital, drain the joint, treat with nonsteroidal anti-inflammatory drugs (NSAIDs), consider antibiotic coverage while cultures are pending, and avoid use of glucocorticoid agents.

5. The answer is B ANA test results are positive in more than 90% of patients with SLE. ANA may also be present—but generally in lower titer—in other diseases (e.g., scleroderma) and in the asymptomatic elderly. An elevated ESR in an older patient with a headache is suggestive of temporal arteritis. In some patients with SLE, the ESR correlates with disease activity.

6. The answer is A There is no clear benefit to administering glucocorticoids in the treatment of scleroderma except for certain specific indications, such as pericarditis and myositis. Most treatment is supportive and symptomatic. However, hypertension needs to be managed aggressively, and ACE inhibitors have been shown to reverse hypertension, renal function impairment, and peripheral ischemia.

7. The answer is A Ibuprofen is a common over-the-counter and prescription nonsteroidal anti-inflammatory drug (NSAID) that uncommonly causes urticaria or bronchospasm. The theorized mechanism for the adverse effects is through the arachidonic acid pathway.

8. The answer is D Intravenous drug users have a propensity to develop infection with *P. aeruginosa.* In the vast majority of cases, a rheumatic joint will be infected with *S. aureus.* A young adult with skin lesions and a hot, swollen knee most likely has a gonococcal infection, although Gram-negative organisms or *Haemophilus influenzae* are remotely possible causes. Infected prosthetic joints are infected with *S. aureus* in 40% of cases, and with *S. epidermidis* in 20% of cases. Sepsis in an elderly, immunocompromised patient may be caused by *E. coli* or other Gram-negative organisms.

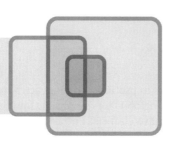

chapter **11**

Dermatologic Emergencies

JOAN SURDUKOWSKI

I APPROACH TO THE PATIENT WITH DERMATOLOGIC LESIONS

A **Patient history**   Answers to the following questions should be sought:

1. **General questions**
   a. How long have the lesions been present?
   b. What did the lesions look like originally?
   c. Does anything exacerbate the rash?
   d. Has the patient traveled anywhere recently?

2. **Questions about symptoms**
   a. Does the rash itch?
   b. Is the rash painful?
   c. Are there any associated symptoms?

3. **Questions about the past medical history**
   a. Is the patient taking any medications?
   b. What is the patient's occupational and social history?
   c. Is there a family history of skin disease?

B **Physical examination**   The patient's entire body should be examined, and the lesion should be palpated.

1. **Types of lesions**
   a. **Macules** are flat lesions, measuring less than 1 cm in diameter, that are different in color from the normal skin tone (e.g., measles).
   b. **Papules** are circumscribed, palpable elevations of the skin measuring less than 1 cm in diameter (e.g., scabies).
   c. **Nodules** are circumscribed, palpable elevations of the skin measuring greater than 1 cm in diameter (e.g., erythema nodosum).
   d. **Patches** are flat lesions greater than 1 cm in diameter (e.g., pityriasis rosea).
   e. **Plaques** are raised lesions measuring greater than 1 cm in diameter (e.g., psoriasis).
   f. **Pustules** are raised lesions greater than 0.5 cm in diameter that contain yellow fluid (e.g., abscesses).
   g. **Vesicles** are raised lesions up to 0.5 cm in diameter that contain clear fluid (e.g., herpes simplex).
   h. **Bullae** are vesicles that are greater than 0.5 cm in diameter (e.g., pemphigus).
   i. **Crust** is a dried exudate (e.g., impetigo).

2. **Location of lesions**
   a. **Site.** The location of the lesions on the body may offer a clue to the diagnosis. For example, varicella spares the palms and soles; scabies favors the finger-web spaces.
   b. **Extent.** Are the lesions localized or generalized?
   c. **Arrangement.** Are the lesions in a group or solitary?

3. **Appearance of lesions**
   a. **Margins** can be raised (as in psoriasis) or more active peripherally (as in tinea).
   b. **Color.** Melanin and hemoglobin are responsible for the colors of lesions.
   c. **Shape.** Annular lesions have clear or contrasting centers (e.g., the target lesions of Stevens-Johnson syndrome).
   d. **Scale.** The epidermis is replaced every 28 days. In psoriasis, the basal cells are mitotically active and produce epidermis or scale.

C **Differential diagnoses**   Many **systemic diseases** have cutaneous manifestations. For example:

1. Necrobiosis lipoidica diabeticorum, an oval, yellowish, shiny plaque with sharp borders, is a characteristic lesion usually located on the shins of patients with diabetes.
2. Erythema nodosum lesions may be seen in patients with ulcerative colitis.
3. Erythema multiforme can be associated with acute leukemia.

D **Evaluation**

1. **Microscopic examination.** An ordinary microscope can be used to examine scrapings from skin lesions.
   a. A **potassium hydroxide (KOH) slide preparation** is used when dermatophyte infections are suspected.
      (1) The lesion is wiped with alcohol and dried, and the border of the lesion is scraped with a #15 scalpel onto a slide.
      (2) One drop of 10% KOH is added to the slide, and the slide is covered with a coverslip. The slide is then heated over an alcohol flame lamp. Alternatively, a solution of 20% KOH and 40% dimethylsulfoxide can be used; this solution dissolves keratin in 5 minutes and does not require heating.
      (3) The slide is examined for long, thin, branching hyphae.
   b. A **Tzanck slide preparation** can confirm the diagnosis of herpes infections.
      (1) Vesicle contents are smeared on a slide, and Wright's stain or methylene blue is used for staining. Alternatively, the slide can be sent for direct fluorescent assay or enzyme-linked immunosorbent assay (ELISA).
      (2) Multinucleated giant cells are characteristic for herpes infection.

2. **Wood's light examination.** A Wood's light is an ultraviolet lamp that emits radiation at a wavelength of 360 nm.
   a. In the presence of tinea capitis infection, the hair shaft will fluoresce bright green under a Wood's light.
   b. Cutaneous corynebacterial infections fluoresce coral pink under a Wood's light.

3. **Skin biopsy** can be performed with basic surgical tools (e.g., forceps, scalpel, curette, scissors, a needle holder) and is best performed by a dermatologist. A specific section of the lesion must be biopsied to obtain a satisfactory specimen for pathology. In addition, the specimen may need to be sent for immunofluorescence studies, electron microscopic examination, or culture.

II DISORDERS CHARACTERIZED BY VESICULAR LESIONS

A **Herpes simplex,** an eruption of a painful group of vesicles usually occurring on the genitals or around the mouth, is discussed in Chapter 5 V B and Chapter 6 IV F.

B **Varicella (chickenpox)**

1. **Discussion.** Chickenpox is caused by the varicella-zoster virus, a member of the herpes family. The disease is spread by air-borne droplets or contact with vesicle fluid and is highly contagious; patients are no longer contagious when all of the lesions have crusted over. The incubation period is 14–21 days.

2. **Clinical features**
   a. Papules progress to vesicles that crust over. Lesions of various stages are seen simultaneously. The rash starts on the trunk and spreads to the face and extremities, sparing the palms and soles.
   b. Adults may experience fever, chills, headache, and malaise 2–3 days before the eruption.

3. **Differential diagnoses** include herpes simplex, bullous impetigo, and disseminated herpes zoster.

4. **Evaluation.** Diagnosis in the emergency department (ED) is usually made on the basis of the patient history and physical examination findings. However, a Tzanck smear of vesicle fluid or serologic titers can confirm the diagnosis.

5. **Therapy**
   a. **Diphenhydramine** (25 mg orally four times daily for adults; 5 mg/kg every 24 hours divided in four doses for children) can be administered to relieve itching. **Menthol lotion** can also provide relief from itching.
   b. **Intravenous acyclovir** (10 mg/kg every 8 hours for 7–10 days) is indicated for immuno-suppressed patients.
   c. **Oral antibiotics** (e.g., cloxacillin) can be prescribed for patients with secondarily infected lesions.

6. **Disposition.** Hospital admission is warranted for patients with complications (e.g., pneumonia, cellulitis, encephalitis, Reye's syndrome).

C **Herpes zoster (shingles)**

1. **Discussion.** Herpes zoster is the reactivation of the varicella virus (chickenpox) along one or two contiguous dermatomes (Figure 11–1). This condition is most common in elderly patients and

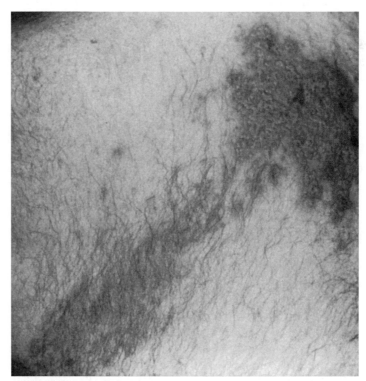

FIGURE 11–1 Herpes zoster on the back. (Reprinted with permission from Shenefelt PD, Fenske NA. The dermatologic examination. In: Schwartz GR, Cayten CG, Mangelsen MA, et al., eds. *Principles and Practice of Emergency Medicine.* 3rd Ed. Baltimore: Williams & Wilkins, 1992:2259.)

is associated with immunosuppression (which occurs with chemotherapy, leukemia, Hodgkin's lymphoma, and other malignancies).

2. Clinical features

   a. Pain, burning, and hyperesthesia precede the eruption of vesicles.

   b. Lesions occur on the face, neck, thorax, lumbosacral area, and tip of the nose. The eruption is limited to one side of the body in most cases.

   (1) Ramsay Hunt syndrome involves cranial nerve VII; vesicles are seen in the ear canal or on the pinna. This syndrome can lead to hearing loss, facial paralysis, and loss of taste in the anterior two thirds of the tongue.

   (2) Serious ocular complications can result from involvement of the trigeminal nerve; lesions are seen on the tip of the nose. Fluorescein stain with slit-lamp eye examination may reveal a dendritic pattern consistent with a serious viral infection of the cornea.

3. Differential diagnoses include herpes simplex, poison ivy, contact dermatitis, and localized bacterial infection. The prodromal pain of herpes zoster can mimic cardiac or pleural disease or an acute abdomen.

4. Evaluation

   a. For lesions involving the nose tip or periorbital area, the eye should be fluorescein-stained to evaluate for herpetic keratitis; consultation with an ophthalmologist is warranted.

   b. A positive Tzanck smear of vesicle fluid and rising viral titers are diagnostic but seldom needed.

5. Therapy

   a. Acyclovir

   (1) Oral acyclovir (800 mg five times daily for 5–10 days) is effective if therapy is initiated within 48 hours of the appearance of lesions.

   (2) Intravenous acyclovir (10 mg/kg over 1 hour every 8 hours for 7 days) is indicated for patients with severe outbreaks, patients with herpes keratitis, and immunosuppressed patients.

   (3) Topical acyclovir can be applied four times daily for 10 days.

   b. Prednisone can be administered orally to shorten the duration of symptoms and is given as a tapered dose, starting at 30 mg.

   c. Analgesics may be needed.

   (1) Acetaminophen with codeine (1 tablet orally every 4–6 hours) may be used.

   (2) Capsaicin cream can be applied topically five times daily and is useful for patients with postherpetic neuralgia.

6. Disposition. Admission is required for immunocompromised patients, patients with ophthalmologic herpes zoster, and patients with complications (e.g., meningitis, peripheral neuropathy, cutaneous dissemination).

III   DISORDERS CHARACTERIZED BY VESICULOBULLOUS LESIONS

A Erythema multiforme

1. Discussion

   a. Definitions

   (1) Erythema multiforme minor is characterized by a skin rash, which may be accompanied by involvement of one mucous membrane site.

   (2) Erythema multiforme major (Stevens-Johnson syndrome) is characterized by severe and extensive mucous membrane involvement and the involvement of multiple organ systems.

   b. Etiology. Erythema multiforme appears to be a **hypersensitivity reaction** to drugs, infectious organisms, and other unknown entities. Causes include:

   (1) Drugs (especially aspirin, penicillins, sulfonamides, phenytoin, rifampin, and phenobarbital)

      (2) Infectious diseases, most commonly herpes simplex, *Mycoplasma* infection, Coxsackie and adenovirus infections, hepatitis B, and histoplasmosis

      (3) Vaccines, including bacille Calmette-Guérin (BCG) and the poliomyelitis vaccine

      (4) Idiopathic (50% of cases)

2. **Clinical features.** The onset is sudden. Fever, malaise, and arthralgias are common. The lesions usually spare the trunk.

   a. Dermal lesions. The rash may present as erythematous macules, papules, wheals, vesicles, or bullae. It appears mostly on the palms, soles, and dorsum of the extremities. The dermal lesions ("target lesions") are papules or vesicles surrounded by a zone of normal skin and then a halo of erythema; they resemble a bull's eye target (Figure 11–2).

   b. Mucosal lesions. Hemorrhagic lesions can be found on the lips and oral mucosa.

   c. A **burning sensation** is present on the skin and mucous membranes. Pruritus is absent.

3. **Differential diagnoses**

   a. The **dermal lesions** must be differentiated from secondary syphilis, contact dermatitis, and meningococcemia.

   b. The **mucosal lesions** must be differentiated from pemphigus and herpetic stomatitis.

4. **Evaluation.** Diagnosis depends primarily on history and physical examination findings. Skin biopsy specimens show edema, extravasated erythrocytes, and necrolysis in the epidermis.

5. **Therapy**

   a. The cause should be treated (e.g., with antibiotics or termination of drug therapy) if it can be identified.

   b. The use of systemic corticosteroids is controversial and has been associated with both remission of the disease and with secondary, fatal, respiratory infections. If steroid treatment is used, prednisone (2 mg/kg/day) is given with subsequent tapering.

6. **Disposition.** Patients with mild cases are treated as outpatients; patients with more severe mucous membrane involvement require hospitalization. Recurrent attacks lasting 2–4 weeks and usually occurring in the spring or autumn have been reported.

B **Stevens-Johnson syndrome** (Figure 11–3)

1. **Discussion.** Stevens-Johnson syndrome is a severe form of erythema multiforme, associated with a mortality rate of 10%. The disease is most common in children and young adults.

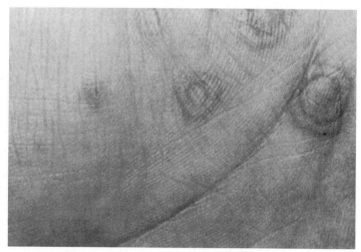

FIGURE 11–2 Target lesions of erythema multiforme on the palm. (Reprinted with permission from Shenefelt PD, Fenske NA. The dermatologic examination. In: Schwartz GR, Cayten CG, Mangelsen MA, et al., eds. *Principles and Practice of Emergency Medicine.* 3rd Ed. Baltimore: Williams & Wilkins, 1992:2258.)

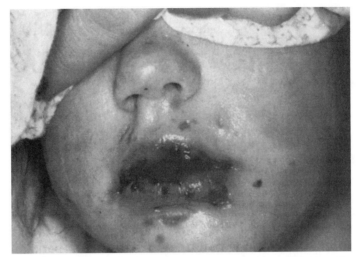

FIGURE 11–3 Sulfonamide-induced Stevens-Johnson syndrome. (Reprinted with permission from Shenefelt PD, Fenske NA. The dermatologic examination. In: Schwartz GR, Cayten CG, Mangelsen MA, et al., eds. *Principles and Practice of Emergency Medicine*. 3rd Ed. Baltimore: Williams & Wilkins, 1992:2286.)

Complications include blindness, renal failure, meningitis, necrotizing tracheobronchitis, dehydration, secondary bacterial infection, arrhythmias, and congestive heart failure (CHF).

2. **Clinical features**
   a. **Upper respiratory tract infection, headache, fever, hematuria, diarrhea,** and **arthralgias** can precede the rash.
   b. **Rash.** Skin lesions are burning but not pruritic.
      (1) **Bullae** appear in 1–14 days on the skin and the mucous membranes of the mouth, genitalia, and anus.
      (2) **Ulcers.** Corneal ulcers can lead to blindness. Ulcerative stomatitis leads to hemorrhagic crusting. Patients are unable to eat or drink, and continuously drool.
      (3) **Vesicles** rupture and leave denuded bases and necrotic epithelium.
   c. **Signs of toxic epidermal necrolysis (TEN)** may develop (see XI A). **Urinary retention** can result from urethral involvement.
3. **Differential diagnoses** include TEN and pemphigus.
4. **Evaluation.** Skin biopsy findings include necrolysis with edema and erythrocytes in the dermis.
5. **Therapy**
   a. **Definitive treatment** entails **treating the cause** if it can be identified (e.g., with antibiotics or termination of drug therapy). The use of steroids is controversial. **Prednisone** (80–120 mg/day in divided doses) can be administered orally with subsequent tapering.
   b. **Supportive treatment**
      (1) **Cool, wet compresses**
          (a) **Aluminum acetate** compresses are applied to blisters.
          (b) Compresses soaked in **potassium permanganate solution** are applied to bullous lesions.
      (2) **Anesthetic troches, 2% viscous lidocaine,** or **10% sodium bicarbonate mouthwashes** can be used to soothe mouth lesions. If the patient cannot tolerate a liquid diet, he or she will require **intravenous rehydration.**
      (3) **Antibiotic therapy** is indicated for patients with secondary bacterial infections.
      (4) **Ophthalmology consult.** An ophthalmologist should be consulted.

6. **Disposition.** Patients with severe mucous membrane involvement require admission to a burn unit for reverse isolation and treatment of fluid and electrolyte imbalances.

C Pemphigus vulgaris

1. **Discussion.** Pemphigus vulgaris is a rare disease that affects elderly patients. The mortality rate is 10%; most deaths result from steroid complications, secondary infection, dehydration, or thromboembolism. Pemphigus vulgaris is caused by the attachment of immunoglobulin G (IgG) autoantibodies to the epidermis. It has been associated with D-penicillamine and captopril administration.

2. **Clinical features**
   a. **Oral erosions** precede skin lesions by weeks or months.
   b. **Nonpruritic, painful, flaccid bullae** appear that rupture easily. Blisters can be extended or new bullae formed by applying firm tangential pressure on intact epidermis.
   c. **Weakness, weight loss,** and **dysphagia** may be presenting complaints.

3. **Differential diagnoses** include erythema multiforme, bullous impetigo, and herpes zoster.

4. **Evaluation.** Biopsy of lesions shows eosinophils, intraepidermal bullae, and acantholysis. Indirect immunofluorescent staining shows IgG antibodies. Serum titers can be followed to evaluate the effectiveness of therapy.

5. **Therapy**
   a. **Prednisone** (200–350 mg/day) for 5–10 weeks is used until cessation of new blister formation occurs. The dosage is then reduced to 40 mg on alternative days and tapered over the course of 1 year.
   b. **Azathioprine** (100 mg/day) is added to the regimen and the dosage is reduced over a 4- to 6-month period. **Methotrexate** and **cyclophosphamide** can be used instead of azathioprine.
   c. **Topical analgesics** (e.g., viscous lidocaine) can be used to alleviate the pain associated with oral lesions.

6. **Disposition.** Patients with severe cases and oral lesions may require hospital admission for intravenous hydration. Others can be treated as outpatients with close follow-up.

IV DISORDERS CHARACTERIZED BY PAPULOSQUAMOUS ERUPTIONS

A Psoriasis

1. **Discussion.** Psoriasis, a hereditary disorder, is a chronic, recurrent disease that is worse in the winter and during periods of stress. Psoriasis is also exacerbated by drugs (especially lithium, β blockers, and systemic steroids) and repeated minor trauma to the skin. Complications include hypo- and hyperpigmented areas and psoriatic arthritis. The incidence of psoriatic arthritis is 7%.

2. **Clinical features.** The clinical presentation can be diverse. Patients have recurring remissions and exacerbations.
   a. Papules and white, scaly lesions are seen most often on the knees, elbows, scalp, gluteal cleft, and nails. Psoriasis affects the extensor surfaces and usually spares the palms, soles, and face.
   b. Removal of the scale results in the appearance of blood droplets (**Auspitz sign).

3. **Differential diagnoses** include tinea corporis, eczema, pityriasis rosea, candidiasis, and seborrheic dermatitis.

4. **Therapy** may be initiated in the ED, but outpatient follow-up and treatment are necessary.
   a. **Triamcinolone acetonide 0.5%,** a corticosteroid, can be applied twice daily for 2 weeks.
      (1) To maximize effectiveness, following topical application, the area should be covered with plastic wrap if possible.
      (2) Prolonged application of corticosteroids can lead to atrophy of the skin, striae, and telangiectasia.

b. **Coal tar,** in the form of a 5% gel, can be applied twice daily to lesions. A tar shampoo can be used for scalp lesions.

c. **Anthralin 0.1%** can be used by patients with chronic plaques. The topical preparation is applied and washed off in 20 minutes.

d. **Ultraviolet light therapy**

(1) **Ultraviolet B light therapy** (twice weekly) is combined with tar therapy for patients with severe psoriasis.

(2) **Ultraviolet A light therapy** is used in combination with **psoralens,** a chemotherapeutic agent. **PUVA** (**P**soralens + **UVA**) is reserved for patients who do not respond to conventional treatments.

e. **Methotrexate** is prescribed by dermatologists in resistant cases.

5. **Disposition.** Most patients are treated as outpatients.

B **Pityriasis rosea**

1. **Discussion.** This skin eruption is seen in patients between 10 and 35 years of age.

2. **Clinical features.** A **herald patch,** a single, oval lesion on the trunk or an extremity, is followed by plaques in 1–2 weeks. Lesions appear in a "Christmas tree" pattern with drooping "branches" that follow skin lines.

3. **Differential diagnoses** include tinea corporis, psoriasis, eczema, a drug eruption resulting from captopril therapy, and secondary syphilis.

4. **Therapy.** Most cases resolve spontaneously in 4–7 weeks.

a. **Diphenhydramine** (25 mg every 6 hours for adults, 5 mg/kg/24 hours in four divided doses for children) can be used to relieve pruritus.

b. **Triamcinolone acetonide 0.1% cream** can be applied twice daily.

c. **Ultraviolet B light** treatments hasten resolution.

5. **Disposition.** Patients are treated on an outpatient basis.

V **DERMATITIS**

A **Contact dermatitis**

1. **Discussion.** Inflammation of the skin is caused by a primary irritant or allergen.

a. **Irritant dermatitis** is caused by caustic industrial solvents and detergents.

b. **Allergic contact dermatitis** involves a delayed hypersensitivity reaction mediated by lymphocytes. Clothing, jewelry, soaps, plants, medicines, and cosmetics commonly cause allergic contact dermatitis.

2. **Clinical features.** Skin lesions appear as red macules and papules. Vesicles or bullae may be present. The lesions are pruritic.

3. **Differential diagnoses** include drug reaction, scabies, syphilis, and herpes.

4. **Evaluation.** Diagnosis is largely on the basis of patient history and physical examination findings. Patch skin testing with allergens can be performed by a dermatologist.

5. **Therapy.** Mild dermatitis resolves in 7–10 days.

a. **Minimization of contact.** An effort should be made to eliminate contact with irritants or allergens.

b. **Supportive therapy** entails relief of pruritus. Measures include:

(1) **Diphenhydramine** (25 mg every 6 hours for adults, 5 mg/kg/24 hours in four divided doses for children)

(2) **Colloidal oatmeal baths**

(3) **Hydrocortisone 1% cream** (applied twice daily)

         (4) Oral prednisone (30–80 mg daily tapered over a few weeks; shorter courses result in rebound) for patients with severe cases of contact dermatitis

    6. Disposition. Patients are treated on an outpatient basis. Complications include hyperpigmentation of skin.

B **Toxicodendron (Rhus) dermatitis**

    1. Discussion

        a. Etiology. Poison ivy, poison oak, and **poison sumac** belong to the genus *Toxicodendron* (*Rhus*) and produce a sensitizing oleoresin, **urushiol.** Cross-sensitivity exists among poison ivy, poison oak, and poison sumac.

        b. Transmission. Eruptions can occur 8 hours to 1 week after exposure, but usually develop within 2 days. The rash is not spread by contact with the blister fluid; rather, scratching with antigen-contaminated fingernails disseminates the dermatitis. A soap and water bath or shower will remove these oils and decrease the contact spread.

    2. Clinical features. Vesicles and blisters can be linear if the leaf or stem was drawn across the skin. Smoke carrying particles of the plant can disseminate the disease and cause mucous membrane involvement. The rash may seem to "spread," but it is due to a variable immune reaction that resolves over several days.

    3. Differential diagnoses include drug reaction, scabies, syphilis, and herpes.

    4. Therapy. Mild cases of *Toxicodendron* dermatitis resolve in 7–10 days.

        a. Minimizing contact. Washing the skin, hands, and fingernails with soap inactivates the oleoresin and is most effective within 30 minutes of exposure.

        b. Supportive therapy is the same as for contact dermatitis (see V A 5 b).

        c. Education. Patients should be shown the appearance of poison ivy so that it can be avoided.

    5. Disposition. Most patients are treated on an outpatient basis. Complications include acute secondary cellulitis and hyperpigmentation of the skin. Several commercial over-the-counter medicines are available that may be applied to the skin prior to possible exposure. These "blocking agents" have a variable degree of protection from future rhus dermatitis.

VI   ERYTHEMA NODOSUM

A **Discussion**

    1. Definition. Erythema nodosum is an inflammatory disease of the skin and subcutaneous tissue characterized by tender red nodules.

    2. Etiology. Causes include:

        a. Bacterial infections (e.g., *Streptococcus, Salmonella, Neisseria gonorrhoeae, Mycobacterium tuberculosis,* and *Chlamydia*)

        b. Deep fungal infections (e.g., histoplasmosis, coccidioidomycosis)

        c. Viral diseases (e.g., mononucleosis)

        d. Drugs (e.g., sulfonamides, oral contraceptives)

        e. Idiopathic

B **Clinical features**

    1. Rash. The pretibial region is most often involved, but the forearms or thighs may be involved as well. Raised, warm, tender red nodules appear that have a bluish discoloration and resemble bruises later on. Healing occurs in 3–6 weeks without scarring, atrophy, or ulcers.

    2. Hilar adenopathy is occasionally noted. Fever, malaise, myalgias, and arthralgia are common.

C **Differential diagnoses** include cellulitis, lymphoma, and superficial thrombophlebitis.

D **Evaluation** An elevated erythrocyte sedimentation rate (ESR) is a common laboratory finding, but the diagnosis is made based on the typical clinical findings. Throat and stool cultures may be indicated. Skin biopsy can be performed but is seldom needed.

E **Therapy**

1. **General measures** include bed rest and elevation of the extremities. Causative drugs should be discontinued, and underlying disease treated.
2. **Pain relief** can be achieved by administering naproxen (500–1000 mg/day in two divided doses) or enteric aspirin (350 mg, 8–12 tablets per day).
3. **Potassium iodide** is administered (400–900 mg daily in three divided doses for 3–4 weeks).
4. **Corticosteroids** are used in patients with severe, refractory disease.

F **Disposition** Most patients are treated as outpatients.

VII   FUNGAL SKIN INFECTIONS

A **Candidiasis**

1. **Discussion.** *Candida albicans* is part of the normal flora but can become pathogenic in pregnant women, infants, elderly patients, diabetic patients, immunosuppressed patients (e.g., patients with AIDS, patients taking steroids), patients who are using oral contraceptives, and patients who are taking antibiotics.
2. **Clinical features**
   a. **Oral candidiasis (thrush)** appears as a white exudate or adherent plaque on the buccal mucosa, tongue, or esophagus. Dysphagia can occur.
   b. **Cutaneous candidiasis** favors warm, moist areas like skinfolds, the diaper area, the axilla, and the groin. It appears as a glistening red plaque. Satellite lesions are vesicles or pustules peripheral to the main area.
3. **Evaluation.** KOH slide preparations show hyphae or blastospores (oval yeast forms).
4. **Therapy**
   a. **Oral candidiasis.** Treatment options include:
      (1) **Nystatin oral suspension** (1 mL applied to the inside of each cheek four times daily for 10 days in children, 4–6 mL four times daily for 10 days in adults)
      (2) **Clotrimazole troches** (dissolved in the mouth five times daily for 14 days)
      (3) **Oral ketoconazole** (200 mg for 2 weeks for adults, 6.6 mg/kg/24 hours for children), used for severe cases of oral thrush
   b. **Cutaneous candidiasis** is treated with **miconazole nitrate,** applied twice daily. **Wet aluminum acetate compresses** can be used first to help dry the lesions. **Talcum powder** can be used to keep the area dry throughout treatment.
5. **Disposition.** Patients are followed as outpatients.

B **Tinea**

1. **Discussion**
   a. **Etiology.** The many types of tinea (dermatophytoses) are caused by fungi from the genera *Microsporum, Epidermophyton,* and *Trichophyton.*
   b. **Pathogenesis.** Dermatophyte infections can be acquired from another person, from fomites, from pets, and, rarely, from soil. The fungi invade the stratum corneum and liberate a toxin. They can also produce an allergic reaction.
2. **Clinical features**
   a. **Tinea pedis ("athlete's foot").** Blisters or dry scales are noted on the soles and sides of the feet and between the toes.

   b. Tinea unguium results in thick, opaque, crumbled nails that can detach laterally.

   c. Tinea cruris ("jock itch") is characterized by red scaly patches with a sharp raised border on the perineum, thighs, and buttocks. The scrotum is usually spared.

   d. Tinea corporis (ringworm) is common in children. Ringworm is characterized by round, scaly patches with a raised border and can occur anywhere on the body.

   e. Tinea capitis. Gray, scaly, round patches occur on the scalp; the hairs in the areas of the lesions are broken off, and the patches may become bald. A **kerion** is an inflammatory reaction with a boggy, indurated mass that exudes pus.

3. Differential diagnoses include eczema, psoriasis, erythema migrans, and cellulitis.

4. Evaluation

   a. Wood's lamp examination. *Microsporum* or *Trichophyton* species invade hair shafts. Infected hairs will appear bright green when illuminated with a Wood's lamp.

   b. KOH preparation. In patients with tinea corporis, a KOH slide preparation of the scaly, red border will show hyphae.

5. Therapy

   a. Tinea pedis, tinea corporis, and **tinea cruris**

     (1) Topical treatment

       (a) Miconazole cream applied twice daily for 1 month is effective.

         (i) **Wet aluminum acetate compresses** should be applied to macerated skin for 30 minutes twice daily before applying antifungal creams.

         (ii) After the inflammation has resolved, **tolnaftate powder** can be applied to keep the area dry.

         (iii) **Cotton** should be placed between the toes.

       (b) Clotrimazole–betamethasone dipropionate cream contains steroids and should only be used for short periods in the groin area, because it can cause striae.

     (2) Oral treatment may be necessary for treating resistant infections (except tinea pedis).

       (a) Griseofulvin (250 mg twice daily in adults, 10 mg/kg/day in children) for 6–8 weeks is used. Side effects include headache, urticaria, photosensitivity, and stomach upset.

       (b) Ketoconazole (200 mg twice daily for adults, 6.6 mg/kg/24 hours for children) for 4 weeks is an alternative to griseofulvin. In rare cases, hepatotoxicity occurs; therefore, patients being treated with ketoconazole should have their liver function assessed at the beginning of therapy and at frequent intervals throughout therapy.

   b. Tinea unguium

     (1) Toenails. Tinea unguium of the toenails is rarely cured. **Debridement** of the affected nails and application of **clotrimazole lotion** four times daily may help if less than half the nail is affected. **Griseofulvin** (500 mg twice daily) is administered for 6–9 months.

     (2) Fingernails. Tinea unguium of the fingernails is treated for 6–9 months with **griseofulvin. Ketoconazole** (200 mg daily) is an alternative to griseofulvin.

   c. Tinea capitis is treated with **griseofulvin microcrystalline** (10 mg/kg/day twice daily for 6–12 weeks). If no improvement is seen after 1 month, the dose can be increased to 15 mg/kg/day. **Selenium sulfide 2.5% shampoo** may also be used. Shaving or cutting the hair is not necessary.

6. Disposition. Patients are treated on an outpatient basis. Patients given griseofulvin and other similar medicines need to have routine hepatic blood tests to monitor for possible liver inflammation.

VIII   PARASITIC SKIN INFECTIONS

A   Scabies

1. Discussion. The mite *Sarcoptes scabiei* causes a hypersensitivity reaction ("scabies") as it burrows into the skin and lays eggs. Scabies is associated with poor hygiene and is transmitted by direct contact with an infested person or infested clothing or bedding. Primary infections have an incubation period of 1 month.

2. **Clinical features.** Excavations and "S"-shaped burrows (2–15 mm) occur on the waist, buttocks, back, axilla, pubic area, breasts, extremities, and finger webs (Figure 11–4). Vesicles and papules are often present. Severe itching occurs at night.

3. **Differential diagnoses** include herpes simplex, pediculosis pubis, and syphilis.

4. **Evaluation.** Mites, eggs, and feces are visible when scrapings from the lesion are mounted on a slide with mineral oil and viewed using a microscope. The mite is a third of a millimeter long, is oval, and has eight legs.

5. **Therapy**
   a. **Topical therapy.** Options include:
      (1) **Permethrin 5% cream** is applied and washed off after 14 hours. Application can be repeated in 7 days if symptoms are not improved.
      (2) **Crotamiton** can be applied once daily for 5 days and washed off 48 hours after the last application.
      (3) **Lindane lotion** can be used, but is associated with neurotoxicity.
   b. **Supportive therapy**
      (1) **Diphenhydramine** (25 mg for adults, 5 mg/kg/24 hours in four divided doses for children) can be administered every 6 hours to relieve itching, which can persist even after successful eradication of the parasite.
      (2) **All bedding, towels,** and **clothes should be washed in hot water.**
      (3) **Antibiotics** may be necessary to treat secondary infections, a common complication.

6. **Disposition.** Most patients are treated on an outpatient basis. Close contacts and sexual partners may be co-infected and should be counseled to seek medical care.

B Pediculosis

1. **Discussion.** Lice, wingless insects with six legs, are spread by close personal contact or by sharing combs, linen, or clothing with an infested person. Lice feed on human blood five times a day.

2. **Clinical features.** Lice should be suspected when a patient complains of itching in a localized area, but no rash is present. Uninfected bites present as red papules and can be seen on the axilla, groin, trunk, or scalp.

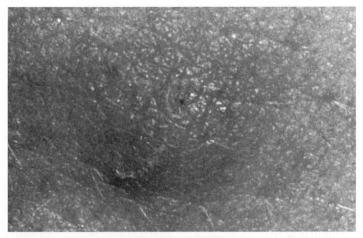

FIGURE 11–4 Scabies burrow. (Reprinted with permission from Shenefelt PD, Fenske NA. The dermatologic examination. In: Schwartz GR, Cayten CG, Mangelsen MA, et al., eds. *Principles and Practice of Emergency Medicine*. 3rd Ed. Baltimore: Williams & Wilkins, 1992:2261.)

a. **Pediculosis capitis** (infestation of the scalp and eyelashes) is common in children. Lice eggs (nits) are found on hair shafts. Scratching produces infection characterized by pustules, crusting, and cervical adenopathy.

b. **Pediculosis pubis** (infestation of the pubic area) results in pruritus and adenopathy. Nits are visible in the pubic hair. Gray-blue macules (maculae caeruleae) are seen.

c. **Pediculosis corporis** (infestation of the buttocks, shoulders, and waist) is most often seen in patients unable to change or launder clothing.

3. **Differential diagnoses** include scabies, dermatitis, eczema, tinea, impetigo, and folliculitis.

4. **Evaluation.** Lice and nits can be seen under a microscope. Live nits fluoresce when viewed under a Wood's light.

5. **Therapy**

a. **General measures.** Clothing, towels, and bedding should be laundered in hot water.

b. **Pediculosis capitis** and **pediculosis pubis**

(1) A **permethrin cream rinse** is applied, saturating the hair and scalp, and washed out after 10 minutes. **Formic acid 8%** is then applied and left in for 10 minutes before being washed out. The hair is then combed with a **metal nit removal comb.**

(2) Eyelashes can be treated with **petroleum jelly** or **baby shampoo** rubbed into the lids and brows three times daily for 5 days.

(3) Resistant head lice in adults can be treated with **co-trimoxazole** (1 tablet twice daily for 3 days).

c. **Pediculosis corporis.** Body lice are treated with pyrethrin or permethrin, which is applied to the affected areas and washed off after 10 minutes. Treatments should be repeated in 7 days.

6. **Disposition.** Patients are followed as outpatients.

IX   VIRAL EXANTHEMS

A   Measles (rubeola)

1. **Discussion.** Measles is spread by respiratory droplets. The incubation period is 10–14 days. The patient ceases to be a source of infection 5 days after the rash appears.

2. **Clinical features**

a. **Cough, coryza, conjunctivitis,** and **fever** occur 3–4 days before the rash.

b. **Koplik's spots** (blue-white papules with a red halo) appear on the buccal mucosa 2 days before the rash develops.

c. **Rash.** Elevated red maculopapules appear on the fourth or fifth day behind the ears, spreading to the face, trunk, and extremities. Discrete lesions become confluent on the upper body. The rash fades within 5–10 days.

3. **Differential diagnoses** include scarlet fever, German measles, infectious mononucleosis, roseola, and secondary syphilis.

4. **Therapy** is with supportive care only (i.e., fluids, rest, antipyretics).

5. **Disposition.** Patients with complications (e.g., pneumonia, otitis media, encephalitis) may need to be admitted to the hospital.

B   German measles (rubella)

1. **Discussion**

a. Rubella is an RNA virus that is spread by respiratory droplets. The incubation period is 14–21 days.

b. Complications include encephalitis and arthritis. In pregnant women, rubella exposure during the first trimester can result in fetal cardiac defects, cataracts, and deafness. Spontaneous abortion, premature delivery, and growth retardation are also common complications of rubella exposure during pregnancy.

2. **Clinical features**
   a. **Malaise, headache,** and a **low-grade fever** precede the rash. **Adenopathy** of the posterior auricular, suboccipital, and cervical lymph nodes is present.
   b. **Rash.** The rash consists of small, round, red macules and papules that begin on the neck and face and spread to the trunk and extremities. The rash resolves in 3 days.

3. **Differential diagnoses** include measles, scarlet fever, and drug eruption.

4. **Therapy** is supportive care only.

5. **Disposition.** Most patients are treated on an outpatient basis.

C Erythema infectiosum

1. **Discussion.** Erythema infectiosum is a parvovirus infection that affects children between the ages of 5 and 14 years. The incubation period is 13–18 days. Complications include polyarthritis.

2. **Clinical features**
   a. **Malaise, sore throat,** and a **low-grade fever** are present.
   b. **Rash.** Red papules appear on the face, sparing the nose and mouth. This **"slapped cheek" appearance** fades in 4 days.
   c. **Erythema.** A fishnet-like pattern of erythema appears on the extremities and spreads to the trunk and buttocks. The eruption fades in 6–14 days but may reappear in the next 2–3 weeks.

3. **Differential diagnoses** include measles, rubella, and scarlet fever.

4. **Therapy** is supportive care only, with fluids, rest, and antipyretics.

5. **Disposition.** Patients are treated on an outpatient basis.

D Roseola infantum

1. **Discussion.** Roseola infantum is caused by herpesvirus 6. Children between the ages of 6 months and 4 years are most often affected. The incubation period averages 12 days.

2. **Clinical features**
   a. The sudden onset of a **high fever** (103°F–106°F) occurs with few symptoms other than **vomiting;** patients usually appear well despite the high temperature. **Febrile seizures** can occur. **Occipital adenopathy** may be present.
   b. **Rash.** Pale pink, almond-shaped macules appear on the trunk and neck as the fever subsides. The rash clears in 1–2 days.

3. **Differential diagnoses** include measles, scarlet fever, and infectious mononucleosis.

4. **Therapy** is supportive. Acetaminophen (15 mg/kg every 4 hours) can be administered to reduce the fever.

5. **Disposition.** Most patients are treated on an outpatient basis.

E Hand-foot-and-mouth syndrome

1. **Discussion.** Hand-foot-and-mouth syndrome is caused by a **coxsackievirus.**

2. **Clinical features.** A **maculopapular confluent rash** is seen on the palms and soles, and **vesicles** are seen in the mouth. **Fever, vomiting, diarrhea,** and a **sore throat** may be present.

3. **Differential diagnoses** include measles, scarlet fever, infectious mononucleosis, and drug eruption.

4. **Therapy** is with supportive care only.

5. **Disposition.** Patients with complications (e.g., myocarditis, meningitis, pneumonia) need to be admitted.

X BACTERIAL SKIN INFECTIONS

A Scarlet fever

1. **Discussion.** Children are most often affected. The rash results from infection with a group A β-hemolytic streptococcus, which produces an erythrogenic toxin. The infection usually originates in the pharynx or the skin and the incubation period is 2–4 days. Complications include glomerulonephritis, rheumatic fever, pneumonia, otitis media, and peritonsillar abscess.

2. **Clinical features.** A syndrome characterized by **fever, pharyngitis, vomiting,** and **headache** is followed in 48 hours by the development of a **rash. Lymphadenopathy** and **palatal petechiae** are usually present. A white coating on the tongue sheds in 2 days to leave a red **"strawberry tongue"** with prominent papillae.
   a. The rash consists of fine, pinhead-sized macules that feel like sandpaper. It spares the palms, soles, and circumoral region. **Linear petechiae (Pastia's sign)** can be found in skinfolds in the antecubital area.
   b. **Desquamation** begins on the face and trunk and spreads to the palms and soles. The desquamation lasts as long as 8 weeks.

3. **Differential diagnoses** include measles, drug eruption, rubella, and infectious mononucleosis.

4. **Evaluation.** A throat culture should be obtained.

5. **Therapy.** Antibiotic therapy is necessary to reduce the risk of developing rheumatic fever.
   a. **Penicillin G benzathine** (1.2 million U in adults; 600,000 U in children) can be administered intramuscularly as a one-time dose.
   b. **Penicillin VK** (250 mg four times daily in adults; 50 mg/kg/day in four divided doses for children) or **erythromycin** (40 mg/kg/day) can be used for patients who are allergic to penicillin.

6. **Disposition.** Most patients are treated on an outpatient basis.

B Impetigo

1. **Discussion.** Impetigo is commonly seen in children and is caused by group A β-hemolytic streptococci or *Staphylococcus aureus* infection of the skin. Lesions are very contagious. Poor hygiene, malnutrition, and antecedent dermatoses (e.g., scabies, varicella, contact dermatitis) predispose patients to impetigo. Complications include glomerulonephritis and cellulitis.

2. **Clinical features.** Vesicles erode into honey-colored crusts. A bullous form is caused by *S. aureus.* Regional lymphadenopathy is present, and fever is rare.

3. **Differential diagnoses** include tinea, contact dermatitis, varicella, and herpes simplex.

4. **Evaluation.** Cultures of the pharynx and skin lesions can be tested for group A streptococci.

5. **Therapy**
   a. **Topical therapy.** Skin should be cleansed daily with **antibacterial soap,** and crusts removed daily. **Mupirocin** is applied three times daily to the lesions.
   b. **Oral antibiotics.** Pediatric dosages of cloxacillin (50–100 mg/kg/day) or cephalexin (25–50 mg/kg/day) for 10 days result in higher cure rates than topical therapy.

6. **Disposition.** Patients are treated on an outpatient basis.

C Cutaneous abscesses

1. **Discussion.** *S. aureus* and *Streptococcus* are the most common causes of cutaneous abscesses. Methicillin-resistant *S. aureus* (MRSA) is increasing in prevalence and should be considered as a possible etiology. Abscesses may form in association with hair follicles or sweat glands, in perineal and perirectal areas, under skin lesions, and following transcutaneous drug use.

2. **Clinical features**
   a. **Hidradenitis suppurativa** is a disorder of recurrent abscess formation of apocrine sweat glands in the axilla and groin.

    b. Folliculitis is inflammation of the hair follicle caused by infection, physical injury, or chemical irritation.

    c. Furuncle (**abscess** or **boil**). A furuncle is a walled-off collection of pus that forms a painful fluctuant mass. Furuncles are characterized by a greater degree of inflammation than folliculitis; the inflammation extends from the follicle into the surrounding dermis.

    d. Carbuncle. A carbuncle is a collection of infected hair follicles that have multiple follicular openings on the skin surface. Therefore, a carbuncle is a collection of furuncles. Malaise, chills, and fever may be present.

3. Differential diagnoses include acne, tinea, molluscum contagiosum, and warts.

4. Evaluation. Gram stain and culture of abscess aspirate may be considered.

5. Therapy

    a. Warm compresses should be applied three times daily.

    b. Incision, drainage, and **packing** of the abscess with iodoform gauze is the treatment of choice. The skin over the abscess is anesthetized with lidocaine and incised with a surgical blade. The abscess should be irrigated; it may be necessary to break up loculations.

    c. Antibiotic therapy is not indicated unless the infection is recurrent, cellulitis or septicemia is present, or the patient has diabetes or is immunocompromised. If antibiotic therapy is necessary, **dicloxacillin** (500 mg orally four times daily for 10 days) can be used. If MRSA is suspected, clindamycin or trimethoprim-sulfamethoxazole should be used.

6. Disposition

    a. Discharge. Most patients can be followed up as outpatients at 24 hours.

    b. Admission

        (1) Patients with diabetes, immunocompromised patients, or patients with abscesses on the hands and face should be admitted to the hospital for intravenous antibiotic therapy.

        (2) Intravenous drug users at risk for septicemia or endocarditis require admission.

D Erysipelas

1. Discussion. Erysipelas is an infection of the dermis and the subcutaneous tissues caused by group A β-hemolytic streptococci. Skin that is inflamed, traumatized, or ulcerated is at risk. Immunocompromised individuals and those with diabetes are also at risk. The lymphatics are dilated and infiltrated with lymphocytes.

2. Clinical features

    a. Malaise, fever, headache, vomiting, and chills appear first.

    b. A red patch appears acutely on the face or lower extremities. It is pruritic and has a sharply demarcated border. Desquamation and vesicle formation can occur.

3. Differential diagnoses include contact dermatitis, lupus, and scarlet fever.

4. Evaluation. The white blood cell (WBC) count may be elevated. An antistreptolysin O titer may be positive. It may be possible to culture streptococci from exudates or blood.

5. Therapy

    a. Antibiotics

        (1) Penicillin (500 mg every 6 hours for adults, 25–50 mg/kg/day in four divided doses for children) is administered for 10 days.

        (2) Cephalosporins or **erythromycin** can also be used.

    b. Bed rest, hydration, antipyretics, and **cold compresses** are also helpful.

6. Disposition. Most patients can be treated as outpatients. In patients with severe disease, admission for the intravenous administration of antibiotics (e.g., penicillin, 1.2 million U every 6 hours) is warranted. Complications include meningitis, bacteremia, abscess, and pneumonia.

XI   LIFE-THREATENING DERMATOSES

A   TEN

1. **Discussion**
   a. **Definition.** TEN is a severe form of erythema multiforme where complement–immunoglobulin complexes are deposited in the cutaneous microvasculature. TEN is more common in adults.
   b. **Etiology.** Common causes include **drugs** (e.g., aspirin, penicillins, sulfonamides, phenytoin, phenobarbital) and **infections** (e.g., *Mycoplasma,* herpesvirus). TEN can also develop **following vaccination** against polio, measles, diphtheria, and tetanus.
   c. **Complications** include secondary bacterial infection, dehydration, pneumonia, blindness, renal failure, and gastrointestinal hemorrhage.
   d. **Mortality.** The mortality rate associated with TEN in elderly patients approaches 25%.

2. **Clinical features**
   a. Headache, fever, and a sore throat can precede skin lesions by 1 week. Myalgias, arthralgias, vomiting, and diarrhea also occur.
   b. Diffuse, painful, warm erythema develops. The skin separates easily into sheets (**Nikolsky's sign**). Pigment is removed from the skin as it desquamates.
   c. Mucous membranes blister and form erosions. Severe conjunctivitis is present.

3. **Differential diagnoses**
   a. **Early presentations** may be confused with an early drug eruption, toxic shock syndrome (TSS), or scarlet fever.
   b. **Late presentations** resemble staphylococcal scalded skin syndrome (SSSS) or erythema multiforme.

4. **Evaluation.** Skin biopsy shows separation at the dermoepidermal junction.

5. **Therapy**
   a. **Fluids and electrolytes** should be replaced as necessary.
   b. **Debridement.** Loose or necrotic skin and blisters are surgically débrided and covered with porcine xenografts.
   c. **Applying dressings soaked in 0.5% silver nitrate** and bathing the affected skin in **potassium permanganate** are useful. Silver sulfadiazine should be avoided because it delays reepithelialization.
   d. **Antibiotic therapy** is indicated to treat the conjunctivitis. An ophthalmologist should be consulted. Erythromycin ointment is usually used.
   e. **Corticosteroids.** The role of systemic corticosteroids (e.g., prednisone, 300 mg/day) is controversial.

6. **Disposition.** Admission for intravenous fluid therapy is indicated. Isolation in a burn unit is needed for patients with greater than 10% skin loss to protect them from developing septicemia or Gram-negative pneumonia.

B   SSSS (see also Chapter 6 VI A)

1. **Discussion.** SSSS is caused by *S. aureus* phage group II exotoxin, which cleaves the epidermis in the stratum granulosum. It is common in children younger than 6 years.

2. **Clinical features.** Painful erythema and blistering of the skin are seen in association with fever. There is no mucous membrane involvement. The skin wrinkles and peels off in large sheets, leaving a moist, glistening surface. **Nikolsky's sign** is present.

3. **Differential diagnoses** include scarlet fever, TEN, and erythema multiforme. SSSS and TEN are compared in Table 11–1.

TABLE 11–1 Comparison of Staphylococcal Scalded Skin Syndrome (SSSS) and Toxic Epidermal Necrolysis (TEN)

	Population	Pathology	Cause
SSSS	Children younger than 6 years	Split in epidermis	*Staphylococcus aureus*
TEN	Adults	Split in dermis	Drug reaction (most common)

4. **Evaluation.** Biopsy of the skin shows splitting of the epidermis. Cultures from the lesions, the throat, and the blood should be taken.

5. **Therapy.** Intravenous fluids should be administered to combat dehydration from fluid loss. Nafcillin (50–100 mg/kg/day) can be administered intravenously. Unaffected skin should be moisturized with Nutraderm; bathing should be kept to a minimum. Steroids are contraindicated.

6. **Disposition.** Patients with extensive disease should be hospitalized for the admission of intravenous antibiotics.

Study Questions

Directions: *Each of the numbered items or incomplete statements in this section is followed by answers or by completions of the statement. Select the ONE lettered answer or completion that is BEST in each case.*

1. A 7-year-old boy is brought to the emergency department (ED) for evaluation. His mother reports that the rash that is now visible on his trunk and extremities started on his face. She says that the rash was preceded by a high fever; a cough; red, watery eyes; and a runny nose. Physical examination reveals that the rash is maculopapular. What is the most likely diagnosis?

- [A] Roseola
- [B] Rubella
- [C] Rubeola
- [D] Varicella
- [E] Scarlet fever

2. What is the recommended treatment for a patient with *Toxicodendron* contact dermatitis and wide-spread inflammation?

- [A] Oral diphenhydramine
- [B] Colloidal oatmeal baths
- [C] Calamine lotion
- [D] Oral prednisone
- [E] Topical corticosteroids

3. A herald patch precedes the generalized rash in which of the following disorders?

- [A] Pityriasis rosea
- [B] Psoriasis
- [C] Tinea corporis
- [D] Drug eruption
- [E] Molluscum contagiosum

4. Which one of the following drugs could cause Stevens-Johnson syndrome?

- [A] Phenytoin
- [B] Carbamazepine
- [C] Cephalexin
- [D] Ciprofloxacin
- [E] Gentamicin

5. A 4-year-old girl is brought to the emergency department (ED) because her mother is concerned about the development of golden brown, weeping lesions on her arm. The child is afebrile and otherwise appears well. There is no lymphadenopathy present. Which one of the following statements about this disorder is correct?

- [A] Acute rheumatic fever is a common complication.
- [B] Acute glomerulonephritis occurs in 20% of patients.
- [C] Antibiotic therapy should cover *Staphylococcus* and *Streptococcus*.
- [D] Penicillin is the oral antibiotic of choice.
- [E] Topical antibiotic therapy with mupirocin is the most effective therapy.

6. A 38-year-old woman with leukemia develops a painful rash involving her left eyebrow, her left eyelid, the left side of her forehead, and her nose. The patient is undergoing chemotherapy for the leukemia. What is the most appropriate treatment for this patient?

- [A] Corticosteroids
- [B] Antibiotic eyedrops
- [C] Intravenous antibiotics
- [D] Oral acyclovir
- [E] Intravenous acyclovir

7. A 50-year-old man comes to the emergency department (ED) complaining of itching and a rash. Upon physical examination, multiple healing excoriations are noted. Two red, linear lesions are present on his feet. No cellulitis is present. The patient states that he had been in the ED 5 days previously with the same complaint, and he had been prescribed lindane lotion, which he used. The patient insists the lotion is not working and wants another prescription. What would be the next appropriate step?

- [A] Another course of lindane should be prescribed.
- [B] Permethrin should be prescribed.
- [C] Erythromycin (500 mg orally every 8 hours for 10 days) should be prescribed.
- [D] Diphenhydramine (25 mg orally every 6 hours) and calamine lotion should be prescribed.
- [E] Oral prednisone should be prescribed.

8. Which one of the following statements concerning the treatment of tinea is true?

- [A] Tinea unguium of the toenails can be cured with a 6- to 9-month course of oral griseofulvin.
- [B] Tinea capitis is treated with a tar shampoo.
- [C] Ketoconazole, used as an alternative to griseofulvin in the treatment of tinea corporis, can cause hepatotoxicity.
- [D] Topical antifungals are poorly absorbed through nails and should not be used.

9. Which one of the following clinical features is associated with roseola infantum?

- [A] Febrile seizures
- [B] Age less than 6 months
- [C] Conjunctivitis
- [D] Concurrent maculopapular rash and high fever
- [E] Maculopapular rash preceded by a high fever

Answers and Explanations

1. The answer is C The child most likely has rubeola (measles). This childhood disease is characterized by a maculopapular rash that starts on the face and spreads to the extremities and trunk. There is a prodromal syndrome of cough, coryza, conjunctivitis, and fever. The rash of rubella (German measles) is also maculopapular with a similar distribution, but the fever is low-grade and lymphadenopathy is prominent. Roseola affects younger children (between the ages of 6 months and 3 years) and is characterized by a high fever followed by a macular rash that lasts only 2 days. Varicella appears as a vesicular rash that begins on the trunk, not the face. Scarlet fever begins abruptly with fever, malaise, and a sore throat; these symptoms are followed in 12–48 hours by the development of a papular rash. The papules are pinhead-sized and sandpapery. The perioral area is spared.

2. The answer is D In a patient with a severe case of *Toxicodendron* contact dermatitis and widespread inflammation, oral prednisone can be administered, tapering the dose over 2–3 weeks. Shorter courses of prednisone result in rebound. Diphenhydramine, colloidal oatmeal baths, and calamine lotion provide symptomatic relief of the pruritus that accompanies poison ivy, but are too conservative for use in a patient with a severe case. Topical corticosteroids can be used in situations where the dermatitis is mild and limited to a few anatomic areas.

3. The answer is A Pityriasis rosea begins as a single, oval lesion 2–10 mm in diameter on the trunk of a proximal extremity. This lesion is known as a herald patch and is commonly confused with the lesion of tinea corporis (ringworm). However, the scaly ring of pityriasis rosea does not reach the edge of the red border as it does in tinea corporis. In pityriasis rosea, a generalized eruption of red plaques follows the herald patch in 1–2 weeks. The generalized eruption follows the skin lines and resembles a Christmas tree with drooping branches.

4. The answer is A Stevens-Johnson syndrome, a severe form of erythema multiforme, can be caused by many drugs, including phenytoin, phenobarbital, penicillin, sulfonamides, phenothiazines, quinidine, and salicylates. As the list of commonly implicated drugs would suggest, patients treated for seizure disorders are particularly prone to the development of Stevens-Johnson syndrome. It also can be caused by infections (e.g., *Mycoplasma*, herpesvirus).

5. The answer is C Impetigo, a skin disorder often seen in children and characterized by vesicles that erode into honey-colored crusts, is caused by *Streptococcus* and *Staphylococcus aureus*. Penicillinase-resistant antibiotics (e.g., cloxacillin, cephalexin) would be effective against both *Streptococcus* and *S. aureus*. Oral antibiotics produce a higher cure rate: mupirocin is used in the treatment of impetigo, but may not be effective in all cases. Rheumatic fever is a complication of streptococcal throat infections, not skin infections. Glomerulonephritis can develop following streptococcal impetigo, but only in 1% of patients.

6. The answer is E Herpes zoster (shingles) is caused by reactivation of the varicella virus and is most common in elderly patients and immunosuppressed patients. This woman, as a result of her chemotherapy for leukemia, is immunosuppressed, and has most likely developed herpes zoster that is affecting the trigeminal nerve (as suggested by the lesions on her nose). Involvement of the trigeminal nerve is associated with serious ocular complications. Furthermore, patients who are immunosuppressed are at risk for dissemination of herpes. Therefore, the intravenous administration of acyclovir is appropriate for this patient. Consultation with an ophthalmologist is also necessary.

7. The answer is D The lesions and itching of scabies persist even after successful eradication of the parasite. Antipruritic agents (e.g., diphenhydramine) and analgesics can provide relief. Retreatment with scabicidal medication should not be considered for 1 week after initial treatment. Lindane has been associated with neurotoxicity and seizures. Antibiotics are needed only if a secondary infection is present. Corticosteroids have no role in the treatment of scabies.

8. The answer is C Ketoconazole, used as an alternative to griseofulvin in the treatment of tinea corporis, tinea cruris, and tinea unguium of the fingernails, is associated with hepatotoxicity and hepatitis; therefore, liver function should be assessed before treatment and at frequent intervals during treatment. Tinea unguium of the toenails is a highly resistant infection and is rarely cured. Tinea capitis is treated with selenium sulfide 2.5% shampoo and ultra-micronized griseofulvin. Topical antifungals are effective for onychomycosis if less than half the nail is affected.

9. The answer is A Roseola infantum is seen in children between the ages of 6 months and 4 years. Febrile seizures may occur. A high fever that persists for 3–4 days precedes the development of a maculopapular rash on the trunk, buttocks, extremities, and face. The rash begins as the fever subsides and fades in 1–2 days. Associated symptoms include cough, lymphadenopathy, coryza, and anorexia. Conjunctivitis is a clinical feature of rubeola (measles). The maculopapular rash of measles appears concurrently with the high fever and the peak intensity of the symptoms of cough, coryza, and photophobia. The rash peaks in 3 days and fades over 5–10 days.

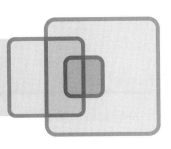

chapter 12

Eye, Ear, Nose, Throat, and Dental Emergencies

THOMAS WIDELL

I   EYE

A Examination of the eye

1. **Evaluation of visual acuity** is analogous to evaluation of a patient's vital signs during a general physical examination.
   a. **Snellen eye chart.** The patient is asked to read the chart from a distance of 20 feet.
      (1) First one eye is covered, and the patient reads the lines with the open eye. The smallest line the patient can read with only a few mistakes is recorded, and then the procedure is repeated with the other eye.
      (2) The "large E" is clear with 20/400 vision and the smallest line on the chart is clear with 20/10 vision. A normal or average eye would see the "large E" from a distance of 400 feet and the smallest line on the chart from a distance of 10 feet.
   b. **Finger test.** If a patient is unable to see the chart, the examiner should hold his or her hand 3 feet away from the patient and the patient should be asked to count the number of fingers that the examiner is holding up. If the patient accurately reports the number of fingers, "counts fingers at 3 feet" should be recorded in the patient's chart.
   c. **Motion and light perception**
      (1) **Motion.** If a patient is unable to count fingers at a distance of 3 feet, then the examiner should wave his or her hand from side to side in front of the patient, asking the patient if he can "see hand motion."
      (2) **Light.** The patient should also be asked if he or she can perceive light; the ability to do so is recorded as "light perception" in the patient's chart.
      (3) **Peripheral vision.** The patient's peripheral vision should be checked and documented.

2. **Inspection of the soft tissues**
   a. The **brows, eyelashes,** and **eyelids** are evaluated for swelling, redness, discharge, or abnormal appearance.
   b. The **conjunctivae** are inspected for redness, infection, papillae, follicles, or discharge.

3. **Inspection of the pupils**
   a. **Appearance.** The roundness and size of the pupils should be evaluated.
   b. **Reaction to light.** Both direct and consensual constriction should be evaluated.
   c. **Accommodation.** The patient is asked to watch the examiner's finger as the examiner brings his or her finger toward the patient's nose. The patient's eyes should converge and the pupils should constrict.

4. **Evaluation of extraocular motion.** The **six eye movements** are controlled by three cranial nerves and six muscles (Table 12–1).

TABLE 12–1 Eye Movements

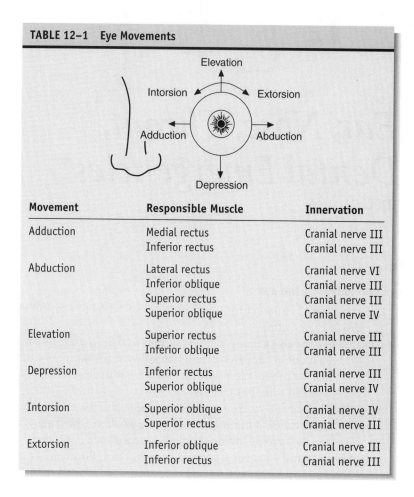

Movement	Responsible Muscle	Innervation
Adduction	Medial rectus	Cranial nerve III
	Inferior rectus	Cranial nerve III
Abduction	Lateral rectus	Cranial nerve VI
	Inferior oblique	Cranial nerve III
	Superior rectus	Cranial nerve III
	Superior oblique	Cranial nerve IV
Elevation	Superior rectus	Cranial nerve III
	Inferior oblique	Cranial nerve III
Depression	Inferior rectus	Cranial nerve III
	Superior oblique	Cranial nerve IV
Intorsion	Superior oblique	Cranial nerve IV
	Superior rectus	Cranial nerve III
Extorsion	Inferior oblique	Cranial nerve III
	Inferior rectus	Cranial nerve III

5. **Inspection of the cornea.** The cornea should be inspected for clarity and smoothness, and the depth of the anterior chamber should be noted. If injury to the cornea is suspected, fluorescein stain should be placed in the eye and then the cornea should be examined for abrasions using a slit lamp under cobalt blue light.

6. **Inspection of the iris.** The iris should be examined for any irregularity.

7. **Examination of the fundus** is performed with an ophthalmoscope and is best accomplished after instilling a mydriatic (e.g., tropicamide 0.5%) to dilate the pupil.
   a. The **optic disc** is inspected for cupping, inflammation, and edema.
   b. The **retina** is inspected for abnormalities (e.g., hemorrhages, exudates, cotton wool spots).
   c. The **arteries** and **veins** are inspected for arteriovenous nicking, copper wiring, and engorgement or paucity of blood.

8. **Evaluation of intraocular pressure.** A Schiötz tonometer, the applanation tonometer on the slit lamp, or a noncontacting tonometer can be used to record the pressures in both eyes.

B **Disorders characterized by severe ocular pain**

1. **Angle closure glaucoma**
   a. **Discussion**
      (1) **Pathogenesis.** Angle closure glaucoma occurs when the outflow of aqueous humor through the trabecular meshwork is obstructed by forward displacement of the iris.

- (a) Forward displacement of the iris narrows the angle between the iris and the cornea and usually occurs when increased intraocular pressure causes the lens to push against the pupillary opening, forcing the iris forward.
- (b) The pressure in the eye continues to increase. Unless the condition is treated, damage to the optic nerve can lead to blindness.
- (2) **Predisposing factors.** Blacks, Asians, and women are at increased risk.
- b. **Clinical features.** The presentation may be chronic, subacute, or acute.
  - (1) **Symptoms**
    - (a) **Chronic angle closure glaucoma.** Patients may be asymptomatic, or they may report a dull ache and blurred vision.
    - (b) **Subacute angle closure glaucoma.** Patients present with a dull ache in one eye and mildly blurry vision. They often report that the symptoms worsen while watching television or reading, or when they are fatigued.
    - (c) **Acute angle closure glaucoma.** Patients report severe ocular pain, blurred vision, seeing halos around lights, lacrimation, nausea, vomiting, and headache.
  - (2) **Physical examination findings** vary according to presentation.
    - (a) **Chronic angle closure glaucoma.** The patient's pupils are normal. The intraocular pressure is normal to elevated and the cup:disc ratio is increased.
    - (b) **Subacute angle closure glaucoma.** The pupils are enlarged. The intraocular pressure is usually normal and the anterior chamber is shallow.
    - (c) **Acute angle closure glaucoma** is characterized by lid edema, conjunctival hyperemia, and circumcorneal infection.
      - (i) The cornea appears cloudy as the result of microcystic edema.
      - (ii) The anterior chamber is shallow and cell, and flare (i.e., hazy fluid), secondary to an inflammatory reaction, is noted on slit-lamp examination.
      - (iii) The pupil is midsized, fixed, and often ovoid.
      - (iv) The intraocular pressure is markedly elevated.
- c. **Differential diagnoses** include anterior uveitis, miotic-induced glaucoma, neovascular glaucoma, and traumatic glaucoma.
- d. **Evaluation.** The diagnosis is usually based on the clinical scenario.
- e. **Therapy**
  - (1) **Chronic** or **subacute angle closure glaucoma** is treated with **peripheral iridectomy** or **laser iridotomy** on an outpatient basis.
  - (2) **Acute angle closure glaucoma** is an emergency. The main goal of treatment is to reduce the intraocular pressure.
    - (a) **Hyperosmotic agents** are used to draw fluid back into the blood by increasing the osmolarity of the blood. These agents must be used with caution in patients with congestive heart failure (CHF) or renal failure.
      - (i) **Oral agents** include **50% glycerin** (0.1–0.15 g/kg) or **isosorbide** (1.5–2 g/kg).
      - (ii) **Intravenous agents** include **mannitol 20%** (1–2 g/kg over 45 minutes).
    - (b) **Carbonic anhydrase inhibitors** are used to reduce the production of aqueous humor by the ciliary body. **Acetazolamide** (500 mg) is administered intravenously, followed by 500 mg orally, then 250 mg orally every 6 hours.
    - (c) **β Blockers** increase aqueous outflow. These agents must be used with caution in patients with CHF, chronic obstructive pulmonary disease (COPD), or asthma. Agents include:
      - (i) **Timolol 0.5%** (1 drop every 12 hours)
      - (ii) **Betagan 0.5%** (1 drop every 12 hours)
      - (iii) **Betaxolol 0.5%** (1 drop every 12 hours)
    - (d) **Miotics** constrict the pupil and increase the flow of aqueous humor through the trabecular meshwork. **Pilocarpine 2%–4%** solution (1 drop) is the agent of choice, except in the setting of recent eye surgery.

> (e) **Corticosteroids** are used to reduce inflammation. **Prednisolone acetate 1%** (1 drop every 4–6 hours) is the agent of choice.
>
> (f) **Antiemetics** may be needed to control nausea and vomiting.

   f. Disposition

> (1) **Chronic** and **subacute angle closure glaucoma.** Patients can be discharged with instructions to consult an ophthalmologist for treatment.
>
> (2) **Acute angle closure glaucoma.** Patients must be admitted to the hospital for treatment.

2. Anterior uveitis

   a. Discussion

> (1) **Definitions.** Anterior uveitis is inflammation of the anterior segment of the eye.
>
> > (a) **Iritis** is inflammation that involves only the iris.
> >
> > (b) **Iridocyclitis** is inflammation of both the iris and ciliary body.
>
> (2) **Etiology.** The causes of uveitis are many:
>
> > (a) **Infection** (e.g., tuberculosis, syphilis)
> >
> > (b) **Systemic disease,** including autoimmune disorders and immune complex–mediated disorders [e.g., sarcoidosis, Lyme disease, ankylosing spondylitis, Reiter's syndrome, systemic lupus erythematosus (SLE), Sjögren's syndrome, interstitial nephritis]
> >
> > (c) **Idiopathic**
> >
> > (d) **Trauma**

   b. Clinical features

> (1) **Symptoms** include the acute onset of deep eye pain and decreased visual acuity. Patients often develop photophobia.
>
> (2) **Physical examination findings**
>
> > (a) **Funduscopic examination. Ciliary flush** (i.e., circumcorneal perilimbal injection of the episcleral and scleral vessels) and **conjunctival injection** are noted. **Flare and cells** may also be present.
> >
> > (b) **Pupils.** The pupil on the affected side is small. Testing both the direct and consensual light reflex will cause the pain in the affected eye to increase.

   c. Differential diagnoses include conjunctivitis, episcleritis, scleritis, keratitis, and acute angle closure glaucoma.

   d. Evaluation. Because more than 50% of cases are the result of systemic disease, the underlying disease should be sought. A complete evaluation is best left for the primary care physician because the work-up to rule out potential causes can be extensive.

   e. Therapy

> (1) **Treatment of the underlying disease process** should be initiated by the emergency physician if the diagnosis is obvious.
>
> (2) **Symptomatic treatment**
>
> > (a) **Cycloplegics.** A cycloplegic agent should be administered to reduce pain and photophobia by dilating the pupil and relaxing the ciliary muscles. The formation of synechia (i.e., adhesions between the iris and lens) is prevented by dilatation as well. Cycloplegia can be accomplished using one of the following agents:
> >
> > > (i) **Homatropine hydrobromide 2%** (1 drop twice daily)
> > >
> > > (ii) **Scopolamine hydrobromide 0.25%** (1 drop twice daily)
> > >
> > > (iii) **Cyclopentolate hydrochloride 1%** (2 drops twice daily)
> >
> > (b) **Steroids.** The administration of steroids to reduce inflammation is best left to the ophthalmologist, because the use of steroids can exacerbate infectious causes. However, if an infectious cause has been ruled out, **prednisolone acetate 1%** (2 drops every hour, then tapered to 2 drops four times daily) can be considered.

   f. Disposition. Follow-up should be arranged with an ophthalmologist as soon as possible.

C **Disorders characterized by vision loss**

1. **Central retinal artery occlusion (CRAO)**

   a. **Discussion.** Occlusion of the central retinal artery (e.g., by a thrombus, thromboemboli, cholesterol plaque, talc, calcium, or vasospasm) interferes with the major supply of blood to the retina, causing vision loss. In 25% of individuals, the cilioretinal arteries supply the macula as well; in these people, some central vision is spared in the event of CRAO.

   b. **Clinical features**

      (1) **Symptoms.** CRAO is characterized by a **sudden, painless, monocular loss of vision.** Occasionally, it is preceded by **amaurosis fugax** (i.e., episodes of transient vision loss).

      (2) **Physical examination**

         (a) **Visual acuity.** The patient is often only able to perceive light.

         (b) **Examination of the pupils** shows a relative afferent pupillary defect (i.e., **Marcus Gunn pupil;** Figure 12–1).

         (c) **Funduscopic examination**

            (i) A **pale retina** with a **red spot** is visible on funduscopic examination. The red spot is the pigment of the choroid showing through the thin macula. In individuals with retinal blood supply from the cilioretinal vessels, some preservation of macular blood flow may also be noted.

            (ii) The appearance of **emboli** may help identify the cause of the CRAO: **yellow** = cholesterol plaque, **white** = calcium plaque or talc (the latter is most often seen in intravenous drug abusers), **fluffy** = platelet fibrin, and **red** = sickle cells, thrombus, or thromboembolism.

   c. **Differential diagnoses** include other causes of painless visual loss, including central retinal vein occlusion (CRVO), retinal detachment, retrobulbar neuritis, snowblindness, and hysteria.

   d. **Evaluation**

      (1) If thrombi are seen, the work-up should include evaluation of the carotids, heart, and especially the cardiac valves as a source of the thrombi.

      (2) In elderly patients, a sedimentation rate should be ordered. If the sedimentation rate is elevated, giant cell arteritis or temporal arteritis is the likely underlying cause.

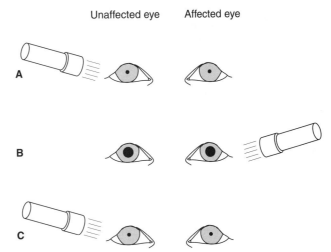

FIGURE 12–1 Relative afferent pupillary defect (Marcus Gunn pupil). **(A)** A penlight directed at the unaffected eye causes constriction of both pupils because both direct and consensual constriction occurs. **(B)** As the light is directed at the affected eye, which does not detect light, the direct and consensual responses do not occur and both eyes dilate. **(C)** When the light is swung back toward the unaffected eye, both pupils again constrict.

e. **Therapy** is usually not particularly effective but should be attempted emergently to try to save the patient's sight. An attempt must be made to **reduce the intraocular pressure,** thereby increasing the pressure gradient in the artery. Increasing the pressure gradient in the artery may force the embolus further along in the artery, leading to the restoration of some vision. Methods to decrease the intraocular pressure include the following:

   (1) **Application of digital pressure** to the cornea through the closed eyelid may help force aqueous fluid into the canals of Schlemm, reducing the intraocular pressure. Pressure should be applied for 30 seconds, then released and repeated.

   (2) **Pharmacologic intervention**

      (a) **Carbonic anhydrase inhibition** with **acetazolamide** (500 mg orally) reduces aqueous humor production.

      (b) **β Blockade** (e.g., with timolol 0.5%, 1 drop every 12 hours) increases the flow of aqueous humor out of the anterior chamber.

   (3) **Paracentesis** of the anterior chamber is performed by introducing a 25- or 27-gauge needle through the edge of the cornea and removing some of the aqueous humor from the anterior chamber. This is not a commonly performed procedure in the emergency department (ED).

f. **Disposition.** Admission to the hospital is necessary, both for treatment and for work-up of the underlying cause.

2. **Branch retinal artery occlusion (BRAO).** A painless partial loss of vision may result if an embolus lodges in a branch retinal artery (either originally, or following treatment for CRAO). The patient complains of loss of peripheral vision and, if the macula is involved, of the loss of central vision as well. Visual field confrontation reveals a visual field deficit opposite the retinal artery occlusion. Funduscopic examination reveals a pale area on the retina distal to the embolus in the branch retinal artery. Treatment is the same as for CRAO.

3. **Central retinal vein occlusion (CRVO)**

   a. **Discussion.** The major cause of CRVO is an atheromatous artery that, because of increasing size and rigidity, presses on the vein, leading to collapse of the vein wall and occlusion of the vein.

   b. **Clinical features**

      (1) **Symptoms.** The patient notes a **painless, monocular decrease in vision.** Because some vision often remains, the history helps differentiate CRVO from CRAO.

      (2) **Physical examination findings**

         (a) **Examination of the pupils.** A relative afferent pupillary defect may be noted. Many times, enough light perception remains to allow both direct and consensual light reflex.

         (b) **Funduscopic examination** can reveal anything from a few scattered flame hemorrhages and cotton wool spots to a florid, hemorrhagic blood-streaked retina with prominent dilated veins. The optic disc is often edematous.

   c. **Differential diagnoses** include CRAO, BRAO, retinal detachment, retrobulbar neuritis, and stroke.

   d. **Evaluation** is mainly by history and physical examination.

   e. **Therapy.** Little can be done to reverse the damage that has occurred. Often, there is only branch retinal vein occlusion; in this case, laser photocoagulation by an ophthalmologist can reduce the incidence of later complications (e.g., neovascular glaucoma, vitreous hemorrhage).

   f. **Disposition.** Urgent follow-up with an ophthalmologist is required.

4. **Retinal detachment**

   a. **Discussion.** A tear in the retina allows vitreous fluid to seep behind the retina, detaching it from the underlying choroid.

b. Clinical features

    (1) Symptoms

        (a) Prodromal symptoms (e.g., flashing lights in the peripheral visual field, especially at night; floating "spider webs" moving across the visual field) are often part of the patient history.

        (b) The patient may report that the **actual detachment** was like **"having a curtain drawn up or down"** the visual field.

    (2) Physical examination

        (a) Visual acuity. The blindness will be in the peripheral fields unless the macula is involved, in which case, central vision will be affected as well.

        (b) Funduscopic examination will reveal an undulating, pale, detached retina. Vitreous hemorrhages from the vessels that bridge the retina and underlying choroid may be noted.

c. Differential diagnoses include CRAO, CRVO, retrobulbar neuritis, and strokes in the visual pathway.

d. Evaluation is by physical examination. A good funduscopic examination is essential.

e. Therapy is with **photocoagulation** and is carried out by an ophthalmologist.

    (1) If the detachment is inferior, the patient should rest with his or her head elevated.

    (2) If the detachment is superior, then the patient's head should not be elevated while resting.

f. Disposition. Prompt evaluation and treatment by an ophthalmologist are essential. If the patient's central vision is intact, there is an excellent chance of preserving the vision.

5. Optic neuritis

  a. Discussion

    (1) Definitions

        (a) Papillitis is involvement of the optic nerve head.

        (b) Retrobulbar neuritis is involvement of the optic nerve.

    (2) Etiology. Optic neuritis can have multiple causes, the most common being **multiple sclerosis**. Other causes include **sarcoidosis, leukemia,** a **previous viral illness, syphilis, collagen vascular disease, tuberculosis,** and **heavy metal intoxication.**

    (3) Predisposing factors. Women are more often affected than men.

  b. Clinical features

    (1) Symptoms

        (a) The **loss of visual acuity** can occur over hours, but generally worsens over the course of 1 week. **Central scotomata** are quite common, and **color vision is more affected.**

        (b) Patients often report **pain** in the region of the globe, especially with movement.

    (2) Physical examination. There may be no findings in retrobulbar neuritis, hence the expression, "The patient sees nothing, and the doctor sees nothing." However, a relative afferent pupillary defect may be noted, and funduscopic examination may reveal optic disc swelling or papillitis.

  c. Differential diagnoses include other causes of painless loss of vision. Because the onset of visual loss is usually gradual, the differential diagnosis list also includes papilledema, ischemic optic neuropathy, orbital tumors or tumors compressing the optic nerve, and severe systemic hypertension.

  d. Evaluation is usually focused on identifying systemic underlying causes, such as multiple sclerosis, viral infections, granulomatous inflammations (e.g., syphilis, tuberculosis, sarcoidosis, *Cryptococcus* infection), and toxic causes (e.g., lead poisoning, chloramphenicol toxicity).

  e. Therapy is directed toward the underlying cause. Systemic steroids seem to work best in retrobulbar neuritis, shortening the course of recovery. The recovery period can be as short as 1 week or as long as 2–3 months, but is generally approximately 6 weeks.

  f. Disposition is according to the underlying illness.

D **Eye infections**

1. **Blepharitis**
   a. **Discussion.** Blepharitis is chronic inflammation of the lid margins.
      (1) **Infectious blepharitis** is caused by *Staphylococcus aureus* or *Staphylococcus epidermidis.*
      (2) **Seborrheic blepharitis** is associated with *Pityrosporum ovale* infection, but may occur in the absence of *P. ovale.*
   b. **Clinical features**
      (1) **Symptoms** are irritation, burning, and itching of the lid margins.
      (2) **Physical examination** reveals red-rimmed eyelids, with scale and debris clinging to the lashes.
         (a) In the **staphylococcal type,** the scales are dry, the lashes tend to fall out, and occasionally tiny ulcerations are found along the lid margin.
         (b) In the **seborrheic type,** the scales are greasy and the margins are not as inflamed.
   c. **Differential diagnoses** include conjunctivitis, hordeolum, dacryocystitis, allergic conjunctivitis, and foreign bodies.
   d. **Evaluation** is by history and careful physical examination.
   e. **Therapy**
      (1) **Cleansing.** The eyebrows and lid margins should be cleaned daily using baby shampoo and a cotton swab to remove the debris on the lid margin.
      (2) **Antibiotics.** Staphylococcal blepharitis is treated with **sulfacetamide ophthalmic drops.**
   f. **Disposition.** The patient may be sent home with instructions to follow up with a primary care physician in 1–2 weeks.

2. **Hordeola**
   a. **Discussion**
      (1) **Definition.** A hordeolum is an infection (abscess) of the glands of the eyelid.
         (a) An **internal hordeolum** is an infection of the deep **meibomian glands.**
         (b) A **superficial hordeolum (sty)** is an infection of the smaller, more external and superficial **Zeis** or **Moll's glands.**
      (2) **Etiology.** Most hordeola are caused by *S. aureus.*
   b. **Clinical features**
      (1) **Symptoms** include pain, redness, and swelling of the eyelid.
      (2) **Physical examination** reveals redness, swelling, and, often, pointing of the abscess on the lid.
         (a) **Internal hordeola** may point to the skin or conjunctival surface.
         (b) **Superficial hordeola** always point to the skin.
   c. **Differential diagnoses** include blepharitis and tumors of the eyelid.
   d. **Evaluation** is by physical examination.
   e. **Therapy**
      (1) **Conservative measures** include the application of warm compresses to increase blood supply and facilitate spontaneous drainage. In adults, application of an erythromycin-containing ophthalmic ointment every 3 hours may hasten resolution.
      (2) **Complicated cases**
         (a) If cellulitis develops, systemic antibiotics may be needed.
         (b) An abscess that does not resolve in 48 hours may need to be surgically drained.
            (i) Incisions made on the conjunctival surface must be vertical to avoid the other meibomian glands.
            (ii) Incisions made on the skin surface must be horizontal to follow the lines of the face and to reduce scarring.

      f. Disposition. The patient should be sent home with instructions to follow up in 2 days if the abscess has not spontaneously drained. If cellulitis develops, the patient should be advised to return to the ED immediately.

3. Dacryocystitis

    a. Discussion

        (1) Definition. Dacryocystitis is an infection of the lacrimal sac.

        (2) Etiology

            (a) Acute infections

                (i) *Haemophilus influenzae* is the most common cause in infants.

                (ii) Acute infections in adults most often occur in postmenopausal women and are usually caused by ***S. aureus.*** Occasionally, **β-hemolytic streptococci** are the culprits.

            (b) Chronic infections are usually the result of ***Streptococcus pneumoniae*** or ***Candida albicans.***

    b. Clinical features

        (1) Symptoms

            (a) In **acute dacryocystitis,** the patient experiences tearing and discharge as well as swelling and pain in the medial canthus.

            (b) In **chronic dacryocystitis,** tearing is the usual complaint.

        (2) Physical examination findings. The lacrimal sac is tender, and purulent material can often be expressed from the duct.

    c. Differential diagnoses include blepharitis, hordeolum, and conjunctivitis.

    d. Evaluation is by physical examination. Cultures are needed if therapy fails.

    e. Therapy

        (1) Warm compresses are used to increase blood supply.

        (2) Antibiotic therapy

            (a) Children. Oral antibiotics are used in children:

                (i) Amoxicillin–clavulanate (40 mg/kg/day, divided, three times daily)

                (ii) Second- or third-generation cephalosporin, such as **cefaclor** (20–40 mg/kg/day, divided, twice daily) or **cefixime** (8 mg/kg/day, divided, twice daily)

                (iii) Trimethoprim–sulfamethoxazole (8 mg/kg/day, divided, twice daily), for patients who are allergic to penicillin

            (b) Adults

                (i) Acute infections can be treated with oral **dicloxacillin** (250 mg orally four times daily) or **erythromycin** (250 mg orally four times daily, for patients who are allergic to penicillin).

                (ii) Chronic infections. Antibiotic eyedrops are usually necessary to prevent recurrence.

4. Cellulitis

    a. Periorbital (preseptal) cellulitis occurs anterior to the orbital septum, a broad layer of fascia that separates the orbit from the eyelids.

        (1) Clinical features

            (a) Symptoms include warmth, redness, swelling, and tenderness over one or both of the eyelids. There should never be eye pain.

            (b) Physical examination findings

                (i) Inflammation of the conjunctiva and swelling of the eyelids are noted. Chemosis is often seen.

                (ii) Fever is common, but its absence does not rule out the diagnosis.

                (iii) Extraocular motions are full and no pain is elicited on motion. On palpation of the globe, there should be no tenderness.

(2) Differential diagnoses. It is important to differentiate between preseptal cellulitis and orbital cellulitis (see I D 4 b).

(3) Evaluation

   (a) Computed tomography (CT). A CT scan should be performed to look for evidence of orbital involvement.

   (b) Blood cultures may help identify an organism but are often negative, even with orbital cellulitis.

   (c) Needle aspirations of the orbit are of **no value** and may actually spread the infection posteriorly.

(4) Therapy. It is advisable to assume that the cellulitis is orbital and treat it aggressively [see I D 4 b (5)] unless it can be proven that the cellulitis is confined to the preseptal tissues.

   (a) Oral antibiotics. If one is certain that the cellulitis is periorbital, then outpatient therapy can be initiated with one of the following agents:

   (i) A **second-** or **third-generation cephalosporin,** such as **cefaclor** (40 mg/kg/day, divided, three times daily) or **cefixime** (8 mg/kg/day, divided, twice daily)

   (ii) Amoxicillin–clavulanate (40 mg/kg/day, divided, every 6 hours)

   (iii) Trimethoprim–sulfamethoxazole (8 mg/kg/day, divided, twice daily)

   (b) Intramuscular antibiotics. Often, an intramuscular injection of a cephalosporin (e.g., ceftriaxone, 50 mg/kg) is given before discharge.

(5) Disposition. Next-day follow-up and re-examination are mandatory. The patient should be instructed to return to the ED immediately if he or she experiences pain in the eye, double vision, or other vision problems.

b. Orbital cellulitis extends deep to the fascia and into the orbit.

(1) Discussion

   (a) Etiology. *H. influenzae* is the most common organism, found in over 50% of cases. Other causative organisms include *S. aureus, S. epidermidis, S. pneumoniae* and other streptococci, *Corynebacterium diphtheriae,* and *Pseudomonas.*

   (b) Predisposing factors. Approximately 75% of patients with orbital cellulitis have recently had sinusitis, an upper respiratory tract infection, or otitis media with effusion.

(2) Clinical findings. In addition to the findings of periorbital cellulitis, **ocular pain** and **limitation of eye movement** are noted. Other physical examination findings may include:

   (a) Lid edema, erythema, and even ecchymoses

   (b) Proptosis and marked tenderness of the globe

   (c) Decreased visual acuity, possibly even to the point of blindness

   (d) Pupillary paralysis

   (e) Increased ocular pressure

   (f) Loss of sensation along the trigeminal nerve distribution (rare)

(3) Differential diagnoses include the less serious periorbital (preseptal) cellulitis and the often fatal cavernous sinus thrombosis. Dilatation of the episcleral vessels is the first sign of extension into the cavernous sinus. Late signs are pupillary fixation and venous engorgement of the fundus.

(4) Evaluation

   (a) CT. A CT scan of the orbit is important to identify orbital involvement and locate any abscesses that need to be drained.

   (b) Blood cultures are only positive approximately one third of the time, but they can help identify the organism.

   (c) Lumbar puncture is indicated if the patient has altered mentation or nuchal rigidity [which may suggest spread to the central nervous system (CNS)].

(5) Therapy. Orbital cellulitis is a true emergency and **intravenous antibiotics** should be started as soon as the diagnosis is entertained, even before CT evaluation.

- (a) **Children**
  - (i) The regimen of choice is **cefuroxime** (100 mg/kg/day, divided, every 6 hours) **plus** a **penicillinase-resistant synthetic penicillin** (e.g., nafcillin, 50 mg/kg/day, divided, every 4–6 hours).
  - (ii) Children who are allergic to penicillin can be treated with **chloramphenicol** (50–100 mg/kg/day, divided, every 6 hours) or **trimethoprim–sulfamethoxazole** (8 mg/kg/day, divided, twice daily).
- (b) **Adults.** A **first-generation cephalosporin** (e.g., cefazolin, 1 g every 6 hours) or a **penicillinase-resistant synthetic penicillin** (e.g., nafcillin, 1–2 g every 4 hours) should be administered. **Vancomycin** can be used in adults who are allergic to penicillin.

5. **Conjunctivitis**
   a. **Viral conjunctivitis** can be caused by adenoviruses, coxsackieviruses, enterovirus, and herpesviruses.
   - (1) **Clinical features**
     - (a) **Symptoms.** The most common symptoms are itching, profuse tearing, and redness of the eyes. In most patients, the infection is bilateral, but unilateral viral conjunctivitis does occur. Many patients have associated systemic symptoms of fever, neuralgia, and pharyngitis.
     - (b) **Physical examination findings**
       - (i) The conjunctiva is injected, with minimal exudate.
       - (ii) Follicles are noted on the tarsal plate. Pharyngeal follicles may be noted if pharyngitis is present.
       - (iii) Preauricular lymphadenopathy is often noted.
   - (2) **Differential diagnoses** include bacterial conjunctivitis, foreign bodies, iritis, corneal ulcer, and keratoconjunctivitis. **Fluorescein staining** should be performed to rule out keratitis of herpes infection.
   - (3) **Evaluation. Gram** or **Giemsa staining** reveals mononuclear cells (lymphocytes).
   - (4) **Therapy** mainly consists of the application of warm compresses. If the diagnosis is in doubt or one wishes to prevent secondary bacterial infection, an antibacterial agent (e.g., neomycin, polymyxin, gramicidin, gentamicin) in the form of an ointment or solution can be prescribed. Frequent hand washing is advised to prevent spread to others.

   b. **Bacterial conjunctivitis** is most commonly caused by *S. aureus, H. influenzae, S. pneumoniae,* and *Neisseria gonorrhoeae.*
   - (1) **Clinical features.** The infection is usually in one eye but may have been spread to the other eye by auto-infection.
     - (a) **Symptoms** include pruritus, the sensation of a foreign body, tearing, and photosensitivity. A mucopurulent discharge is usually present and may be profuse when *N. gonorrhoeae* is the causative organism. Matting of the lashes is usually noted.
     - (b) **Physical examination findings** include conjunctival hyperemia or chemosis and tarsal plate papillae (seen on eversion of the eyelid).
   - (2) **Differential diagnoses** include viral conjunctivitis, foreign bodies, iritis, corneal ulcer, and keratoconjunctivitis. **Fluorescein staining** should be undertaken for patients with suspected bacterial infection to look for corneal ulcers or keratitis.
   - (3) **Evaluation. Gram** and **Giemsa staining** reveal polymorphonuclear neutrophils (PMNs) and bacteria. If Gram-negative intracellular diplococci are seen, gonorrhea is the diagnosis.
   - (4) **Therapy**
     - (a) *S. aureus* is the most common cause of bacterial conjunctivitis in children; therefore, **bacitracin** or **gentamicin ointment** is indicated.
     - (b) *S. pneumoniae* is the most likely cause in adults; **bacitracin ointment** is a good choice for these patients.

(c) *N. gonorrhoeae.* **Systemic ceftriaxone** is administered. Frequent eye irrigation is indicated to remove bacteria. Inadequate treatment can lead to ulceration and penetration of the cornea, which, in turn, can lead to infection within the globe of the eye.

(5) **Disposition**

(a) **Admission.** Patients with gonorrhea conjunctivitis need to be admitted for intravenous antibiotic therapy and irrigation.

(b) **Discharge.** Patients with other types of bacterial conjunctivitis are treated on an outpatient basis with instructions to follow up in 24 hours if the infection has not improved.

6. **Corneal ulcers**

a. **Discussion**

(1) **Etiology.** Corneal ulcers occur when an infective organism invades the cornea and breaks down the protective epithelial layer. Commonly implicated organisms include:

(a) **Bacteria**

(i) Gram-positive organisms (e.g., staphylococci, streptococci, bacilli)

(ii) Gram-negative organisms [e.g., *Pseudomonas* (common among contact lens wearers), diplococci, bacilli, anaerobes]

(iii) Anaerobes (e.g., cocci, bacilli)

(b) **Viruses** (e.g., herpesvirus)

(c) **Fungi**

(2) **Predisposing factors.** Ulceration is often secondary to infection following burns, abrasions, extended-wear contact lens overuse, or inappropriate use of topical anesthetics.

b. **Clinical features**

(1) **Symptoms** include a foreign body sensation, blurred vision (especially if the ulcer is in the line of vision), light sensitivity, and mucopurulent discharge.

(2) **Physical examination findings** include conjunctival injection and irregularity of the cornea. Fluorescein staining reveals uptake of dye in the denuded area of cornea.

c. **Differential diagnoses** include corneal abrasions, foreign bodies, and conjunctivitis.

d. **Evaluation**

(1) **Staining.** Scrapings should be sent for staining to attempt to identify the organism.

(2) **Cultures** should be taken and plated to culture media directly.

e. **Therapy.** Covering the eye or administering steroids can worsen the infection.

(1) **Topical antimicrobial therapy** should be instituted immediately.

(a) **Gram-negative infections** are treated with **gentamicin 0.3%** or **tobramycin 0.3%** in an ointment or solution applied every 1–6 hours.

(b) **Gram-positive infections** are treated with a **cephalosporin** (e.g., cefazolin, 50 mg/mL every 6 hours).

(c) **Herpesvirus infections** are treated with **antiviral agents** [see I D 7 e (1) (a)] and **prophylactic topical antibiotics** to cover Gram-negative and Gram-positive organisms.

(d) **Fungal infections** are treated with **intravenous amphotericin B.**

(2) **Cycloplegia** with **homatropine 2.5%** (2 drops every 6–24 hours) reduces pain and photophobia.

f. **Disposition.** Prompt consultation with an ophthalmologist is advised.

7. **Herpes infections**

a. **Discussion.** Any of the herpesviruses can infect the eye.

(1) In neonates, **herpes simplex virus-type 2 (HSV-2)** is most common, but **herpes simplex virus-type 1 (HSV-1)** is becoming more prevalent. HSV-1 and HSV-2 infections cause **conjunctivitis** or **keratoconjunctivitis.**

(2) In adults, **varicella-zoster virus** is the most common viral cause of eye infections and should be suspected if there is a lesion at the tip of the nose (nasociliary branch of cranial

nerve V), or if the eyelid is involved. Herpes zoster infection usually occurs in older patients and may be recurrent.

    (3) Epstein-Barr virus may cause **conjunctivitis** or **keratitis in association with mononucleosis.**

    (4) Cytomegalovirus can cause a **severe retinitis** in patients with AIDS.

b. Clinical features

    (1) Symptoms include pain, foreign body sensation, photophobia, decreased visual acuity, and tearing. Constitutional symptoms, especially malaise, may also be present.

    (2) Physical examination reveals marked conjunctival injection and possibly vesicles on the inner aspect of the lid.

c. Differential diagnoses include bacterial keratoconjunctivitis, *Chlamydia* (inclusion) conjunctivitis, corneal abrasion, uveitis, and recurrent corneal erosion.

d. Evaluation

    (1) Slit-lamp examination. Fluorescein staining reveals the characteristic dendritic ulcers on the cornea in HSV-1 or -2 infection.

    (2) Scrapings

        (a) Rose bengal staining is positive in herpes zoster and HSV-1 or -2 infection.

        (b) Giemsa staining of scrapings will show multinucleated giant cells.

    (3) Cultures can help identify the virus.

e. Therapy

    (1) Antiviral agents

        (a) HSV-1 or -2 infection. Acceptable regimens include:

            (i) Vidarabine 3% (0.5 inch applied five times daily)

            (ii) Trifluridine 1% (2 drops every 2 hours while awake)

            (iii) Idoxuridine 0.5% ointment (applied every 4–6 hours)

        (b) Varicella-zoster virus infection is treated with **oral acyclovir,** 800 mg five times daily.

    (2) Cycloplegia. Cyclopentolate 1% solution applied three times daily may relieve some of the photophobia.

    (3) Debridement reduces the viral load and hastens healing in patients with HSV-1 or -2 infection. Patients should be referred to an ophthalmologist for this procedure.

    (4) Steroids have been shown to be beneficial, but prescribing them should be left to the ophthalmologist. They are particularly helpful for reducing inflammation in the anterior chamber.

f. Disposition

    (1) Discharge. The patient can usually be discharged with instructions to consult an ophthalmologist.

    (2) Admission. Patients with severe or systemic infections should be admitted, especially if the patient is immunocompromised.

E Trauma

1. Corneal abrasion

    a. Etiology. Causes include **foreign bodies** under the eyelid, **accidental self-inflicted wounds** (e.g., babies often scratch their own corneas with their fingernails), and **contact lenses,** which may leave multiple abrasions in the central cornea.

    b. Clinical features

        (1) Symptoms include a sharp, stabbing pain or a foreign body sensation aggravated by lid movement, tearing, and photophobia.

        (2) Physical examination findings

            (a) The conjunctival fornices should be inspected for a foreign body. The eyelid should also be everted to check for a foreign body.

        (b) A drop of tetracaine instilled in the eye will cause a burning sensation at first, but then the pain will be temporarily relieved. The relief of pain points to a corneal problem. In addition, the relief of pain facilitates the rest of the examination.

        (c) Instillation of fluorescein stain and examination under a cobalt blue light source will reveal the abrasion.

  c. Differential diagnoses include corneal abrasions, corneal ulcers, corneal laceration, foreign bodies, and keratoconjunctivitis.

  d. Evaluation. Physical examination findings should be adequate for diagnosis.

  e. Therapy

    (1) Foreign body removal. If a foreign body is identified, it should be removed by irrigation or by wiping the everted eyelid with a moistened cotton swab. If the foreign body is impeded in the cornea, removal with a corneal spud or a hypodermic needle (guided by the slit lamp) may be necessary.

    (2) Cycloplegia with **cyclopentolate 1%** or **homatropine 5%** (2 drops) will help relieve photophobia and pain.

    (3) Antibiotic therapy. An antibiotic ophthalmologic ointment such as **bacitracin** should be applied and the eye covered with a patch for 24 hours. The patch should be removed by an ophthalmologist the next day.

    (4) Analgesia. The patient can be advised to take an **over-the-counter pain medication** (e.g., acetaminophen, ibuprofen) to relieve pain once the anesthetic has worn off. Anesthetic drops should not be prescribed for use on an outpatient basis because repeated use can soften the cornea and lead to corneal ulcer.

  f. Disposition. The patient can be discharged with instructions to make an appointment with an ophthalmologist for an examination within 24 hours.

2. Corneal laceration

  a. Etiology. Corneal lacerations can result from impeded foreign bodies, high-energy injuries to the cornea, or intraocular foreign bodies (see I E 3).

  b. Clinical features

    (1) Symptoms are similar to those of corneal abrasion.

    (2) Physical examination findings. Care should be taken to avoid applying pressure to the cornea or the globe, because doing so will express aqueous fluid through the laceration.

        (a) The pupil may be shaped like a teardrop as a result of prolapse of the iris through the cornea. The prolapsed tissue may look like a foreign body at the edge of the cornea.

        (b) On fluorescein staining, streaming of aqueous fluid from a corneal abrasion may be noted, signifying that fluid is flowing through the laceration.

  c. Differential diagnoses include foreign bodies, intraocular foreign bodies, and corneal abrasion.

  d. Evaluation

    (1) Laboratory studies are not routinely needed, unless required for evaluation in anticipation of operative management.

    (2) Imaging studies. Orbital radiographs or CT scans may be needed to rule out an intraocular foreign body.

  e. Therapy. A rigid eye shield should be placed over the orbit to protect the eye, and the patient should be referred emergently to an ophthalmologist for surgical repair. Antibiotics should be initiated after consultation.

3. Intraocular foreign body

  a. Etiology. Penetration of the globe by a foreign body is usually associated with a history of an object propelled at high velocity (e.g., a pellet from an airgun, a projectile from hammering).

  b. Clinical features

    (1) Symptoms. The initial injury may be painful, but often there may not be much pain after the object is imbedded. A **dull, nonlocalizing ocular ache** and **decreased vision** are often the first complaints.

        (2) Physical examination findings. Care should be taken to avoid applying pressure on the globe.

            (a) Pupils. The presence of a **"teardrop pupil"** suggests laceration and protrusion of the iris near the limbus.

            (b) Sclera. Small points of hemorrhage in the sclera may represent a penetration. If bright light is directed in the pupil and a glow is seen at the site of hemorrhage, penetrating injury is likely.

            (c) Slit-lamp examination is performed to search for minute perforations.

            (d) Funduscopic examination should be performed through a dilated pupil. The retina and the area immediately in front of the retina should be examined for foreign bodies.

    c. Differential diagnoses include corneal abrasion, corneal laceration, subconjunctival hemorrhage, foreign body on the cornea or on the conjunctiva, and a nonpenetrating impeded foreign body.

    d. Evaluation. Radiographs, tomograms, or a CT scan of the orbit may be necessary to locate the foreign body. Magnetic resonance imaging (MRI) is contraindicated because if the foreign body is ferrous, attraction of the foreign body by the magnet can be disastrous.

    e. Therapy is **surgical removal** of the foreign body by an ophthalmologist.

    f. Disposition. An ophthalmologist should be consulted as soon as possible.

4. Hyphema

    a. Etiology and pathogenesis. Blunt injury to the eye (e.g., by a direct hit from a ball or a fist) can cause small tears in the vessels supplying the iris, leading to the accumulation of blood in the anterior chamber. The blood then forms a layer (i.e., a hyphema) in the lower pole of the chamber. Complications of blood in the anterior chamber are staining of the corneal epithelium with blood and blockage of the trabecular meshwork, which can lead to the development of glaucoma.

    b. Clinical features

        (1) Symptoms include blurred vision and ocular pain.

        (2) Physical examination may reveal a cloudy anterior chamber. Slit-lamp examination will reveal the layer of blood in the lower portion of the anterior chamber.

    c. Differential diagnoses include conjunctival hemorrhage, traumatic iritis, corneal abrasion, and lens dislocation.

    d. Evaluation is by the patient history and careful slit-lamp examination. Laboratory tests are not needed.

    e. Therapy

        (1) Bed rest is mandatory.

        (2) Cycloplegia is usually instituted with homatropine 5% drops.

        (3) Monitoring. The affected eye should be re-examined daily for evidence of rebleeding (which occurs in approximately 20% of patients in the first 3 days after the injury). The intraocular pressure should be measured to monitor for the development of glaucoma.

        (4) Minimization and treatment of complications

            (a) Rebleeding. Some ophthalmologists use **aminocaproic acid** (100 mg orally every 4 hours) to reduce the risk of rebleeding by stabilizing the clot.

            (b) Glaucoma should be treated with β blockers, acetazolamide, and hyperosmotic agents. If pressures remain high, the clot may need to be surgically removed.

    f. Disposition. Patients should be admitted to the hospital for treatment.

5. Orbital fractures

    a. Discussion. Blunt trauma to the globe transmits forces to the entire orbital cavity. The bones of the floor and medial wall are particularly fragile. When the floor fractures, the orbital fat and inferior rectus muscle can prolapse through the fracture and become entrapped. The infraorbital nerve also traverses the floor and may be involved in injury.

b. Clinical features

(1) **Symptoms** include orbital pain, episodes of double vision, and, possibly, tingling along the distribution of the infraorbital nerve (i.e., the cheek and along the side of the nose).

(2) **Physical examination findings** may include:

(a) Swelling and ecchymoses about the eye

(b) Enophthalmos

(c) Restricted extraocular movement, especially upward and laterally, accompanied by diplopia in these gazes

(d) Sensory deficits in the infraorbital nerve distribution

(e) Signs of hyphema

c. Differential diagnoses include globe rupture, hyphema, lens dislocation, and zygomatic arch fracture.

d. Evaluation

(1) **Orbital radiographs.** A Water's view usually demonstrates the fracture.

(2) With the cost of **CT scans** now approaching the cost of radiographs, a CT scan may be a better primary imaging study because it provides more information that is useful when planning treatment.

e. Therapy is usually conservative and most ophthalmologists wait until the swelling and edema have subsided before attempting surgical repair. If repeat examinations show no improvement, surgery is undertaken to repair the defect. It is also important to watch for delayed development of hyphema.

f. Disposition

(1) **Discharge.** If no hyphema is present, the patient can usually be discharged with instructions to follow up with an ophthalmologist. Obviously, other consequences of trauma should be addressed before the patient is discharged.

(2) **Admission.** If the patient develops hyphema, admission is usually required.

6. Chemical burns

a. Etiology and pathogenesis. Burns to the eye can occur with both acids and alkalis. The substance does not necessarily have to be a liquid; some powders and solids (e.g., lye, lime, potassium hydroxide, magnesium hydroxide) mix with water to form alkali, and the wet eye is a source of water.

(1) **Alkali burns** are generally worse than acid burns. Alkali burns cause saponification of tissues, leading to liquefaction necrosis. Therefore, these substances can penetrate deeper (i.e., they can penetrate the globe).

(2) **Acid burns** cause a protein coagulation, which often limits deeper acid penetration.

b. Clinical features

(1) **Symptoms** are ocular pain and blurred vision.

(2) **Physical examination findings.** The eye can be quickly assessed to rule out frank rupture, but immediate irrigation should be instituted. Assessment of the degree of damage should be carried out after therapy.

(a) **Minor burns** are characterized by:

(i) Erythema and edema of the eyelid

(ii) Superficial punctate keratitis of the corneal epithelium

(iii) Chemosis, hyperemia, and hemorrhages

(iv) Possibly, a mild anterior chamber reaction and hazy appearance of fluid on slit-lamp examination

(b) **Moderate to severe burns** are characterized by:

(i) Second- or third-degree burns of the eyelids

(ii) Corneal edema, opacification, and epithelial defects on fluorescein staining

(iii) Chemosis and perilimbal blanching of the conjunctiva

        (iv) A marked anterior chamber reaction and clouding of the fluid

        (v) Possibly, increased intraocular pressures

  c. Differential diagnoses include a foreign body, corneal ulcers, and chemical conjunctivitis.

  d. Evaluation is mainly by patient history. Therapy should not be delayed for a thorough physical examination if the cause of the patient's complaint is obvious.

  e. Therapy

    (1) Irrigation. It is **impossible to overirrigate.** Irrigation can be done with a Morgan lens, a cuplike device that is placed on the eye and attached to a saline intravenous bag. Alternatively, saline can be directly irrigated into the eye using intravenous tubing.

      (a) pH. During irrigation, the pH of the inferior cul-de-sac should be repeatedly checked with an indicator test strip until it registers neutral. After irrigation is completed, it should be rechecked in 5–10 minutes to ensure that the pH has remained neutral.

      (b) Visual acuity. Following irrigation, the visual acuity is checked and the eye is inspected by both direct and slit-lamp examination. Provided the pH remains stable and there is not a penetrating injury, additional therapy can be undertaken.

    (2) Supportive therapy

      (a) Cycloplegics (e.g., cyclopentolate 1%, three times daily) help reduce photophobia.

      (b) Broad-spectrum antibiotic ointment or **drops** should be prescribed prophylactically.

      (c) Tear substitutes should be prescribed as well.

      (d) Ascorbic acid (vitamin C) can be administered (500 mg orally four times daily) to facilitate tissue repair.

      (e) Steroids, both topical and systemic, are helpful, but are probably best prescribed by the ophthalmologist.

    (3) Treatment of complications. If glaucoma develops, it should be treated by the usual methods.

  f. Disposition

    (1) Discharge. Patients with mild burns can be discharged with instructions to follow up the next day with an ophthalmologist.

    (2) Admission. Patients with more severe burns may need to be admitted. If the globe has been penetrated, the ophthalmologist needs to see the patient in the ED.

II   EAR

A Infections

  1. Otitis externa

    a. Discussion

      (1) Definition

        (a) Otitis externa is inflammation of the auditory canal.

        (b) Necrotizing (malignant) otitis externa is a severe form of otitis externa that involves the surrounding tissues. It is almost always caused by *Pseudomonas* and occurs in patients with diabetes and other debilitating diseases.

      (2) Etiology. Otitis externa is usually caused by a bacterial infection (most often *Pseudomonas, Staphylococcus, Streptococcus,* or a Gram-negative rod). Other, less common causes include fungal infection (most commonly *Aspergillus*) and eczema.

      (3) Predisposing factors include trauma to the epithelium; swimming; hot, humid weather; cotton ear swabs; and the use of a hearing aid.

    b. Clinical features

      (1) Symptoms include otalgia, pruritus, plugging of the ear and decreased hearing.

      (2) Physical examination findings

        (a) The canal is erythematous, often with a purulent discharge.

(b) The preauricular lymph nodes may be swollen.
(c) When the tragus pinna is pulled to open the canal for visualization, there is often pain.

c. Differential diagnoses include eczematous otitis externa, necrotizing otitis externa, otitis media, mastoiditis, and a foreign body.

d. Evaluation. Diagnosis is usually made on the basis of the physical examination. The only time additional testing is warranted is if necrotizing otitis externa is suspected; in this situation, a CT scan to evaluate the deep tissues may be appropriate.

e. Therapy
(1) Cleansing. The canal should be cleaned of debris by gentle irrigation with tepid water or 2% acetic acid solution (vinegar).
(2) Antimicrobial therapy
(a) Uncomplicated otitis externa. A topical antibiotic with steroids (e.g., **polymyxin B otic suspension**) should be instilled in the ear (4 drops three times daily for 10 days).
(b) Necrotizing external otitis media is treated intravenously with **ciprofloxacin** (400 mg every 12 hours) or **ceftizoxime** (2 g every 8 hours).
(c) Fungal infection. Amphotericin B should be used in consultation with an infectious disease specialist.

f. Disposition. Patients with uncomplicated otitis externa can be sent home with instructions to follow up with a primary care physician in 3–5 days. Patients with necrotizing otitis externa must be admitted for intravenous antibiotic therapy. The ear should be kept clean and dry and the patient should be educated about minimizing use of cotton swabs.

2. Otitis media
a. Discussion
(1) Definition. Otitis media is a bacterial infection of the middle ear.
(2) Etiology. The organisms that usually cause otitis media are *S. pneumoniae, H. influenzae, Moraxella catarrhalis,* and group A streptococci.
(3) Predisposing factors. Otitis media is often preceded by a viral upper respiratory infection that produces eustachian tube dysfunction secondary to swelling of the mucous membranes. The middle ear then fills with fluid, which becomes infected with bacteria.

b. Clinical features
(1) Symptoms
(a) In young patients, the only symptoms may be fever and irritability. Infants may bat at or play with the affected ear.
(b) Older children and adults complain of pain and fullness in the ear and trouble hearing.
(2) Physical examination findings
(a) Fever is often present but not necessary for diagnosis.
(b) The tympanic membrane will be bulging and erythematous and is often yellow in color. A poor light reflex on the tympanic membrane is noted. If the eardrum has ruptured, pus may be noted in the canal. Pneumatic insufflation reveals an immobile tympanic membrane.

c. Differential diagnoses include otitis media, otitis externa, malignant otitis externa, and a foreign body. If there is swelling behind the ear, mastoiditis should be considered.

d. Evaluation. In general, no additional testing is needed. If a pediatric patient appears very ill or dehydrated, then additional work-up may be warranted to rule out septicemia and bacteremia.

e. Therapy
(1) Nonsteroidal anti-inflammatory drugs (NSAIDs). Acetaminophen (15 mg/kg every 4 hours in children, 1000 mg every 6 hours in adults) or **ibuprofen** (10 mg/kg every 6 hours in children, 400 mg every 6 hours in adults) is indicated to treat fever and pain.
(2) Antibiotics
(a) Children. Acceptable regimens include:

(i) **Amoxicillin** (40 mg/kg, divided, every 8 hours), the drug of choice, except in patients who are allergic to penicillin and those with recently recurrent infections

(ii) **Trimethoprim–sulfamethoxazole** (40–80 mg/kg/day, divided, every 12 hours)

(iii) **Erythromycin–sulfisoxazole** (40 mg/kg/day, divided, every 6 hours)

(iv) **Cefixime** (8 mg/kg/day, divided, every 12 hours)

(b) **Adults.** Acceptable regimens include:

(i) **Amoxicillin** (500 mg every 8 hours)

(ii) **Double-strength trimethoprim–sulfamethoxazole** (800/160 mg every 12 hours)

(iii) **Erythromycin** (250 mg every 6 hours)

f. **Disposition**

(1) **Discharge.** Most patients can be discharged with instructions to return to a primary care physician in 2 weeks for a follow-up examination. However, if the patient still has a fever or other symptoms after 3 days of therapy, a return visit to the ED or follow-up with the patient's own physician is advised.

(2) **Admission.** Very ill or dehydrated children with otitis may require admission to the hospital.

(3) **Referral.** Patients with recurrent infections may need to be referred to an otolaryngologist, who can evaluate whether tympanostomy tube placement is an appropriate option for the patient.

3. **Mastoiditis**

a. **Discussion.** Mastoiditis is an inflammatory process in the mastoid air cells.

(1) **Acute mastoiditis** is a suppurative process that is usually preceded by an acute episode of otitis media.

(2) **Chronic mastoiditis** is usually associated with a cholesteatoma or chronic ear disease.

b. **Clinical features**

(1) **Symptoms** include otalgia, fever, and pain behind the ear. Hearing may be impaired.

(2) **Physical examination findings**

(a) Fever is almost always present.

(b) The tympanic membrane is bulging and erythematous, except when perforation has occurred; with perforation, otorrhea is seen.

(c) Postauricular erythema, edema, swelling, and tenderness may be seen.

(d) The auricle may be protruded forward, causing the ear to "stick out."

(e) Altered mental status or meningeal signs may be present.

c. **Differential diagnoses** include otitis externa, malignant otitis externa, otitis media, and a foreign body.

d. **Evaluation**

(1) **Laboratory studies.** A complete blood count (CBC) shows elevation of the white blood cell (WBC) count with a left shift in the differential.

(2) **Imaging studies**

(a) A **radiograph** of the mastoid air cells may show clouding or an air–fluid level.

(b) A **CT scan** is more definitive and may reveal thickening of the mastoid air cell epithelial membrane, air–fluid levels, and a subperiosteal abscess.

(3) **Other studies.** In a patient with altered mental status or signs of meningeal irritation and no evidence of an abscess on the CT scan, a lumbar puncture should be performed to rule out meningitis, which can result from progression of the mastoiditis. Immediate antibiotic therapy directed at an abscess or meningitis (ceftriaxone or cefotaxime in children and adults and high-dose penicillin in elderly patients) should be instituted without awaiting the results of testing.

e. **Therapy**

(1) **Antibiotic therapy**

        (a) Adults. Appropriate regimens include intravenous:
          (i) Ampicillin (1–2 g every 6 hours)
          (ii) Ampicillin–sulbactam (750 mg every 8 hours)
          (iii) Cefuroxime (750 mg every 8 hours)
        (b) Children. Appropriate regimens include intravenous:
          (i) Ampicillin (200 mg/kg/day, divided, every 6 hours)
          (ii) Cefuroxime (75 mg/kg/day, divided, every 8 hours)

    (2) Myringotomy with **tube placement** is performed by an otolaryngologist.
        (a) Following the procedure, **daily cleaning** of the ear is necessary to ensure patency.
        (b) Topical antibiotics (e.g., polymyxin B otic suspension) are often instilled after cleaning.
    (3) Mastoidectomy is reserved for patients who do not respond to treatment and patients with meningeal signs.

  f. Disposition. Admission to the hospital and consultation with an otolaryngologist in the ED are indicated.

B Foreign body

1. **Discussion.** Foreign bodies in the ear are a common presenting complaint in the ED. Children and mentally handicapped patients often present with objects such as beads, erasers, and small toys lodged in the ear canal. Insects in the ear, usually cockroaches and often alive, are also seen in a number of cases.

2. **Clinical features**
   a. **Symptoms**
      (1) If the foreign body has been present for a relatively long time, the presenting complaint may be discharge from the ear. Children often deny the presence of a foreign body because they are afraid of punishment.
      (2) Live insects can cause pain and patients are often anxious to have something done immediately.
   b. **Physical examination findings**
      (1) Signs of otitis externa may be present if the foreign body has been in the ear for some time.
      (2) The object may be impacted in cerumen. A live or dead insect may be seen.

3. **Differential diagnoses** include otitis externa, malignant otitis externa, and otitis media with perforation.

4. **Evaluation** is by physical examination.

5. **Therapy**
   a. **Object removal.** Children need to be restrained or sedated to prevent struggling while attempting removal. If the foreign body is a live insect, mineral oil or lidocaine solution can be instilled in the ear to kill the insect prior to attempting removal.
      (1) **Irrigation.** Often, objects can be flushed out with warm water and an irrigating bulb or a syringe attached to an 18-gauge angiographic catheter.
      (2) **Alligator forceps** can be used to remove objects. Care should be used not to perforate the tympanic membrane. Beads often have a hole and can be rotated to allow easier grasping with the forceps.
      (3) A **whistle-tip suction catheter** can sometimes be used to remove beads or other round objects. Care should be taken to avoid indiscriminate suctioning, which can lead to perforation of the tympanic membrane.
   b. **Supportive care.** After removal, an antibiotic with steroid (e.g., polymyxin B otic suspension, 4 drops three times daily) may be used to prevent infection and reduce inflammation. Re-examination after the object is removed may reveal abrasions, otitis externa, or both, in which case proper therapy should be instituted.

6. **Disposition.** In most cases, patients can be discharged with instructions to follow up with a primary care physician in 3–5 days. If attempts in the ED to remove the object are unsuccessful, the object may need to be surgically removed, which requires admission.

C **Tympanic membrane rupture** Disarticulation of the ossicles and rupture of the round or oval windows may be seen in addition to tympanic membrane rupture.

1. **Etiology**
   a. **Increased pressure in the external ear canal,** such as can result from a slap to the ear, while scuba diving, or from an explosion, can lead to rupture of the tympanic membrane.
   b. **Penetrating injuries** can result from overambitious cleaning of the external ear canal with a cotton swab and from flying debris (e.g., explosions, welding sparks).

2. **Clinical features**
   a. **Symptoms** include otalgia, hearing loss, and bloody otorrhea.
   b. **Physical examination findings**
      (1) The perforation may range from small and linear to stellate.
      (2) Inflammation of the underlying epithelium may occur as a result of infection. Infection is more likely to occur in association with diving and welding accidents.
      (3) Rhine-Weber (tuning fork) hearing tests reveal conductive hearing loss. Bone conduction is better than air conduction.
      (4) Evidence of vertigo or spontaneous nystagmus must be sought. These findings could represent a more serious injury to the inner ear.

3. **Evaluation** is by physical examination. In patients with evidence of vertigo, severe hearing loss, or facial nerve palsy, immediate consultation with an otolaryngologist is indicated.

4. **Therapy**
   a. **Simple, noncontaminated perforations.** The patient should be advised to keep water out of the affected ear until the perforation heals spontaneously.
   b. **Simple, contaminated perforations** are treated with **polymyxin B otic suspension** (4 drops three times daily). Patients should be advised to avoid getting water in the affected ear.
   c. **Complicated perforations.** Patients with marked destruction of the tympanic membrane and debris in the middle ear should be seen by an otolaryngologist for debridement.

5. **Disposition.** Most patients can be discharged with instructions to follow up with an otolaryngologist. If marked destruction of the tympanic membrane or vertigo is present, consultation with an otolaryngologist in the ED is appropriate.

III **NOSE**

A **Sinusitis**

1. **Discussion**
   a. **Definition.** Sinusitis is an inflammation of the paranasal (ethmoid, frontal, maxillary, or sphenoid) sinuses. It is classified as acute or chronic, depending on how long the infection has been present.
   b. **Etiology and pathogenesis.** Sinusitis occurs when pus is trapped in the sinus and is unable to drain completely through the ostia into the nasal cavity.
      (1) **Bacterial causes** include *H. influenzae, S. pneumoniae,* streptococci, and *M. catarrhalis.*
      (2) **Fungal causes** are most common in patients with diabetes. Mucormycosis is particularly life-threatening.
   c. **Predisposing factors** include chronic nasal edema, nasal polyps, nasal allergies, preceding upper respiratory tract infection, and upper tooth abscess.

2. **Clinical features**
   a. **Symptoms**
      (1) **Pain.** Nasal congestion increases the **pressure** in the sinus, leading to pain that often worsens when the patient bends over. Patients may complain of a **headache. Facial pain** often corresponds to the affected sinus:
         (a) Cheeks and upper teeth—maxillary sinus
         (b) Eyebrow area—frontal sinus
         (c) Eyes or behind the eyes—ethmoid sinus
      (2) **Generalized malaise** and **periorbital edema** are common complaints.
      (3) **Nasal discharge** is often blood-tinged and purulent. A postnasal drip may cause **coughing** and a **sore throat.**
   b. **Physical examination findings**
      (1) **Fever** is often present in acute sinusitis but is rare in chronic sinusitis.
      (2) **Tenderness to percussion** may be present over the affected sinus.
      (3) **Opacity of the affected sinus** may be evident on **transillumination.** A negative transillumination does not rule out sinusitis, because the test is only positive when the sinusitis is advanced.

3. **Differential diagnoses** include viral rhinitis, allergic rhinitis, vasomotor rhinitis, tumors, foreign bodies, and Wegener's granulomatosis.

4. **Evaluation**
   a. **Laboratory studies.** In acute sinusitis, a CBC may reveal an elevated WBC count with a leftward shift of the differential.
   b. **Cultures** taken from the ostia may help identify the organism.
   c. **Imaging studies**
      (1) **Radiographs.** Plain sinus films may reveal air–fluid levels, cloudiness, or thickening of the sinus mucosa. Radiographs of the apices of the teeth are required in patients with chronic maxillary sinusitis to exclude a periapical abscess.
      (2) **CT scans** may identify an underlying predisposing anatomic condition (e.g., abnormally narrowed outlets, tumorous or cystic obstructions).
      (3) **Endoscopy** or **sinoscopy** may be appropriate.

5. **Therapy**
   a. **Supportive measures**
      (1) An effort should be made to **avoid air-borne irritants** (e.g., smoke, pollen).
      (2) Although steam inhalation and environmental humidification are useful adjuncts, **aggressive systemic rehydration** is essential to mobilize and prevent reaccumulation of the thickened secretions.
      (3) **Analgesics, decongestants, antihistamines,** and **steroids** may also be helpful.
         (a) **Analgesics. Acetaminophen** (1000 mg orally every 6 hours) or **ibuprofen** (400 mg orally every 6 hours) helps relieve pain and fever.
         (b) **Decongestants** reduce inflammation and edema of the tissues, allowing better drainage of the sinuses. Agents include **oxymetazoline** (2 sprays in both nares twice daily for 3 days), **phenylephrine** (2 sprays in both nares every 4 hours for 3 days), and **pseudoephedrine** (60 mg orally every 6 hours for 3 days).
         (c) **Antihistamines** reduce the inflammation and swelling that lead to obstruction of the ostia. Agents include **diphenhydramine** (25–50 mg orally four times daily for 3 days), **terfenadine** (60 mg orally twice daily for 3 days), and **astemizole** (30 mg orally on the first day, 20 mg on the second day, and 10 mg every day after for 3 days).
         (d) **Steroids.** If there is a history of allergic rhinitis, topical nasal steroids may help.
   b. **Antibiotic therapy.** Acceptable regimens include:
      (1) **Amoxicillin** (250–500 mg three times daily for 14 days)

(2) Amoxicillin clavulanate (500 mg three times daily for 2–3 weeks)

(3) Trimethoprim–sulfamethoxazole (double strength, twice daily for 14 days)

c. **Surgery.** Surgical drainage of the sinus may be indicated if medical treatment fails. Surgery may also be indicated to correct underlying anatomic defects.

6. **Disposition.** All patients diagnosed with sinusitis should be followed up until clinically cured.

a. **Discharge.** In the absence of complications (e.g., orbital cellulitis, osteomyelitis, septic cavernous thrombosis, contiguous spread to involve the nervous system), acute sinusitis is associated with favorable outcomes if treated aggressively and in a timely fashion. Patients can be sent home with instructions to follow up in 1–2 days.

b. **Admission** is indicated for extremely ill patients, patients with orbital edema, and patients with nuchal rigidity or altered mental status.

B Foreign body

1. **Discussion.** Nasal foreign bodies are seen most often in children.

2. **Clinical features**

a. **Patient history.** Sometimes, a parent brings the child to the ED after witnessing the child or the child's sibling place an object (e.g., a bead, bean, sponge, toy) in the child's nose. However, more often the parent brings the child to the ED after noticing a foul-smelling, purulent discharge from the child's nose. ·

b. **Symptoms.** The patient may be asymptomatic, or foul, purulent rhinorrhea or epistaxis may be present.

c. **Physical examination findings.** Often, the foreign body can be identified using a nasal speculum and a headlamp. It may be necessary to suction the nares to clean away purulent secretions in order to visualize the foreign body.

3. **Differential diagnoses** include sinusitis and rhinitis.

4. **Evaluation.** Physical examination is usually adequate for diagnosis. Fiberoptic evaluation may be necessary if the object is in the posterior or turbinate areas.

5. **Therapy**

a. **Object removal.** Pediatric patients need to be restrained in a papoose or rolled in a sheet to minimize movement during examination and removal. Some children may require sedation.

(1) **Forceful expulsion.** One method that often works is to have the parent seal off the opposite naris and blow into the child's mouth in a manner similar to that used during mouth-to-mouth resuscitation. The result is the expulsion of the object and a fair amount of mucus through the other naris (it is helpful to cover the face with a towel).

(2) A **suction catheter** with the tip cut off flat can be introduced into the nasal passage until the tip contacts the object, at which point suction is applied. This method works best with smooth objects that can form a seal with the catheter tip.

(3) **Alligator forceps** can be used to grab the object. With beads, it is best to rotate the bead so that the hole can be grasped with the forceps.

b. **Supportive care.** After removal of the object, saline drops can be instilled to moisten the nasal passage. If pus is present, a course of amoxicillin or erythromycin should be prescribed to treat possible purulent rhinitis or sinusitis.

6. **Disposition.** If attempts at removing the object in the ED are successful, the patient can be sent home. If the object cannot be removed in the ED, an otolaryngologist should be consulted because the patient may need admission to the hospital for surgical removal of the object.

C Epistaxis

1. **Discussion**

a. **Etiology.** There are many causes of nosebleeds; most can be classified as belonging to one of the following three groups.

(1) **Local causes** include trauma (e.g., nose picking, foreign bodies, nasal fractures), inflammation, upper respiratory tract infection, and environmental irritants.

(2) **Regional causes** include vascular abnormalities, neoplasms, and ectopic endometriosis.

(3) **Systemic causes** include intrinsic and drug-induced coagulopathies, thrombocytopenia, leukemia, hepatic disease, and infections. Hypertension is not in itself a cause of epistaxis, because the relative frequency in patients with hypertension is the same as in the general population. However, the elevated blood pressure may make it more difficult to stop a nosebleed once one has started.

b. **Location.** It is important to differentiate anterior bleeds from posterior bleeds, because anterior bleeds are generally easy to treat, whereas posterior bleeds are more difficult.

(1) **Anterior bleeds** usually occur in Kiesselbach's plexus on the anterior nasal septum and account for 90% of all nose bleeds. They may also occur on the anterior inferior turbinate.

(2) **Posterior bleeds** occur from the sphenopalatine artery or in the nasopharynx, often from branches of the carotid arteries.

2. **Clinical findings**

a. **Anterior bleeds** are almost always unilateral, unless the nasal septum is perforated. Asking the patient to pinch his nose (thereby applying pressure to Kiesselbach's plexus) will tamponade most anterior bleeds, whereas posterior bleeds will continue to bleed unabated.

b. **Posterior bleeds.** Because posterior bleeds occur behind the septum, the blood will often exit both nares and large clots can accumulate in the nasopharynx.

3. **Evaluation.** Most patients with nasal bleeds do not require any laboratory testing. However, additional studies may be indicated in patients with a history of bleeding problems, oral anticoagulant use, possible hepatic disease, or bleeding that is difficult to control. In these patients, useful tests would include:

a. A **CBC** to check hemoglobin and look for thrombocytopenia or leukemia

b. A **prothrombin time (PT)** and **partial thromboplastin time (PTT)** to look for overanticoagulation or hepatic dysfunction

c. A **blood type and crossmatch** in case transfusion is necessary to compensate for ongoing blood loss

d. An **angiogram** to identify the source of bleeding and to perform embolization if all attempts to stop the bleeding fail

4. **Therapy**

a. **Initial stabilization.** In a patient who presents with hypotension and tachycardia, an intravenous line should be started, blood samples should be drawn, and fluid resuscitation should be initiated immediately. An adequate airway should be ensured in all patients. Pulse oximetry and a cardiac monitor should be used in elderly and complicated patients.

b. **Terminating bleeding**

(1) **Preliminary preparations.** Hospital staff should be gloved, gowned, and wearing protective eyewear. The following equipment should be readied:

(a) A bright light source

(b) Suction (turned on and connected)

(c) A nasal speculum, Bayonet forceps, $4'' \times 4''$ gauze pads, cotton swabs, cotton balls, a medication cup, silver nitrate sticks, Surgicel or a nasal tampon, petroleum jelly gauze strips, and two #10 Foley catheters

(d) Cocaine 4% solution or viscous solution, lidocaine 1% solution, and phenylephrine 1% solution

(2) **Clearing the nasal passages.** The patient should be seated in a protective gown with a basin to collect blood. While waiting for treatment, the patient should pinch his or her nose to attempt to slow the bleeding. Once the necessary equipment is assembled, the patient should be asked to gently blow his or her nose and clear his or her throat to get as much blood and clot out of the nasal cavity as possible.

(3) Anesthesia. Cocaine-soaked pledgets or cotton swabs are placed in the nares to anesthetize the mucous membranes and cause vasoconstriction. (These effects usually occur after 5–10 minutes.) Alternatively, a mixture of lidocaine and phenylephrine can be used.

(4) Inspection. When adequate anesthesia has been obtained, a headlamp with a bright light source is used to insert the nasal speculum in the nares. The anterior septum should be inspected for the source of the bleeding (a clot may be seen if the bleeding has stopped). Suctioning may be necessary to visualize the source. The absence of an anterior bleed and continued epistaxis point to a more serious posterior bleed.

    (a) If the bleeding has stopped, the patient should be observed for 15–30 minutes. No additional treatment is necessary.

    (b) If the bleeding has not stopped, the evaluation must continue.

(5) Tamponade and cautery. When the source of the bleeding is found, an attempt to tamponade the bleeding with an applicator or phenylephrine should be made. If an anterior bleed cannot be stopped by applying pressure, cautery can be attempted with the silver nitrate stick.

(6) Anterior packing. If both tamponade and cautery fail, it will probably be necessary to pack the anterior nose. Often both nares need to be packed to get adequate tamponade with any of the following three common methods:

    (a) Commercially available nasal tampons saturated with a clotting agent can be placed in the nares. As blood fills the sponge, it expands, stopping the bleeding (a small amount of saline can be added to the sponge to hasten the expansion).

    (b) A commercially available balloon pack can be used. The pack is placed in the nares and the balloon is inflated as instructed in the insert.

    (c) A $0.5'' \times 72''$ strip of petroleum jelly–impregnated gauze can be placed in the nares using a bayonet forceps. After placing the end in the nares, the next length is inserted, repeating the process until the nares are packed. The average patient will require the entire $72''$ strip.

(7) Posterior packing is necessary for posterior bleeds.

    (a) There are two common methods:

        (i) Commercially available posterior packing balloons can be inserted in both nares and inflated as per the insert instructions.

        (ii) The alternative is posterior gauze packing (Figure 12–2).

    (b) Failure to control the posterior bleeding may require operative management or angiography and embolization.

5. Disposition

a. Discharge

(1) Bleeds controlled by pressure tamponade. Patients should be observed for 15–30 minutes to ensure that rebleeding does not occur. The patient can be discharged with "nosebleed instructions" (i.e., no picking or blowing the nose, no sneezing through the nose, no bending forward or lifting). Patients should be advised to use a humidifier and to coat the nares with petroleum jelly the next day.

(2) Bleeds controlled by anterior packs. Patients should be observed for 15–30 minutes to ensure tamponade. An antibiotic (e.g., amoxicillin) should be prescribed to prevent sinusitis and the patient should have an appointment with an otolaryngologist 2–3 days later to have the packing removed.

b. Admission

(1) Patients with **multiple recent bleeds, severe anemia, debilitating illnesses, or hepatic dysfunction,** or those who are taking **anticoagulants** probably need to be admitted for observation.

(2) Patients with **posterior bleeds** require hospital admission, usually in a monitored setting [i.e., the intensive care unit (ICU) or a step-down unit]. These patients are at risk of

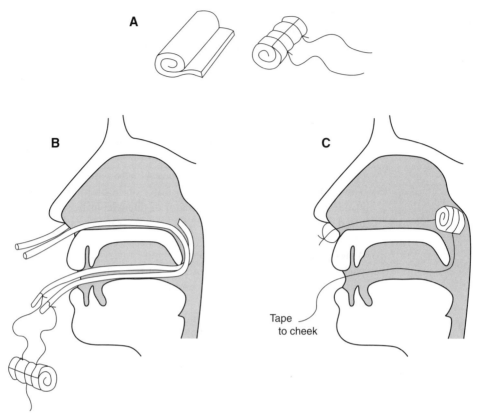

FIGURE 12–2 Placement of posterior gauze packing. **(A)** A 1-0 silk suture is tied around each end of a 4″ × 4″ gauze pad that has been rolled up. A third suture is tied around the middle of the gauze pack. **(B)** Two #10 Foley catheters are placed in each nares, advanced to the oral pharynx, grasped with a forceps, and brought out of the mouth. The ends of the sutures on the ends of the gauze roll are tied to the tips of the Foley catheters; the end of the third suture around the middle of the roll is left hanging. **(C)** Both Foley catheters are pulled back out of the nares. The sutures are then pulled until the pack ascends the nasopharynx to tamponade the posterior nares. The sutures exiting both nares are tied to each other over a piece of gauze around the columna of the nares to hold the posterior pack in place. The third suture should be hanging out of the patient's mouth and can be taped to the face for later removal of the pack. To complete the process, both nares require anterior nasal packing with 0.5″ strips of petroleum jelly–impregnated gauze (not shown). (Redrawn with permission from Rosen P. *Emergency Medicine: Concepts and Clinical Practice.* 3rd Ed. St. Louis: Mosby-Year Book, 1992:2467.)

rebleeding, airway obstruction, and, for a not clearly understood reason, profound hypoxemia. Prophylactic antibiotics should be administered to prevent sinusitis and toxic shock syndrome (TSS).

D Nasal fractures

1. **Discussion.** Nasal fractures are the most common fractures of the face and are often misdiagnosed. Nasal fractures are often associated with epistaxis and septal hematomas.

2. **Clinical features** include pain in the nasal bridge with swelling, ecchymosis, and deformity. A septal hematoma should be ruled out by directly visualizing the septum.

3. **Differential diagnoses** include more severe fractures involving the cribriform plate, ethmoidal bones, or lacrimal bones. More severe fractures may be associated with the leakage of cerebrospinal fluid (CSF) into the nasal cavity.

4. **Evaluation.** Usually, the clinical findings of pain, crepitance, and deformity are adequate for diagnosis. Radiographs can be used if uncertainty regarding the diagnosis remains. A Waters' view is useful for diagnosing septal deviation, and lateral views will show displacement of nasal bone.

5. **Therapy**
  a. **Repair**
    (1) **Minimally displaced fractures** are usually treated with an external splint.
    (2) **More severely displaced fractures** are treated with immediate or delayed reduction.
      (a) **Immediate reduction** is recommended if the patient is hemorrhaging or if there is marked deformity. If waiting to reduce the fracture is unacceptable, the nose can be repositioned early and rebroken later and formed (using an old photograph as a basis for comparison) to achieve a better end result.
      (b) **Delayed reduction.** Often, delayed reduction is preferable because it is performed after the swelling has subsided, facilitating evaluation of outcome.
  b. **Supportive care.** Epistaxis must be controlled, and septal hematomas require evacuation. A patient requiring packing should be given prophylactic antibodies to prevent sinusitis.

6. **Disposition**
  a. **Discharge.** Most patients with nasal fractures can be discharged with instructions to follow up with an otolaryngologist.
  b. **Admission.** Indications for admission include:
    (1) Failure to control hemorrhage
    (2) The presence of other injuries requiring hospitalization
    (3) The presence of a CSF leak associated with deeper fractures in the nasal cavity, the cribriform plate, or the ethmoidal bones

IV THROAT

A **Pharyngitis** and **tonsillitis** are discussed in Chapter 6 V A.

B **Peritonsillar cellulitis** and **peritonsillar abscess**

1. **Discussion**
  a. **Definitions.** When an acute bacterial tonsillitis is present, there is always the possibility of spread to surrounding tissue in the pharynx.
    (1) **Peritonsillar cellulitis** is an infection that has spread to the surrounding area, causing inflammation and edema in the peritonsillar area.
    (2) **Peritonsillar abscess** is present when the infection progresses to form an abscess or collection of pus in the pharyngeal pillar.
  b. **Etiology.** The most common cause is β-hemolytic *Streptococcus,* but often the infection is polymicrobic, involving *S. pneumoniae, H. influenzae,* and *Staphylococcus,* as well as anaerobes such as *Bacteroides fragilis.*
  c. **Complications.** Local extension of the cellulitis or abscess can lead to more serious conditions:
    (1) Extension of the abscess into contiguous neck spaces, including the retropharynx, subglossal spaces, and mediastinum
    (2) Erosion into the carotid artery, leading to life-threatening hemorrhage, or into the internal jugular vein, leading to septic thrombosis

2. **Clinical features**
  a. **Symptoms**
    (1) The **classic features of tonsillitis—fever, sore throat, and odynophagia**—are present for 2–3 days. The throat pain localizes to one side. The patient may drool because of an inability to swallow.
    (2) The patient may also complain of **dysphagia, dysphonia,** and **referred pain to the ear.**
  b. **Physical examination findings**
    (1) **Trismus** (spasm of the muscles of mastication) may be present and the patient may have difficulty opening the mouth.

       (2) Marked swelling of the pharyngeal pillar displaces it downward. The uvula is pushed to the opposite side.

         (a) In **peritonsillar cellulitis,** the pillar will be soft and not as enlarged as it is in patients with a peritonsillar abscess.

         (b) In **peritonsillar abscess,** the pillar is larger and firm or fluctuant.

  3. Differential diagnoses

    a. Epiglottitis does occur in adults, and an absence of pharyngeal findings or the presence of stridor should warrant consideration of this diagnosis.

    b. If a noninfectious asymmetrical swelling is present, squamous cell carcinoma, lymphoma, a vascular lesion, or other neoplasms should be considered.

    c. Mononucleosis and other viral infections, as well as diphtheria, must be ruled out.

  4. Evaluation

    a. Needle aspiration of the tonsillar pillar allows differentiation between cellulitis and an abscess. Failure to aspirate pus in a soft pillar will indicate cellulitis, whereas the diagnosis is peritonsillar abscess if pus can be aspirated.

    b. Laboratory studies are of little value in the diagnosis. However:

      (1) In a septic, dehydrated, or diabetic patient, additional work-up, including a CBC, serum electrolyte panel, and a glucose level, may be appropriate.

      (2) If mononucleosis is suspected, a mono spot test may be of value.

    c. Imaging studies. If there is any suggestion of airway compromise, a lateral soft tissue film of the neck can rule out epiglottis or retropharyngeal abscess.

  5. Therapy

    a. Abscess drainage. If an abscess is present, it needs to be drained. There is some debate as to how this is best accomplished.

      (1) Needle aspiration without opening the abscess is advocated by some.

      (2) Incision and **drainage** by opening the abscess with a scalpel and gently opening the space with a forceps is the second option.

      (3) Acute tonsillectomy to remove the tonsil and open the abscess has its proponents. Supporters of this approach believe that it treats the abscess and also removes the possibility of recurrence should subsequent infection occur.

    b. Antibiotic therapy

      (1) Patients who are able to swallow and are not dehydrated or toxic can be administered **intramuscular** or **oral antibiotics.** Acceptable regimens include:

         (a) Benzathine penicillin G (1.2 million U intramuscularly)

         (b) Benzathine penicillin G plus penicillin G procaine (1.2 million U intramuscularly)

         (c) Clindamycin (600 mg orally every 6 hours for 10 days), which is better for coverage against anaerobes

      (2) Dehydrated patients who are unable to swallow should receive **intravenous fluids** and **antibiotics.**

         (a) Penicillin (1–2 million U every 4 hours)

         (b) Clindamycin (600 mg every 6 hours)

    c. Supportive therapy

      (1) Salt-water gargles often help soothe the throat and rinse the incised pillar. Mouthwashes should be avoided because they are irritating.

      (2) An **analgesic/antipyretic agent** should be prescribed.

         (a) Acetaminophen (1000 mg every 6 hours)

         (b) Acetaminophen plus codeine (2 tablets every 6 hours)

         (c) Ibuprofen (400 mg every 6 hours)

  6. Disposition

   a. Discharge. Patients who are discharged after initiating intramuscular or oral antibiotic therapy should be seen in 24 hours for re-evaluation. These patients should be instructed to return to the ED if they experience trouble swallowing or breathing.

   b. Admission is required for any patient who is unable to swallow, dehydrated, toxic, or immunocompromised.

   c. Referral. Consultation with an ear, nose, and throat specialist should be arranged if the patient was not seen by a specialist in the ED.

C Ludwig's angina

1. **Discussion**

   a. Definition. The fascial planes within the head and neck are potential spaces for abscess formation. Ludwig's angina is abscessation of the submaxillary, sublingual, and submental spaces accompanied by elevation of the tongue.

   b. Etiology. The lower second and third molars are the usual source of infection. The usual causes are β-hemolytic streptococci, staphylococci, and mixed anaerobic and aerobic infection.

   c. Pathogenesis. Ludwig's angina is a serious infection that can lead to airway compromise. There is also the potential for the infection to spread inferiorly and invade the mediastinum.

2. **Clinical features**

   a. Symptoms. The patient presents with swelling in the jaw, stiffness of tongue movements, and trismus, accompanied by fever, chills, and difficulty swallowing.

   b. Physical examination findings

   (1) There is swelling beneath the chin, which is often tense and brawny without fluctuance.

   (2) The tongue is displaced up and posteriorly. Often, trismus makes opening the mouth for examination difficult.

   (3) The second and third lower molars are often carious.

   (4) If the presentation is late, airway obstruction and edema of the larynx may be present.

3. **Differential diagnoses**

   a. Other causes of swelling in the area of the tongue include tumors of the tongue and salivary glands, and salivary duct obstructions.

   b. Other causes of neck swelling include mumps, salivary duct obstructions, tuberculous cervical lymphadenitis (scrofula), and Sjögren's syndrome of the salivary glands.

4. **Evaluation** should be carried out after airway patency is ensured.

   a. Radiographs. The extent of swelling and airway compromise can be assessed with a lateral soft tissue radiograph of the neck.

   b. CT scans of the neck and chest may be necessary to determine the extent of abscess formation and extension into the neck and mediastinum.

5. **Therapy**

   a. Initial stabilization. Ensuring airway competence should be the first concern. Often oral intubation is not possible; therefore, cricothyrotomy may be required.

   b. Abscess drainage is by incision and drainage. An otolaryngologist should be consulted as soon as the diagnosis is made.

   c. Intravenous antibiotic therapy should be instituted as soon as possible.

   (1) **Penicillin G** (2 million U every 4 hours) is one acceptable regimen; **metronidazole** (500 mg every 6 hours) may be added to provide anaerobic coverage against *B. fragilis.*

   (2) **Clindamycin** (600–900 mg every 8 hours) provides better anaerobic coverage than penicillin alone.

   (3) **Cefoxitin** (1–2 g every 8 hours) is a third alternative.

6. **Disposition.** Patients are generally sent to the operating room for incision and drainage. If an abscess is not yet present, admission to a monitored setting is appropriate. The airway should be closely watched and intubation performed before trouble develops.

D **Parapharyngeal abscess**

1. **Discussion**
   a. **Definition.** Pharyngeal abscess is abscessation of the lateral pharyngeal space, which lies lateral to the pharynx and medial to the masticator space. It extends from the base of the skull to the hyoid bone. The space is lateral to the superior pharyngeal constrictor muscle and medial to the mandible and internal pterygoid muscle.
   b. **Pathogenesis.** Airway compromise can occur as well as spread to the mediastinum.

2. **Clinical features** include the rapid onset of a high fever, chills, and swelling. The swelling in the neck can proceed rapidly and swallowing may be difficult. Trismus is usually present and there is marked pain as the space distends.

3. **Differential diagnoses** include posterior pharyngeal abscess, masticator space abscess, Ludwig's angina, and angioedema.

4. **Evaluation.** Because the abscess can spread to the mediastinum, CT scans of the neck and chest are often needed prior to incision and drainage.

5. **Therapy**
   a. **Initial stabilization.** Airway patency is the first concern and oral intubation or cricothyrotomy may be necessary.
   b. **Incision and drainage** are usually performed in the operating room after making an external incision.
   c. **Antibiotic therapy** is the same as for Ludwig's angina (see IV C 5 c).

6. **Disposition.** Patients are generally sent to surgery for incision and drainage.

E **Retropharyngeal abscess**

1. **Discussion**
   a. **Definition.** The retropharyngeal space is the fascial plane between the posterior pharyngeal muscles and the paraspinous muscles.
   b. **Etiology and pathogenesis**
      (1) **Children.** Retropharyngeal abscess is mostly a pediatric problem because there are lymph nodes in the retropharyngeal space that can become suppurative.
      (2) **Adults.** The lymph nodes in the retropharyngeal space involute in adolescence. Infections in adults are usually secondary to trauma (e.g., foreign body perforations from chicken or fish bones, iatrogenic injuries from intubation or endoscopy).

2. **Clinical features.** The patient usually appears ill and presents with a fever, sore throat, and neck pain. The neck is often stiff and motion at the neck is painful. The voice may be muffled and airway compromise is possible. If the abscess extends into the mediastinum, chest pain is a likely symptom.

3. **Differential diagnoses.** The lack of trismus helps differentiate retropharyngeal abscess from Ludwig's angina and parapharyngeal abscess.

4. **Evaluation.** Imaging studies may be indicated after ensuring a patent airway.
   a. **Lateral soft tissue radiographs** of the neck will show swelling posterior to the airway.
   b. **CT scans** of the neck and chest are needed to identify the extent of the abscess.

5. **Therapy**
   a. **Initial stabilization.** An open airway must be ensured.
   b. **Incision and drainage** are carried out in the operating room.
   c. **Antibiotic therapy** is administered intravenously. Regimens include:
      (1) **Penicillin G plus metronidazole** for *B. fragilis*
         (a) The **adult dosage** is penicillin G, 2–4 million U every 4 hours, and metronidazole, 500 mg every 6 hours.

(b) The **pediatric dosage** is penicillin G, 75,000–100,000 U/kg/day, divided, every 6–8 hours, and metronidazole, 30 mg/kg/day, divided, every 12 hours.

   (2) **Clindamycin**

      (a) The **adult dosage** is 600–900 mg every 6 hours.

      (b) The **pediatric dosage** is 25–40 mg/kg/day, divided, every 6 hours.

   (3) **Cefoxitin**

      (a) The **adult dosage** is 2 g every 8 hours.

      (b) The **pediatric dosage** is 80–160 mg/kg/day, divided, every 6 hours.

6. Disposition is to the operating room for incision and drainage.

V   TEETH, MAXILLA, AND MANDIBLE

A **Dental anatomy**   The tooth consists of a crown and root. The crown consists of the enamel, dentin, and pulp above the gingiva. The root has no enamel and the dentin is fixed to the periodontal ligament by the cementum. The neurovascular bundle leaves the root at the apex. **Identification** of the teeth for charting purposes is illustrated in Figure 12–3.

B **Dental caries (cavities)** result from bacterial erosion through the enamel into the dentin and pulp.

  1. Clinical features

    a. Symptoms. The chief complaint is usually a "toothache" or jaw pain. The pain is exacerbated by hot and cold liquids or food. The tooth is often sensitive to touch as well. Pain can be referred to the jaw or ear.

    b. Physical examination reveals pitting of the tooth surface. Percussion of the tooth or probing of the caries may elicit pain.

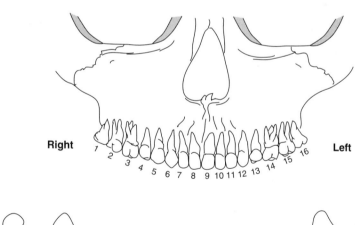
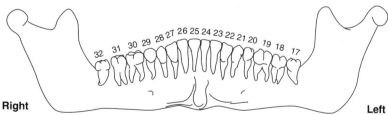

FIGURE 12–3 In adults, the teeth are numbered starting with the right upper molar (wisdom tooth) and proceeding to the left upper molar. Numbering resumes with the left lower molar and ends with the right lower molar. In children, the approach is the same, but letters are used instead of numbers (A–J for the top, K–T for the bottom). Older children will have a mixture of numbers and letters, representing the presence of both deciduous and permanent teeth. (Redrawn with permission from Harwood-Nuss AL, Linden CH, Luten RC, et al. *The Clinical Practice of Emergency Medicine.* 2nd Ed. Philadelphia: Lippincott-Raven, 1996:56.)

2. **Differential diagnoses** include apical abscess, periodontal abscess, and fracture of the tooth. Myocardial infarction (MI) can present as tooth or jaw pain and should be considered in a patient who is short of breath or ill-appearing and in whom no caries can be readily identified.

3. **Evaluation.** Physical examination is the sole means of evaluation.

4. **Therapy.** Definitive therapy is placement of a filling by a dentist. In the ED, supportive care can be provided (e.g., analgesics, local anesthesia with a lidocaine or mepivacaine injection at the root of the tooth, and placement of dental wax in the cavity to reduce sensitivity).

5. **Disposition.** Patients are discharged with instructions to see a dentist as soon as possible.

C **Dental abscesses**

1. **Discussion.** A tooth that has caries is susceptible to infection.
   a. **Apical abscesses** occur when the pulp is infected and the infection progresses along the root to form an abscess at the apex of the tooth.
   b. **Periodontal abscesses** result from infection of the gum or periodontium.

2. **Clinical features**
   a. **Symptoms.** The chief complaint is usually a "toothache" or pain in the gums.
   b. **Physical examination findings.** A fluctuant, tender gingival area at the base of the infected tooth is palpable. The tooth may feel loose as a result of an abscess at the base of the root.

3. **Differential diagnoses** include caries, gingivitis, and gingival foreign bodies.

4. **Evaluation** is by physical examination.

5. **Therapy**
   a. **Drainage of the abscess** is best performed by incision with a #15 scalpel blade. A small piece of Penrose drain can be sutured into the incision to help maintain drainage.
   b. **Antibiotic therapy.** An antibiotic effective against anaerobes, such as penicillin VK (250 mg four times daily) or clindamycin (300 mg four times daily), should be administered.

6. **Disposition.** Patients can be discharged with instructions to follow up with a dentist.

D **Trauma**

1. **Dental trauma**
   a. **Tooth fractures.** Dental trauma can lead to a tooth being chipped or broken. The Ellis classification scheme is used to classify dental fractures (Figure 12–4).
      (1) **Clinical features**
         (a) **Ellis class I fractures.** Patients complain of a chip or a sharp edge, but no pain. Physical examination will reveal the chip.
         (b) **Ellis class II fractures.** Patients often complain of sensitivity to changes in temperature or to air. On physical examination, a yellow spot (i.e., the dentin) in the center of the fracture is visible.
         (c) **Ellis class III fractures** can be painful because the nerve is exposed. On physical examination, the fracture has a pink center (representing bleeding from the disturbed blood vessels and nerves in the pulp). Class III fractures that occur at the root are often missed because the tooth may seem to be intact. Therefore, any tooth that is loose or painful after trauma should be evaluated by a dentist.
      (2) **Evaluation** entails careful inspection. The tooth should be blotted (to improve visibility), but never probed, because probing can introduce bacteria to exposed pulp.
      (3) **Therapy**
         (a) **Ellis class I fractures** are a minor problem and often do not require any treatment. If there is a bothersome sharp edge, it can be rounded with an emery board.
         (b) **Ellis class II fractures** in older children and adults should be covered with calcium hydroxide and a dressing. In children, some class II fractures require emergent treatment by a dentist to reduce the risk of infection.

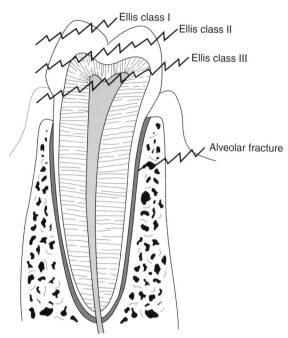

FIGURE 12–4 Ellis classification scheme for dental fractures. In Ellis class I fractures, the enamel is fractured. In Ellis class II fractures, the enamel and dentin are fractured. In Ellis class III fractures, the enamel, dentin, and pulp are fractured. (Modified with permission from Amsterdam JT, Rose LF. Dental alveolar trauma. *Curr Top Emerg Med* 1981;2(9):1.)

> > **(c) Ellis class III fractures** should be treated emergently by a dentist to reduce the risk of infection. Often a root canal must be performed.
>
> **(4) Disposition.** Generally, patients with Ellis class I or II fractures are referred to a dentist for follow-up the next day. Patients with class III fractures, children with class II fractures, and patients with suspected root fractures should be referred emergently to the dentist.

> **b. Tooth subluxation or intrusion**
>
> > **(1) Discussion**
> >
> > > **(a) Subluxation** occurs when an injured tooth is loose or displaced in the socket.
> > >
> > > **(b) Intrusion** occurs when a tooth is impacted in the socket.
> >
> > **(2) Clinical features.** The tooth may be loose, painful, and maloccluded. On physical examination, the tooth will be loose and it may be impacted into the gum. Often there is blood in the gingival crevice.
> >
> > **(3) Differential diagnoses.** Subluxation must be differentiated from root fracture and avulsion.
> >
> > **(4) Evaluation** often requires dental radiographs, which are not available in most EDs.
> >
> > **(5) Therapy**
> >
> > > **(a) Reduction** is often painful and anesthesia (provided by a lidocaine injection at the root) may facilitate the process. Once reduced, the tooth can be immobilized with dental wax.
> > >
> > > **(b) Analgesia** should be provided.
> >
> > **(6) Disposition.** Patients should be referred to a dentist for definitive treatment as soon as possible.

> **c. Tooth avulsion** occurs when a tooth is knocked out of its socket.
>
> > **(1) Differential diagnoses.** Avulsion must be differentiated from an alveolar fracture.
> >
> > **(2) Therapy.** An avulsed tooth is a true emergency and must be reimplanted as soon as possible. Each minute that the tooth remains out of its socket reduces the likelihood of the tooth surviving by approximately 1%.

(a) It is important to determine whether the tooth is a primary (baby) tooth or a secondary tooth. Primary teeth are not reimplanted because they often ankylose or fuse to the bone, causing permanent deformity.

(b) The avulsed tooth should only be handled by the enamel to avoid disturbing the periodontal ligament, which is still attached to the tooth. The tooth should be rinsed with sterile water but not scrubbed.

   (i) In alert patients, the tooth can be placed under the tongue to bathe it in saliva.

   (ii) Alternatively, the tooth can be placed in milk or a commercially available tooth preservative or wrapped in moist gauze.

(c) The tooth is replaced in the socket and stabilized with dental wax. The patient should be seen in the ED or immediately referred to a dentist or oral surgeon for definitive treatment, which entails wiring the tooth into place.

2. **Maxillary fractures**

   a. **Discussion**

   (1) **Etiology.** Most maxillary fractures are the result of motor vehicle collisions.

   (2) **Types** include:

   (a) **Simple alveolar fractures,** which run through the alveolar portion of the maxilla, where the teeth are implanted

   (b) **Antrum fractures,** which are fractures of the maxilla at the base of the nose

   (c) **Le Fort's fractures** (Figure 12–5)

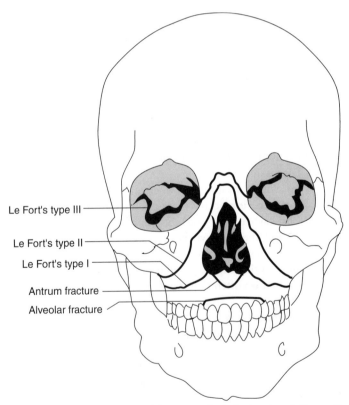

FIGURE 12–5 Le Fort's fractures are fractures of the midface. In Le Fort's fracture type I, the maxilla is separated from the upper face by a horizontal fracture though each nostril above the hard palate. In Le Fort's fracture type II, the fracture is oblique and runs from the nasomaxillary area through the orbit, separating the zygoma and orbits from the nose. Leakage of cerebrospinal fluid (CSF) can occur if the cribriform plate is involved. In Le Fort's fracture type III (craniofacial dysjunction), the facial bones are separated from the cranium. The fracture runs through the maxillary sinus, orbits, and zygoma. (Redrawn with permission from Rosen P. *Emergency Medicine: Concepts and Clinical Practice.* 3rd Ed. St. Louis: Mosby-Year Book, 1992:366.)

b. Clinical features. Le Fort's fractures are usually a combination of the three types (e.g., one type may be seen on one side of the face and another type may be seen on the other).

  (1) Le Fort's type I fractures

    (a) Symptoms include malocclusion (manifested as an inability to bite) and facial tingling (as a result of infraorbital nerve involvement).

    (b) Physical examination findings include a bilateral epistaxis, a long-appearing face, a mobile hard palate, and crepitance. Airway obstruction may occur secondary to swelling in the area of the soft palate.

  (2) Le Fort's type II fractures

    (a) Symptoms include malocclusion, facial tingling, and often diplopia.

    (b) Physical examination findings

      (i) Bilateral epistaxis, periorbital ecchymosis, and a long-appearing face are noted.

      (ii) The central region of the face will be mobile between the bridge of the nose and teeth, and crepitance is present.

      (iii) A step-off defect at the inferior orbital rim, a medial canthal deformity, enophthalmos, and restricted extraocular motion (resulting from entrapment of the inferior oblique muscle) may be noted.

      (iv) Airway obstruction can occur as a result of swelling in the nasopharynx.

  (3) Le Fort's type III fractures

    (a) Symptoms include malocclusion, tingling in the face, diplopia, and facial pain.

    (b) Physical examination findings

      (i) Bilateral epistaxis and CSF rhinorrhea are noted.

      (ii) The face is unstable, moving laterally through the orbits with stress.

      (iii) Marked facial swelling, ecchymosis, a medial canthal deformity, a lateral orbital rim defect, and enophthalmos may be noted.

      (iv) Significant retropharyngeal swelling can lead to airway obstruction.

c. Differential diagnoses include orbital blow-out fractures, orbital tripod fractures, fracture of the antrum of the maxillary sinus, and Le Fort's type I and type II fractures.

d. Evaluation

  (1) CT. A CT scan yields the most information because the three-dimensional image allows clear visualization of the fracture.

  (2) Radiographs

    (a) Radiographs can identify the fracture but are more difficult than a CT scan to interpret. A lateral view should be ordered to evaluate the pterygoid plates and to check for the presence of a retropharyngeal hematoma. A Waters' view should be ordered to evaluate the maxillary sinus, orbits, and frontal sinus.

    (b) Because a Le Fort's type III fracture represents the application of major forces to the face, the cervical spine should be evaluated radiographically to rule out injury.

e. Therapy

  (1) Airway control is the most important priority and should be accomplished early, before airway obstruction is present. It is much easier to intubate a patient when the airway is moderately swollen—when the airway is obstructed, cricothyrotomy often becomes necessary.

  (2) Control of epistaxis is often difficult. If packing is unsuccessful, emergent reduction of the fracture may be needed to control the bleeding.

  (3) Fracture reduction and **internal fixation** are accomplished by an ear, nose, and throat specialist.

  (4) Antibiotic therapy is needed to minimize the risk of CNS infection.

f. Disposition

  (1) Alveolar fractures should be stabilized using dental wax or arch wires. Urgent follow-up with an oral surgeon is necessary.

  (2) Antrum fractures can be repaired on an outpatient basis if no other injuries are present.

(3) **Le Fort's fractures.** Patients require admission for open reduction and internal fixation. Often these patients have other injuries and require a complete trauma evaluation anyway.

3. **Mandibular fractures**
   a. **Discussion.** Mandibular fractures (Figure 12–6) are relatively common and are usually the result of a direct blow.
   b. **Clinical features**
      (1) **Symptoms** include pain, the inability to open the mouth, malocclusion, and tingling of the lip if the inferior alveolar nerve is affected.
      (2) **Physical examination findings**
         (a) Trismus, deviation of the jaw, an inability to bite down, and malalignment of the teeth are usually noted. Lip and chin sensation may be impaired.
         (b) In patients with a condylar fracture, blood may be noted in the external auditory canal.
         (c) The teeth should be inspected. Bleeding at the base of a tooth signifies an open fracture through the socket.
   c. **Differential diagnoses** include an alveolar fracture, dislocation of the jaw, and trismus from a zygoma fracture.
   d. **Evaluation** is by radiographs.
      (1) A **Panorex view** is best because it enables visualization of the entire mandible.
      (2) A **posterior-anterior (PA) view** is useful for evaluating the ramus, body, and angle.
      (3) A **lateral oblique view** allows assessment of the body, ramus, condyle, and coronoid process.
      (4) An **occlusal view** allows evaluation of the symphysis.
   e. **Therapy**
      (1) **Fractures that displace the mandible forward** are more amenable to treatment because the muscles help to stabilize the fracture. These fractures can be stabilized with arch wire supports to the teeth. The patient should be placed on a diet of soft foods.
      (2) **Fractures that displace the mandible backward** are more difficult to treat, because the masseter, medial pterygoid, and temporalis muscles displace the fracture. These fractures often require open reduction and internal fixation.

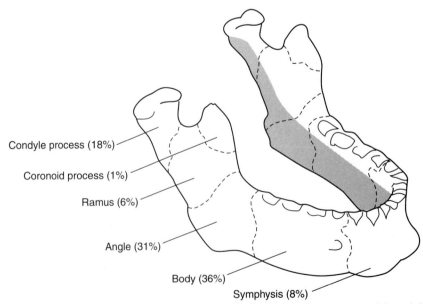

Condyle process (18%)
Coronoid process (1%)
Ramus (6%)
Angle (31%)
Body (36%)
Symphysis (8%)

FIGURE 12–6 The most common locations of mandibular fractures are the body, the angle, the condyle, and the symphysis. In more than 50% of patients, the mandible is broken in two places. (Redrawn with permission from Rosen P. *Emergency Medicine: Concepts and Clinical Practice.* 3rd Ed. St. Louis: Mosby-Year Book, 1992:368.)

        (3) Open fractures. Prophylactic antibiotics must be prescribed to prevent infection of the bone. Penicillin G (2 million U administered intravenously every 4 hours) or cefazolin (1 g administered intravenously every 6 hours) can be used.

  f. Disposition

      (1) Discharge. Patients with closed fractures amenable to treatment can be discharged with instructions to follow up with an ear, nose, and throat specialist.

      (2) Admission. Patients with open fractures that are amenable to treatment require admission for prophylactic antibiotics and open irrigation of the wound. Patients with complicated fractures also require admission, for open reduction and internal fixation.

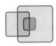

Study Questions

Directions: *Each of the numbered items or incomplete statements in this section is followed by answers or by completions of the statement. Select the ONE lettered answer or completion that is BEST in each case.*

1. What is the single most important step in the evaluation and treatment of chemical burns to the eye?
    - (A) Antibiotic therapy to reduce the likelihood of a secondary infection
    - (B) Copious irrigation with saline or water as soon as the patient presents to the emergency department (ED)
    - (C) Slit-lamp examination to assess the depth of the burn
    - (D) Cycloplegia to dilate the pupil to increase flow of aqueous humor into the anterior chamber and decrease pain
    - (E) Evaluation of visual acuity

2. Which one of the following statements regarding epistaxis is true?
    - (A) Hypertension is a risk factor for developing nose bleeds.
    - (B) Posterior bleeds occur in Kiesselbach's plexus.
    - (C) Anterior bleeds are easier than posterior bleeds to control but are less common.
    - (D) Patients with posterior bleeds require packing and admission to the hospital.
    - (E) A complete blood count (CBC), prothrombin time (PT), and partial thromboplastin time (PTT) should be sent for all patients with epistaxis.

3. Which one of the following statements regarding acute sinusitis is true?
    - (A) Plain sinus radiographs provide more information than a computed tomography (CT) scan of the sinuses.
    - (B) Ciprofloxacin is the antibiotic of choice for the treatment of acute sinusitis.
    - (C) Maxillary sinusitis is often preceded by an apical abscess of an upper molar.
    - (D) The commonly cultured organism is *Mycoplasma*.
    - (E) The use of decongestants and steroids in the treatment of acute sinusitis is strongly discouraged.

4. Which one of the following statements regarding the treatment of dental injuries is true?
    - (A) An avulsed tooth should be scrubbed to remove debris and replaced in the socket as soon as possible.
    - (B) A fractured tooth that bleeds from the center of the fracture should be cleaned with a dental pick and then filled and covered with dental wax.
    - (C) An avulsed tooth should be handled only by the enamel.
    - (D) An apical abscess is best treated with oral antibiotics and follow-up in 2–3 days.
    - (E) A fractured tooth that has a yellow center and does not bleed can be treated at the next available dental appointment without any treatment in the emergency department (ED).

5. A 65-year-old female complains of losing vision in her right eye suddenly. Which of the following approaches is NOT useful in the treatment of central retinal artery occlusion (CRAO)?
    - (A) Applying digital pressure to the globe
    - (B) Anterior chamber paracentesis
    - (C) Administering mannitol or glycerol
    - (D) Administering acetazolamide
    - (E) Administering calcium channel blockers

6. Uveitis resulting from which one of the following general causes should NOT be treated with steroids?

   (A) Autoimmune disease
   (B) Trauma
   (C) Idiopathic uveitis
   (D) Infection

7. Which one of the following statements regarding acute mastoiditis is true?

   (A) Altered mental status is common and usually due to the severe pain.
   (B) In a patient with altered mental status, treatment with intravenous antibiotics effective against the agents most often responsible for meningitis and brain abscesses should be started after obtaining a computed tomography (CT) scan of the brain.
   (C) A CT scan is not a reliable imaging study to diagnose mastoiditis.
   (D) Radiographs of the mastoids are not reliable for ruling out mastoiditis.
   (E) Complex mastoiditis with abscess formation is usually treated with myringotomy tube placement and oral antibiotics.

Answers and Explanations

1. The answer is B The single most important measure to take when evaluating and treating a patient with chemical burns to the eye is copious irrigation. The more irrigation, the better; inadequate irrigation allows additional damage to occur, especially in alkali burns. The administration of prophylactic antibiotics to help prevent secondary infections is appropriate, but it is not the first priority. A thorough examination, including evaluation of visual acuity and slit-lamp examination, should follow therapy and is useful in gauging the severity of the burn. The administration of a cycloplegic may reduce photophobia but is certainly not a priority when treating chemical burns to the eye.

2. The answer is D In patients with epistaxis resulting from a posterior bleed, packing the posterior pharynx is associated with hypoxemia and respiratory arrest, and rebleeding can occur. For these reasons, patients with posterior bleeds need to be admitted to the hospital [usually to an intensive care unit (ICU) or monitored area]. Posterior bleeds often involve branches of the carotid artery, not Kiesselbach's plexus. Kiesselbach's plexus is the site of most anterior bleeds, which account for 90% of cases of epistaxis and are usually easy to control. A CBC, PT, and PTT are indicated in patients with a history of anticoagulant use, a bleeding disorder, cancer, leukemia, lymphoma, or AIDS, and in patients with difficult-to-control nosebleeds who may have one of these disorders that has not yet been diagnosed. Because posterior bleeds are often difficult to control and bleed more profusely, a CBC, PT, PTT, and blood type and crossmatch are appropriate parts of the inpatient work-up for these patients. However, most patients with nosebleeds do not require laboratory evaluation. In patients with hypertension, nosebleeds may be more difficult to control, but hypertension is not a risk factor for the development of nosebleeds.

3. The answer is C Maxillary sinusitis is often preceded by an abscess in an upper molar or by an upper respiratory tract infection. Other predisposing factors include allergic rhinitis, nasal edema, and polyps. Radiographs of the sinuses may be of use, but a computed tomography (CT) scan of the sinuses is more sensitive and gives more information about the affected sinus. The most commonly cultured organisms are *H. Influenzae* and *S. pneumoniae*. Amoxicillin clavulanate or trimethoprim–sulfamethoxazole is the preferred antibacterial agent. Amoxicillin alone is less expensive, but it is not as effective against *H. Influenzae.* The use of steroids is particularly helpful in infections preceded by allergic rhinitis. Decongestants used on a short-term basis help to reduce swelling and open the ostia for better drainage of the sinus.

4. The answer is C Avulsed teeth should only be handled by the enamel. The dental ligament attached to the root is delicate and must remain on the root in order for the tooth to survive when it is replanted. The sooner the tooth is replaced, the better the chance it has for survival. Until it can be reimplanted, the tooth should be placed under the patient's tongue (if the patient is alert) or in milk or a commercially available preservative to keep it viable. Patients with dental fractures that involve the dentin (yellow) and pulp (red) need to be seen as soon as possible by a dentist for root canal or capping. It is best to just cover the tooth with dental wax or aluminum foil until the patient can see a dentist. Apical abscesses, like all other abscesses, are treated by incision and drainage. Antibiotics can be used after the abscess is drained.

5. The answer is E When the central retinal artery is occluded, blood supply to the retina is lost. By decreasing the intraocular pressure, the pressure head in the artery is increased. The clot or embolus can then at times be forced further down the artery, restoring blood flow to some extent. If performed early enough, some of the lost vision may be restored. Intraocular pressure can be reduced by applying digital pressure to the globe through a closed eyelid, forcing aqueous humor into the canals of Schlemm. Performing anterior paracentesis after applying digital pressure removes aqueous humor from the anterior chamber, further reducing the intraocular pressure. Mannitol administered intravenously increases the oncotic pressure of the blood, causing fluids (including those in the eye) to move from the third space into the blood. Acetazolamide is a carbonic anhydrase inhibitor that minimizes production of aqueous humor. Calcium channel blockers, on the other hand, would reduce the blood pressure, causing the pressure head in the artery to decrease and lessening the chance that the embolus would be forced out of the artery.

6. The answer is D Uveitis secondary to infection should not be treated with steroids, because steroids can exacerbate the infection. Noninfectious causes of uveitis tend to improve more rapidly with the use of steroids, which reduce inflammation. Generally, infections of the eye should not be treated with steroids and the prescribing of steroids for use in patients with ophthalmologic conditions is best left to an ophthalmologist.

7. The answer is B In a patient with suspected mastoiditis and signs of meningeal irritation or mental status changes, one should assume meningitis or a brain abscess is present. Failure to treat these infections immediately can increase the likelihood of complications; therefore, one should not delay treatment until a CT scan is obtained. Cerebrospinal fluid (CSF) cultures will not be affected for up to 6 hours after antibiotics are given because the blood–brain barrier delays entry of the antibiotic into the CSF. A CT scan of the mastoid air cells is much better than a radiograph for diagnosing mastoiditis, because radiographs can be normal and therefore cannot be used to rule out the diagnosis. Simple mastoiditis can be treated with myringotomy tube placement and intravenous antibiotics.

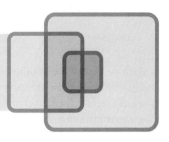

chapter 13

Psychiatric Emergencies

ERIC C. MILLER

I · ORGANIC BRAIN DISORDERS AND PSYCHOSIS

A **Discussion and clinical features**

1. **Organic brain disorders** are characterized by impaired orientation and cognitive brain function.

   a. **Dementia.** These patients are usually elderly with a known history of diminished cognition. They are often agitated or violent due to inability to understand their surroundings or the intentions of other people. They may have an overlying component of psychosis or delirium.

   b. **Delirium,** usually caused by a metabolic abnormality, drug intoxication, or structural lesion, is characterized by the rapid onset of impaired orientation and cognition. These patients may have a readily treatable and reversible condition (e.g., hypoglycemia) as the cause of their delirium.

2. **Psychosis** is typically characterized by abnormal thought patterns, often with intact cognition. These patients often have the ability to perform calculations, memorize items, or converse, but they have bizarre ideas and thoughts. Psychosis is usually secondary to one of the mental disorders listed below but may be a result of acute drug intoxication or chronic abuse (e.g., methamphetamine abuse).

   a. **Schizophrenia** is characterized by delusions and hallucinations, and is the most common cause of psychosis. Mood is usually unaffected and often very flat. These patients may present to the emergency department (ED) in a quiet and withdrawn state, or they may be violent, paranoid, and suspicious of healthcare workers. Neuroleptics are the mainstay of treatment, both emergently and on a chronic basis. These patients often present to the ED because they have stopped taking their medications.

   b. **Mania** is usually associated with bipolar disorder, wherein patients have cyclical mood swings that vary from depression to mania. Mania is characterized by elevated mood and energy. Acutely manic patients will exhibit fast and pressured speech, agitation, grandiose delusions, and insomnia. They may be violent in the ED, feeling that people are interfering with their plans. Sedating neuroleptics are often needed in the emergency setting to control the patient. Lithium is often used to prevent manic episodes, but it has no place in acute management.

   c. **Depression.** Patients may present with psychotic features, although this is rare. Delusions are the most common psychotic feature seen in depressed patients; these patients are not usually violent or agitated.

B **Evaluation** EDs should have a defined plan for dealing with violent or abusive patients. If the patient is threatening, evaluation and treatment should always take place with several people in the room.

1. **History and physical examination.** An attempt should be made to obtain as much information about the patient's condition as possible from the patient's relatives, friends, paramedics, and other healthcare workers. It is best to perform as much of the history or physical examination as possible before restraining or sedating the patient (see I D 1).

2. **Laboratory studies** and other studies (e.g., radiography) should be guided by the history and physical examination findings. Patients with known psychiatric disorders or dementia may

require minimal work-up. Standard tests for these patients often include an **ethanol level, drug screen,** and **basic electrolyte evaluation.**

C **Therapy**

1. **Restraint and sedation.** The first priority in dealing with patients with organic brain disorders or psychosis is ensuring the safety of both healthcare workers and the patient. This can be accomplished in several ways.
    a. **Environmental seclusion.** Placement of the patient in a quiet, darkened room will often prevent escalation of agitation in patients who are mildly agitated.
    b. **Physical restraint.** Violent and severely agitated patients may require physical restraints. At least five or six ED personnel must be present to restrain each of the patient's limbs and his or her trunk in unison. A mask may be placed on the spitting patient.
    c. **Chemical restraint (sedation)** may be required if the patient remains agitated. Quick and safe sedatives to use include **droperidol** or **haloperidol** (2–5 mg intravenously or intramuscularly every 30 minutes) or **lorazepam** (2 mg intramuscularly or intravenously every 30 minutes) until control is achieved. Care must be taken to avoid oversedation and hypotension, especially in elderly patients.
        (1) Patients on phencyclidine or methamphetamines may require substantial doses (e.g., 10 mg droperidol, 10–15 mg lorazepam) before control is achieved.
        (2) Because some neuroleptics may lower the seizure threshold, the use of benzodiazepines may be more appropriate in certain circumstances (e.g., cocaine intoxication).
        (3) Patients with acute uncontrolled psychosis often require the rapid administration of neuroleptics to gain control. High-potency neuroleptics (e.g., haloperidol) are best suited for this purpose, usually in doses of 2–5 mg intravenously, intramuscularly, or orally every 15–30 minutes until control is achieved.
2. **Glucose, oxygen, thiamine, naloxone,** and **flumazenil** should be considered for patients with delirium. These agents may rapidly correct treatable causes of delirium.

D **Disposition**

1. Acutely psychotic patients usually need inpatient psychiatric care. An involuntary psychiatric hold may need to be invoked.
2. Patients with delirium should be admitted to the hospital unless a readily reversible or minor cause is found in the ED.
3. Many patients with drug or alcohol intoxication can be observed in the ED until they are sober enough to discharge.

II **ANOREXIA NERVOSA AND BULIMIA NERVOSA**

A **Discussion**   Approximately 90% of patients are women younger than 25 years of age.

1. **Anorexia nervosa** is a syndrome of self-starvation.
2. **Bulimia nervosa** is characterized by frequent episodes of binge eating. The patient usually consumes large amounts of food during a defined period of time (e.g., less than 2 hours) and then uses compensatory measures (e.g., laxatives, diuretics, induced vomiting) to prevent weight gain.

B **Clinical features**

1. **Anorexia nervosa.** The patient usually weighs less than 85% of the expected weight.
    a. The patient may present with **life-threatening malnutrition, hypotension,** or **bradycardia.**
    b. Endocrine abnormalities are present, usually **amenorrhea.**
2. **Bulimia nervosa.** These patients are often of normal or excessive weight for their size (as opposed to patients with anorexia).

      a. Serious complications of repeated vomiting (e.g., **esophageal rupture, Mallory-Weiss tears**) may be the presenting complaint.

      b. Electrolyte imbalances (e.g., hypokalemia) are fairly common secondary to repeated vomiting or laxative or diuretic abuse.

C **Differential diagnoses**

1. **Medical causes** of excessive weight loss (e.g., **diabetes, Crohn's disease, cancer, hyperthyroidism**) must be excluded.

2. **Depression** or **schizophrenia** can lead to profound weight loss in a small number of patients.

D **Evaluation**

1. **History and physical examination** form the basis for the diagnosis of these disorders.

    a. There is often a family history of eating disorders or job pressures to be thin (e.g., professional dancers, gymnasts).

    b. The patient is often evasive about purging or the use of laxatives or diuretics. Friends or family members are more likely to mention these behaviors with regard to the patient.

2. **Laboratory studies.** Appropriate studies include a **serum electrolyte panel** and **glucose level** and **renal and thyroid function tests.**

3. **Electrocardiography.** An **electrocardiogram (ECG)** may be warranted.

E **Therapy** **Intensive psychiatric therapy** and frequent monitoring of weight are the cornerstones of treatment for patients with these disorders. Antidepressants have been shown to be effective in treating patients with bulimia, but no medications have proven useful for the treatment of anorexia.

F **Disposition**

1. **Discharge.** Most patients will require only outpatient treatment.

2. **Admission** to the hospital is indicated for any patient with substantial electrolyte imbalances or signs of cardiac abnormalities. Patients with severe malnutrition or those who fail to gain weight with outpatient treatment should also be admitted.

III   PANIC DISORDER

A **Discussion** Panic disorder is a form of anxiety that is characterized by recurrent **panic attacks** (i.e., sudden episodes of intense fear or impending doom associated with a variety of somatic symptoms).

1. Panic attacks are often unpredictable, although they may occur commonly in certain situations.

2. Panic attacks are rarely seen in patients older than 45 years.

B **Clinical features**

1. Symptoms associated with panic attacks may mimic life-threatening conditions:

    a. Palpitations or a pounding heart

    b. Diaphoresis

    c. A sensation of shortness of breath or choking

    d. Chest pain or discomfort

    e. Nausea, dizziness, or light-headedness

    f. Numbness, tingling, or chills

2. Some symptoms are not associated with panic attacks and always require medical evaluation, such as true vertigo, loss of consciousness, loss of bowel or bladder control, headaches, slurred speech, and temporary weakness.

TABLE 13–1 Differential Diagnoses for Panic Disorder
Acute myocardial infarction
Cardiac arrhythmias
Pulmonary emboli
Hyperthyroidism
Pheochromocytoma
Mitral valve prolapse
Alcohol withdrawal
Use of central nervous system (CNS) stimulants
Hypoglycemia

C **Differential diagnoses** Many medical conditions can mimic the symptoms of panic disorder and need to be considered (Table 13–1), especially in patients older than 45 years.

D **Evaluation**

1. **Patient history.** A careful history of recurrent, short-lived episodes of panic will usually lead to the correct diagnosis.

2. **Laboratory studies** should be guided by the patient history and may include a **serum electrolyte panel** and **glucose level,** a **drug screen,** and an **arterial blood gas (ABG)** report. Older patients or those with atypical symptoms should have a thorough work-up to detect conditions with a medical basis.

3. **Electrocardiography and radiology.** An ECG or chest radiograph may be warranted.

E **Therapy** Generally, both **medications** and **behavioral therapy** are used for patients with panic disorder. Usually, medical therapy for panic attacks should be started by the patient's primary care physician, not in the ED. However, commonly used medications include the following:

1. **Imipramine** has been shown by many studies to be efficacious in panic disorder, although weeks of therapy may be required before symptomatic improvement occurs.

2. **Alprazolam** and **clonazepam** are both useful for panic attacks and usually produce a response within several days of beginning the medication.

F **Disposition** Patients with risk factors for significant cardiopulmonary disease should be admitted to the hospital to rule out a life-threatening condition.

IV **CONVERSION REACTIONS**

A **Discussion** A **conversion reaction** is the transformation of a stressor into a physical symptom. To diagnose a conversion reaction, the following **five elements** must be present:

1. There is a physical dysfunction or symptom that suggests a neurologic or medical condition.

2. The onset of the symptom is preceded by a stressful situation or conflict.

3. The patient does not knowingly produce the symptom.

4. The symptom cannot be explained by a known medical condition.

5. The symptom is not limited to sexual dysfunction or pain, and is not explained by another psychiatric disorder.

B **Clinical features** The symptom associated with a conversion reaction is usually a neurologic complaint, but other systems may be affected. Typical symptoms include blindness, paralysis, sensory loss, seizures, vomiting, or diarrhea.

TABLE 13–2	Differential Diagnoses for Conversion Reaction
Multiple sclerosis	Dystonia
Myasthenia gravis	AIDS
Guillain-Barré syndrome	Subdural hematoma
Brain tumor	Myopathy

C **Differential diagnoses** In some studies, up to 25% of patients diagnosed with conversion reactions eventually are found to have a medical cause of their symptoms. Therefore, it is important to consider organic causes for the patient's symptoms (Table 13–2).

D **Evaluation** The evaluation of a possible conversion reaction necessitates a complete **neurologic** or **symptom-related examination.**

1. A patient with conversion reaction will often have an inconsistent examination over brief periods of time.

2. A patient with conversion reaction will often fail tests designed to evaluate the symptom. For example, a patient who has symptoms of paralysis or anesthesia may avoid painful stimuli, or a patient who complains of blindness may avoid a visual threat.

E **Therapy** in the ED entails **reassurance** that there is no serious disease process present and the assurance that the symptom will resolve with time. The patient should not be confronted with the suspicion that his or her symptoms are completely psychogenic; patients respond poorly to this approach. Long-term counseling may be required.

F **Disposition** With a supportive, nonconfrontational approach, 90%–95% of patients will experience relief of their symptoms in a short period of time. Patients should be discharged to a supportive environment.

V DEPRESSION AND SUICIDE

A **Discussion** Depression and suicide attempts or ideation are often seen together.

1. **Depression** is the most common psychiatric disorder, occurring in approximately 2%–3% of the population at a given time. Major depression is defined as a persistent dysphoric mood or loss of interest in activities for at least 2 weeks.

2. **Suicide** is the second leading cause of death among adolescents and young adults. In general, women attempt suicide more often than men, but men are more likely to be successful in the attempt.

B **Clinical features**

1. **Psychiatric symptoms of depression.** Depressed patients usually express feelings of guilt, worthlessness, and hopelessness, and report that they have thoughts of death or suicide.

2. **Physiologic symptoms that may accompany depression** include:
   a. A change in appetite or weight
   b. Insomnia or excessive sleep
   c. Fatigue
   d. Difficulty concentrating

C **Differential diagnoses**

1. **Medical causes** of depression include hypothyroidism, drug and alcohol abuse, and certain medications.

2. **Situational/loss depression.** Depression may also be situational (e.g., related to the death of a spouse or parent, related to the loss of a job).

D **Evaluation**

1. **Patient history.** The patient's past medical and psychiatric problems and medication history should be carefully reviewed.

2. **Risk assessment.** In patients who are brought to the ED because of an attempted suicide, the physician should assess the patient's risk of successfully carrying out a suicide attempt in the future.

    a. **High risk.** Patients who have attempted to commit suicide by hanging or present with a self-inflicted gunshot wound are classified as high risk. Patients at high risk for successfully carrying out plans of suicide generally make the attempt in an isolated area and fail to call or leave notes for family members or friends.

    b. **Low risk.** Patients who have attempted to overdose with over-the-counter medications or present with superficial cuts to the wrists are classified as low risk. These patients often want to be rescued; they tend to make immediate calls to friends or relatives and their attempt is usually in a highly visible location.

E **Treatment**   Therapy with antidepressant medications is best initiated by the patient's regular physician, not by the ED physician.

F **Disposition**

1. **Admission.** Patients who have attempted suicide and meet any of the following criteria should be admitted to an inpatient psychiatric facility:

    a. Acute psychosis
    b. Age over 45 years
    c. High risk:rescue suicide ratio
    d. Moderate risk with poor social support system

2. **Discharge.** Patients who present to the ED as the result of a low-risk suicide attempt and who have good social support can usually be treated as outpatients with early follow-up. To be treated as an outpatient, the patient should no longer exhibit any active suicidal ideation.

Study Questions

Directions: *Each of the numbered items or incomplete statements in this section is followed by answers or by completions of the statement. Select the ONE lettered answer or completion that is BEST in each case.*

1. What is a distinguishing feature of psychosis (as opposed to delirium)?

   (A) Agitation
   (B) Impaired cognition
   (C) Fever
   (D) Aural hallucinations
   (E) An acute onset

2. What is the initial priority in dealing with physically violent patients?

   (A) Establishing intravenous access
   (B) Restraining the patient to ensure safety
   (C) Obtaining a pulse oximetry reading
   (D) Obtaining a urine drug screen
   (E) Checking the glucose level

3. Which one of the following electrolyte disturbances is most likely in a bulimic patient?

   (A) Hypernatremia
   (B) Hypermagnesemia
   (C) Hypoglycemia
   (D) Hypercalcemia
   (E) Hypokalemia

4. Which one of the following medical conditions can easily be mistaken for panic disorder?

   (A) Gastroenteritis
   (B) Supraventricular tachycardia
   (C) Peptic ulcer
   (D) Grand mal seizure
   (E) Cerebrovascular accident

5. Where does suicide rank on the list of causes of death in young adults?

   (A) Last
   (B) First
   (C) Second
   (D) Third
   (E) Fourth

6. Which one of the following patients is at the highest risk for completing a suicide attempt?

   (A) A 20-year-old stewardess who took 20 acetaminophen tablets and then called a friend
   (B) A 35-year-old accountant who slashed his wrists in the hall at work
   (C) A 50-year-old housewife who states that she wants to die but has no plan for achieving this goal
   (D) A 14-year-old teenager who drinks 12 sodas and vomits on the carpet
   (E) A 65-year-old, unemployed, single man who attempted to hang himself in the woods

7. It is necessary to sedate an agitated older patient without intravenous access. Which one of the following is the best regimen to use?

- (A) Haloperidol, 2–5 mg intramuscularly every 30 minutes to a maximum dose of 20 mg
- (B) Diazepam, 10 mg intramuscularly every 15 minutes to a maximum dose of 50 mg
- (C) Droperidol, 5 mg intramuscularly every 15 minutes to a maximum dose of 30 mg
- (D) Lorazepam, 1 mg orally every 45 minutes to a maximum dose of 5 mg
- (E) Trazodone, 100 mg orally every 30 minutes to a maximum dose of 1 g

8. Which symptom is not usually experienced by patients with panic disorder?

- (A) Dysarthria
- (B) Sweating
- (C) Palpitations
- (D) Tingling in an extremity
- (E) Chest pain

Answers and Explanations

1. The answer is D Psychosis is seen with primary psychiatric disorders (e.g., schizophrenia), as opposed to delirium, which usually has an organic basis. Aural hallucinations are a hallmark of psychosis. Although hallucinations may also occur with delirium, hallucinations associated with delirium are usually visual.

2. The answer is B When dealing with a violent patient, it is important to ensure everyone's safety by sedating or restraining the patient before proceeding with the examination. Physical restraint is a cooperative effort that requires assistance from three to four emergency department (ED) personnel. Chemical restraint with haloperidol, droperidol, or benzodiazepines may be required if the patient remains combative or violent in physical restraints.

3. The answer is E Bulimic patients generally use vomiting, laxatives, or diuretics to lose weight after binge eating. With each of these methods, there is usually a loss of potassium-rich fluids. The levels of most other electrolytes are not dramatically affected. Hypokalemia may cause profound weakness, respiratory difficulty, and some cardiac dysrhythmias.

4. The answer is B The symptoms associated with panic attacks often mimic those of life-threatening conditions and are short-lived (e.g., 10–30 minutes in duration). Supraventricular tachycardia, like a panic attack, often occurs for brief periods of time, producing chest tightness and shortness of breath. The symptoms of gastroenteritis, peptic ulcer, and cerebrovascular accident usually persist over a longer period of time. Seizures produce a loss of consciousness not seen with panic attacks.

5. The answer is C Suicide is the second leading cause of death in teenagers and young adults.

6. The answer is E The 65-year-old man who attempted to hang himself in the woods is most at risk for completing a second suicide attempt. Pertinent risk factors in this patient include his age (older than 45 years), his gender (male), his marital status (single), and the fact that he is unemployed. Social isolation is also a risk factor. In addition, people who leave little chance of rescue from the attempt—as evidenced by choosing a method with a high success rate (e.g., shooting, hanging) and carrying out the attempt in an isolated location (e.g., in the woods)—are at high risk for completing a second suicide attempt, if they fail the first time.

7. The answer is A The patient in question is elderly and has no intravenous access. Therefore, it would be advisable to use a medication that is rapidly absorbed from the intramuscular route and that has minimal serious side effects. Haloperidol is an excellent medication for use in elderly patients because it is rapidly absorbed and produces very few side effects. The suggested dose is 2–5 mg every 30 minutes to a maximum dose of 20 mg. Diazepam is poorly absorbed via the intramuscular route, and droperidol can cause significant hypotension, especially in the elderly. Lorazepam and trazodone work slowly when administered orally.

8. The answer is A Patients with panic disorder usually experience hypersympathetic-type symptoms or nonspecific neurologic symptoms. Dysarthria (slurred speech) is not associated with panic disorder and usually is a feature of a significant medical condition. Any patient suspected of having panic disorder but who has focal neurologic complaints needs a thorough medical work-up.

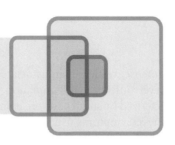

chapter 14

Obstetric and Gynecologic Emergencies

DANA A. STEARNS

I PELVIC PAIN

A Discussion   There are two types of pelvic pain.

1. **Visceral pain** results from stimulation of the nerves innervating the splanchnic organs and is vague, dull, and poorly localized.

2. **Somatic pain** results from stimulation of the peripheral somatic nerves. The pain is dermatomal or localized, is sharp, and usually involves the skin, muscle, or parietal peritoneum.

B Clinical features   There are four patterns of pelvic pain that can be helpful to know when trying to isolate the cause of the pain.

1. **Mild visceral pain** results from visceral inflammation due to infection or distention. Causes include the following:

   a. **Pelvic inflammatory disease (PID)** is characterized by vague lower abdominal pain and diffuse cervical, uterine, and adnexal tenderness.

   b. **Early appendicitis** is characterized by diffuse abdominal pain, primarily epigastric or periumbilical, with right lower quadrant tenderness on direct palpation. Symptoms include fever, nausea, and anorexia, usually evolving over 24–48 hours.

   c. **Vaginitis** or **cervicitis** can cause diffuse, lower abdominal pain focused around the suprapubic region. Tenderness is appreciated on vaginal and cervical examination with no adnexal findings. Other symptoms include vaginal discharge, dyspareunia, and dysuria.

   d. **Urinary tract infection (UTI)** is characterized by suprapubic fullness and crampy pain, possibly referred to the flank. Patients may describe dysuria or hematuria associated with painful, burning urethral irritation.

   e. **Ovarian cyst.** Symptoms usually occur around midcycle or during the postovulatory phase. Fluid engorgement and distention cause dull, constant, achy pain in the lower abdominal adnexal region. Adnexal tenderness may be noted around the affected ovary.

   f. **Early ectopic pregnancy.** The growing trophoblast causes distention at the implantation site, vague lower abdominal pain, and adnexal tenderness. Other findings include vaginal bleeding and a positive pregnancy test (see II).

   g. **Menstrual cramps** are a diagnosis of exclusion.

   h. **Uterine fibroids** are associated with pubic pressure, pain, and dysmenorrhea or menorrhagia. Uterine tenderness may be noted and tender fibroids may be palpable.

   i. **Endometriosis.** Growth of ectopic endometrial tissue may cause a dull, constant ache that worsens late in the menstrual cycle due to hormone shifts and tissue breakdown. Pain may intensify during menstruation as the lesions "slough," causing local inflammation. Examination may note adnexal or cul-de-sac tenderness without cervical motion tenderness.

2. **Severe visceral pain** is an intense, restless pain associated with fever, nausea, and vomiting. Underlying causes include severe infection, inflammation, obstruction, and visceral ischemia.
   a. **Ovarian torsion** is characterized by sudden, severe pain that is out of proportion to the concomitant adnexal tenderness. Symptoms usually occur around midcycle, but can also occur in pregnant patients. The patient may have a history of ovarian cysts.
   b. **Nephrolithiasis** is characterized by colicky, intermittent, restless pain that usually begins in the flank but may progress or radiate to the lower quadrant, suprapubic, and groin regions. Associated nausea, vomiting, and hematuria are possible. Examination may reveal flank and/or lower quadrant tenderness without peritoneal signs.
   c. **Bowel obstruction** is associated with diffuse, crampy pain, bloating, nausea, and vomiting. Examination may reveal a distended abdomen, decreased or high-pitched bowel sounds, and diffuse tenderness without peritoneal signs. Previous abdominal surgery is a risk factor.
   d. **Dysmenorrhea** is cyclic, painful menstruation thought to be mediated by prostaglandins. The patient may describe a dull, progressive pelvic ache that radiates to her back or thighs. Primary dysmenorrhea is idiopathic, whereas secondary dysmenorrhea may be related to endometriosis, uterine fibroids, pelvic adhesions, or ovarian cysts.

3. **Visceral pain progressing to somatic pain.** Organ inflammation causes the adjacent peritoneum to become progressively irritated. The inflamed parietal peritoneum may produce localized, somatic pain sensation.
   a. **Appendicitis.** Progression of appendiceal inflammation may induce parietal peritoneal inflammation. The patient describes diffuse, crampy pain that becomes progressively more localized to the right lower quadrant. Tenderness in that region becomes more sharp, intense, and focal. The incidence of appendicitis is unchanged during pregnancy, but the location of pain and tenderness may vary due to uterine displacement.
   b. **Complicated PID.** Extension of salpingeal infection to involve the parietal peritoneum can produce local peritonitis. Gonococcal seeding of Glisson's capsule (in the liver) may produce severe, right upper quadrant pain and tenderness and right pleuritic chest pain due to diaphragmatic irritation (Fitz-Hugh–Curtis syndrome).
   c. **Advanced ectopic pregnancy.** As trophoblastic tissue erodes the implantation site, hemorrhage can occur, causing local peritoneal pain, progressive adnexal and cul-de-sac tenderness, abdominal distention, diffuse peritonitis, and shock.

4. **Sudden somatic pain.** Parietal peritoneal inflammation from blood, cystic fluid, pus, urine, or feces can induce severe local abdominal pain that can progress to diffuse peritonitis.
   a. **Ruptured ectopic pregnancy.** Small amounts of hemorrhage may produce sudden, severe, localized abdominal pain and tenderness. As bleeding continues, the peritoneum becomes diffusely involved, causing significant peritoneal findings on examination.
   b. **Ruptured ovarian cyst.** Cyst rupture spills fluid or blood onto the adjacent parietal peritoneum, producing sudden, significant unilateral adnexal pain and tenderness that may become diffuse.
      (1) **Follicular cysts** rupture midcycle; rupture is associated with ovulatory pain (**mittelschmerz**).
      (2) **Luteal cysts** rupture late in the menstrual cycle and may be associated with significant hemorrhage and shock.

C **Evaluation**

1. **Stabilization.** Airway, respiratory, and cardiovascular status should be assessed, and shock should be treated immediately before making a diagnosis.
2. **Patient history.** It is imperative to obtain a menstrual history in all women of childbearing age.
3. **Physical examination.** Consider the type of pain and tenderness the patient is experiencing. Is there an associated fever, abdominal distention, or vaginal discharge? Peritonitis is best demon-

strated by percussion, gentle motion of the bed, or asking the patient to cough. Rebound tenderness can be deceiving.

4. **Laboratory studies**
   a. **Pregnancy test.** All women of childbearing age should undergo a pregnancy screen to rule out ectopic pregnancy or miscarriage.
   b. **Blood work.** A blood type and screen and a complete blood count (CBC) should be obtained.
   c. **Urinalysis** should be performed on a sample obtained by catheterization.
   d. **Culture.** Cervical and vaginal swabs are sent for culture and smeared on microscope slides for analysis as indicated. Blood and urine cultures should be considered in patients with fever.

5. **Other diagnostic tools**
   a. **Abdominal** and **pelvic ultrasonography** may be indicated to search for free fluid in the cul-de-sac, ectopic pregnancy, ovarian cyst, ovarian torsion, tubo-ovarian abscess, or an inflamed appendix.
   b. **Laparoscopy** and **biopsy** are necessary to definitively diagnose endometriosis.

D **Therapy** addresses the underlying cause. Therapies for gynecologic causes of pelvic pain are summarized here; therapies for other causes of pelvic pain are discussed in Chapter 4 ("Gastrointestinal Emergencies") and Chapter 5 ("Urogenital Emergencies").

1. **Vaginitis, cervicitis,** and **PID.** Therapy is discussed in VII A 5, B 5, and C 5, respectively.

2. **Ectopic pregnancy.** Therapy is discussed in II E.

3. **Ovarian cyst.** A patient with lower abdominal tenderness and sonographic evidence of free fluid in the cul-de-sac may be observed without intervention. Patients with any suggestion of hemorrhage or hemodynamic instability should undergo exploratory laparoscopy or laparotomy.

4. **Ovarian torsion.** Patients with suggestive history, examination, and sonographic findings should undergo laparoscopy or laparotomy for exploration and attempted salvage.

5. **Endometriosis.** Oral contraceptive regimens, danazol, methyltestosterone, or progesterone may be used to suppress ectopic endometrial growth. Surgical excision is performed to cure refractory cases.

6. **Dysmenorrhea.** Oral contraceptive therapy may be attempted to suppress endometrial growth. Pain control is attempted using nonsteroidal anti-inflammatory drugs (NSAIDs) such as ibuprofen (400–600 mg orally four times daily), naproxen (275 mg orally four times daily), or ketorolac (10 mg orally two to three times daily). Narcotic derivatives are avoided.

E **Disposition**

1. Hemodynamically unstable patients are treated with aggressive fluid resuscitation and taken to the operating room.

2. Hemodynamically stable patients are admitted for observation and treatment when an evolving surgical disease is suspected or the patient is at risk for systemic toxicity. Patients unable to tolerate oral fluids are admitted for intravenous hydration.

3. All patients must have follow-up arranged and verified prior to discharge from the ED.

II ECTOPIC PREGNANCY

A **Discussion**   Ectopic pregnancy is the development of a fertilized ovum outside of the uterine cavity (e.g., in the fallopian tube, ovary, cervix, or abdominal cavity). The ectopic site can rarely sustain the pregnancy beyond several weeks, at which time the implantation site ruptures. Ruptured ectopic pregnancies account for 10% of maternal deaths in the United States.

1. **Pathogenesis.** The fertilized ovum implants at the ectopic site, stimulating a persistent corpus luteum. The resultant elevated estrogen levels stimulate endometrial growth, and progesterone maintains this lining for a conception that never arrives. The ectopic pregnancy continues to

proliferate until it outgrows its blood supply and involutes or ruptures. The following are possible results of such growth:

a. **Conception and fallopian tube rupture.** Early erosion through the walls of the implantation site occurs, causing bleeding and peritoneal irritation followed by rupture, heavy bleeding, and shock.

b. **Tubal abortion** with extrusion into the abdominal cavity causes acute peritonitis.

c. **Tubal blood mole.** Spontaneous bleeding distends the chorionic sac, causing the conception to rupture into the fallopian tube lumen, producing transient vaginal bleeding. If rupture of the sac occurs early, the conceptus is reabsorbed and extruded, manifesting clinically as an abnormal menstrual period.

2. **Risk factors** are, for the most part, related to tubal dysfunction or injury and include:

a. **Tubal anomalies** (e.g., hypoplasia, diverticula)

b. **Salpingitis** (characterized by inflammation, scarring, and lumen narrowing)

c. **Tubal adhesions** (e.g., from infection or endometriosis)

d. **Previous tubal surgery** (e.g., salpingostomy, tubal ligation)

e. **Intrauterine device (IUD) use**

f. **Previous ectopic pregnancy**

B **Clinical features** The "classic triad" of a missed period, abdominal pain, and a palpable mass on examination is present in fewer than 30% of patients. Important historical and clinical findings include the following:

1. **Menstrual history.** A history of amenorrhea or a late period is common in patients with ectopic pregnancy. Only 10% of patients describe a normal last menstrual period (LMP).

2. **Abdominal pain or tenderness.** Ninety percent of patients complain of abdominal or pelvic pain, possibly localized to a lower quadrant.

a. Pain usually begins as colicky and diffuse (as a result of ectopic distention and inflammation) and later becomes localized (as a result of inflammation of the adjacent abdominal wall and local bleeding).

b. Peritoneal symptoms may be noticed if the bleeding causes diffuse peritoneal irritation. With severe bleeding and peritonitis, the abdomen will be rigid, distended, and tender.

3. **Cervical motion tenderness** or **adnexal tenderness** is highly suggestive of a pathologic process.

4. **Vaginal bleeding.** Fifty to ninety percent of patients will note abnormal bleeding, ranging from spotting to heavy flow with large clots.

5. **Uterine enlargement.** In pregnancy, the uterus normally softens and grows in response to hormonal stimulation, regardless of the site of conceptus implantation. One cannot assume the pregnancy is intrauterine on the basis of uterine size.

6. **Palpable mass.** Experienced examiners may note a unilateral or cul-de-sac mass, although the absence of such a mass does not rule out an ectopic pregnancy. A recent study noted a significant incidence of ectopic pregnancies found by ultrasound or by laparoscopy on the side opposite the examined mass.

7. **Shoulder pain.** A ruptured ectopic pregnancy with hemoperitoneum can cause diaphragmatic irritation and pain referred to the shoulder.

8. **Volume depletion.** Tachycardia, orthostatic hypotension, near-syncope, abdominal pain, and a positive pregnancy test in an otherwise healthy woman are indicative of a ruptured ectopic pregnancy until proven otherwise; these patients require acute obstetric and surgical intervention.

C **Differential diagnoses** include threatened miscarriage, inevitable miscarriage, ovarian cyst, vaginitis, cervicitis, salpingitis, PID, combined pregnancy (i.e., intrauterine and ectopic, may be seen in patients taking infertility medications), normal intrauterine pregnancy, appendicitis, UTI, acute nephrolithiasis, enteritis, and diverticulitis.

D **Evaluation**   A woman of childbearing age is pregnant until proven otherwise. Pregnant patients in the first trimester have ectopic pregnancies until proven otherwise. The incidence of detected ectopic pregnancies has increased fivefold over the last 20 years due to sensitive screening aids, including quantitative β-human chorionic gonadotropin (β-hCG), pelvic sonography, and new research involving serum progesterone levels.

1. **Stabilization.** It is important to establish the airway, respiratory, and cardiovascular status immediately before making a diagnosis. Two large-bore peripheral lines are secured for fluid and blood resuscitation.

2. **Laboratory studies**
   a. **Urine pregnancy test.** A urine sample can provide a quick **qualitative β-hCG screen** and most screens are sensitive to 20 mIU, or approximately 4 weeks' gestational age. Serum quantitative levels, however, provide an estimation of gestational age that is comparable to age by date since the patient's LMP.
   b. **Blood work. Blood typing and screening, Rh sensitivity, quantitative β-hCG level,** and a **CBC** are sent **immediately.** β-hCG levels normally double every 36–48 hours. Levels in abnormal pregnancies do not increase as rapidly and may plateau or decline over this time frame. Thus, if they are available, serial levels are useful in establishing a growth pattern.

3. **Ultrasonography.** A distinct fetal body and fetal cardiac activity can be detected ultrasonographically by 6 weeks' gestation (transvaginal) or 7 weeks' gestation (transabdominal), making the search for the ectopic site a bit easier at this stage. Younger gestations can be difficult to detect. The transvaginal method is more sensitive than the transabdominal approach.
   a. There must be two distinct echogenic layers (i.e., the decidua vera and the decidua capsularis) surrounding the gestational sac before the diagnosis of intrauterine pregnancy can be made. **Inability to identify the dual decidual sac sign** infers an ectopic pregnancy, even if the ectopic site is not identified sonographically.
   b. Sonographically detectable ectopic pregnancies are classified as follows:
      (1) **Type 1:** Living ectopic pregnancy, unruptured with identifiable decidual sacs or fetal heart activity
      (2) **Type 2:** Nonviable gestation or blood clot
         (a) Nonviable gestations are older than 6 weeks by dates (i.e., from the date of the LMP) and have a heart but no cardiac activity.
         (b) Blood clots noted in a patient with a fetal gestational age of less than 6 weeks by dates continue to be considered type 1 ectopic pregnancies.
      (3) **Type 3:** Ruptured, bleeding ectopic pregnancy with cul-de-sac fluid accumulation

4. **Culdocentesis** (i.e., aspiration of intra-abdominal fluid from the pelvic cul-de-sac) is used to identify hemoperitoneum in patients who are too unstable to undergo a sonographic study or when ultrasound is unavailable.
   a. **Nonclotting blood** (0.5 mL or more) is diagnostic.
   b. **Serous fluid** (0.5 mL or more) is considered a negative result.
   c. **Clotting blood** or **no fluid** is indeterminate.

E **Therapy**

1. **General therapy.** All Rh-negative mothers are given **RhoGAM** in a single intramuscular dose to prevent potential maternal Rh antibody formation.

2. **Specific therapy**
   a. **Unruptured (type 1) ectopic pregnancy.** These patients are hemodynamically stable. Treatment options include:
      (1) Laparoscopic salpingostomy and ectopic excision
      (2) Nonsurgical treatment with oral, intramuscular, or intravenous methotrexate and alternate-day leucovorin rescue or single-dose methotrexate without leucovorin
      (3) Salpingocentesis (i.e., transvaginal needle aspiration of the gestational sac)
      (4) Direct injection of methotrexate or potassium chloride

    b. Ectopic pregnancy without cardiac activity (type 2 ectopic pregnancy). Patients with serial decline of β-hCG levels and no evidence of erosion or rupture on repeat sonography can be followed with no intervention. Sonograms are repeated regularly to document embryonic reabsorption. Laparotomy or laparoscopic salpingostomy is performed if there is any sign of erosion or rupture.

    c. Ruptured (type 3) ectopic pregnancy. These patients are hemodynamically unstable and therefore require aggressive fluid and blood resuscitation and control of bleeding. Laparoscopic ectopic excision via salpingostomy or salpingectomy is indicated.

F Disposition

1. A hemodynamically stable patient with a pregnancy of less than 6 weeks' gestation (as determined by dates and quantitative β-hCG); a history of abdominal pain, vaginal bleeding, or both; a benign examination; and ultrasound revealing no clear evidence of ectopic or intrauterine pregnancy may be discharged. These patients should see an obstetrician in 48 hours for a repeat examination and quantitative β-hCG levels. Ultrasound is repeated in 2–7 days to search for pregnancy.

2. A hemodynamically stable patient with a pregnancy of less than 6 weeks' gestation (as determined by dates and quantitative β-hCG); a history of abdominal pain, vaginal bleeding, or both with abdominal or adnexal tenderness on physical examination; and evidence of cul-de-sac fluid accumulation on ultrasound but no clear evidence of intrauterine pregnancy should be admitted for observation, serial abdominal examinations, repeat quantitative β-hCG levels (in 36–48 hours), and repeat sonography.

3. A hemodynamically stable patient with a pregnancy of greater than 6 weeks' gestation (principally determined by dates), with or without abdominal or adnexal tenderness and sonographic evidence of ectopic pregnancy, is admitted for observation, serial examinations, and repeat ultrasound to determine a safe treatment.

4. A hemodynamically unstable patient with a pregnancy documented by qualitative β-hCG requires aggressive resuscitation en route to the operating room for laparotomy and hemorrhage control.

III VAGINAL BLEEDING DURING PREGNANCY

A First-trimester bleeding

1. **Ectopic pregnancy** is discussed in II.

2. **Miscarriage**
    a. Discussion. Approximately 20% of all pregnancies terminate and 80%–90% of these end as miscarriage during the first trimester (weeks 1–14). Risk factors include previous miscarriage, increased maternal parity, and increased maternal age.
    b. Clinical features. Fetal demise usually occurs 2–3 weeks prior to the onset of clinical symptoms. Miscarriage is described in the following forms:
        (1) Threatened miscarriage is seen commonly in emergency medicine. The patient complains of vaginal bleeding, which may or may not be accompanied by abdominal pain. Examination reveals blood in the vaginal vault, a closed internal cervical os, and an enlarged, tender uterus. Quantitative β-hCG levels may not correlate with the gestational age according to the LMP.
        (2) Inevitable miscarriage presents in the same manner as threatened miscarriage, except the internal cervical os is open on examination.
        (3) Incomplete miscarriage may yield findings similar to inevitable miscarriage, except blood or gestational products are noted in the cervical canal and vaginal vault on examination. The internal cervical os is open.
        (4) Completed miscarriage is rarely diagnosed in the emergency department (ED) and not without obstetric consultation. The patient may report a history that would suggest that

threatened miscarriage had occurred at some point, followed at a later date by the vaginal passage of large amounts of blood and gestational products. Upon examination, the uterus is nontender and the internal cervical os is closed. Diagnosis cannot be made unless the patient actually miscarries in the ED, allowing identification of an intact gestational sac and products (e.g., chorionic villi).

(5) Missed miscarriage occurs when fetal products are retained in utero despite their demise. Fetal products may remain for as long as 2 months. The patient may complain of frequent episodic abdominal cramping and vaginal spotting. Examination reveals a closed internal cervical os. Quantitative β-hCG levels are low for the gestational age and ultrasound reveals no fetal cardiac activity.

(6) Septic miscarriage usually begins as an inevitable miscarriage complicated by intrauterine infection due to prolonged os opening, repeated examinations, or instrumentation. The patient is febrile with cervical motion tenderness and uterine tenderness noted on examination.

c. Differential diagnoses. Although 15% of first-trimester pregnancies terminate as miscarriage, **ectopic pregnancy** must top the differential list until it can be ruled out by examination, ultrasonography, or surgical or cytopathologic findings. Other differential diagnoses include **normal intrauterine pregnancy, molar pregnancy, vulvovaginitis, cervicitis, UTI, PID,** and **vaginal foreign body.**

d. Evaluation

(1) Patient history. The date of the LMP must be identified. The patient should be questioned about the amount, character, and time course of the bleeding. A history of trauma, bleeding during pregnancy, and associated pain should be sought.

(2) Laboratory studies. The work-up should proceed as for ectopic pregnancy (see II D).

(3) Microscopic examination. All expulsed products of conception must be examined microscopically for the presence of a gestational sac, chorionic villi, or fetal material before miscarriage can be diagnosed.

e. Therapy

(1) A hemodynamically stable patient with no clinical evidence suggesting inevitable or incomplete miscarriage and no clinical or sonographic evidence supporting ectopic or intrauterine pregnancy has an ectopic pregnancy until proven otherwise. These patients must remain on limited activity and undergo repeated quantitative β-hCG levels every 48 hours and sonograms every week until the pregnancy is located and β-hCG levels dictate viability or demise.

(2) Intrauterine miscarriage may occur spontaneously and requires little intervention.

(a) Patients with clinical evidence of inevitable or incomplete miscarriage may require **dilatation and curettage** to reduce the risk of retained products, continued bleeding, and infection. **Oxytocin** (10–20 U in 1 L normal saline infused over 1 hour) is sometimes used after dilatation and curettage to induce uterine contraction and reduce bleeding.

(b) Patients who are hemodynamically unstable despite an aggressive resuscitative effort require surgical intervention (e.g., dilatation and curettage, hysterectomy). Patients with clinical, sonographic, or culdocentesis data suggesting pelvic intraperitoneal hemorrhage must undergo surgical exploration.

f. Disposition

(1) Hemodynamically stable patients with no evidence of ongoing hemorrhage, pelvic bleeding, or intraperitoneal bleeding and no findings suggesting inevitable or incomplete miscarriage may be discharged after obstetric follow-up has been arranged. These patients should see an obstetrician within 24–48 hours for repeat quantitative β-hCG and sonography.

(2) Hemodynamically unstable patients are admitted for definitive operative therapy and observation.

3. **Normal intrauterine pregnancy** may be associated with vaginal bleeding, especially during the first trimester. Patients may experience abdominal cramping with vaginal spotting but on examination, the cervical os is closed and the uterus is nontender.

   a. Serial quantitative β-hCG levels increase normally (i.e., they double every 36–48 hours, peaking at 100,000 mIU by 8–11 weeks).

   b. After 6 weeks' gestation, ultrasound reveals an intrauterine pregnancy with fetal heart activity.

B **Second- and third-trimester bleeding**

1. **Discussion**

   a. **Placenta previa**

      (1) **Pathogenesis.** Placenta previa occurs when a portion of the placenta implants on the lower uterine segment. Placenta previa is classified as marginal (24%), partial, (29%), or total (47%), depending on the amount of encroachment on the internal cervical os. As the uterus grows or as the cervix dilates, more or less of the os may be covered by placenta.

      (2) **Risk factors** include increasing maternal age, increasing maternal parity, and prior uterine scarring from surgery.

   b. **Placental abruption (abruptio placentae, ablatio placentae,** or **accidental hemorrhage)** occurs when the placenta separates from the decidua basalis of the uterus beyond 20 weeks' gestation but prior to stage III of labor. Separation can be partial or complete. Vaginal bleeding may occur, or the hemorrhage may be concealed under the placenta away from the cervical os.

      (1) **Pathogenesis.** Abruption is associated with defective placental vasculature.

      (2) **Risk factors** include multiparity, increased maternal age, previous abruption, pregnancy-induced hypertension, a short umbilical cord, trauma, smoking, and cocaine abuse.

   c. **Molar pregnancy (hydatidiform mole)** is defined as placental proliferation without fetal tissues.

      (1) **Pathogenesis.** Hydatidiform mole is associated with chromosomal anomalies producing trophoblastic hyperplasia and vascular, grape-like chorionic villi. Hydatidiform mole carries the risk of subsequent choriocarcinoma.

      (2) **Risk factors** include maternal age greater than 40 years or less than 20 years.

2. **Clinical features**

   a. **Placenta previa.** Patients present with spontaneous, painless, bright red vaginal bleeding, either slight or profuse. Initial bleeding may cease suddenly, only to recur.

   b. **Placental abruption**

      (1) Sudden abdominal or pelvic pain is seen in 90% of patients; bleeding occurs in 80% of patients. Shock is variably present.

      (2) The uterus may be tender, hypertonic, or enlarged for gestational age (due to bleeding). Premature labor may be present. Fetal compromise is variably present.

   c. **Molar pregnancy.** Symptoms include painless vaginal bleeding, most commonly before 20 weeks' gestation. Uterine size is large for gestational age. Rarely, patients may exhibit symptoms of pre-eclampsia before they reach the 20-week gestation mark.

3. **Differential diagnoses** include trauma, blood dyscrasias and cirrhosis, and estrogen excess state.

4. **Evaluation**

   a. **Stabilization.** Maternal resuscitation is the highest priority. Once the patient's airway, breathing, and circulatory status have been stabilized, historical information should be obtained. Blood typing and screening (including ABO and Rh sensitivity), quantitative β-hCG studies, a CBC, and coagulation profile are sent immediately. Fetal monitoring is established as appropriate for gestational age.

   b. **Physical examination** of patients with second- or third-trimester bleeding should be performed in consultation with an obstetrician in the operating room to minimize the potential for hemorrhagic catastrophe.

    c. **Laboratory studies**
      (1) **Quantitative β-hCG levels** are abnormally high (500,000–1,000,000 mIU; the normal peak is 100,000 mIU) in molar pregnancy.
      (2) **Coagulation studies** may reveal low fibrinogen, diminished factors V and VIII, and a low platelet count in patients with placental abruption.
    d. **Ultrasonography.** Uterine ultrasound can make the distinction between placenta previa and placental abruption. Its use is paramount, especially in patients with second- or third-trimester bleeding, because complete pelvic examination is contraindicated in these patients until placenta previa and placental abruption are ruled out.
      (1) **Placenta previa.** Ultrasound is the diagnostic test of choice to document the location and extent of previa. The placental margin covers part or all of the os.
      (2) **Placental abruption.** Ultrasonography reveals retroplacental clots and fetal distress.
      (3) **Molar pregnancy.** Ultrasound is usually diagnostic, revealing a "snowstorm" intrauterine pattern and absence of fetal heart activity.

5. **Therapy**
    a. **Hemodynamically stable patients with no evidence of fetal distress.** Strict **bed rest** and **observation** with frequent fetal checks until the fetus reaches maturity are indicated for hemodynamically stable patients with no evidence of fetal distress, but who have ultrasonographic evidence of placenta previa or abruption. Fetal maturity is documented by dates, sonography, and amniotic phospholipid ratios [see VI B 1 c (2)].
    b. **Hemodynamically unstable patients with or without evidence of fetal distress. Aggressive fluid and blood resuscitation,** positioning of the mother in the **left lateral decubitus position,** and emergent delivery by **cesarean section** if the fetus is older than 24 weeks are indicated. A fetus younger than 24 weeks cannot survive outside of the uterus and is considered a second-trimester miscarriage. **Oxytocin** is administered after placental delivery to reduce further bleeding. **RhoGAM** is given to all Rh-negative mothers experiencing hemorrhage in pregnancy to prevent maternal Rh antibody formation and risk of hydrops fetalis with future pregnancy.
    c. **Molar pregnancy.** After sonographic documentation, dilatation and curettage is necessary to ensure complete removal, which reduces the risk of subsequent choriocarcinoma. Follow-up serial β-hCG levels should be obtained.

6. **Disposition.** Patients with second- or third-trimester bleeding should be admitted for further sonographic evaluation, fetal maturity studies, maternal–fetal monitoring, bed rest, and observation.

IV   HYPERTENSION IN PREGNANCY

A **Discussion**   Untreated hypertensive disorders are associated with fetal compromise resulting in growth retardation, progressive placental insufficiency, placental abruption, and fetal demise. Hypertension may complicate 10% of all pregnancies (20% of nulliparous pregnancies and 40% of twin gestations).

B **Clinical features**   The American College of Obstetrics and Gynecology (ACOG) has classified hypertensive disorders in pregnancy on the basis of the onset of clinical findings, associated symptoms, and previous (prepregnancy) hypertension.

1. **Gestational hypertension** occurs after the 20-week gestation mark. Patients develop a mean arterial pressure (MAP) greater than 100–106 mm Hg but have no associated edema or proteinuria. The blood pressure returns to baseline postpartum.

2. **Chronic hypertension** is defined by a blood pressure that exceeds 140/90 mm Hg or a MAP greater than 100–106 mm Hg that was present prepregnancy or before the 20-week gestation mark. Chronic hypertension is not associated with edema or proteinuria.

3. **Pre-eclampsia** is similar to worsened gestational hypertension. It is noted after the 20-week gestation mark and is associated with peripheral edema, proteinuria, and any of the following findings: hepatic dysfunction, hypoalbuminemia, coagulation abnormalities, hemoconcentration, or hyperuricemia. The disorder usually improves within 48 hours of delivery, but may persist for days to weeks.

   a. **Risk factors** include nulliparity, diabetes mellitus, multiple gestations, extremes of age, a family history of pre-eclampsia, hydrops fetalis, and hydatidiform mole. The rollover test can be used to predict the patient's risk of developing pre-eclampsia: beginning at 26–32 weeks, blood pressures are taken in the left lateral decubitus position and compared to those taken when the patient is supine. Ninety percent of patients with recurrent documented diastolic pressures greater than 15 mm Hg will develop pre-eclampsia.

   b. **Classification.** Pre-eclampsia is classified as follows:

      (1) **Mild pre-eclampsia** is characterized by recurrent, elevated diastolic pressures (i.e., greater than 15 mm Hg) before pregnancy or during the first trimester. The elevated blood pressures are accompanied by edema and proteinuria.

      (2) **Moderate pre-eclampsia.** A systolic pressure greater than 30 mm Hg and a diastolic pressure greater than 15 mm Hg are noted after 20 weeks' gestation. The elevated pressures are accompanied by significant edema of the lower extremities and proteinuria.

      (3) **Severe pre-eclampsia** is characterized by markedly elevated blood pressures (greater than 160/110 mm Hg) or a MAP that exceeds 120–126 mm Hg, generalized edema, and symptoms of headache, blurred vision, epigastric pain or tenderness, pulmonary edema, significant proteinuria (greater than 5 g/24 hours), and oliguria.

      (4) **Atypical pre-eclampsia** is severe pre-eclampsia complicated by HELLP syndrome (**h**emolytic anemia, **e**levated **l**iver enzymes, and **l**ow **p**latelet count). As the plasma volume is reduced, vasoconstriction (and, therefore, blood pressure) is enhanced.

4. **Pre-eclampsia superimposed on chronic hypertension.** Hypertension develops before the 20-week gestation mark and is accompanied by proteinuria and edema later in the pregnancy. This disorder is found in 10% of patients with hypertension despite continued treatment during pregnancy.

5. **Eclampsia** is severe pre-eclampsia complicated by generalized seizures. Eclampsia carries the risk of aspiration and maternal–fetal hypoxia.

C **Differential diagnoses**

1. **Chronic hypertension** caused by renal artery stenosis, chronic renal insufficiency, systemic lupus erythematosus (SLE), pheochromocytoma, primary aldosteronism, essential hypertension, and anxiety should be considered.

2. **Seizures.** In addition to being caused by eclampsia, generalized seizures can be caused by drugs, substance intoxication or withdrawal, epilepsy, cerebrovascular accident, or trauma.

D **Evaluation**

1. **Patient history.** Important questions to address include:

   a. What was the patient's prepregnancy or first-trimester blood pressure?

   b. Is the patient on an antihypertensive regimen?

   c. Has a cause for the patient's hypertension been identified?

   d. Has the patient noted progressive swelling of the feet or hands?

   e. Has the patient experienced headache, visual changes, or abdominal pain?

2. **Physical examination**

   a. **Vital signs.** A systolic pressure greater than 30 mm Hg and a diastolic pressure greater than 15 mm Hg above expected baseline should raise concern.

   b. **General examination.** Generalized, pitting edema may be noted, especially of the extremities and face. A petechial rash or ecchymosis suggests hepatic dysfunction.

    c. Ocular examination. Findings may range from the "retinal sheen" of pregnancy to arteriovenous nicking, "copper wire" arteries, or spot hemorrhages and exudates.

    d. Abdominal examination may reveal epigastric, right upper quadrant tenderness and ascites.

    e. Neurologic examination. The patient may have hyperreflexia.

3. Laboratory studies

    a. Blood work

      (1) A CBC may reveal an elevated hematocrit, suggesting hypovolemia and worsening of pre-eclampsia. A low platelet count (less than 100,000/μL) is suggestive of HELLP.

      (2) Smears may show evidence of hemolysis.

      (3) Elevated liver transaminases and lactic dehydrogenase (LDH) and a prolonged prothrombin time (PT) or partial thromboplastin time (PTT) are indicative of hepatic dysfunction in patients with severe pre-eclampsia.

    b. Urinalysis reveals significant proteinuria, more than 1 g/L with random collection.

E **Therapy**

1. Chronic hypertension. A careful balance must be maintained between controlling the blood pressure and minimizing the side effects and teratogenic risk of antihypertensive agents.

    a. Methyldopa, a central α-adrenergic agonist, reduces the effects of norepinephrine, thereby lowering arterial resistance without seriously affecting uterine blood flow.

      (1) Side effects include postural hypotension, depression, liver dysfunction, and hemolytic anemia.

      (2) Dose. The dose is 250–500 mg orally every 8 hours, to a maximum dose of 2 g/day.

    b. β Blockers cause arterial dilatation directly and are generally used in the second and third trimesters.

      (1) Side effects include a potential reduction in uterine blood flow, bronchospasm in patients with asthma, and hepatotoxicity.

      (2) Dose

        (a) Labetalol. The initial dose is 10 mg intravenously with subsequent doubling of the previous dose every 10 minutes until the desired pressure is attained or the maximum dose of 300 mg is reached.

        (b) Propranolol may be given orally, 20–40 mg every 6 hours.

    c. Hydralazine acts by direct vasodilatation and is usually given with methyldopa or a β blocker, because reflex tachycardia is a common complication of hydralazine use when it is used alone. Other side effects include headache, nausea, and diarrhea. The dose is 5 mg intravenously over 1–2 minutes, followed by 5- to 10-mg doses every 30 minutes to effect or until the maximum dose of 20 mg is reached. If the patient does not respond to hydralazine, a second agent (e.g., labetalol) is added.

    d. Diuretics, used in combination with methyldopa, reduce vascular volume and resistance. This regimen is recommended only for patients with pulmonary edema or congestive heart failure (CHF). **Furosemide** (10–20 mg intravenously every 6–12 hours) or **hydrochlorothiazide** (25–50 mg intravenously every 24 hours) may be used.

    e. Calcium channel blockers (e.g., **nifedipine**) have been used for short-term therapy with good results but are not currently recommended due to limited data.

    f. Angiotensin-converting enzyme (ACE) inhibitors have been shown to reduce uterine blood flow and are not recommended.

2. Pre-eclampsia. Definitive treatment is by **fetal delivery,** but treatment of maternal blood pressure and end-organ pathology prior to fetal maturity is paramount. The following regimens may be considered:

    a. Magnesium sulfate has a direct vasodilator effect as well as anticonvulsant properties and is usually reserved for patients with severe pre-eclampsia or those patients who are unresponsive to other regimens.

       (1) Dose. The loading dose is 4–6 g intravenously over 20 minutes, followed by 2–3 g/hour.

       (2) Side effects include those of hypermagnesemia (i.e., serum magnesium levels greater than 9 µg/dL): muscle relaxation and hyporeflexia. Hypermagnesemia can lead to depressed deep tendon reflexes and apnea. Treatment of magnesium toxicity is calcium gluconate, 1 g administered intravenously.

   b. Labetalol and **hydralazine** may be used as described for chronic hypertension (see IV E 1 b).

   c. Diazoxide, a direct arterial vasodilator, is considered for use in patients who are refractory to hydralazine. The dose is 30 mg intravenously every 5 minutes until the desired response is achieved.

   d. Diuretics are used only in patients with CHF or pulmonary edema.

   e. Sedation (to reduce patient activity, thereby reducing the blood pressure and seizure activity) may be appropriate. **Phenobarbital** (30–60 mg orally every 6 hours), **secobarbital** (100 mg orally each evening), or **hydroxyzine** (50–100 mg orally or intramuscularly every 6 hours) may be used.

3. Atypical pre-eclampsia

   a. Volume expansion is provided slowly to maintain urine output at 0.5–1 mL/kg/hour while avoiding volume overload and pulmonary edema.

   b. Albumin or **Plasmanate administration,** to maintain plasma volume, may be considered.

   c. Transfusion. In patients with severe thrombocytopenia (less than 20,000/dL), a platelet transfusion can be considered. Patients with coagulopathy may require fresh frozen plasma or plasmapheresis.

4. Eclampsia is managed acutely by maintaining adequate oxygenation and monitoring cardiovascular status. Fluid input and output are monitored carefully to avoid overload.

   a. Seizures are treated initially with a **benzodiazepine** (e.g., diazepam, 5–10 mg or midazolam, 2–5 mg intravenously) or a **barbiturate** (e.g., phenobarbital, 100–200 mg intravenously).

   b. When the convulsions have ceased, **magnesium sulfate infusion** is initiated as described in IV E 2 a (therapeutic levels are 4–7 mEq/L).

F | **Disposition**

1. Chronic hypertension. Patients with a history of chronic hypertension are screened for superimposed pre-eclampsia and admitted for blood pressure control as needed.

2. Pre-eclampsia. All patients displaying criteria for pre-eclampsia are admitted to obstetrics and screened for fetal growth retardation, oligohydramnios, and maternal end-organ damage.

3. Eclampsia. Patients require emergent treatment and admission to obstetrics for continued monitoring and treatment.

V | **EMERGENCY DELIVERY**

A | **Discussion**   Delivery in the ED may be indicated when a patient presents in labor with complete cervical dilatation and a fetal presenting part pressing on the perineal verge.

B | **Clinical features**   Cardinal movements of a vertex-presenting fetus include the following sequence: pelvic engagement, descent, flexion, internal rotation, extension, external rotation, and expulsion.

C | **Evaluation**   Examination of the fetal head, fontanelles, and cranial sutures serves to verify fetal position. Meconium-stained vaginal discharge suggests the strong possibility of fetal/newborn meconium aspiration.

D | **Therapy**

1. Countertraction of the head will allow a controlled progression, reducing risk of vaginal laceration. If the perineum is tearing, a midline or left mediolateral episiotomy is performed to reduce the risk of urethral or anal trauma.

2. Once the head is delivered, the infant's nasopharynx and hypopharynx must be suctioned. If meconium-stained vaginal discharge was noted, direct laryngoscopy may be necessary following delivery to remove meconium from the cords or trachea.

3. Gentle downward traction is applied to the head and neck together, allowing for anterior shoulder delivery. Upward traction is then applied to deliver the posterior shoulder.

4. The umbilical cord is clamped in two sites side by side and cut between the two clamps to prevent severe newborn or maternal hemorrhage.

5. The infant is dried, warmed, and stimulated. The physician should observe the infant for spontaneous respiratory efforts, color, heart rate, and muscle tone. If Apgar scores remain less than 6 after stimulation, bag-mask ventilation or intubation may be required.

6. The placenta delivers spontaneously within 30 minutes of fetal delivery. Placental structures should deliver intact; irregularity suggests retained contents.

7. All Rh-negative mothers are given a single intramuscular injection of RhoGAM to prevent maternal Rh antibody formation.

E **Disposition** All mothers are admitted to the Labor and Delivery unit for continued maternal and fetal monitoring. Newborns are evaluated by the pediatrician or neonatologist for admission to the neonatal intensive care unit (NICU) or to the nursery.

VI COMPLICATIONS OF PARTURITION

A **Approach to the pregnant patient with complications of labor** Upon presentation of a mother after 24 weeks' gestation, one is dealing with two patients. Both maternal and fetal monitoring are indicated, searching for potential hemodynamic compromise.

1. Maternal resuscitation is paramount to maintaining fetal stability—the greatest cause of fetal demise is failure to treat the mother first. Administration of supplemental oxygen, positioning in the left lateral decubitus position (to relieve cord compression, ensure venous return, and maximize placental perfusion), and establishment of peripheral intravenous access should be carried out immediately.

2. A blood type and screen, Rh sensitivity screen, and CBC should be sent as quickly as possible.

3. The fetal heart rate is recorded continuously. The normal basal rate is approximately 150 beats/min, with beat-to-beat variability. During uterine contractions, a quick return to the baseline rate should be observed after each contraction deceleration. Variable deceleration is a sign of head or cord compression, and late decelerations or persistent fetal bradycardia is a sign of fetal hypoxia.

4. Vaginal and cervical examinations are performed with sterile technique to reduce the risk of infection. The cervix is examined for effacement and dilatation and the fetal presenting part is checked for position relative to the cervix (station).

5. Fetal ultrasonography is useful in evaluating fetal activity, amniotic fluid volume, uterine anatomy, and placental abnormalities.

B **Complications of labor**

1. **Premature rupture of membranes**
   a. **Discussion.** Premature membrane rupture complicates less than 5% of pregnancies but **causes 30%–40% of premature births** (see V B 2). At term, 90% of mothers go into labor within 24 hours of membrane rupture. However, preterm rupture may not induce labor immediately and carries a **high risk of maternal and fetal infection** prior to delivery. Chorioamnionitis is a common complication that is directly related to both delay of labor onset and the number of digital cervical examinations the patient has undergone.

b. **Clinical findings.** The patient usually reports a sudden leak or gush of vaginal fluid. The fluid may be clear, cloudy (indicating the presence of pus), or green (indicating the presence of meconium). Symptoms of early infection may include malodorous, cloudy discharge, maternal fever, tachycardia, uterine tenderness, frequent contractions, and fetal distress.

c. **Evaluation**
  (1) Amniotic fluid will cause an **alkaline reaction on Nitrazine paper** (i.e., the color changes from yellow to blue), and **ferning** (i.e., the development of fern-like crystals) will be apparent when the fluid sample is smeared on a microscope slide.
  (2) If the gestational age is less than 38 weeks, amniotic phospholipid testing must be used to evaluate lung maturity. **Lecithin:sphingomyelin ratios** of less than 2.0 suggest pulmonary immaturity.

d. **Therapy**
  (1) **Antibiotic therapy.** Fever, tachycardia, malodorous vaginal discharge, and cervical or uterine tenderness all suggest chorioamnionitis and, therefore, antibiotic therapy may be appropriate. Prophylactic antibiotics are controversial but may be advocated to lengthen the latent interval prior to labor (in an attempt to give the fetus more time to mature).
  (2) **RhoGAM.** All Rh-negative mothers are given a single intramuscular injection of RhoGAM to prevent maternal Rh antibody formation.

2. **Premature labor**
  a. **Discussion.** Premature labor (i.e., preterm uterine contractions leading to progressive cervical effacement and dilatation) complicates 8%–10% of pregnancies and is associated with high neonatal morbidity and mortality rates. If the gestational age is less than 37 weeks, a cause must be identified and tocolysis considered if initial treatment fails to cease cervical dilatation. Causes include:
    (1) **Premature membrane rupture** (see VI B 1)
    (2) **Genitourinary tract infections**
    (3) **Placenta previa** or **placental abruption**
    (4) **Maternal hypertension**
    (5) **Diabetes mellitus** (long-standing or gestational)
    (6) **Uterine** or **fetal anomalies**
  b. **Clinical features.** Patients may complain of progressive frequency, intensity, and duration of contractions. Complaints of vaginal discharge or dysuria are possible. Vaginal bleeding or abdominal pain suggests placental previa or abruption.
  c. **Evaluation.** Preterm labor requires close maternal–fetal monitoring.
    (1) A maternal **leukocyte count with differential, urinalysis,** and **cervical culture** are obtained to screen for **infection.**
    (2) In patients with ruptured membranes and a gestational age of less than 38 weeks, **fetal lung maturity** should be evaluated using **phospholipid testing of amniotic fluid.**
  d. **Therapy**
    (1) **Supportive therapy** entails control of the underlying cause (e.g., hypertension, hyperglycemia).
    (2) **Corticosteroid therapy** may be required to enhance fetal lung maturity.
    (3) **Tocolysis** is not attempted without consultation with an obstetrician. Therapy consists of **β agonists** (e.g., terbutaline, 0.25–0.5 mg subcutaneously every 2 hours; ritodrine, 0.05 mg/min intravenously; or isoxsuprine, 10–20 mg intramuscularly every 2–4 hours), followed by **magnesium sulfate** (4–6 g administered as an intravenous load over 30 minutes and 3–6 g/hour as a maintenance infusion).
    (4) **RhoGAM.** All Rh-negative mothers are given a single intramuscular injection of RhoGAM to prevent maternal Rh antibody formation.

3. **Prolapsed umbilical cord**
   a. **Discussion.** Prolapse of the umbilical cord may occur with uterine contractions and low intrauterine volumes following membrane rupture. The cord may pass through the cervix before the fetal presenting part, causing cord compression and compromising fetal circulation.
   b. **Clinical findings.** The mother usually presents in labor after membrane rupture with increasingly frequent uterine contractions. The cord is noted on vaginal or cervical inspection. Deep variable decelerations or persistent bradycardia on fetal monitoring are concerning signs.
   c. **Therapy.** Prolapsed umbilical cord is an obstetric emergency. Observation of cord prolapse warrants prompt elevation of the presenting part and maternal positioning to the left lateral decubitus or knee–chest position. The examiner's hand must remain in position, maintaining countertraction until the fetus is delivered by **cesarean section.**

4. **Abnormal presentation**
   a. **Discussion**
      (1) **Shoulder dystocia** is a rare presentation, occurring in 0.5% of patients, in which the fetal shoulder breadth exceeds the anterior-posterior pelvic diameter. The fetal shoulder is caught behind the pelvic outlet, while the head is engaged or presenting, leading to fetal hypoxia. Retraction of the head after its delivery (the turtle sign) is highly suggestive.
      (2) **Breech** (i.e., presenting with the buttocks), **frank breech** (i.e., presenting with hip flexion and knee extension), **shoulder presentation,** and **transverse lie** are other abnormal presentations.
   b. **Therapy.** Shoulder dystocia is an obstetric emergency requiring emergent consultation.
      (1) **McRoberts maneuver** (i.e., hyperflexion of the mother's hips) and the **application of suprapubic pressure** are performed to dislodge the shoulder from under the pubic symphysis.
      (2) **Other procedures,** including **episioproctotomy, posterior shoulder delivery, Wood's maneuver** (i.e., axis rotation of the shoulders), or **Zavanelli maneuver** (i.e., restitution with cesarean section), may be performed with obstetric supervision.

5. **Postpartum hemorrhage**
   a. **Discussion.** Postpartum hemorrhage can be profuse and, in 90% of patients, is caused by uterine atony. Postpartum hemorrhage can also be caused by vaginal lacerations or retained placental structures.
   b. **Clinical features.** Complete inspection of the vault will reveal reparable lacerations. A soft, boggy uterus despite direct massage suggests atony.
   c. **Therapy**
      (1) Prompt fluid and blood resuscitation is indicated.
      (2) The patient should be examined for signs of vaginal trauma and any damage should be surgically repaired promptly.
      (3) Missing portions of the placenta suggest retained contents, which must be removed.
      (4) Direct palpation of the uterus may stimulate its contraction and reduce bleeding. Oxytocin (20–40 U in 0.9% NaCl) is infused over 30 minutes to stimulate uterine contraction. Methyl ergonovine (0.2 mg) or prostaglandins (250 µg administered intramuscularly) are also considered to enhance uterine contraction.

C **Disposition**   All mothers are admitted to the Labor and Delivery unit for continued maternal and fetal monitoring. Newborns are evaluated by the pediatrician or neonatologist for admission to the NICU or to the nursery.

VII   VAGINITIS, CERVICITIS, AND PELVIC INFLAMMATORY DISEASE

A **Vaginitis**

1. **Discussion.** Vaginitis is inflammation of the vulva and vaginal vault.
   a. **Predisposing factors** include multiple unprotected sexual exposures, high estrogen states (e.g., use of oral contraceptives, pregnancy), antibiotic use, and immunosuppression.

    b. **Etiology**
- (1) **Infection** is the leading cause of vaginitis.
  - (a) *Candida albicans,* a fungus, is not usually sexually transmitted.
  - (b) *Trichomonas vaginalis* is a sexually transmitted, protozoal infection involving the cervical and vaginal epithelium.
  - (c) **Gardnerella (Haemophilus) vaginalis,** a bacterium, is not generally sexually transmitted, although this infection is common in sexually active women. Symptoms occur when there is overgrowth of normal flora in the vaginal vault (e.g., in immunocompromised or diabetic patients).
- (2) **Foreign bodies** (e.g., tampons, sanitary napkins) may produce vaginal irritation and a malodorous discharge.
- (3) **Chemical irritation** (e.g., from medications, douches, perfume) can cause local irritation and acute tenderness during intercourse (dyspareunia). Physical examination may reveal an erythematous, inflamed vaginal vault without discharge or cervical motion tenderness.
- (4) **Reduced estrogen levels** in postmenopausal women result in a more friable vaginal mucosa, leading to **atrophic vaginitis** (characterized by pruritus, erythema, and tenderness).

2. **Clinical features.** Inflammation of the vulva and vaginal vault leads to itchy, tender, erythematous tissues and increased vaginal discharge. Patients may also complain of dyspareunia or dysuria. A thorough physical examination, including a rectal examination, should be performed.
    a. *C. albicans vaginitis* is characterized by a **"cheesy" discharge** on the cervix and in the vaginal vault. The patient may have mild cervical motion tenderness, but no uterine or adnexal tenderness.
    b. **Trichomoniasis.** Patients complain of a **thin, "frothy," malodorous discharge, vaginal pruritus, dysuria,** and **dyspareunia.** Examination reveals an erythematous, tender vagina and cervix (**"strawberry cervix"**).
    c. **Bacterial vaginitis.** Patients complain of a **thin, foul-smelling discharge, vaginal pruritus,** and **dyspareunia. Cervical motion tenderness** may be present.

3. **Differential diagnoses** include pinworm infection, acute cystitis, cervicitis, and sexually transmitted diseases (STDs), such as gonorrhea and chlamydia.

4. **Evaluation**
    a. **Patient history.** It is important to obtain a complete gynecologic and menstrual history.
    b. **Laboratory studies**
- (1) **Culture.** Vaginal and cervical discharge should be cultured and evaluated microscopically.
  - (a) **C. albicans vaginitis.** A potassium hydroxide (KOH) preparation, NaCl preparation, or Gram staining may reveal yeast buds.
  - (b) **Trichomoniasis.** A NaCl microscope slide preparation reveals round, flagellated, motile protozoa.
  - (c) **Bacterial vaginitis.** A NaCl preparation may reveal "clue" cells (i.e., epithelial cells studded with bacteria).
- (2) **Syphilis serologies** should be sent when a sexually transmitted agent is suspect.
- (3) **Urinalysis** (on a sample obtained by catheterization) **and culture** should be performed to rule out concurrent urinary tract involvement.

5. **Therapy**
    a. **Infectious vaginitis**
- (1) **Fungal vaginitis**
  - (a) **C. albicans vaginitis** is treated with **miconazole suppositories** (200 mg each evening for 3 days), **oral clotrimazole** (200 mg daily for 3 days), or **terconazole suppositories** (80 mg each evening for 3 days).
  - (b) **Other fungal agents of vaginitis** (e.g., *Torulopsis glabrata*) may be resistant to conventional antifungal agents. Yeast infections refractory to conventional therapy are treated with **gentian violet** (2% solution every other day for 10 days).

(2) Trichomoniasis is treated with **oral metronidazole** (2 g administered in a single dose). In pregnant patients, **clotrimazole suppositories** (inserted each evening for 7 days) are used; treatment with metronidazole may be initiated after delivery.

(3) Bacterial vaginitis is treated with **metronidazole** (2 g administered in a single oral dose or 250 mg orally every 8 hours for 7 days). Treatment with **clotrimazole suppositories** can be considered for pregnant patients with severe infections.

b. Foreign object vaginitis. Following **removal of the object,** a **povidone–iodine douche** should be administered.

c. Contact vaginitis is treated by terminating exposure to the offending agent.

d. Atrophic vaginitis is improved by applying **topical estrogen cream** daily for 5–10 days.

6. Disposition. All patients require follow-up with a gynecologist within 24–48 hours of evaluation in the ED.

B Cervicitis

1. Discussion. Cervicitis involves inflammation of the cervix, producing dyspareunia and cervical motion tenderness on examination. The infectious agents responsible for vaginitis can also cause concomitant cervicitis. In addition, the following micro-organisms can cause cervicitis:

a. *Neisseria gonorrhoeae* is a Gram-negative diplococcus that infects up to 90% of patients after a single sexual encounter with an infected partner.

b. *Chlamydia trachomatis,* the most common sexually transmitted organism in the United States, is an obligate, intracellular bacterium. It may cause cervicitis (nongonococcal cervicitis) as it "ascends" the reproductive tract, producing acute PID (see VII C).

c. Herpes simplex virus (HSV) is a DNA virus of two serotypes. Type 2 is predominantly associated with genital lesions, although type 1, more commonly causing stomatitis, may be found in 20% of patients. Transmission is via direct mucous membrane contact, most commonly sexual.

2. Clinical features

a. Gonococcal cervicitis. The incubation period is 2–5 days, although up to 75% of patients with gonococcal cervicitis are asymptomatic for many months. Patients with symptoms note abnormal vaginal discharge, lower abdominal pain, and dyspareunia. Examination reveals a yellowish, mucopurulent discharge from the cervix and tenderness on digital manipulation. No adnexal tenderness is noted.

b. Nongonococcal cervicitis. The incubation period for *Chlamydia* is 6–21 days, and 60%–70% of patients may have an asymptomatic "latent" period. Patients with acute cervicitis may complain of an abnormal vaginal discharge. Examination reveals an erythematous, friable cervix with motion tenderness.

c. Viral cervicitis. Most patients have localized lesions involving the vulvovaginal and cervical region. The development of hyperesthetic tissues and red, papular eruptions, which evolve into ulcerating vesicles that eventually crust and heal, occurs after an incubation period of 3–7 days. Constitutional symptoms include malaise, fever, myalgias, and headache. Herpetic lesions are exquisitely tender to touch, making pelvic examination difficult. Symptoms may persist for 7–20 days with gradual resolution.

3. Differential diagnoses include bacterial or protozoal vaginosis, PID, and cervical cancer.

4. Evaluation

a. Gonococcal cervicitis. Gram stain of the discharge may show Gram-negative intracellular and extracellular diplococci.

b. Nongonococcal cervicitis. Gram stain of the discharge is rarely revealing. Diagnosis is usually confirmed with a cervical culture. Over 90% of patients with chlamydial cervical infection will have concomitant gonococcal infection.

c. Viral cervicitis. Tzanck smear of an ulcer crater may reveal multinucleated giant cells.

5. **Therapy.** Appropriate regimens for gonococcal infection followed by chlamydial infection include the following:

   a. Ceftriaxone, 125 mg in one intramuscular dose plus doxycycline (100 mg orally every 12 hours for 7 days) *or* tetracycline or erythromycin (500 mg orally every 6 hours for 7 days) can be used. Doxycycline should be avoided in pregnant women.

   b. Ciprofloxacin or ofloxacin, 500 mg administered in a single oral dose, followed by azithromycin, 1 g administered in a single oral dose, can be used.

   c. Spectinomycin (2 g) can be administered in a single, intramuscular injection followed by doxycycline.

C PELVIC INFLAMMATORY DISEASE (PID)

1. **Discussion.** PID is an ascending infection (from the lower genital tract) that involves acute infection of the uterus and fallopian tube. PID rarely occurs during pregnancy because the cervical mucus plug prevents infection from traveling beyond the cervix.

   a. **Incidence.** The incidence is 1 in 100 women of childbearing age (i.e., between the ages of 15 and 40).

   b. **Risk factors** include unprotected intercourse, multiple partners, prior infection, pelvic procedures (e.g., dilatation and curettage), and IUD use.

   c. **Etiology.** Over 75% of infections are sexually transmitted. Causative organisms include *C. trachomatis, N. gonorrhoeae,* and *Mycoplasma hominis.* Normal vaginal flora may also ascend through the cervix, causing symptoms.

   d. **Complications** include infertility (20% risk after first infection), ectopic pregnancy, recurrent infection, and chronic pelvic pain. PID may also be complicated by gonococcal perihepatitis (Fitz-Hugh–Curtis syndrome) or the development of tubo-ovarian abscess.

2. **Clinical features.** PID is characterized by vague, lower abdominal pain with diffuse cervical, uterine, and adnexal tenderness. A vaginal or cervical discharge and a fever may also be noted.

3. **Differential diagnoses** include pyelonephritis, appendicitis, ovarian cyst, ovarian torsion, endometritis, enteritis, inflammatory bowel disease, cholecystitis, and diverticulitis.

4. **Evaluation.** Standardized criteria are in place to make a correct diagnosis of PID.

   a. All of the following must be found on physical examination: lower abdominal tenderness, cervical motion tenderness, and unilateral or bilateral adnexal tenderness

   b. One of the following must also exist:

      (1) Body temperature higher than 38°C

      (2) Leukocyte count greater than 10,000/μL

      (3) Mucopurulent discharge on culdocentesis or laparoscopy

      (4) Inflammatory mass on examination or ultrasound

      (5) Evidence of endocervical *C. trachomatis* infection on a monoclonal antibody screen or *N. gonorrhoeae* infection on Gram stain

5. **Therapy**

   a. **Outpatient therapy.** Appropriate regimens include:

      (1) Ceftriaxone, 125 mg administered in a single, intramuscular injection plus doxycycline

      (2) Cefoxitin, 2 g administered in a single intramuscular injection plus probenecid, 1 g administered in a single oral dose and doxycycline

      (3) Ciprofloxacin or ofloxacin, 500 mg administered in a single oral dose plus doxycycline, 100 mg administered orally every 12 hours for 10–14 days or tetracycline, 500 mg administered orally every 6 hours for 10–14 days

   b. **Inpatient therapy.** Appropriate regimens include:

      (1) A cephalosporin (e.g., ceftriaxone, 1 g every 24 hours; cefotetan, 2 g every 12 hours; ceftizoxime or cefotaxime, 1 g every 8 hours; or cefoxitin, 2 g every 6 hours) plus doxycycline (100 mg every 12 hours) administered intravenously.

      (2) Clindamycin (900 mg every 8 hours) plus gentamicin (an initial loading dose of 2 mg/kg followed by a maintenance infusion of 1.5 mg/kg every 8 hours intravenously)

6. **Disposition.** Admission criteria include severe, systemic toxicity; an inability to tolerate oral antibiotic or pain medications; an inability to rule out a surgical disease process; suspected tubo-ovarian abscess; failed outpatient treatment; and concomitant pregnancy. Inpatient therapy should be considered for patients who have no history of PID and for infected nulliparous patients who desire pregnancy at a later date.

VIII   ABNORMAL VAGINAL BLEEDING IN NONPREGNANT PATIENTS

A **Discussion**   Bleeding that differs in cyclic interval, duration, or flow from the patient's normal menstrual pattern must be evaluated. Infection, trauma, or hormonal imbalances may explain bleeding in premenarchal girls. Causes of abnormal vaginal bleeding in nonpregnant patients include:

1. **Bleeding disorders**

2. **Trophoblastic disease (molar pregnancy)**

3. **Trauma** to genital structures may occur from straddle injuries, coitus, vaginal delivery, self-manipulation, or sexual assault. Perineal or periurethral ecchymosis or vaginal vault or perianal lacerations, abrasions, and excoriations should raise suspicion.

4. **Neoplasia,** either benign or malignant, can cause significant bleeding. The most common sites are the cervix, uterus, and ovary.
   a. **Malignant neoplasia.** Malignancy is most common in older patients.
      (1) **Cervical cancer** has a prevalence of 1 per 1000 women and carries a high mortality rate if left untreated. It is difficult to distinguish the lesions of cervical cancer from those caused by infection. Risk factors include unprotected intercourse and multiple partners.
      (2) **Endometrial carcinoma.** Although more common in perimenopausal women, endometrial carcinoma has a 25% incidence in the reproductive age group. Diabetes mellitus, hypertension, obesity, and history of anovulation are risk factors.
      (3) **Ovarian carcinoma** is most common in postmenopausal women. Common symptoms include abnormal vaginal bleeding, increased abdominal girth, and weight loss. Endometrial hyperplasia may be present due to hormone excess from the tumor. A palpable mass is highly suggestive.
   b. **Benign neoplasia**
      (1) **Cervical polyps** may produce metrorrhagia (i.e., noncyclic bleeding), especially after intercourse. The polyps are red, ulcerated lesions that protrude from the cervical os. They rarely become malignant.
      (2) **Uterine leiomyomas (fibroids)** are benign lesions affecting 20% of women older than 35 years. Submucosal or interstitial lesions commonly cause menorrhagia (i.e., painfully prolonged or heavy menses). Fibroids may be palpated during pelvic examination.
      (3) **Adenomyosis,** more common in older women, results in hyperplastic, benign, globular infiltration of the myometrium, producing heavy menses, dysmenorrhea, local uterine enlargement, and tenderness.

5. **Ovarian cysts** can result from anovulatory cycles (follicular cysts) or occur following ovulation (luteal cysts).
   a. **Follicular cysts** enlarge due to continued hormonal stimulation as a result of failed ovulation. They are usually multiple, bilateral, and associated with endometrial hyperplasia (leading to breakthrough bleeding).
   b. **Luteal cysts** may persist long after successful conceptus implantation. Continued hormonal secretion from the cyst maintains an amenorrheic state. Cyst enlargement and hemorrhage can occur, producing a tender, adnexal mass or peritonitis from cyst rupture. Symptoms may mimic those of ectopic pregnancy; however, a β-hCG screen will be negative.

6. **IUD use** may cause irregular and/or excessive bleeding due to local inflammation or erosion of an endometrial vessel.

7. **Endogenous** or **exogenous anovulation** may cause **dysfunctional uterine bleeding.**
   a. **Endogenous anovulation** is caused by unopposed estrogen inducing endometrial hyperplasia. These patients may be amenorrheic for several months followed by episodes of moderate to heavy breakthrough bleeding. Estrogen excess may be due to central hypothalamic or pituitary dysfunction, satellite tumor secretion, or androgen aromatization (seen in some patients with liver disease).
   b. **Exogenous anovulation** can be caused by failure to comply with an oral contraceptive regimen. Variable hormone levels are attained with different oral contraceptive preparations. Hormone excess or deficiency may induce endometrial hyperplasia or withdrawal bleeding.

B **Clinical features**   Use of an increased number of tampons or the passage of blood clots suggests an abnormality. Changes in the nature of menstrual cramping also increase suspicion of a pathologic process.

C **Differential diagnoses** include pregnancy, endometriosis, molar pregnancy, cystitis, bladder tumor, hemorrhoids, diverticulosis, hemorrhagic enteritis, inflammatory bowel disease, gastrointestinal tumors, bleeding disorders, liver diseases, and hypertension.

D **Evaluation**

1. **Stabilization.** Attention should be directed to the patient's airway, respiratory, and cardiovascular status, and shock should be treated before making a diagnosis.

2. **Patient history.** After initial resuscitation, a detailed gynecologic history should be obtained:
   a. When was the patient's last "normal" period and the period prior to that?
   b. What is different regarding this episode?
   c. When was the patient's most recent sexual contact?
   d. Which, if any, contraceptive method does the patient use?

3. **Physical examination.** The presence of clotting blood (abrupt, acute hemorrhage) and vaginal or cervical lesions should be noted during the pelvic examination. An open internal cervical os suggests a uterine process. Is the uterus firm, tender, or enlarged? Is a mass or tenderness noted in the adnexa? Is there cul-de-sac tenderness, a palpable mass, or bloody stool on rectal examination?

4. **Laboratory studies**
   a. **Blood work.** A blood type and screen, CBC, coagulation profile, and β-hCG should be sent immediately.
   b. **Urinalysis.** A urine specimen should be obtained via catheterization (to avoid contamination with vaginal flora).
   c. **Vaginal** and **cervical cultures** and a **Papanicolaou smear** are sent from the ED.

5. **Other diagnostic tools**
   a. **Ultrasound** may be helpful in locating a pelvic mass or free pelvic fluid.
   b. **Culdocentesis** is reserved for the hemodynamically unstable patient who cannot wait for an ultrasound. The procedure should be performed with gynecologic consultation.
   c. **Biopsy.** Hemodynamically stable patients with identified sources of hemorrhage may have the lesion biopsied in the ED with close gynecologic follow-up.

E **Therapy**

1. **Acute therapy**
   a. Hypotensive patients are resuscitated using a **crystalloid solution** (0.9% sodium chloride or lactated Ringer's solution). A fluid bolus of 20 mL/kg is provided and repeated if the patient's blood pressure has not improved.
   b. **Blood products** are infused if the hypotension is refractory to crystalloid infusion. Blood type O Rh-negative is infused if type-specific products are pending (i.e., not yet available). Boluses of 10 mL/kg are infused and titrated to the desired pressure.

2. **Definitive therapy**
   a. **Ruptured ovarian cysts** require operative repair to terminate severe bleeding.
   b. **Intra-abdominal hemorrhage.** All patients with significant hemodynamic compromise and examination findings consistent with intra-abdominal hemorrhage are taken to the operating room without delay.
   c. **Uterine leiomyomas.** Dilatation and curettage may be required. All material removed is evaluated for dysplasia or malignant changes.
   d. **Dysfunctional uterine bleeding** may require curettage followed by prophylactic hormone therapy. Such a regimen should be chosen with gynecologic consultation.
   e. **Exogenous anovulation.** Hemodynamically stable patients with minimal bleeding may receive progesterone in oil (100 mg administered intramuscularly) to stabilize the endometrium. Administration of progesterone in oil will be followed by a shortened period of withdrawal bleeding. This therapy is performed only after gynecologic consultation and adequate follow-up have been arranged.

F **Disposition**

1. Hemodynamically unstable patients are admitted to the Gynecology service for observation and work-up.

2. Hemodynamically stable patients with no evidence of surgical emergency or continued bleeding may be discharged. Follow-up with a gynecologist within 24 hours should be arranged.

IX **AMENORRHEA**

A **Discussion**

1. **Types**
   a. **Primary amenorrhea** is present when a woman never experiences menarche.
   b. **Secondary amenorrhea** is present when a woman with a previous history of periodic menses misses menses for more than 6 months.

2. **Etiology.** There are three broad causes of amenorrhea—anatomic defects, ovarian failure, and chronic anovulation.
   a. **Anatomic defects**
      (1) **Vaginal defects** include **imperforate hymen, transverse vaginal septae, vaginal hypoplasia** (müllerian agenesis, seen in the XX karyotype), and **blind vagina** (occurring in XY genetic males with testicular feminization or agenesis).
      (2) **Uterine defects** include cervical stenosis or endometrial scarring and destruction from curettage (Asherman's syndrome).
   b. **Ovarian failure**
      (1) **Genetic defects,** such as **Turner's syndrome** (gonadal dysgenesis and an absence of germ cells seen in XO genetic females) and **X chromosomal mosaicism** can cause amenorrhea.
      (2) **Resistant ovaries.** The ovarian follicles are arrested in development and resistant to follicle-stimulating hormone (FSH).
      (3) **Infection** or **environmental processes** in utero may cause gonadal streak destruction.
      (4) **Chemotherapy** or **radiation therapy** for malignancy may destroy germ cells.
      (5) **Autoimmune phenomena** can produce polyglandular failure in otherwise normal women, producing premature menopause as well as adrenal insufficiency and hypothyroidism.
   c. **Chronic anovulation**
      (1) **Estrogen-sufficient patients** experience withdrawal bleeding in the presence of progesterone therapy.
         (a) **Polycystic ovarian disease** may account for chronic anovulation despite estrogen presence. Menarche occurs on time but the irregular onset, duration, and amount of bleeding eventually culminate in amenorrhea. Patients have high adrenal and ovarian

estrogen levels. These estrogens stimulate the release of luteinizing hormone (LH) but suppress FSH, resulting in ovarian stromal proliferation without follicular development. The ovaries become sclerotic with multiple "frozen" follicles in various stages of atresia.

    (b) Ovarian tumors may also produce excessive estrogen and androgens, causing amenorrhea, and therefore appear clinically similar to polycystic ovarian disease.

  (2) Estrogen-insufficient patients fail to have withdrawal bleeding in the presence of progesterone therapy. These patients often have underlying hypothalamic–pituitary dysfunction. **Hypothalamic destruction** by **tumor, infection, central nervous system (CNS) trauma,** or **radiation therapy** can lead to impaired synthesis or release of luteinizing hormone–releasing hormone (LHRH).

  (3) Functional causes, including **anxiety, depression, grief reaction,** and **excessive weight loss,** can lead to altered hormone release and amenorrhea.

B Clinical features

1. **Anatomic defects**
   a. Women with imperforate hymen or transverse vaginal septae may have cyclic, predictable lower abdominal cramping but no bloody show (as a result of blood accumulating behind the obstruction).
   b. Patients with müllerian agenesis experience normal ovulation and have a functional endometrium, but the associated vaginal hypoplasia prevents menstruation. One third of such patients will also have urologic or spinal abnormalities.
   c. Patients with testicular feminization or agenesis have a blind vagina and no uterus but exhibit female breasts and paucity of pubic hair.

2. **Ovarian failure.** Patients with Turner's syndrome have short stature, a webbed neck, shield chest, and cardiovascular problems.

3. **Chronic anovulation**
   a. **Polycystic ovarian disease.** Circulating androgens produce excessive body hair (hirsutism). Obesity may be factorial in enhancing extraglandular estrogen levels.
   b. **Mass effect** or **trauma** may cause headache or visual field deficits.

C Differential diagnoses include pregnancy and total abdominal hysterectomy with bilateral oophorectomy.

D Evaluation

1. **Patient history.** An extensive gynecologic, obstetric, and medical history should be obtained.

2. **Physical examination.** Attention should be directed toward breast development, maturity, and the presence and quality of the vaginal discharge. Does the patient have pubic and axillary hair? Are the external genitalia fully developed? Is there evidence of an anatomic defect (e.g., imperforate hymen, cervical scarring)? Does the patient have a uterus?

3. **Laboratory studies**
   a. **Pregnancy testing** is paramount in all patients.
   b. **Serum estrogen** and **prolactin levels** may be sent to determine the need for a progestogen trial, estrogen plus progestogen therapy, and/or CNS work-up for a tumor. (These studies are performed at a later date by a specialist.)

4. **Other diagnostic tools**
   a. **Ultrasonography** may demonstrate abnormal reproductive organs, including polycystic ovaries.
   b. **Computed tomography (CT).** A history of headache, sinus pressure, or visual changes may warrant a head CT to rule out a pituitary mass lesion.

E **Therapy**

1. **Anatomic barriers** may be surgically corrected.

2. **Hypothalamic–pituitary disorders** (e.g., neoplasia) are treated with bromocriptine and/or surgical excision.

3. **Polycystic ovarian disease.** Goals include:

   a. Decreasing ovarian androgen production (with oral contraceptive regimens or ovarian wedge resection)

   b. Decreasing peripheral estrogen production (with weight reduction)

   c. Enhancing FSH secretion (with clomiphene or gonadorelin)

4. **Ovarian tumors** are treated with chemotherapy, surgical excision, or both, reducing the clinical features of polycystic ovarian disease.

5. **Functional causes** of chronic anovulation may be treated with reduction of stress, improved diet, and limited exercise.

F **Disposition**   All patients must be referred to a gynecologist or reproductive endocrinologist for follow-up on the tests drawn in the ED, and for further evaluation and treatment. CNS mass lesions require immediate neurosurgical consultation and admission.

X   SEXUAL ASSAULT

A **Discussion**

1. **Definitions**

   a. **Criminal sexual assault** is defined as genital, anal, or oral penetration by a part of the accused's body or by an object without the victim's consent.

   b. **Aggravated criminal sexual assault** occurs when force, physical violence causing bodily harm, or a threat of physical violence is used.

2. **Incidence.** The National Crime Victimization Survey, published in August 1995, estimates that 500,000 women and 50,000 men are sexually assaulted annually. However, many victims refuse or postpone medical care after assault. Physicians are obligated to report all cases of child and adolescent sexual assault to local police or protective services.

B **Clinical features**   When patients admit to sexual assault, they have been victimized. Patients may be incapable of admitting that they have been assaulted. **Somatic symptoms** suggestive of sexual assault may include anxiety, agitation, vomiting, diarrhea, sweating, palpitations, chest discomfort, dyspnea, abdominal pain, and focal or diffuse weakness. Family or friends may describe the patient as exhibiting **"bizarre behavior"** (e.g., amnesia, emotional lability or flat affect, mood swings, flashbacks, or traumatic stress symptoms).

C **Evaluation**   The first priority when evaluating a victim of sexual assault is to assess the patient's overall medical and psychological status. The second priority is to procure and preserve physical evidence.

1. **Stabilization.** Victims of sexual assault may have other internal injuries. Therefore, immediate attention should be directed toward stabilizing the patient's airway, respiratory, hemodynamic, and neurologic status.

2. **Patient history.** A thorough patient history (including a medical, drug, obstetric, and gynecologic history) must be obtained. Important questions to ask include the following:

   a. Does the patient have any allergies?

   b. When was the patient's last tetanus immunization?

    c. When was the date of the patient's last menstrual period?

    d. Has the patient ever been diagnosed as having an STD?

    e. What contraceptive method, if any, has been used?

    f. When was the patient's last sexual encounter?

    g. Did the patient voluntarily use drugs or alcohol prior to the assault?

    h. Has the patient bathed, urinated, defecated, or taken any drugs since the assault?

    i. When and where did the assault take place?

    j. How many attackers made physical contact with the patient?

    k. What acts were involved (e.g., kissing; fondling; attempted oral, vaginal, or anal penetration; ejaculation)?

    l. Did the attacker spit, bleed, urinate, or defecate on the victim?

    m. Did the attacker use force? Were restraints, a weapon, or another object used? How?

3. **Physical examination.** A physical examination must be performed within 72 hours of the assault in order to yield legally valid evidence. Positive and negative findings should be noted. The state **Rape Kit Protocol** is used to properly document and maintain evidence of the assault. The results are not available for physician use; therefore, one must anticipate the need for duplicate samples for clinical care.

    a. **Sample collection.** The following samples are collected: the patient's clothing; blood samples for blood type and DNA analysis; saliva samples for prostatic acid phosphatase analysis; fingernail scrapings; vaginal, cervical, and anal swabs; and pubic (and other hair) combings.

    b. **Wood's light inspection** of the skin should be performed to detect semen on the skin.

    c. **Documentation of physical injuries.** All physical injuries are assessed and documented using a traumagram to depict their location. A written description of the size, color, and location of all wounds should accompany the traumagram.

4. **Laboratory studies**

    a. **Testing for STDs**

        (1) The Centers for Disease Control and Prevention (CDC) recommends that all patients be tested for **gonorrhea, chlamydia, trichomoniasis, bacterial vaginosis,** and **syphilis.**

        (2) Testing for *Giardia lamblia* and *Entamoeba histolytica* infection is suggested when anal penetration has occurred.

        (3) Screening for **hepatitis B** viral antigen or antibody must also be considered.

        (4) Although the CDC notes that the risk of **HIV** transmission from sexual assault is low, cases have been well documented. Baseline testing is part of the rape protocol in some states. If an HIV test is performed, follow-up testing and counseling must be arranged. Repeated testing occurs at 3, 6, and 12 months.

    b. **Pregnancy testing.** Women of childbearing age must have a pregnancy test during the evaluation.

D Treatment

1. **Treatment** and **prophylactic therapy for STDs and HIV** should be initiated (e.g., arrangements for outpatient vaccination with hepatitis B immunoglobulin should be made) with consideration of postexposure HIV prophylaxis after counseling of the risks and benefits.

2. **Pregnancy prophylaxis.** If the patient was not pregnant prior to the assault, counseling is indicated for postcoital contraceptive medication. Prophylactic regimens are 97% effective if initiated within 24 hours of the assault. Regimens include **ethinyl estradiol-norgestrel** (2–4 tablets administered orally and repeated in 12 hours) or **conjugated estrogens** (30 mg administered orally daily for 5 days or 50 mg administered intravenously daily for 2 days).

E **Disposition**

1. Women are referred to a gynecologist for follow-up on the culture screens and examination findings. STD screening performed during the initial evaluation and compared to follow-up screening results will differentiate pre-existing infection from that resulting from the assault.

2. Men are referred to an internist.

3. **Counseling.** Arrangements should be made to have the victim evaluated and counseled by appropriate mental health and psychological support agencies.

4. **Law enforcement.** Appropriate agencies should be contacted early in the evaluation as required by law to report victims of violent crime.

Study Questions

Directions: Each of the numbered items or incomplete statements in this section is followed by answers or by completions of the statement. Select the ONE lettered answer or completion that is BEST in each case.

1. A 34-year-old nulliparous woman comes to the emergency department (ED) complaining of abdominal cramping that has been present for the past 2 days and spotting that started 6 hours previously. The patient's last menstrual period (LMP) was 12 weeks ago. The menses prior to that occurred 4 weeks earlier and was normal. The patient's vital signs are stable and she is not orthostatic. There is suprapubic tenderness on abdominal examination. Pelvic examination reveals a small amount of cervical bleeding, but the os is closed. Tenderness is noted in the left adnexa. No mass is palpated. The patient states that she and her husband have attended an infertility clinic for 6 months and that 3 months prior to the onset of symptoms, she began taking a new medication. A urine β-human chorionic gonadotropin (β-hCG) screen is positive, and the quantitative level is 1200 mIU (suggesting a gestation of 5 weeks). A transvaginal sonogram reveals a dual sac in the uterus consistent with an intrauterine pregnancy of 5 weeks' gestation. What is the most likely diagnosis?

- **A** Inevitable miscarriage
- **B** Molar pregnancy
- **C** Threatened miscarriage
- **D** Ectopic pregnancy
- **E** Torsed ovary

2. A 21-year-old woman is brought to the emergency department (ED) because she has been experiencing abdominal pain for the past 12 hours that has been getting progressively worse. The date of her last menstrual period (LMP) was 8 weeks ago. The patient is found by the paramedics to be pale and lethargic, with a systolic blood pressure of 70 mm Hg. Upon arrival in the ED, her blood pressure is unchanged. The patient's abdomen is distended and rigid with percussion tenderness. What is the most likely diagnosis?

- **A** Threatened miscarriage
- **B** Intrauterine pregnancy
- **C** Ectopic pregnancy
- **D** Incomplete miscarriage
- **E** Torsed ovary

3. A 17-year-old primigravida, determined to be at 16 weeks' gestation by dates and ultrasound, complains of an itchy, abnormal vaginal discharge. She denies pain, bleeding, or dysuria. Examination reveals no fever and no abdominal findings, but a thin, watery vaginal discharge is present and the cervix is erythematous and tender. The cervical os is closed. The uterus is grapefruit-sized and nontender. There is no adnexal tenderness. Microscopic evaluation reveals a motile organism. What is the most likely diagnosis?

- **A** Pelvic inflammatory disease (PID)
- **B** Bacterial vaginosis
- **C** Foreign body
- **D** Trichomoniasis
- **E** Gonorrhea

4. A 28-year-old multiparous woman, at 30 weeks' gestation by dates, arrives in the emergency department (ED) because she is concerned about the sudden onset of bright red vaginal bleeding and the passage of blood clots. She denies a history of trauma or pain. Her vital signs are stable on arrival. How should the emergency physician proceed?

[A] An immediate and thorough pelvic examination is indicated.
[B] Vaginal delivery should be induced.
[C] A cesarean section should be performed.
[D] The patient should be transferred to the operating room to undergo examination.
[E] The patient should be referred to an obstetrician.

5. A 40-year-old mother, determined to be at 30 weeks' gestation by an ultrasound performed 5 days previously, arrives in the emergency department (ED) because she is alarmed by the sudden onset of an abnormal vaginal discharge. The patient has been healthy and has had no complications associated with the pregnancy. Her vital signs are stable. Examination reveals thin, clear vaginal fluid in the vault and a closed cervical os. A Nitrazine test is positive. Ferning is noted microscopically. Fetal monitoring reveals a normal heart rate range with good beat-to-beat variability. What is the appropriate next step?

[A] Phospholipid screening and admission for immediate delivery
[B] Phospholipid screening, cervical cultures, and admission for fetal monitoring
[C] Phospholipid screening, cervical cultures, and follow-up with the onset of uterine contractions
[D] Cervical cultures, antibiotics, and admission for fetal monitoring
[E] Cervical cultures, fetal monitoring, and discharge

6. A 21-year-old college coed comes to the emergency department (ED) complaining of fever, abdominal pain, and an abnormal vaginal discharge that has been present for 2 days. She has lost her appetite and is even refusing fluids because of the pain. Her last menstrual period (LMP) was 1 week ago and on time. She has never been pregnant or had any vaginal infections. She is sexually active with one partner and uses oral contraceptives. Examination reveals a fever of 39°C and lower abdominal tenderness, but no peritoneal signs. Mucopurulent cervical discharge is noted from a closed os that is exquisitely tender. Marked bilateral adnexal tenderness is also appreciated. The pregnancy test is negative. Her leukocyte count is 15,000/μL. Gram stain of the discharge reveals no bacteria. What is the most likely diagnosis and appropriate management?

[A] Cervicitis; outpatient oral antibiotics and follow-up
[B] Pelvic inflammatory disease (PID); inpatient intravenous antibiotics
[C] PID; outpatient oral antibiotics and follow-up
[D] Salpingitis; intravenous antibiotics in the ED followed by an outpatient oral regimen and follow-up
[E] Salpingitis; outpatient oral antibiotics and follow-up

7. A 35-year-old pregnant woman, determined to be at 40 weeks' gestation by dates and ultrasound, presents in active labor. She reports that a sudden "gush" of a greenish, watery vaginal discharge occurred several hours before arrival. Examination reveals fetal head presentation, bulging the perineum. What is the most appropriate action for the physician to take at this time?

[A] Applying countertraction to the baby's head
[B] Performing an episiotomy
[C] Having the patient transferred to the Labor and Delivery suite
[D] Suctioning the neonatal nasopharynx and pharynx
[E] Asking the mother to push

8. A healthy, 30-year-old pregnant woman, determined to be at 31 weeks' gestation by dates and ultrasound, presents to the emergency department (ED) because she has been experiencing progressive headaches, blurred vision, and upper abdominal pain for 7 days. She also complains that her wedding ring no longer fits, and her shoes seem to be too tight. Examination reveals a blood pressure of 140/110 mm Hg, retinal arteriovenous nicking, mild epigastric abdominal tenderness, and diffuse, pitting edema. What is the clinical diagnosis and treatment?

[A] Mild pre-eclampsia; begin therapy with methyldopa and arrange for outpatient follow-up.
[B] Moderate pre-eclampsia; begin therapy with magnesium sulfate and labetalol or hydralazine and admit.

C Severe pre-eclampsia; begin therapy with magnesium sulfate and labetalol or hydralazine and admit.

D Pre-eclampsia; begin therapy with magnesium sulfate, hydralazine, and furosemide and admit.

E Eclampsia; begin therapy with magnesium sulfate, hydralazine, and furosemide and admit.

9. A 35-year-old mother of two arrives complaining of vision problems. The patient states that she has been well until 3 mornings ago, when she says she "woke up seeing double." The patient denies blurred vision, loss of vision, headache, and other focal neurologic findings. Her past medical history is notable for a lack of menstrual periods for the last 6 months. Her pregnancies were uncomplicated. "Tunnel vision" (loss of peripheral vision) is noted on ocular examination. The patient visited her gynecologist last week and had "some blood tests drawn"; the results of the tests are obtained and reveal that the patient has low prolactin, estrogen, and gonadotropin levels. What is the most likely diagnosis?

A Genetic defect

B Tumor

C Asherman's syndrome

D Polycystic ovarian disease

E Pregnancy

10. An 18-year-old college coed is brought to the emergency department (ED) on a Sunday night by her roommate. The roommate says that the patient has been acting "strange." The roommate had gone home for the weekend and had returned to find the patient crying on the floor. The patient is subdued, distracted, and intermittently tearful, and has said repeatedly, "I want to get tested. He touched me." What is the most appropriate course of action?

A Psychiatric consultation in a quiet area

B Complete pelvic examination with rape protocol

C History and physical examination searching for evidence of trauma

D Immediate notification of the police or children protective services agency

E Immediate notification of the patient's parents

Answers and Explanations

1. The answer is D Although the dual decidual sac sign, which is highly suggestive of an intrauterine pregnancy, is present on the ultrasonogram, a concomitant ectopic gestation cannot be definitively ruled out. Concern for an ectopic pregnancy is increased because the patient is taking an infertility medication, which can induce multifollicular maturation and ovulation. Multiple ova may be fertilized simultaneously but not all will necessarily implant in the uterus. The adnexal tenderness also supports the suspicion of a concomitant ectopic pregnancy. The β-hCG levels do not correlate with the menstrual dates, which is also suggestive of an abnormal pregnancy. The data may also support a threatened miscarriage, but ectopic pregnancy must be ruled out and is more likely in light of the patient's medication history. The patient's cervical os is closed; therefore, inevitable miscarriage, which occurs when the os is open (leading to expulsion of the uterine contents), is impossible. In molar pregnancy, the quantitative β-hCG levels are extremely high (i.e., greater than 100,000 mIU at 12 weeks' gestation), the uterus is unusually large according to the date of the LMP, and a snowstorm pattern is observed on ultrasound. Patients with ovarian torsion present with severe unilateral pain.

2. The answer is C A woman of childbearing age with hypotension, abdominal distention, and abdominal pain has a ruptured ectopic pregnancy until proven otherwise. An intrauterine pregnancy complicated by placental abruption or uterine rupture may produce similar symptoms, but these disorders would occur later (i.e., in the second or third trimester). A threatened miscarriage could cause hypotension (as a result of vaginal bleeding), but threatened miscarriage is not associated with peritoneal symptoms such as those seen in this patient. Incomplete miscarriage may be associated with hypotension but does not cause intraperitoneal hemorrhage. Ovarian torsion does not typically cause hypotension.

3. The answer is D *Trichomonas vaginalis* is a sexually transmitted protozoal infection. The flagellated, motile organism infects the cervix and vagina, producing local tenderness and erythema ("strawberry cervix") and a thin, malodorous discharge. Bacterial vaginosis produces similar symptoms, but microscopic evaluation reveals clue cells (epithelial cells coated with bacteria), not a motile, flagellated organism. A vaginal foreign body may also produce local irritation and vaginal discharge, but the offending agent would be seen during the pelvic examination. PID, commonly caused by *Chlamydia trachomatis* or *Neisseria gonorrhoeae,* is rare in pregnant patients due to changes in the vaginal pH and cervical mucus that are induced by pregnancy. Specific diagnostic criteria exist in order to make the diagnosis of PID, including fever, lower abdominal tenderness, and adnexal tenderness.

4. The answer is D Vaginal bleeding in the second or third trimester is assumed to be placenta previa or placental abruption until proven otherwise. Stabilization of the patient is the highest priority; however, because this patient's vital signs are stable, the next step would be to transfer the patient to the operating room for evaluation. Pelvic examination (beyond inspection of the introitus) is contraindicated in the ED due to the risk of previa disruption and catastrophic hemorrhage. Therefore, evaluation is performed in the operating room because the operating room is more amenable to performing immediate maternal resuscitation and fetal delivery should the need arise. Fetal delivery is indicated for patients with hemodynamic compromise in the setting of continued maternal hemorrhage. Cesarean section, not vaginal delivery, is performed because delivery is more rapid and often the cervix has not dilated or a previa is occluding the outlet. Referral to an obstetrician would lead to delayed care, which could have disastrous consequences.

5. The answer is B The patient has experienced premature rupture of membranes, documented by the finding of alkalinity on the Nitrazine test and ferning. Phospholipid testing of amniotic fluid is indicated to document fetal lung maturity. Steroids, to enhance lung development, may be indicated if the lecithin:sphingomyelin ratio is less than 2.0. Cervical cultures are sent because the patient is at increased risk for infection (e.g., chorioamnionitis) and the neonate is at increased risk of sepsis when the onset of labor is prolonged after the rupture of membranes. Frequent cervical examinations also increase the risk for infection. The use of prophylactic antibiotics remains controversial. Admission for maternal and fetal monitoring, not discharge with follow-up, is indicated because the majority of mothers will go into labor within 24 hours of membrane rupture. There is no fetal distress; thus, immediate delivery is not indicated.

6. The answer is B This young woman has several diagnostic criteria for PID: lower abdominal tenderness, cervical motion tenderness, bilateral adnexal tenderness, a fever of 38°C, a leukocyte count greater than 10,000/μL, and a mucopurulent cervical discharge. In addition, the patient is unable to eat or drink, making successful outpatient therapy unlikely. Some centers use the history of nulliparity as an admission criterion as well. Therefore, this patient should be admitted for intravenous antibiotic therapy. Salpingitis, an upper genital tract infection that can lead to PID, is a possible diagnosis, but the patient appears too ill for outpatient management. Cervicitis is not associated with adnexal tenderness.

7. The answer is A The patient is in active labor with imminent delivery of the fetal head. Countertraction of the baby's head will reduce the risk of rapid head expulsion and damage to the perineal structures. Episiotomy is performed if the perineal structures appear at risk despite careful countertraction. Airway suctioning is performed immediately after the fetal head is delivered. Ordering transfer of the patient to the Labor and Delivery suite or asking the mother to push may result in an uncontrolled, unmonitored delivery, compromising both mother and child.

8. The answer is C The patient's diastolic blood pressure and symptoms suggest that the most likely diagnosis is severe pre-eclampsia. Admission of the patient (for treatment and fetal evaluation) is imperative. Treatment must be initiated with magnesium sulfate, labetalol, and hydralazine to stabilize the patient's blood pressure. Furosemide therapy is appropriate only for patients with severe pre-eclampsia accompanied by pulmonary edema. The mild form of pre-eclampsia is characterized by elevated diastolic pressures (i.e., 15 mm Hg above baseline), accompanied by minimal edema and proteinuria. Moderate pre-eclampsia is characterized by elevated systolic and diastolic pressures (i.e., 30 mm Hg and 15 mm Hg above baseline, respectively), accompanied by significant edema and proteinuria of the lower extremities. Patients with moderate pre-eclampsia do not have vision changes, abdominal discomfort, or pulmonary congestion. Eclampsia is defined by the presence of seizures.

9. The answer is B The patient's history and examination findings strongly suggest a lesion involving the optic chiasm resulting in the loss of peripheral vision and diplopia. Low levels of prolactin and gonadotropins implicate a hypothalamic–pituitary process as the cause of this patient's amenorrhea. The patient has delivered two children, ruling out a genetic defect. Anatomic defects (e.g., endometrial scarring from curettage) may cause menstrual problems, but the patient has no such history. Polycystic ovaries are associated with elevated estrogen levels, which ultimately suppress follicle-stimulating hormone (FSH), preventing ova maturation and secretion. Pregnancy does not cause tunnel vision.

10. The answer is C The presenting complaints strongly suggest sexual assault. Victims may sustain other internal injuries during the assault. Such injuries should be sought and addressed (by obtaining a patient history and performing a physical examination) before procurement of evidence, in accordance with the state rape protocol, is initiated. Psychiatric consultation may be indicated, but only after the patient's physical status has been addressed. Notification of local authorities or services is done after the patient's physical and psychological status has been addressed. Because the patient is no longer a minor, her parents should not be called unless requested by the patient.

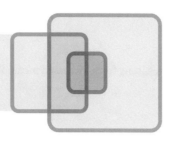

chapter **15**

Pediatric Emergencies

C. JAMES CORRALL

I   **APPROACH TO THE ILL PEDIATRIC PATIENT**

A **Discussion**   Approximately 30%–35% of patients seen in the emergency department (ED) are within the pediatric age range. Most of these children require urgent care or office care for self-limited illnesses but are unable to gain access to the primary provider's office. Thus, they present for care in the ED. Between 3% and 6% of ED visits are true emergencies in which children could suffer death or serious disability if not cared for in a timely and appropriate fashion.

B **Clinical features**   Children in rapid need of assessment are often referred to as "septic" or "sick" by experienced pediatricians, who rapidly make the assessment based on a constellation of symptoms and signs that are difficult to teach without first-hand experience. These signs and symptoms include:

1. Lethargy with little or no apprehension to examination or painful procedures
2. Irritability, particularly when held by parents, with inability to be comforted
3. Poor feeding associated with weak suck and poor interest in feeding
4. Weak cry or no cry when painful procedures or examination maneuvers are performed
5. Elevated temperature or hypothermia
6. Poor capillary refill with mottled skin appearance and poor turgor
7. Persistent vomiting with or without feedings
8. Complaint of headache and photophobia (in older children); not a reliable sign in children younger than 18 months
9. Seizures, which may be prolonged or focal in nature and are often associated with fever
10. Altered mental status, particularly with combativeness or inappropriate thoughts
11. Respiratory distress, particularly with nasal flaring, grunting respirations, tachypnea, intercostal and subcostal retractions, or diaphragmatic breathing
12. Drooling or stridor with severe air hunger
13. Cyanosis of lips and extremities with poor perfusion and absent pulses in the lower extremities
14. Extreme hypotension with gross hematuria
15. Any presentation of trauma that may be associated with a blunt injury to the head or thorax or with a penetration injury to the chest
16. Petechiae or purpura associated with fever

C **Differential diagnoses**   Children who suffer true, life-threatening emergencies fall into several distinct categories of illness. Children with any of the following life-threatening emergencies usually have initial respiratory compromise resulting from increased metabolic demands and cardiac compromise as a secondary event:

1. Acute respiratory distress
2. Cardiovascular disorders
3. Shock syndromes
4. Traumatic disorders
5. Environmental injuries
6. Injuries and emergencies with altered states of consciousness

D Evaluation

1. A **primary survey** should be performed immediately.
   a. **Airway.** The airway should be assessed for patency.
      (1) The airway should be opened with external maneuvers to relieve tongue obstruction.
      (2) Obstruction from foreign bodies should be recognized and relieved.
      (3) Gas exchange should be assessed and optimized.
      (4) Aspiration of gastric or oral contents should be prevented.
      (5) An artificial airway should be provided if no protective reflexes exist.
   b. **Breathing.** The adequacy of ventilation should be assessed, including the equality of chest rise and breath sounds.
      (1) A determination of whether air entry is impaired from a central or pulmonary cause should be made.
      (2) Ventilation should be enhanced if necessary with mouth-to-mouth breathing, bag-mask ventilation, or endotracheal intubation with or without bag assistance.
      (3) A surgical airway should be provided if an oral or endotracheal airway cannot be established.
   c. **Circulation** should be assessed, including the quality and intensity of pulses in the upper and lower extremity and blood pressure.
      (1) Hemorrhage should be controlled with direct pressure until surgical intervention can be accomplished.
      (2) Intravenous vascular access and a resuscitative fluid bolus should be provided.
      (3) External cardiac massage should be provided if no pulse exists.
      (4) Pharmacologic management of circulation should be provided if fluid status is adequate and cardiac output is impaired because of either vascular or pump instability.
      (5) Conversion of dangerous cardiac rhythm disturbances should be provided if hypotension and unresponsiveness ensue.
   d. **Neurologic examination.** A preliminary assessment should be made according to the following simple scale:
      (1) Alert and responsive to verbal stimuli
      (2) Responsive to verbal stimuli but no spontaneous alertness
      (3) Responsive only to painful stimuli
      (4) Unresponsive to any stimuli
   e. **Overall examination.** Infants should be unclothed and examined rapidly for injuries. Passive heat loss should be prevented by removing wet clothing and by providing external warmth. The patient's core temperature should be obtained to monitor for hypo- or hyperthermia.
2. A **secondary survey,** entailing a detailed physical examination and history, is then performed.
   a. **Head**
      (1) Evidence of trauma is determined by palpating bony prominences and the maxillae and by inspecting the nose and ears for drainage of cerebrospinal fluid (CSF).
      (2) The existence of dehydration is determined by inspecting the mucosae for evidence of decreased tearing or moisture or sunken eyes.

        (3) The eyes should be inspected for pupillary size and extraocular movements. A funduscopic examination should be performed to assess for central nervous system (CNS) or toxic involvement.

        (4) The oral cavity should be inspected for odor or discoloration that may imply a toxicologic basis for the condition.

b. Neck

        (1) The neck should be palpated for midline tenderness or deformity.

        (2) Flexion, extension, and rotation should be performed only after injury has been excluded either clinically or by radiographic means.

c. Chest

        (1) The chest wall should be inspected for symmetric expansion or disarticulation.

        (2) Palpation for change in respiratory fremitus or inequality should be performed.

        (3) Auscultation of the chest for breath sounds and for evidence of adventitial sounds such as rales, rhonchi, or wheezes should be performed.

        (4) Penetrating or blunt chest trauma is treated immediately.

d. Abdomen

        (1) The abdominal wall should be inspected for bruising, penetration, or hematoma.

        (2) Palpation for trauma, masses, or guarding and rigidity, which may indicate peritonitis, should be performed.

        (3) Palpation of the flanks to search for hematoma or an expanding mass should be performed.

e. Pelvis

        (1) The pelvis should be palpated laterally and in an anterior-posterior position for tenderness or instability.

        (2) The perineum should be inspected for lacerations, active bleeding, or hematoma. The urethra and rectum should be inspected for trauma or blood.

        (3) In age-appropriate females, a pelvic and rectal examination should be performed, and pregnancy should be excluded.

f. Extremities

        (1) The extremities should be inspected for signs of abrasion, hematoma, laceration, or deformity.

        (2) Palpation of the bones for instability, tenderness, or deformity should be performed.

g. Neurologic assessment

        (1) Attention should be focused on cranial nerve function, motor function, and sensory function, along with the patient's level of consciousness.

        (2) The presence or absence of reflexes should be noted.

        (3) A serial examination for changes in level of consciousness or loss of neurologic function should be performed.

3. Additional studies are often nonspecific but may provide clues to the diagnosis.

a. Laboratory studies

        (1) Complete blood count (CBC) and differential

        (2) Electrolytes and bicarbonate

        (3) Blood urea nitrogen (BUN) and creatinine

        (4) Immediate fingerstick glucose and serum glucose

        (5) Aerobic and anaerobic cultures of blood

        (6) Arterial blood gas (ABG) determination

        (7) Serum acetone determination

        (8) Urinalysis and urine culture

        (9) Stool culture

b. Radiologic studies

        (1) Chest radiography

        (2) Abdominal radiography

      (3) Abdominal ultrasonography

      (4) Computed tomography (CT)

  c. Ancillary studies

      (1) Echocardiography

      (2) Electrocardiography

      (3) Urine for toxicologic analysis

      (4) Lumbar puncture

E Therapy

1. **Stabilization** is the first priority. Prior to admission or transport, all life-threatening conditions (in particular, tenuous airway or circulatory dysfunction) must be addressed fully.

  a. Any possibility of airway compromise must be addressed and stabilized prior to admission or transport, and endotracheal intubation must be secured, if in question.

  b. Circulatory status must be addressed fully; resuscitative fluid boluses or blood transfusions may be indicated.

  c. Vasoactive drugs (e.g., dopamine, dobutamine) should be administered only in the presence of a physician or of a nursing staff qualified in critical care. The environment should be monitored and should have intravenous pump capabilities.

2. **Supportive care** is essential.

  a. Fluid resuscitation. A fluid bolus of 20 mL/kg should be provided to establish blood volume and increase efficiency of the heart. Care must be taken to avoid cerebral edema when vascular volume is restored.

  b. Anticonvulsant therapy is indicated to control seizures.

  c. Assisted ventilation may be necessary to control cerebral edema or respiratory failure.

  d. Surgical consultation should be obtained promptly in all cases of suspected trauma or when the diagnosis is in doubt in a critically ill infant with nonspecific physical signs.

3. **Antibiotic therapy** should be initiated for children with presumed sepsis, meningitis, or pneumonia.

  a. Agent selection. The patient should be treated with an antibiotic that is effective against the pathogens that most often cause disease in the patient's age group.

    (1) Neonates and infants younger than 2 months are usually given ampicillin sodium and either an aminoglycoside or cefotaxime.

    (2) Infants and older children may be treated with ceftriaxone in single or daily divided doses, or cefotaxime.

  b. Duration of therapy is based on the patient's age and the causative organism.

    (1) Infants with sepsis but without meningitis are usually treated with intravenous antibiotics for 7–10 days.

    (2) Infants with meningitis receive 10–14 days of parenteral therapy depending on the causative organism. Meningitis caused by *Neisseria meningitidis* may be treated for fewer than 7 days under certain circumstances.

4. **Corticosteroid therapy** is indicated for patients with meningitis to reduce the incidence of hearing loss. These drugs also may augment survival in children with sepsis or meningitis, but the effective dosage is unknown.

F Disposition

1. **Critically ill infants** must be evaluated and treated in a timely manner and admitted to the hospital for further treatment.

  a. Such children should be cared for by the highest level of provider available, preferably a pediatrician able to care for critically ill infants.

b. When higher-level care is unavailable, transport should be arranged to a referral center with the capability to care for critically ill children.

2. Seriously ill infants who may have the possibility of a bacterial process should not have antibiotics withheld pending hospital admission or transfer. All seriously ill infants should be accompanied by the admitting physician to the admitting ward or be attended by another physician during transfer and transport.

II PAIN

A Discussion

1. Definition. Pain is a **subjective experience** of superficial or visceral sensation that is sensory as well as emotional and relates to the degree of the injury or anticipation of a procedure and often has preceding emotional lability. Pain can be defined as what the patient describes as hurting and exists when the patient perceives it to be so.

2. Misconceptions about pain and its management in children include:
   a. Children will not remember painful events.
   b. Pain sensation is decreased because of neurologic immaturity.
   c. Children are more sensitive to analgesics, particularly when parenterally administered.

3. Quantitation of pain in children is difficult because of neurologic immaturity and expressive immaturity, but it can be partially characterized by facial expression, excess motor activity, and autonomic responses (e.g., diaphoresis, intensity of cry). Pain can be measured roughly, depending on the age of the patient.
   a. In children **younger than 3 years,** no good visual guideline is available.
   b. In children **older than 3 years,** a visual analog scale consisting of drawn facial expressions may be useful.
   c. In **older children and adolescents,** a numerical scale may be used relative to pain that the child has perceived prior to this episode. Numerical pain scales are not useful for small children and may have limited validity for adolescents because of their emotional and psychologic lability.

B Clinical features
Pain may be made evident by withdrawal of the injured parts, fleeing the immediate treatment situation, extreme facial expressions, crying, or excess verbal or motorically aggressive behavior.

C Differential diagnoses

1. Preoperative pain from a painful injury

2. Postoperative pain following a difficult procedure

3. Chronic pain syndromes associated with malignancy or chronic conditions

D Evaluation

1. Prompt intervention to prevent loss of life or limb should take place, including:
   a. Airway support and control
   b. Assessment of quality of breathing
   c. Support of circulation and control of hemorrhage with replacement of fluid loss

2. A **thorough secondary survey** is performed following the initial assessment and stabilization of the patient.
   a. An appropriate **physical examination** is necessary to assess the degree of injury or the site of pain as it may relate to visceral pathology (e.g., appendicitis).
   b. An **analog scale** appropriate to the patient's age should be used to assess the severity of pain.

E Therapy   Treatment of pain should be instituted based on the injury and emotional distress. Throughout treatment, monitoring is necessary to assess the quality of intervention and the potential side effects of medications.

1. **Local anesthesia** is a safe and effective method of pain relief during painful procedures or injuries, particularly those involving lacerations or fractures. Toxicity is determined by the total amount of drug absorbed into the circulation and the rapidity of administration. Local anesthetic may be applied topically to provide minimal anesthesia for simple procedures.

   a. **Eutectic mixture of local anesthetics (EMLA),** such as lidocaine 2.5% and prilocaine 2.5%
      (1) EMLA must be applied 60–90 minutes before procedures.
      (2) EMLA requires an overlay of occlusive dressing.
      (3) Safety in open wounds is not established.

   b. **Tetracaine, adrenaline,** and **cocaine (TAC) solution**
      (1) Mixture concentrations are variable from institution to institution.
      (2) TAC solution may be applied to open wounds.
      (3) Contact with the eyes, nose, and mouth must be avoided to prevent absorption.
      (4) Effectiveness of anesthesia is visible by the appearance of skin blanching.

   c. **Subcutaneous infiltration** may be used to effect regional anesthesia at the site of the injury. Buffering of the injected agent with **sodium bicarbonate** may lessen the sensation of pain caused by the acidic nature of the anesthetic. **Epinephrine hydrochloride** may be added to increase the duration of a block but should not be used in areas supplied by end arteries (e.g., the distal digits, nose, pinna, penis).
      (1) **Lidocaine (2% or 4%)** can be infiltrated locally.
      (2) **Bupivacaine** may be used for prolonged anesthesia.

   d. **Peripheral nerve block** is achieved by local infiltration of a nerve supplying a wounded or painful area. Usually, 2%–4% lidocaine is used without adrenaline. A peripheral nerve block should be used only by skilled personnel with prior training.

   e. **Regional nerve block** is achieved by local infiltration of a nerve supplying an extremity. Usually, 2%–4% lidocaine is used without epinephrine. This method is attempted by specially trained individuals to control painful procedures.

2. **Sedation**

   a. **Nitrous oxide** calms the emotional reaction to pain perception. It requires patient cooperation in the form of holding the mask to the face and is usually not indicated for children younger than 3 years of age. Nitrous oxide should be used only with continuous (transcutaneous) monitoring of the oxygen tension and cardiorespiratory function monitoring. Because nitrous oxide is a mixture of gases, its administration requires prior training.

   b. **Ketamine** is a dissociative anesthetic that interrupts electrophysiologic perceptions between higher thalamocortical centers and limbic and medullary centers. Ketamine is most often used in combination with either local or regional anesthesia to induce amnesia during painful procedures. It is also useful for children with anxiety-induced bronchospasm. Ketamine may be associated with emergence phenomena that can manifest as psychosis.

   c. **Midazolam** may be used intranasally, orally, parenterally, or rectally. It is useful as an anxiolytic and has no analgesic effect. It may be used in combination with other narcotics (e.g., fentanyl, meperidine) to achieve a combination effect. **Midazolam** plus **fentanyl** is extremely useful for very painful procedures (e.g., reduction of a fracture or dislocation).
      (1) Continuous monitoring is necessary for patients receiving combination therapy because of the degree of anesthesia. After the painful procedure is completed, care must be taken not to forget about the patient because a lack of pain drive afterward can result in profound respiratory depression.
      (2) At the bedside, midazolam plus fentanyl should be used only with the narcotic antagonist naloxone and the benzodiazepine antagonist flumazenil.

d. **Propofol** is useful for rapid and deep induction of anesthesia within 40 seconds of injection but requires maintenance infusion for continued sedation. The incidence of apnea in 5%–7% of patients necessitates cardiorespiratory monitoring and airway equipment at the bedside. There is a rapid emergence of alertness (within 3–5 minutes) after cessation of anesthesia. Propofol must be used only by physicians skilled in its usage; dosage guidelines are usually individualized to patient need.

e. **Chloral hydrate** cannot be recommended because of its safety profile. The dosage is far too speculative for safety and usually provides for excessive recovery times in children. Chloral hydrate has been associated with aspiration syndromes.

f. **Demerol (meperidine), Phenergan (promethazine),** and **Thorazine (chlorpromazine) [DPT]** were used in the past because of a lack of any other agent. Its use causes prolonged sedation and unpredictable results. It is no longer indicated for usage in children.

g. **Hydroxyzine** plus **meperidine** is used extensively in adults but minimal studies have been performed in children. Hydroxyzine may not be used intravenously and therefore requires administration either orally or intramuscularly.

h. **Iontophoretic fentanyl** is still in the investigational phase for adults. Its mechanism of action is controlled by the amount of stimulus applied to the extremity with electrical current across the topically applied agent. The result is exquisite control of depth of analgesia and sedation that is not obtained with usual intravenous formulation. Rapid drug elimination allows for gradual or rapid emergence by adjusting electrical current.

F Disposition

1. **Discharge.** Patients who have received anesthetics or sedatives may be discharged, provided that all immediate life threats have been addressed and the following have taken place:

   a. **Stable airway and cardiorespiratory function** are documented after careful monitoring.

   b. The patient has **full function** of the injured area and neurologic assessment of the area reveals **no deficits.**

   c. The patient is **neurologically intact** and has demonstrated **protective airway reflexes.**

   d. The patient is **able to function** commensurate with age and **able to walk** without staggering or falling.

   e. The patient has **full truncal control** consistent with growth and development, is able to **sit unaided** (if age appropriate), and is able to **take liquids.**

2. **Additional monitoring** or **admission.** Any patient who does not return to functional baseline responsiveness should be monitored for additional time or admitted for further evaluation.

III SUDDEN INFANT DEATH SYNDROME (SIDS)

A Discussion

1. **Definition.** SIDS is the sudden death of any infant or child that is unexpected by history and not explained by findings on postmortem examination, examination of the past medical history, or a review of the death scene.

2. **Statistics**

   a. SIDS accounts for 40%–60% of infant deaths between the ages of 1 month and 12 months and is the **most common cause** of postneonatal infant death in developed countries.

      (1) Approximately 6000 deaths occur each year with a peak age of incidence of 2–4 months.

      (2) Between 95% and 98% of all cases occur before or by 6 months of age, with almost no cases seen prior to 1 month of age.

   b. The rate in the general population in the United States is 1.3–2.5/1000 live births.

B **Clinical features**

1. **History**

   a. Children are usually discovered by parents or caregivers in the early morning hours lifeless and cyanotic with no cardiorespiratory effort. Most infants show signs of struggle and are often wrapped in bed clothing, suggesting entanglement. Vomitus is often found in the mouths of infants with SIDS, which suggests aspiration and apnea induced by secretions in the oral cavity.

   b. SIDS has been associated with nonspecific illnesses in the last 2 weeks of life and increased incidence of gastrointestinal illness preceding death. Fatigue during feedings in the week prior to death and profuse sweating during sleep are often present. Lethargy in the 24 hours preceding death is frequently seen and is associated with an intercurrent upper respiratory tract infection.

C **Differential diagnoses**

1. **Infectious disorders** include misdiagnosed primary or secondary meningitis or sepsis.

2. **Cardiovascular disorders** include undiagnosed critical coarctation of the aorta, severe tetralogy of Fallot, prolonged QT syndrome, or unrecognized arrhythmia.

3. **Environmental disorders** include hypothermia and hyperthermia or hyperthermia associated with undiagnosed cystic fibrosis.

4. **Inborn errors of metabolism** not previously diagnosed include branched-chain aminoacidopathy and many forms of fatty-acid metabolic defects, including medium-chain acetylcoenzyme A (acetyl CoA) dehydrogenase deficiency.

5. **CNS disorders** include prolonged idiopathic seizures, unrecognized CNS hemorrhage due to arteriovenous malformation, or aneurysm rupture.

6. **Traumatic disorders** include particularly nonaccidental trauma that results in CNS events such as intraventricular and intracerebral hemorrhages and subarachnoid and subdural collections of blood.

7. **Asphyxiating injuries** can occur in infants who sleep with large, overweight parents who inadvertently roll onto the infant during sleep.

8. **Fluid and electrolyte disorders,** particularly following gastrointestinal illnesses, include hyponatremia, hypernatremia, hyperkalemia secondary to adrenal insufficiency, or profound dehydration with renal vein thrombosis.

9. **Toxicologic disorders** include inadvertent or purposeful administration of prescription drugs, such as diphenoxylate hydrochloride and atropine for diarrhea, or accidental ingestion of or poisoning with illicit drugs (e.g., cocaine, heroin).

10. **Idiopathic disorders** include Ondine's curse and other hypoventilation syndromes.

D **Evaluation**

1. **Antemortem evaluation.** Survivors of an aborted or near-miss SIDS episode should be evaluated as follows:

   a. **Physical examination.** A careful physical examination should be performed to search for signs of nonaccidental trauma, such as unexplained bruising, retinal hemorrhages, strangulation marks, or handprints on the neck.

   b. **Laboratory studies** should include a CBC; serum electrolyte panel; creatinine phosphokinase determination; prolactin serum concentration; ABG determination; urinalysis for microscopic and amino acid analysis; and culture of blood, CSF, and urine. Urine should also be obtained for toxicologic analysis.

   c. **Radiologic studies** should include a long bone series and a single lateral skull radiograph for occult fractures. A single-view chest radiograph to ascertain the presence of pneumonia or a rib fracture is also helpful.

2. **Postmortem examination.** A thorough postmortem examination must be performed on all infants who are suspected to have died of SIDS. The emergency physician should not allow attending physicians of the deceased infant to take responsibility for the death, even in children with chronic and protracted neonatal illnesses such as bronchopulmonary dysplasia. **Autopsy findings** in patients with SIDS have been inconclusive and have been most consistently associated with the following:
   a. Mild pulmonary edema
   b. Intrathoracic petechia
   c. Evidence of chronic asphyxia
   d. Brain stem dendritic spines with reactive astrocytosis
   e. Elevated substance P, which is a neurotransmitter
   f. Hypoplasia of the arcuate nucleus in the medulla
   g. Prenatal and postnatal growth retardation

E **Therapy**

1. **Resuscitation.** Most infants found cold and with dependent lividity are essentially dead at the scene, and all resuscitation attempts are futile.
   a. Infants who respond to maternal or first-responder **cardiopulmonary resuscitation (CPR)** are salvageable in 80%–90% of cases, when provided with adequate pediatric emergency care.
   b. No medications are effective in preventing SIDS. **Theophylline** and **caffeine** are administered to infants with apnea of prematurity as a respiratory stimulant and are effective for improving the arousal responsiveness in some, but not all, infants.

2. **Monitoring.** Survivors of an aborted or near-miss SIDS episode should be offered home monitoring after risks and benefits are fully explained to parents. Children should be monitored under the direction of a specialist with expertise in SIDS. Monitoring should be discontinued only under the direction of the primary physician and never by an emergency physician.

F **Disposition** In all cases, the appropriate authorities should be notified, including police and child protective agencies. A thorough investigation of the death scene should be performed by individuals skilled in such investigations. Photographs should be taken for later correlation with findings on postmortem examination.

1. **Survivors** of an apparent life-threatening event should be admitted to the hospital for a thorough and complete medical and cardiorespiratory evaluation and monitoring.
   a. Prior to hospital discharge, **parents of infants who have survived** an initial apparent life-threatening event should fully understand home monitoring and should be taught CPR according to American Heart Association standards.
   b. Infants who were under the care of a private physician should be referred back to them. **Private-practice physicians** should be intimately involved in all decisions with regard to monitoring and other apparent concerns of the parents of such children.
   c. Survivors of near-miss events should be fully evaluated in established centers for SIDS with appropriate sleep and awake pneumograms and other studies as clinically indicated.

2. **Infants who do not survive.** Considerations for the remaining family members include the following:
   a. A careful evaluation of other siblings should be performed following the death of the index infant. Similar-aged infant siblings have a 20-fold greater risk of sudden infant death than the general population and should be offered interventional monitoring or further study for risk factors.
   b. Appropriate social services counseling should be offered to the parents and immediate family members following such events and in the weeks after the event.
   c. A follow-up visit for the physician caring for the infant at death as well as the parents and immediate family members should be arranged after the results of all toxicologic and postmortem studies are completed. This meeting is crucial, because many unwarranted fears and concerns may be dispelled by such a meeting.

IV **INGESTED FOREIGN BODIES**

A **Discussion**

1. **Definition.** An ingested foreign body is any aspirated substance that is not natural to the body passage in which it is found. Foreign body ingestion is a common problem because of poor supervision by adults and the normal infant behavior of putting things in the mouth or nasal passages. Approximately 50% of aspiration episodes are unwitnessed by caregivers.

2. **Severity.** Although most foreign objects are expelled immediately by the cough reflex and never require medical attention, foreign body injury is the most common cause of injury-related death in children younger than 1 year of age. Factors that influence the severity of the situation include:
   a. **Size of the foreign body.** Large foreign objects that nearly or completely occlude the upper airway pose an immediate life threat and must be emergently removed.
   b. **Location of the foreign body.** The location is directly related to the size of the pediatric airway. The younger the child is, the greater the chance that the site of obstruction will be more proximal.
      (1) The **larynx** and **cricopharyngeus muscle** are the most common sites of involvement in children younger than 1 year.
      (2) The **trachea** and **bronchi** are the most common sites involved in children between the ages of 15 and 48 months. Despite the acute angle of the left main stem bronchus, the propensity for the object lodging in either side is approximately 50%.
   c. **Composition of the foreign object.** Plant matter usually is much more tenacious and irritating than metal shards.

B **Clinical findings** A high index of suspicion for foreign body aspiration must be held for any child who presents with unexplained respiratory symptoms.

1. Many patients with ingestions may have a **symptom-free interval** during which the body attempts to wall off the object. Walling off leads to definitive symptoms.

2. The **symptoms, physical findings,** and **complication rate** depend on the nature of the aspirated foreign object, the location of the obstruction, and the degree of obstruction.
   a. **Laryngeal foreign bodies** cause an **obstructive cough** that becomes hoarse and brassy, resembling the sound of croup.
      (1) This cough must be recognized quickly and managed correctly.
      (2) Hot dogs and bread are the two most commonly aspirated substances that lodge in the larynx. Bread and peanut butter are particularly irritating and tenacious, making removal difficult.
   b. **Tracheal foreign bodies** cause **cough** and **wheezing, intermittent cyanosis,** and a peculiar **precordial thud,** caused by the object impacting against the subglottic area.
   c. **Bronchial foreign bodies** often present with **blood-streaked sputum, cough,** and **dyspnea** with or without wheezing or absent air sounds.
      (1) Initially, the child may be symptom-free, but later unilateral wheezing or prolongation of the expiratory phase may be noted.
      (2) Edema and lodging of the foreign body in a smaller subsegmental airway may result in obstruction to outflow of air and air trapping or atelectasis and mediastinal shift toward the side of the obstructing foreign body.

C **Differential diagnoses**

1. **Pneumonia syndrome** (see V E). The sudden onset of symptoms will usually not confuse the astute clinician but may well be confused with more protracted symptoms seen in smaller foreign body aspirations. Physical examination findings are helpful only if air trapping or unilateral wheezing is noted.

2. Croup syndrome (see V A). The sudden onset of symptoms is often confused with this entity acutely, but the lack of fever mitigates against the diagnosis.

3. Acute epiglottitis (see V D) usually occurs in older children and is usually heralded by high fever (i.e., greater than 103°F), toxicity, and air hunger. Epiglottitis is rarely seen because of the widespread use of vaccine preparations specific for *Haemophilus influenzae*.

D **Evaluation**

1. **History and physical examination.** A suggestive history and confirmatory physical examination are the most important diagnostic tools initially.

2. **Imaging studies**
   a. **Roentgenographic examination** is truly useful only for radiopaque foreign bodies but may be beneficial for asymmetric lung expansion or collapse.
   b. **Radiographic examination**
      (1) **General considerations**
         (a) The **plane** in which the foreign object lies aids in differential location of the object.
            (i) If the object is in the **sagittal** plane, it is probably in the larynx.
            (ii) If in the **coronal** plane, it is probably in the esophagus.
         (b) The use of **high-kilovoltage films** may enhance recognition of nonopaque foreign objects.
         (c) The **administration of contrast agents** may also guide the location of the foreign object if it is in the esophagus.
      (2) **Plain films** are often helpful for diagnosing bronchial foreign bodies, especially in patients with overinflation syndromes and collapse.
         (a) If an object causes complete obstruction in the expiratory phase but allows air to pass in the inspiratory phase, air becomes trapped and hyperinflation is seen. This appears as a hyperlucency of the involved side.
         (b) If an object causes complete obstruction in both the expiratory and inspiratory phase, then complete atelectasis occurs with shift of the mediastinum to the side of the obstruction.
         (c) If an object causes incomplete obstruction in both the expiratory and inspiratory phase, a ball-valve effect occurs. This may be revealed in a normal plain radiograph of the chest. However, special inspiratory and expiratory films will reveal air trapping on the affected side.
   c. **Bronchoscopy** is usually the only way to definitively diagnose and treat tracheal foreign bodies, although radiographs are helpful for radiopaque objects.

3. **Laboratory studies** are seldom helpful in the management of acute or subacute obstructions with foreign bodies but may be useful with chronic obstructions that were missed. **Blood cultures** are usually not warranted, except for chronic foreign body ingestion of vegetable matter, particularly peanuts, which produces a cough, a septic type of fever, dyspnea, and chronic suppuration.

E **Therapy**

1. **Object removal.** Patients with acute, life-threatening foreign body aspirations should be treated emergently at the scene by either chest blows and thrusts or abdominal thrusts, depending on the age of the patient, while attempting to maintain oxygenation.
   a. In a child who can cough, breathe, or speak, **nonintervention** is essential. A natural cough is more effective than airway or chest-compressive maneuvers. Blind sweeps of the pharynx and hypopharynx in an awake and alert child may induce vomiting and may further lodge the object deeper into the airway, producing complete obstruction.
   b. For a child younger than 1 year of age who is unresponsive, **back blows** and chest thrusts are recommended in concert with attempts at ventilation.

    c. For an unresponsive child older than 1 year, **abdominal thrusts** may be performed in accordance with published standards in addition to attempts at ventilation. Abdominal thrusts are not used for children younger than 1 year of age because of the risk of perforating the abdominal viscus.

    d. Children in whom abdominal thrusts or chest thrusts fail to dislodge the object may require **advanced airway adjuncts** to bypass the site of the obstruction until the object can be removed. Airway adjuncts include:

        (1) Needle cricothyrotomy

        (2) Surgical cricothyrotomy

        (3) Rigid bronchoscopy

        (4) Open bronchotomy

    e. Endoscopy. Children with more distal foreign bodies should undergo endoscopy as soon as practical. A delay doubles the morbidity and mortality.

    f. Surgery may be necessary to remove the object.

  2. Bronchodilator therapy is not recommended because of the risk of dislodging a distal foreign body and having it lodge in a larger airway.

  3. Antibiotic therapy may be indicated if a secondary infection has developed, or in patients with subacute or chronic obstructions. Initiation of antibiotic therapy should not delay the removal of foreign objects.

F **Disposition**

  1. Discharge. Children in whom the foreign body has been expelled may be discharged to home without further intervention or therapy except for accident counseling.

  2. Admission. Children in whom surgical manipulation is necessary to clear obstructions warrant admission to the hospital for 24 hours or less.

  3. Referral. Children with chronic unrecognized aspiration syndromes should have consultation with not only an otolaryngologist, but also a surgeon, with regard for the need for lobectomy.

V **RESPIRATORY TRACT INFECTIONS**

A **Laryngotracheobronchitis (croup syndrome)** is the most common form of non–life-threatening acute upper airway obstruction in childhood.

  1. Discussion

    a. Cause. Nearly all cases of croup are caused by viral pathogens in only three distinct viral groups: influenzae, adenovirus, and parainfluenza viruses.

    b. Incidence. Boys are affected more often than girls. Croup is more common during the colder months of the year, paralleling the prevalence of the most common viral causes of this entity.

    c. Predisposing factors. Approximately 20% of affected children have a strong family history of similar illness, and 5%–10% of children have recurrences of similar symptoms. Recurrences are infrequent with increasing age up to age 7 years, as the size of the airway increases.

  2. Clinical features

    a. Course. Most patients have an **upper respiratory syndrome** for several days preceding the onset of the characteristic symptom complex. The disease is usually prolonged over 7 days. Characteristically, croup syndrome is worse over the first 3 days; then gradual improvement occurs over the next 4 days.

    b. Symptoms and **signs** are characteristically worse at night, with a propensity for 10:00 P.M., and children are most often brought to the ED following the initial event.

      (1) A **"seal-like" barking** or **brassy cough with agitation** is characteristic of croup and is usually diagnosed by parents prior to arrival at treatment facilities. The characteristic cough results from edema in the immediate subglottic region of the trachea.

(2) As obstruction increases, **stridor** develops that is initially expiratory only. With progression of disease, stridor becomes both inspiratory and expiratory in nature.

(3) With worsening disease, the bronchi and bronchioles are affected. The **respiratory effort becomes more labored,** and fatigue ensues. Such worsening is usually seen in younger infants. Most infants are usually comfortable at rest in the caregiver's arms and usually do not display air hunger or drooling.

(4) **Temperature elevations** rarely exceed 102.5°F and usually are not associated early in the illness with toxicity.

3. **Differential diagnosis**

   a. **Acute epiglottitis** (see V D) is characterized by a rapid and fulminant course of high fever with temperatures in excess of 103°F, sore throat, skin mottling, progressive air hunger, and drooling.

   b. **Acute infectious laryngitis** is usually preceded by a viral upper respiratory syndrome (e.g., laryngotracheobronchitis) but with little or no fever. Hoarseness or vocal loss is usually seen without the stridor or brassy cough. Physical examination usually does not demonstrate any accentuation of hoarseness with activity or signs of cardiovascular compromise.

   c. **Acute spasmodic laryngitis** is clinically indistinguishable from acute infectious laryngotracheobronchitis, except for absence of fever. Acute spasmodic laryngitis tends to occur rapidly and is often associated with hoarseness in addition to stridor. Patients usually appear well. Illness usually lasts only 24–36 hours and abates without treatment. Recurrences are common and aid in the diagnosis in most cases.

   d. **Bacterial tracheitis** is associated with high fever in excess of 105°F and profound toxicity shortly after clinical symptoms occur. Initially, bacterial tracheitis usually is indistinguishable from acute laryngotracheobronchitis, but progressive worsening over 48 hours and prostration usually point to the correct diagnosis. Copious, thick purulent secretions are the rule. Occasionally, a cast of the airway may be expectorated with secretions; the cast is composed entirely of purulent necrotic exudate and epithelium. Usually a marked polymorphonuclear response is seen in peripheral blood with immature forms.

   e. **Foreign body aspiration** usually occurs suddenly with choking and coughing and without antecedent upper respiratory infection or fever. Foreign body aspiration may be associated with unilateral or bilateral wheezing or may progress to complete airway obstruction.

   f. **Peritonsillar abscess.** Usually, visible upper airway extrinsic compression is evident. This condition is rare in children younger than 10 years. Drooling is seen that is associated with hoarseness but little or no stridor.

4. **Evaluation**

   a. **Laboratory studies** are rarely needed and are seldom helpful in management. A **CBC** may reveal lymphocytosis and occasionally neutropenia. **Bacterial** and **viral cultures,** although beneficial for epidemiologic inference, are costly and do not affect care.

   b. **Pulse oximetry** is more beneficial for the child who is stridorous at rest and may provide a better guide to respiratory fatigue in the comfortable and nonthreatening environment of a caregiver's arms. **Hypoxemia,** as measured by pulse oximetry, is **usually not a feature** of this disease. If present in an older child, it suggests another diagnosis. Profound hypoxemia, air hunger, drooling, and hypotension suggest another diagnosis and mandate immediate referral for specialty care.

   c. **Radiographic studies** including chest and soft tissue radiography are confirmatory but often do not definitively differentiate any diagnosis, except for epiglottitis.

5. **Therapy**

   a. **Vaporization.** Most children with mild to moderate laryngotracheobronchitis can be managed safely at home if their only manifestation is a brassy cough and stridor with agitation only.

   (1) **Cool mist vaporization** at home is the preferred treatment because of its intrinsic safety and because of its efficacy for providing some humidification to the upper airway. Ultrasonic home nebulizers are best when available, but are cost prohibitive for many families.

    (2) In addition to vaporization, a **bathroom filled with the steam from a hot shower** is often therapeutic and can avert a trip to the hospital. Safety is a concern for the unattended child. Cool or warm mist devices may also be helpful.

    (3) Perhaps the cheapest and easiest home remedy is to **take the child outside into the moist, cool air for a period of 30–60 minutes.** Often the simple act of driving in the family car with the windows down is enough to allay an attack of coughing for several hours.

b. Nebulization. Children with stridor at rest must be seen and evaluated in a hospital by practitioners experienced in the care of such children.

    (1) **Humidified saline.** Children with **mild to moderate stridor at rest** may be initially treated with nebulized, humidified saline. Good results are achieved in more than 50% of these children.

    (2) **Racemic epinephrine.** Children with **moderate to severe stridor** should be treated with nebulized racemic epinephrine (2.25% solution diluted 1:5 or 1:8 with water and given 4 mL nebulized over 15 minutes).

        (a) Children treated in this manner should be observed in the ED for at least 2 hours prior to discharge.

        (b) Past literature suggested that such children may need hospital admission because of the rebound of stridor and potential worsening.

            (i) Most children rebound in 2 hours.

            (ii) Children with extenuating circumstances should be considered for admission, particularly children in poor social situations, for whom shower facilities are unavailable or long commuting distances to the hospital exist.

c. Administration of dexamethasone. Recent literature suggests that all children may benefit from the administration of corticosteroids. Dexamethasone is preferred over prednisone or prednisolone because of its half-life of 36–55 hours, which frequently is all that is necessary for treatment for most cases of stridor.

    (1) Children who received 0.6–1.0 mg/kg of dexamethasone intramuscularly were much improved over children who received cool mist nebulization alone and for longer periods.

    (2) Side effects are very rare and do not warrant additional monitoring with single-dose therapy. Anecdotal reports of corticosteroid use worsening the presentation of common childhood illnesses (e.g., varicella) exist, but have not been substantiated in more rigorous prospective studies.

d. Intubation may be necessary for children who present in marked respiratory distress.

    (1) The endotracheal tube should be one size smaller than the ideal size required for the age of the child.

    (2) The use of paralytic agents for such intubated children is beyond the scope of this text but may be required because of agitation.

    (3) The addition of repeated doses of dexamethasone should be considered in children who require prolonged intubation, but dexamethasone should not be given more frequently than every 48–56 hours.

6. Disposition

  a. Discharge

    (1) Most patients can be managed at home with humidification procedures as outlined above, particularly children who have only **stridor with agitation** or **cough** and are otherwise well. Parenteral dexamethasone (0.6 mg/kg) may markedly improve outcome and prevent worsening.

    (2) Children with **stridor at rest** may be treated with nebulized saline and a single does of dexamethasone 0.6–1.0 mg/kg intramuscularly. Children who worsen or are persistently stridorous after a second nebulization should receive nebulized racemic epinephrine. Such treated children are observed in the department for a minimum of 2 hours and, if free of symptoms, are discharged to close follow-up evaluation within 24–48 hours.

b. Admission

(1) Children who are **worse** or **unchanged** 2 hours after treatment should be considered for hospital admission and further treatment with additional doses of dexamethasone or an inhaled corticosteroid.

(2) Children rarely present in **marked respiratory distress** but may require endotracheal intubation and hospitalization in an intensive care setting.

B **Bronchiolitis** is a common disease of the lower respiratory tract of infants. It is the most common cause of acute respiratory distress and wheezing in small infants and the most common cause of hospitalization for infants between the ages of 6 and 20 months.

1. Discussion

a. **Cause.** Bronchiolitis is predominantly a viral illness.

(1) **Respiratory syncytial virus (RSV)** accounts for more than 50% of cases.

(2) **Parainfluenza virus 3** and **adenovirus** account for 30%–40% of cases.

(3) *Mycoplasma* and *H. influenzae* cause fewer than 5% of all cases.

b. **Incidence.** Bronchiolitis occurs during the first 24 months of life, with a peak incidence in patients between the ages of 6 and 8 months. Incidence is highest in early spring and winter months, but it occurs throughout the year in more temperate climates with less epidemic periodicity.

c. **Predisposing factors.** Bronchiolitis is most common in boys who have not been breast-fed and who live in crowded family quarters with heavy cigarette smokers. Children who develop bronchiolitis usually had an exposure to older children with minor respiratory symptoms 1–2 weeks prior to illness.

d. **Pathogenesis.** Bronchiolitis is characterized by bronchiolar obstruction caused by edema and accumulation of mucus and debris, leading to a dramatic increase in airway resistance.

(1) There is no evidence for bacterial infection as a primary event.

(2) Usually, the course of bronchiolitis is benign but may be severe if it is caused by adenovirus.

(a) **Bronchiolitis obliterans,** a sclerosing bronchiolitis, is most often caused by adenovirus.

(b) **Unilateral hyperlucent lung syndrome** (Swyer-James syndrome), a unilateral variant of bronchiolitis obliterans, results in a radiographic picture that suggests lobar emphysema.

(3) Respiratory rates in excess of 60 breaths/min are directly correlated with hypoxemia and hypercapnia.

2. Clinical features

a. **Symptoms**

(1) Bronchiolitis begins with a **serous nasal discharge, sneezing,** and a **mild fever** (101°–102°F). Gradually, respiratory distress develops that is characterized by **wheezing, cough, intercostal retraction,** and **irritability.**

(2) **Decreased appetite** follows increasing respiratory rates in infants 6 months of age or younger because of obligate nasal breathing patterns and because of the coordinated efforts required to suck and breathe simultaneously.

(3) **Posttussive emesis** may occur and may mimic the postcough whoop or stridor of pertussis.

b. **Physical examination findings** include tachypnea, flaring of the nasal alae, and cyanosis. Rales and expiratory wheeze are common. Artifactual hepatosplenomegaly may be detected because of air trapping with a decrease in the diaphragmatic movement and increased downward excursion of the diaphragm.

3. Differential diagnoses

a. **Reactive airway disease** is the most commonly confused entity. This condition is usually associated with a positive family history of reactive airway disease in immediate family members or parents. Repeated bouts of wheezing in the same infant within the same respiratory season are highly suggestive for reactive airway disease. The onset is sudden without antecedent viral syndrome. Eosinophilia may be evident with peripheral blood staining or nasal washings. One or two treatments of nebulized albuterol sulfate usually produce an immediate response.

b. Congestive heart failure (CHF) is often confused with bronchiolitis initially, but associated other symptoms often guide the clinician. These include the following:

 (1) Slowed feeding for weeks prior to the onset of respiratory symptoms is common in children with CHF.

 (2) True organomegaly is seen and is characterized by not only an increase in the ability to palpate the organ but also by an actual enlargement of the organs caused by stasis that can be demonstrated by percussion of the span on the body surface.

 (3) The history is usually positive for **sweating** during feedings or **cyanosis** with feedings or increased activity.

 (4) Precordial deformity with or without thrill or murmur is often seen with a shift in the point of maximum impulse (PMI) laterally.

 (5) Isolated tachypnea without other respiratory symptoms or fever is often the earliest clinical finding.

c. Foreign body aspiration is usually not difficult to differentiate initially. There is a sudden onset of dyspnea and unilateral or bilateral wheezing without antecedent upper respiratory symptoms and little or no response to nebulized bronchodilator therapy. The history is usually positive for choking immediately preceding the onset of wheezing and dyspnea.

d. Pertussis syndrome. A catarrhal stage of pertussis initially appears similar to early bronchiolitis, but copious secretions that are thick and tenacious are uncommon in bronchiolitis. The characteristic staccato cough and expiratory whoop or stridor usually are not confused with bronchiolitis. Prolonged illness for 4–5 weeks is usual in children with pertussis, with periods of profound apnea seen in infants.

e. Cystic fibrosis is not usually confused with bronchiolitis except in severely affected smaller infants. Family history of a previously affected child may be helpful in differentiation. Recurrent episodes of wheezing and pneumonia associated with failure to thrive suggest the diagnosis, as does a positive sweat chloride test. Cystic fibrosis is rare in black infants.

f. Bronchopneumonia with bronchospasm is commonly confused with bronchiolitis in small wheezing infants. Chest radiography is helpful in 50%–60% of cases with perihilar, segmental, or subsegmental infiltrates. Other signs of consolidation are often seen, such as dullness to percussion, decreased air entry, and diminished breath sounds.

4. Evaluation. Patients with **known cardiac problems** or **bronchopulmonary dysplasia** should be promptly evaluated regardless of the severity of symptoms.

a. Radiographic examination reveals hyperinflation and scattered areas of consolidation in 30%–40% of patients.

 (1) Plate-like or segmental atelectasis is common and is caused by airway collapse and plugging.

 (2) Haziness of the perihilar areas is often seen and cannot adequately exclude an early bacterial pneumonia.

b. Laboratory studies are seldom helpful acutely.

 (1) CBC. A CBC usually reveals a normal white blood cell (WBC) count and differential.

 (2) ABG determinations are seldom indicated; the severe pain associated with the procedure often predisposes to exaggerated hypoxemia due to segmental collapse. **Transcutaneous oximetry** provides a more reliable method of assessing trends in oxygen saturation.

 (3) Nasopharyngeal washings allow retrieval of cells from which a diagnosis of the specific etiologic agent can be made.

 (4) Viral culture is of no cost-effective proven benefit.

 (5) Serology. Increases in specific **antibody titers,** while of epidemiologic importance, may not be of distinct clinical importance. **Immunofluorescence studies** for viral antigen are the most cost-effective diagnostic test and may lead to early treatment.

5. **Therapy.** The most **critical phase** of illness is the first 48–72 hours after the beginning of cough and dyspnea. In infants who are not affected by feeding difficulties at 48–72 hours into the illness, the illness will most likely resolve without consequence.

   a. **Supportive care** is usually all that is indicated, with supplemental intravenous fluids and oxygen based on pulse oximetry results.

   b. **Ribavirin,** an inhalational antiviral with specific activity against RSV, is useful for children with compromised cardiopulmonary status due to either bronchopulmonary dysplasia or congenital heart disease. In some studies, ribavirin was shown to improve arterial oxygen saturation and may shorten the course of illness and avert the need for mechanical ventilation in severely affected infants. Other studies were inconclusive.

   c. **Antibiotics** have no value except when the possibility of a secondary bacterial pneumonia is likely.

   d. **Corticosteroids** have no place in therapy, and no clinical trials of these agents in severe bronchiolitis have been performed.

   e. **Bronchodilators** administered by oral or nebulized routes are often used empirically with no proven effect.

6. **Disposition**

   a. **Discharge.** Infants with **mild wheezing** and **dyspnea** may be evaluated and managed at home with close follow-up evaluation, provided parents are able to understand the illness and the need for appropriate intervention if the condition worsens.

   b. **Admission**

      (1) Infants with **severe dyspnea** or **dehydration** secondary to feeding difficulties should be considered for hospitalization.

      (2) Infants with **moderate symptoms** should be hospitalized because of the propensity for decompensation in such children, even when feeding and alertness are normal and no dehydration is present.

      (3) All infants with **moderate to severe symptoms** associated with decreased oral intake, dehydration, or lethargy should be hospitalized for additional therapy.

C Pharyngitis

1. **Discussion.** Pharyngitis describes any infection of the pharynx, including tonsillitis, pharyngotonsillitis, and uvulitis. The presence or absence of tonsils does not affect one's susceptibility. Most commonly, pharyngitis occurs as part of an upper respiratory tract infection with secondary involvement.

   a. **Incidence.** Pharyngitis is uncommon in children younger than 2 years. There is a peak incidence in children 4–7 years of age.

   b. **Etiology**

      (1) Pharyngitis is caused by **viruses** in approximately 85%–90% of cases.

      (2) **Group A β-hemolytic streptococci** are the only common and significant bacterial pathogens, accounting for approximately 10%–15% of cases. *Mycoplasma* and *Neisseria* species also cause pharyngitis, but usually in adolescents.

2. **Clinical features** differ depending on whether bacteria or viruses are the cause.

   a. **Viral pharyngitis** is a disease of gradual onset usually with malaise, upper respiratory symptoms, and myalgias.

      (1) A **sore throat** usually begins 1–3 days after the onset of symptoms. **Hoarseness, cough, and rhinitis** are common and are the reason for primary medical attention.

      (2) **Inflammation** may be relatively minor.

      (3) **Small ulcerations** may be visible on the palate and posterior pharyngeal wall.

         (a) Ulcerations that start posteriorly and extend anteriorly are usually caused by coxsackievirus.

         (b) Ulceration that begins at the gingival margins is usually caused by herpes simplex.

      (4) Exudates are rarely present, and no uvula edema or palatal petechiae occur.

b. Bacterial (streptococcal) pharyngitis is usually seen in children 2 years of age or older. Associated symptoms include the following:

    (1) Fever in excess of 104°F

    (2) Tonsillar enlargement and exudates; **fetid odor** of breath

    (3) Cervical adenopathy, usually moderate and painful but not fluctuant

    (4) Palatal petechiae and **uvula edema** (40%–60% of cases); diagnostic when present

    (5) Cough, rhinitis, or **hoarseness** (rare)

3. Differential diagnoses

    a. Viral syndrome is associated with hoarseness and cough. The course is usually mild, and often there are no exudates.

    b. Infectious mononucleosis is a nonspecific illness in children younger than 10 years. In adolescents, it is often confused with a streptococcal infection. Associated splenomegaly and generalized adenopathy are helpful in making the diagnosis. The monospot or heterophile antibody tests are not helpful for children younger than 6 years. However, a positive test in young children remains diagnostic.

    c. Diphtheria. In patients with diphtheria, a very adherent membranous exudate is present on the tonsils, posterior pharynx, or palate. This disease may be associated with cardiac symptoms and signs of tachycardia out of proportion to fever.

    d. Herpangina. A tonsillar exudate is not usually seen. However, multiple shallow ulcerations are seen on the pillars, palate, and fauces (throat).

    e. Leukemia is often an initial manifestation of agranulocytosis. A necrotic membrane is present that, when removed, causes the attached tissue to bleed. Associated anemia and abnormal cell morphology on a peripheral blood smear are helpful in making the diagnosis.

4. Evaluation. Laboratory studies are seldom useful. However:

    a. Rapid antigen detection methods for streptococcal infection are accurate in 95%–98% of cases.

        (1) Children with **negative rapid antigen detection** should have a definitive **culture** performed.

        (2) Children with **positive rapid antigen detection** should be considered to have a proven streptococcal infection and should be treated appropriately.

    b. Serologic testing for streptococcal antibody response is not warranted.

5. Therapy

    a. Antibiotic therapy. If antigen detection methods are available, treatment should be guided by results of such testing. Treatment usually results in rapid improvement if it begins before the fifth day of the illness. Reculture is usually not necessary unless symptoms do not abate after 7–10 days of effective therapy.

        (1) Penicillin V potassium (125–250 mg/day, administered four times daily) is usually the cheapest alternative.

        (2) Erythromycin (50 mg/kg/day, divided into three doses) is equally effective for penicillin-allergic patients.

        (3) Intramuscular long-acting benzathine penicillin as a single one-time treatment is indicated when compliance is an issue.

    b. Supportive therapy

        (1) Saline gargles and **cool liquids** are beneficial for relief of symptoms.

        (2) Topical anesthesia with viscous anesthetic agents is usually not warranted, particularly when the possibility for systemic absorption is possible in younger children.

6. Disposition. Most patients with pharyngitis can be managed with conservative antibiotic therapy. Children with a positive family history of rheumatic fever should be followed closely and considered for prophylactic therapy.

D Epiglottitis

1. Discussion

    a. Epiglottitis is a dramatic, potentially life-threatening condition that occurs in children between the ages of 2 and 7 years. Previously, the peak age of incidence was 36–42 months, but the widespread use of the conjugated *H. influenzae* vaccine has shifted the age of incidence toward adolescent and adult age groups. Overall, the widespread use of the conjugated *H. influenzae* vaccine has significantly decreased the incidence of this disease.

  b. Approximately 70% of children who develop epiglottitis have bacteremia caused by *H. influenzae* type b. Children who develop epiglottitis have a qualitatively and quantitatively different antibody response to the causative organism.

2. Clinical features. Epiglottitis has a fulminant course characterized by a high fever, sore throat, dysphagia, progressive dyspnea, and stridor.

  a. Symptoms

  (1) Respiratory symptoms. The characteristic presentation is abrupt onset of high fever, drooling, relative aphonia, and inspiratory stridor. Older children may have only sore throat and dysphagia as the presenting symptoms; as a result, epiglottitis may mimic peritonsillar abscess in that age group. Within 1–2 hours of presentation, airway obstruction becomes more severe and may progress to complete obstruction if not managed properly.

  (2) Posture. Children appear apprehensive, with their posture usually upright and forward in the tripod position (the chin and neck extended forward and mouth open, often with the tongue extruded forward).

  (3) Skin tone. Children may have a mottled or ashen skin coloration, which implies serious illness and, in most instances, bacteremia.

  b. Physical examination findings include moderate to severe respiratory distress with inspiratory and (rarely) expiratory stridor. Retraction of the suprasternal, intercostal, and supraclavicular areas is a sign of impending respiratory failure. Restlessness, agitation, and air hunger follow shortly after retractions and are the earliest, but most severe, signs of impending obstruction.

3. Differential diagnoses

  a. Bacterial tracheitis. Children with bacterial tracheitis are usually profoundly ill with temperature elevation in the range of 106°–107°F. Their cough is productive of thick, purulent secretions that are seen on establishment of an endotracheal airway. Bacterial tracheitis usually is misdiagnosed initially and presents late in a shock-like state.

  b. Diphtheric croup is usually characterized by a gray adherent membrane. There may be evidence of cardiotoxicity.

  c. Measles croup is seen always in conjunction with cough, coryza, conjunctivitis, and the classical morbilliform eruption. The child may have a fulminant course complicated by measles pneumonia.

  d. Acute spasmodic laryngotracheobronchitis occurs in children between the ages of 1 and 5 years. Often, there is a previous history of similar attacks. The child is usually afebrile and not drooling.

  e. Acute infectious laryngotracheobronchitis. Hoarseness and a barking, seal-like cough are seen with mild fever in a well-appearing infant. The hoarseness and loss of voice are out of proportion to the degree of illness.

  f. Foreign body aspiration. There is a sudden onset of symptoms, usually in the daylight hours, after the child has been awake for some time. The age of highest incidence is 6–24 months. Usually there is no fever or other evident signs of infection.

  g. Retropharyngeal abscess is usually a disease of toddlers with a subacute onset of symptoms. Radiographic examination of the lateral cervical airway is often helpful. This condition is usually associated with a muffled voice but not stridor.

  h. Peritonsillar abscess may mimic epiglottitis only in dysphagia, but there usually is no stridor. A muffled voice is characteristic but usually is seen only in the adolescent and older age group.

4. Evaluation. Epiglottitis is a **true medical emergency;** evaluation and treatment must occur in tandem.

  a. Children with **severe symptoms** should not be subjected to routine diagnostic procedures, but should be **evaluated in an operating room** by a team of physicians skilled in airway management, such as:

   (1) Pediatric intensive care physician or skilled pediatrician

   (2) Otolaryngologist with skills in placement of tracheostomy if necessary

   (3) Anesthesiologist capable of intubation of the complicated airway

  b. Laryngoscopy. Definitive diagnosis is by direct visualization of the large edematous epiglottis using **direct laryngoscopy** or **fiberoptic laryngoscopy** in the controlled environment of the operating room. Occasionally, a cooperative child will allow the visualization of a red epiglottis on tongue protrusion, but no attempt should be made to use a tongue blade for visualization. Manipulation of the airway with tongue blades or other instruments should not be attempted without supervision and with airway-adjunctive equipment at the bedside.

  c. Radiography. In children with **mild stridor** who are not acutely ill, a single lateral neck radiograph helps with the diagnosis of epiglottitis. Physical evidence includes:

   (1) Ballooning of the hypopharynx

   (2) Swollen anterior-to-posterior diameter of the epiglottis with the appearance of a thumb (thumb sign)

  d. Laboratory studies

   (1) Culture of the epiglottis and **blood** should be obtained, but only after the airway is secure. Culture and cell analysis of other sites, such as the CSF, are not warranted because no association with meningitis has ever been reported.

   (2) Antigen-detection methods are not useful acutely.

   (3) A **CBC** and **electrolyte determinations** are not beneficial.

 5. Therapy

  a. Airway stabilization. Following visual confirmation of epiglottitis, the child should be intubated and provided with humidified air via a T tube or by ventilator until edema of the upper airway subsides in 2–3 days. Intrinsic lung disease is usually not present, and mechanical ventilation is not usually necessary unless paralysis and sedation are needed.

   (1) Nasotracheal intubation is preferable to orotracheal intubation because it provides anatomic support for the tube and allows the child to feed while it is in place.

   (2) Sedation is necessary while the child is intubated to provide for comfort with the endotracheal tube and to prevent extubation.

  b. Intravenous antibiotic therapy should be instituted in the operating room only after the airway is secure.

   (1) Cefuroxime sodium can be used safely because of the infrequency of secondary infection at sites such as the meninges.

   (2) Ceftriaxone is also highly efficacious and can be used once daily intravenously or intramuscularly.

  c. Corticosteroids are not useful.

  d. Bronchodilators, administered by nebulization, are not warranted unless wheezing is present. **Racemic epinephrine** has no place in therapy, even as a temporizing measure, because any short-term benefit obtained may result in severe rebound after cessation of such therapy.

 6. Disposition. Children with **no evidence of epiglottitis** on direct visualization of the upper airway may be discharged if other causes are not found.

E **Pneumonia syndrome**

 1. Discussion

  a. Definition. Pneumonia is an inflammation of the lung parenchyma including the bronchioles, alveolar ducts and sacs, and the alveoli. The anatomic area of involvement classifies pneumonia as **lobar, lobular,** or **interstitial.**

b. Etiology. There are numerous causes of pneumonia, although most childhood cases are caused by viral pathogens.

   (1) Common respiratory viruses are the most common cause of pneumonia during the first several years of life.

   (2) Bacterial pathogens cause more severe infection and more clinical findings.

   (3) Fungi, parasites, *Mycoplasma,* and **rickettsia** may cause pneumonia but are rare and unusual causes in most children. *Mycoplasma* is the most common cause of nonviral pneumonia in children older than 6 years of age.

2. Clinical features depend on the causative organism.

   a. Bacterial pneumonia presents with mild upper respiratory symptoms followed by abrupt onset of fever, chills, tachypnea, and chest discomfort. A physical examination reveals decreased breath sounds and rales on the affected side. Cough, intercostal retractions, grunting respirations, and nasal flaring may be seen in younger individuals.

   b. Viral pneumonia causes several days of rhinitis and cough followed by fever and coryza but usually no decreased breath sounds and no rales or rhonchi. In younger infants, tachypnea may be the only sign.

   c. Other causes of pneumonia

   (1) *Mycoplasma pneumoniae.* Symptoms including fever and headache have a gradual onset. A nonproductive protracted cough and dyspnea are hallmarks of the disease.

   (2) *Pneumocystis carinii*

   (a) Progressive desaturation with dyspnea may occur in an immunocompromised host.

   (b) Pneumonia caused by *P. carinii* can produce an asymptomatic infection that mirrors viral pneumonia in normal children.

3. Differential diagnoses

   a. Cystic fibrosis (see V B 3 e)

   b. Congenital bronchiectasis

   c. Ciliary dyskinesia syndrome

   d. Tracheoesophageal fistula

   e. Foreign body aspiration (see IV)

   f. Atelectasis

   g. Pulmonary abscess

   h. Allergic bronchitis

4. Evaluation

   a. Physical examination. Diagnosis often is based on the clinical presentation and physical examination findings on chest examination.

   b. Laboratory studies

   (1) A **CBC** reveals leukocytosis but a predominance of neutrophils in bacterial pneumonia.

   (2) Cold agglutinin titer. *M. pneumoniae* may be diagnosed by cold agglutinin titer elevation during the first week of the illness but may be falsely negative in children younger than 5 years.

   (3) Culture or **rapid diagnostic testing.** Specific diagnosis can be made by culture of or rapid diagnostic testing of serum, urine, bronchial wash specimens, or pleural fluid.

   (4) Immunofluorescence or culture. Viral pneumonitis can be specifically diagnosed by immunofluorescence or culture of nasopharyngeal wash.

   (5) Silver staining. The specific diagnosis of *Pneumocystis* pneumonia can be made only by silver staining of specimens from tracheal or bronchial washings, lung aspirate, or lung biopsy.

   (6) Blood cultures are positive in 40%–60% of bacterial pneumonias, but the cost of testing is difficult to justify because it rarely changes therapy acutely.

    c. **Chest radiography.** Dense focal infiltration is noted on chest radiography in bacterial pneumonia. Bilateral, streaking perihilar infiltrates are characteristic of viral pneumonia. Interstitial infiltrates associated with hypoxia in an immunocompromised patient are consistent with *P. carinii* pneumonia (PCP).

5. **Therapy**
    a. **Bacterial pneumonia.** There is no universally accepted antibiotic regimen for presumed pneumonia.
        (1) **Neonates** should be hospitalized and treated intravenously with ampicillin and either an aminoglycoside or cefotaxime.
        (2) **Children older than 3 months** with **mild to moderate illness** and no evidence of desaturation may be treated with oral amoxicillin for presumed bacterial pneumonia.
        (3) **Children with more severe illness,** particularly with respiratory rates in excess of 60 breaths/min and desaturation, should be hospitalized and given intravenous antibiotics.
        (4) **Children older than 6 years** with **mild to moderate illness** and **dyspnea** but no desaturation may be presumed to have *Mycoplasma* illness and should be treated with erythromycin.
        (5) **Immunocompromised children.** Children who are immunocompromised and at high risk for PCP should be treated only after appropriate diagnostic studies.
            (a) **Trimethoprim–sulfamethoxazole** is the drug of choice at a dosage of 20 mg/kg/day of the trimethoprim component.
            (b) Those who do not tolerate trimethoprim–sulfamethoxazole may be treated with **pentamidine isethionate** parenterally or by inhalation after appropriate consultation.
    b. **Viral pneumonia** is usually treated by supportive care alone. Specific antiviral therapy is available for **children with RSV** and should be used for severely infected, confirmed RSV- or **varicella-positive infants** with underlying cardiac or respiratory problems.
        (1) **Ribavirin** is administered by aerosol for a period of 5–7 days.
        (2) **Acyclovir** is useful for varicella zoster or herpes simplex pneumonia.

6. **Disposition**
    a. **Discharge.** Children with **mild to moderate illness** and **no desaturation** may be managed conservatively at home with oral antibiotics appropriate for the likely pathogen according to age.
    b. **Admission**
        (1) Children with **moderate to severe illness,** with failure to feed or take oral therapy, or with desaturation should be admitted for further study and treatment.
        (2) Any **immunocompromised child with pneumonia** should be hospitalized for further evaluation, consultation, and definitive treatment.
        (3) **Neonates up to 3 months of age with pneumonia** should be considered for admission because oral antibiotic therapy is not appropriate.

VI   OTITIS MEDIA

A **Discussion**   Otitis media is a common diagnosis in the ED.

1. **Incidence.** One in three children will have otitis media before his or her sixth birthday. The peak age of incidence is between 6 and 13 months of age. Children with recurrent otitis media frequently have a positive family history for the same type of problems in the mother or father or both.

2. **Clinical forms.** Otitis media is a clinical syndrome consisting of several forms that overlap in pathophysiology and treatment.
    a. **Acute suppurative otitis media.** Acute otitis media can present with purulent drainage from the external canal making differentiation from otitis externa difficult.
    b. **Otitis media with effusion**
    c. **Recurrent acute suppurative otitis media**

3. **Etiology.** Major causative organisms include *Streptococcus pneumoniae*, *H. influenzae*, *Moraxella catarrhalis*, and *Staphylococcus aureus*.

B **Clinical features**

1. **Symptoms**
   a. **Local symptoms.** Children with otitis media complain of ear pain, decreased hearing, and ear discharge. Infants may exhibit ear pulling, head banging or rubbing, or apparent ataxic gait.
   b. **Systemic symptoms** such as fever, abdominal pain, vomiting, irritability, lethargy, and anorexia may be seen.

2. **Physical examination findings.** Marked redness, lack of normal landmarks, splaying, or absent light reflex and lack of (or abnormal) mobility on pneumatic otoscopy are noted.
   a. Children with recurrent otitis media often have only dullness of the tympanic membrane without obvious redness.
   b. Children with surgically placed tympanostomy tubes often present a confusing picture of ear drainage without pain, which can lead to a misdiagnosis of otitis externa.
   c. In a child with a fair complexion who is crying, there is no good diagnostic test except for the lack of mobility of the tympanic membrane. Otitis media cannot be diagnosed without removing cerumen from the canal. Cerumen must be removed by a cerumen loop or gentle ear lavage with warm saline.

C **Differential diagnoses**

1. **Primary ear disease**
   a. **External otitis media,** an inflammatory process of the external canal that produces ear pain and a decrease in hearing, is associated with pain on movement of the pinna of the involved ear.
   b. **External infections** of the auricle, pinna, or helix result in a superficial cellulitis.

2. **Referred pain** along nerves supplying common areas, including:
   a. Pain fibers from the distribution of cranial nerves V, VII, IX, and X, which innervate the posterior pharynx
   b. Pain resulting from postherpetic neuralgia as a result of cutaneous herpes zoster infection

D **Evaluation**

1. **Laboratory studies** are rarely needed and seldom helpful in the diagnosis.

2. **Tympanometry** provides a useful adjunct to diagnosis, as well as a visual confirmation of diagnosis that can be placed in medical records for future reference regarding response to treatment.

3. **Tympanocentesis** may be warranted in special circumstances to aid in the diagnosis of more serious conditions. Indications include:
   a. Intractable pain
   b. The presence of intracranial complications directly related to the otitis media
   c. Fever in an immunocompromised patient
   d. Failure to respond despite an adequate course of therapy

4. **Cultures of the nasopharynx or purulent drainage** from the perforation of an acute suppurative otitis media or from tympanostomy tubes is unrewarding and should be discouraged.

E **Therapy**

1. **Antibiotic therapy**
   a. **Selection of agents.** Many antibiotics are useful for the treatment of otitis media, varying only in interval of dosing and palatability—there is little difference regarding the microbiologic spectrum. The advantage of one antibiotic over another is entirely speculative. Children who have tympanostomy tubes and who develop acute suppurative otitis media should be treated only with an oral antibiotic. There are no studies that support the use of topical antibiotics for otitis media similar to treatment for otitis externa.
      (1) **First-line agents.** Generally, a first-line drug is chosen, with amoxicillin being the drug of first choice. Other first-line drugs may be useful, depending on the presence of sulfa

allergy or prior episodes of otitis media within the past 3 months that have been treated with antibiotics.

(a) **Amoxicillin sodium** (80–90 mg/kg/day, administered every 8 hours) is the most frequently prescribed and cost-effective initial therapy and has an acceptable and safe side effect profile.

(b) **Erythromycin–sulfisoxazole** (30–50 mg/kg/day, administered every 6 hours) is a safe alternative drug with a broad microbial spectrum. However, it is expensive, it requires more doses, and it has side effects inherent to the sulfa class of antibiotics.

(c) **Trimethoprim–sulfamethoxazole** is effective, and it is safe when penicillin allergy exists. However, concern must be raised when administered to black children with regard to glucose-6-phosphate dehydrogenase (G6PD) deficiency and the risk of hepatitis as well as Stevens-Johnson syndrome.

(2) **Second-line agents.** Other, more expensive agents should be considered when failure with a first-line agent or allergy precludes the use of another agent.

(a) **Cefixime** (8 mg/kg/day) is useful for patients with difficulty taking medications. Once-daily dosage is a particular advantage for infants with nausea and vomiting.

(b) **Cefotaxime** (10 mg/kg/day, administered every 12 hours) is an excellent choice with convenient dosing but with an unusual aftertaste that some children may find difficult to overcome.

(c) **Cefaclor** (20–40 mg/kg/day, administered every 8 hours) has the advantage of pleasant taste and good compliance. However, there is a 1%–5% incidence of a painful serum sickness–like reaction, erythema multiforme, and diarrhea.

(d) **Amoxicillin with clavulanate** (90 mg/kg/day, administered every 12 hours) is expensive and is associated with an increased incidence of diarrhea over more conventional amoxicillin.

(e) **Clarithromycin** (15 mg/kg/day, administered every 12 hours) is a macrolide antibiotic that has an acceptable side effect profile and microbiologic spectrum.

(f) **Ceftriaxone** (50 mg/kg, administered intramuscularly in one dose) is attractive to parents and clinicians because of the one-time dosing and a higher than 90% cure rate. Data on recurrences or resolution of serious effusions are not yet available.

b. **Duration of therapy.** Children should be treated for **10 days** for acute suppurative otitis media. Longer treatment courses offer no advantage.

(1) Most patients have no relief of fever before 72 hours of effective antibiotic therapy.

(2) On average, redness decreases substantially by 72 hours of therapy but effusion persists with limited mobility. All children should be reevaluated at 28–42 days after therapy to ensure resolution of effusion. Normally, 50% of children have persistent effusion at 14–21 days after therapy.

(a) Children with persistent effusion after resolution of acute infection should be re-evaluated at monthly intervals for 4–5 months with tympanometry. Based on bacteriologic studies, a prolonged course of antibiotics in excess of 14–21 days may be warranted at the third or fourth month of persistent effusion and may hasten resolution.

(b) Persistent effusion that does not resolve after 4–5 months of observation requires audiometric evaluation and otolaryngologic consultation.

c. **Prophylactic antibiotic therapy.** Children with more than three episodes of recurrent otitis media in 6 months or four episodes in 1 year merit consideration for prophylactic antibiotic therapy daily for 6–8 months.

2. **Decongestants** have no place in the management of either acute otitis media or persistent effusion. Literature suggests that such treatment may actually prolong effusion.

3. **Tympanostomy tube placement.** Despite the frequency of operations for placement of tympanostomy tubes, such devices do not prevent infection. They serve only to improve hearing by allowing better middle ear ventilation. Most children appear to outgrow their episodes of otitis

media because of complex growth of the eustachian tube diameter, the orientation of the tube within the bony skull, and enhanced secretory and cell-mediated immunity.

F **Disposition**   Most patients can be treated on an outpatient basis.

VII   CONGENITAL HEART DISEASE

A **Discussion**   Many types of congenital heart disease are appreciated and are beyond the scope of this text. Only those entities that may present to an ED are covered here.

1. **Incidence.** Congenital heart disease occurs in approximately 8 in 1000 live births; 2–4 of those 1000 newborn infants are symptomatic with heart disease in the first year of life.
   a. The diagnosis is established by 1 week of age in 40%–50% of patients with congenital heart disease.
   b. The diagnosis is made by 1 month of age in 60%–70% of infants with serious congenital heart disease.
2. **Types.** Congenital heart disease can be divided into cyanotic and acyanotic types.
   a. **Acyanotic.** The majority of cases of congenital heart disease involve acyanotic lesions that are usually discovered on examination for other reasons. They usually are not the reason for an ED visit.
   b. **Cyanotic.** The cyanotic congenital heart disease variants are true life-threatening emergencies and often result in such children presenting to the ED in extremis. Cyanosis results when obstruction to right ventricular outflow causes shunting at the cardiac level from right to left or when left ventricular outflow is impeded. Because of decreased ventilatory reserve, profound acidosis is common. Circulatory collapse is imminent after the development of acidosis.

B **Clinical features**

1. **Cyanotic lesions associated with decreased pulmonary blood flow**
   a. **Tetralogy of Fallot** is the most common cyanotic congenital heart defect, accounting for 10% of congenital defects.
      (1) **Pathogenesis.** The primary lesion involves hypoplasia of the infundibulum, resulting in outflow tract obstruction. Variable **right ventricular outflow obstruction** results in functional **pulmonary stenosis.** Dextroposition of the aorta results in overriding of the ventricular septum. Ventricular septal defect and right ventricular hypertrophy may also be evident.
      (2) **Manifestations** reflect the degree of severity of the right ventricular outflow obstruction.
         (a) Cyanosis is variable and may be absent.
         (b) Hypoxemic or "tet spells" characterized by irritability, hyperpnea, cyanosis, and syncope occur and may be fatal if not managed properly.
         (c) A harsh systolic ejection murmur is often heard along the sternal border.
         (d) Because of the functional pulmonary banding that occurs with the anatomy of this syndrome, CHF does not usually develop.
   b. **Pulmonary atresia with or without ventricular septal defect** is an extremely severe form of tetralogy of Fallot.
      (1) **Pathogenesis.** The main pulmonary artery is atretic, and pulmonary blood flow depends entirely on a patent ductus arteriosus or bronchial collateral vessels.
      (2) **Manifestations.** Patients present with findings of severe cyanosis and are usually profoundly ill. Often no murmur is heard, and a single first heart sound (S_1) is all that is appreciated in the syndrome when associated with a ventricular septal defect.
   c. **Transposition of the great vessels with ventricular septal defect and pulmonary stenosis** may mimic tetralogy of Fallot in clinical presentation.

    (1) **Pathogenesis.** This condition is caused by transposition of the vessels; therefore, the obstruction is in the left ventricle instead of the right ventricle. The heart is usually enlarged, and there may be pulmonary congestion, depending on the degree of pulmonary stenosis.

    (2) **Manifestations.** The most common presentation is poor feeding and lethargy, with mild cyanosis present on physical examination.

  d. Epstein anomaly of the tricuspid valve

    (1) **Pathogenesis.** Ebstein anomaly is caused by downward displacement of the right atrium and tricuspid valve into the right ventricle, which results in an enormous right atrium and a regurgitant tricuspid valve.

    (2) **Manifestations.** The severity of symptoms depends on the degree of displacement of the tricuspid valve.

      (a) In most patients, the only complaint is fatigue and cardiac dysrhythmias, of which paroxysmal tachycardia is the most common.

      (b) Some severely affected children may have cyanosis due to the admixture of blood through an open foramen ovale.

      (c) The characteristic murmur is a loud systolic murmur maximal at the right heart border.

2. Cyanotic lesions associated with increased pulmonary blood flow

  a. Total anomalous pulmonary venous return is characterized by partial or complete anomalous drainage of the pulmonary veins with no direct connection with the left atrium. All blood returns to the right atrium or a tributary that drains into it.

    (1) **Types of anomalous drainage**

      (a) **Infracardiac with obstruction of pulmonary venous return** is usually seen in neonates who present with severe cyanosis and tachycardia and marked pulmonary hypertension.

      (b) **Infracardiac or intracardiac pulmonary venous return with only mild to moderate obstruction** results in intermittent bouts of CHF that appear to improve with oxygenation, then recur.

      (c) **Infracardiac or intracardiac anomalous venous return with no obstruction** results in admixture but only mild or no cyanosis and no pulmonary hypertension.

    (2) A **murmur** may be present and depends on the degree of pulmonary obstruction and the degree of pulmonary hypertension.

  b. Truncus arteriosus is characterized by a single outflow vessel arising from the heart to supply systemic, pulmonary, and coronary circulations. It is always associated with ventricular septal defect.

    (1) In **early infancy,** only a murmur and minimal cyanosis are present as pulmonary vascular resistance is high.

    (2) In **later infancy,** when pulmonary resistance falls, signs of CHF predominate but only mild cyanosis is noted. A loud murmur is usually heard at the left sternal border and is usually associated with only a single second heart sound (S_2).

  c. Hypoplastic left heart syndrome is characterized by atresia of the aortic or mitral valve and hypoplasia of the ascending aorta associated with hypoplasia or atresia of the left ventricle. All blood flow to the systemic circulation is via a patent ductus arteriosus. Closure of the patent ductus arteriosus results in immediate and profound shock and hypoperfusion associated with pronounced acidosis.

    (1) A peculiar gray coloration of the lips and skin is seen before frank cyanosis develops.

    (2) Peripheral pulses are either weak or absent.

    (3) A nondescript systolic murmur is often heard but is nondiagnostic.

    (4) If a ventricular septal defect is also present, hypotension is not seen but increasing cyanosis and pulmonary hypertension develop.

C **Differential diagnoses**   Few things present so dramatically as an infant with cyanosis and lethargy. It is imperative to consider all possible differential diagnostic points in critically ill infants and not become fixated on one diagnosis to the exclusion of others. Infants who are profoundly ill should be treated with age-appropriate antibiotics, pending more definitive cardiac evaluation.

1. **Sepsis.** Presentation of infants with sepsis or congenital heart disease often is identical and particularly confusing because of poor perfusion and absent pulses. Pulse pressure that is widened may be very helpful. Frequently, profoundly ill children with congenital heart disease are placed on antibiotics before a primary diagnosis is made.

2. **Inborn errors of metabolism.** Profound acidosis is present in children with inborn errors of metabolism, and ketonuria and aminoaciduria are often present. A family history of similarly affected infants can help differentiate an inborn error of metabolism from a congenital heart defect.

3. **CNS disease**
   a. **Intracranial hemorrhage** accounts for most presentations that are life-threatening.
   b. **Iatrogenic drug administration** or **overdosage** is another possibility, but not in the neonatal period.

4. **Hemoglobinopathies.** Methemoglobinemia resulting in arterial desaturation is a rare cause. The arterial oxygen tension (PaO_2) is usually normal or elevated.

D **Evaluation**

1. **Examination.** Careful physical examination and prolonged observation of breathing patterns should be performed.
   a. **Murmurs.** Location and timing should be carefully noted.
   b. **Upper** and **lower extremity blood pressure** determinations should be made, as well as a **recording of pulses** in the upper and lower extremities, with particular attention to the amplitude and duration of impulse.
   c. **Skin coloration** and **capillary refill** should be noted.
   d. **Associated congenital anomalies** should be sought.

2. **Pulse oximetry** should be performed with the patient breathing room air and 100% oxygen.

3. **Chest radiography** should be performed, focusing on cardiac size and shape as well as pulmonary blood flow.

4. **Electrocardiography** and **two-dimensional echocardiography** are indicated.

5. **Cardiac catheterization** may be required for severely ill infants.

E **Therapy** depends on the diagnosis.

1. **Supportive measures** include:
   a. Supplemental oxygenation
   b. Rapid correction of lactic acidosis
   c. Maintenance of normal temperature
   d. Arrangement for transfer to a center that is equipped to handle such infants
   e. The administration of prostaglandin E_1 (0.05–0.2 µg/kg/min) for suspected ductal-dependent lesions to maintain patency
   f. Dobutamine for patients in CHF who do not have ductal-dependent lesions
   g. Medical stabilization prior to definitive cardiac catheterization or palliative surgery

2. **Tetralogy of Fallot.** Patients require a special form of treatment when hypercyanotic attacks occur, including the following:
   a. Placing the infant on the abdomen in the knee–chest position
   b. Administration of supplemental oxygen

    c. Administration of morphine sulfate subcutaneously in a dose not to exceed 0.2 mg/kg

    d. Rapid correction of metabolic acidosis with administration of sodium bicarbonate

    e. Adrenergic blockade by intravenous administration of propranolol (0.1–0.2 mg/kg) for infants with tachycardia and cyanosis

F Disposition

1. Infants with a **murmur** but **no evidence of CHF** or **cyanosis** may be referred for pediatric cardiology evaluation in a more controlled fashion after initial telephone consultation.

2. Infants with a **murmur** and **signs of CHF** but **no evidence of cyanosis** must be stabilized after initial diagnostic evaluation. The patient should be referred to a tertiary center for cardiology evaluation.

3. Infants with **cyanosis on room air** who **fail to improve following the administration of 100% oxygen** (as determined by pulse oximetry) most likely have a cyanotic congenital heart lesion and are at high risk for deterioration. Transport to the nearest tertiary center should be emergently arranged, with a physician in attendance during the transport.

VIII KAWASAKI DISEASE

A Discussion   Kawasaki disease is a febrile condition associated with vasculitis of the large coronary vessels and marked inflammation of the mucous membranes, especially of the eye and mouth. It is the leading cause of acquired heart disease in children and primarily affects children 5 years of age or younger. The cause is unknown—no putative infectious or autoimmunologic cause has been found. There is no evidence for person-to-person transmission.

B Clinical features

1. **Fever** is abrupt in onset, lasts for at least 5 days, and may be as high as 105°F (the mean temperature is 104°F).

2. **Bilateral nonpurulent conjunctival injection** is present and not associated with discharge or crusting.

3. **Dry, erythematous, fissured lips; injected oral mucosae;** and peculiar **"strawberry tongue"** are noted, which may cause an inappropriate diagnosis as streptococcal infection.

4. **Lymphadenopathy** is present in the cervical and axillary areas. It is usually nonsuppurative and not generalized.

5. **Skin eruptions** are usually present and may be the morbilliform, maculopapular, urticarial, or erythema multiforme type. At times, the skin eruptions may resemble diaper dermatitis.

6. **Swollen feet.** After the third day of the illness, the feet become edematous and painful, with most children refusing to bear weight or walk.

7. **Desquamation.** After several weeks of illness, desquamation of the hands and feet occurs. The first appearance is in the subungual area. Desquamation then spreads to the palms and soles before becoming generalized.

8. **Transient arthritis** is apparent in older children and is characterized by symmetric swelling of the small and large joints of the lower extremities.

9. **Cardiac involvement** is seen in 10%–50% of untreated children and is usually silent. However, cardiac involvement may present as CHF, complete heart block, or an evolving myocardial infarction (MI).

C Differential diagnoses

1. **Scarlet fever.** The "strawberry tongue" of scarlet fever is similar to that of Kawasaki disease, but the characteristic sandpaper-like papular rash of scarlet fever usually allows differentiation of the two entities. Also, children with scarlet fever have no edema of the hands or feet.

2. **Toxic shock syndrome (TSS)** is often difficult to differentiate from Kawasaki disease in severely ill children.

3. **Leptospirosis.** Exposure to a vector is a helpful clue. Profuse conjunctivitis with no other symptoms, along with elevated liver enzymes, often aids in the diagnosis. Hepatitis may mimic infectious mononucleosis.

4. **Epstein-Barr virus infection.** A positive heterophil antibody response in older children or elevation of specific Epstein-Barr complement fixation titers in younger children is common. Splenomegaly is common in adolescents but rare in smaller children.

5. **Juvenile rheumatoid arthritis.** The pauciarticular variety common in small children is difficult to differentiate from Kawasaki disease. Rheumatoid factor is not helpful. The presence of iridocyclitis is helpful diagnostically.

6. **Rocky Mountain spotted fever.** The rash usually begins on the wrists and is petechial and vasculitic in type. It occurs only during the months that the tick vector is active.

7. **Measles** (see Chapter 11 IX A)

8. **Stevens-Johnson syndrome** (see Chapter 11 III B)

D Evaluation

1. **Laboratory studies.** There are no definitive diagnostic laboratory studies available to diagnose Kawasaki disease. Testing for autoimmune disease is unnecessary.
   a. **CBC.** Leukocytosis is marked in the second to third week of the illness with immature forms.
   b. **Sedimentation rate** and **C-reactive protein level** are usually elevated.
   c. **Liver tests.** Enzyme levels may be mildly elevated, but liver tests are nondiagnostic.
   d. **Urinalysis.** Sterile pyuria without bacteriuria is common.

2. **Imaging studies.** A chest radiograph is usually not helpful, but **two-dimensional echocardiography** is essential for the diagnosis. It obviates the need for coronary arteriography in most children and allows rapid assessment of coronary artery size.

3. **Electrocardiography** is usually not helpful.

E Therapy

1. **Intravenous immunoglobulin.** Patients with Kawasaki disease respond dramatically and predictably to the administration of immunoglobulin during the febrile phase. A single dose of 2 g/kg is given over a 12-hour period. Side effects of intravenous immunoglobulin are rare.
   a. Fever abates 24 hours after therapy.
   b. This therapy prevents the formation of coronary artery aneurysms and coronary vasculitis if given within 48 hours of diagnosis. If given after 10 days of illness, the intravenous immunoglobulin ameliorates most symptoms in severely ill infants but will not change coronary vasculitis.
   c. If given within 10 days of onset, aneurysm formation may not be prevented, but further enlargement is prevented.

2. **Salicylate therapy** is indicated during the initial febrile phase of the illness and for 6–8 weeks after active disease subsides.
   a. **Febrile phase.** High doses (80–100 mg/kg/day) may be required to achieve serum concentrations of 30–40 mg/dL.
   b. **Following acute disease.** Salicylate therapy (5–8 mg/kg/day) is continued for its antithrombotic effect. In children with coronary lesions discovered at initial echocardiography, aspirin therapy must be continued until they completely resolve.

3. **Coumadin therapy** is advocated for large, persistent, or multiple nonobstructive aneurysms.

4. **Corticosteroid therapy** has no proven value in therapy.

5. **Thrombolytic therapy** has had limited usage in children with acute coronary thrombosis.

F **Disposition**

1. Children should not be discharged until the acute phase of illness has subsided following salicylate and immunoglobulin therapy.

2. Any child with known coronary artery aneurysms who presents in failure or with chest pain should be considered to have cardiac ischemia until proven otherwise. Acutely ill children should be admitted for monitoring to an intensive care setting until a full evaluation can be performed.

IX   **BACTEREMIA, MENINGITIS, AND SEPSIS**

A **Discussion**

1. **Bacteremia** is defined as the presence of bacteria in the blood; most often, bacteremia is asymptomatic.
   a. **Occult bacteremia** is usually transient and self-limited. It is common in children between the ages of 6 and 30 months and is associated with temperature elevation above 103°F and a leukocyte count of 15,000–20,000/mm³ or more. In 15%–20% of children with occult bacteremia, the leukocyte count is greater than 20,000/mm³, the fever is higher than 103°F, and there is a primary site of infection (e.g., otitis media, pneumonia).
      (1) **Etiology.** *S. pneumoniae* is the most common causative organism. *H. influenzae* is uncommon because of the widespread usage of conjugated *H. influenzae* vaccine.
      (2) **Pathogenesis.** Secondary spread to the meninges occurs in 5%–15% of patients.
   b. **Secondary bacteremia** is caused by spread from a primary site of infection, such as pneumonia or an indwelling medical appliance.

2. **Sepsis** is a life-threatening bacterial invasion of the intravascular compartment that is associated with symptoms of lethargy, irritability, or hypotension and may or may not be associated with a focus of infection. Sepsis is most common in children younger than 3 months of age. It is usually caused by a group B streptococcal infection in children younger than 1 month of age and by *H. influenzae* or *N. meningitidis* in older children.

3. **Meningitis** refers to any inflammation of the meninges and the subarachnoid space. It can be caused by bacterial, viral, or fungal agents. Meningitis is seen most frequently in children older than 6 months of age. It is associated with an increased CSF WBC concentration, variable elevation of CSF protein, and a low level of CSF glucose.
   a. **Bacterial meningitis**
      (1) In **neonates,** the most common cause is group B streptococcus and *Escherichia coli.*
      (2) In **older children,** the most common causative organisms are *H. influenzae, S. pneumoniae,* and *N. meningitidis.*
   b. **Aseptic meningitis** usually is caused by viral agents, predominantly coxsackievirus, echovirus, and the mumps virus. In neonates, herpes simplex should be considered in any child with skin lesions characteristic of the infection and irritability.

B **Clinical features**

1. **Sepsis.** In patients with sepsis, signs and symptoms are usually isolated to a temperature elevation of 103°F or higher and irritability with no obvious focus of infection. Sepsis should be considered in any infant younger than 3 months of age with fever, no obvious source of infection, and ill appearance.

2. **Meningitis** often presents with symptoms of vomiting, poor suck and feeding, lethargy, and irritability.
   a. In **older children,** headache, photophobia, and neck stiffness may be seen.
   b. In **young infants,** a bulging fontanelle may be all that is apparent along with lethargy or irritability.

C **Differential diagnoses** include:

1. CHF

2. Arrhythmia

3. Pericarditis or myocarditis

4. Ductus-dependent cardiac lesions

5. Congenital adrenal insufficiency

6. Electrolyte imbalance (hyponatremia)

7. Inborn errors of metabolism

8. Volvulus

9. Intussusception

10. Leukemia

11. Intoxication

12. Infantile botulism

13. Nonaccidental trauma with CNS sequelae

14. Hemolytic–uremic syndrome

D **Evaluation**

1. **Laboratory studies**
   a. **No child should be excluded from appropriate evaluation or therapy based on the results of a single laboratory test.**
      (1) **Sepsis** is a clinical diagnosis primarily substantiated by laboratory diagnosis and not excluded by a test other than a negative blood culture.
      (2) **Meningitis** is based on analysis of all parameters of the properly performed lumbar puncture, and treatment should not be withheld based on a single test.
   b. **CBC.** The peripheral **WBC concentration** may be remarkable for a leukocytosis in excess of 15,000 cells/mm³ with left shift. Children with sepsis usually have high-grade bacteremia leukocytosis or neutropenia and a shift of the WBC differential concentration to more immature forms. A low WBC of less than 5,000 cells/mm³ is also associated with serious infections.
   c. **Quantitative blood cultures** usually reveal low-level bacteremia in children with occult bacteremia.
   d. **Urinalysis** of an unspun urine sample (obtained by catheterization) is useful for children younger than 1 year of age.
   e. **CSF analysis.** Any child with altered mental status must have an evaluation of the CSF by lumbar puncture to exclude meningitis, which is characterized by the following findings:
      (1) Increased CSF WBC concentration (100–10,000 cells/μL)
      (2) Increased CSF pressure
      (3) Increased protein concentration (greater than 80 mg/dL)
      (4) Decreased CSF glucose concentration (less than 40 mg/dL)
      (5) Positive Gram's stain and positive culture of CSF
      (6) Possibly positive antigen detection tests

2. **Chest radiography** is useful only in children with respiratory symptoms of cough or tachypnea.

E **Therapy**

1. **Antibiotic therapy**
   a. **Occult bacteremia**
      (1) Children who may have occult bacteremia (i.e., those with a WBC count greater than 20,000 mm³ and a temperature higher than 103°F) benefit from a single dose of **ceftriaxone**

given intramuscularly after a complete diagnostic evaluation. These patients should be seen again in 12 hours to ensure that a secondary infection is not present.

(2) Children with occult bacteremia that resolves in 24–48 hours with no clinical findings and no further temperature elevation require no additional therapy.

b. **Sepsis** or **meningitis.** Children with presumed sepsis or meningitis should be treated with an antibiotic that is effective against the common pathogens (as suggested by the patient's age) after a full diagnostic evaluation is completed.

(1) **Neonates and infants younger than 2 months** of age are usually given ampicillin sodium and either an aminoglycoside or cefotaxime.

(2) **Infants and older children** may be treated with a single or daily divided dose of ceftriaxone or with cefotaxime.

c. **Duration of therapy** is based on patient age and the organism treated.

(1) Children with **occult bacteremia** are usually treated with 3 days of intravenous antibiotics followed by oral therapy for 7–10 days.

(2) Infants with **sepsis but without meningitis** are usually treated with intravenous antibiotics for 7–10 days.

(3) Infants with **meningitis** are treated with parenteral antibiotics for 10–14 days, depending on the organism. *N. meningitidis* meningitis may be treated for fewer than 7 days, under certain circumstances (e.g., improving clinical course, afebrile after 3 days of therapy).

2. **Supportive care** is essential and includes:

a. **Fluid resuscitation** to treat shock and hypoperfusion, with care to avoid cerebral edema when vascular volume is restored

b. **Anticonvulsant therapy** to control seizures

c. **Assisted ventilation** to control cerebral edema or respiratory failure

3. **Corticosteroids** are indicated for meningitis to reduce the incidence of hearing loss.

F **Disposition**   Children with **sepsis** or **meningitis** must be admitted for further therapy.

1. Children with stable vital signs may be admitted to a regular-floor bed with close observation and monitoring.

2. Children who are unstable must be admitted to an intensive care unit.

X **GASTROINTESTINAL DISORDERS**

A **Gastroenteritis**

1. **Discussion**

a. **Incidence.** Diarrhea accounts for 3–5 million deaths worldwide yearly and for 25–35 million episodes per year in the United States.

b. The major **mechanism of transmission** of the organisms that cause gastroenteritis is the fecal–oral route. Water-borne and food-borne outbreaks also occur, but they are seasonal. Diarrheal pathogens vary by geographic location and season.

c. **Etiology**

(1) In **underdeveloped countries,** where nutrition is poor, causes are usually diverse and may be bacterial, viral, or parasitic.

(2) In **industrialized countries,** acute or chronic diarrhea is usually caused by bacterial or viral agents that reflect seasonality, local epidemiology, and age.

(a) **Bacterial agents** can cause inflammatory or noninflammatory disease; inflammatory disease is most important in industrialized countries.

(i) *Salmonella* species

(ii) *Shigella* species

(iii) *Campylobacter jejuni*

(iv) *Yersinia enterocolitica*

(b) Viral agents. Most children with diarrhea have a viral etiology for their illness.
  (i) In **young infants, rotavirus** and **enteric adenovirus** can cause severe diarrhea, dehydration, and acidosis, which often necessitates hospitalization.
  (ii) In **older infants** and **adults, Norwalk agent, calicivirus,** and **astrovirus** are associated with a short-lived 3- to 4-day illness that usually does not involve dehydration or acidosis.
(c) Parasitic agents are common in underdeveloped countries. In the United States, *Giardia lamblia* is the most common cause of parasitic diarrhea.

2. **Clinical features.** Enteric infections have local (gastrointestinal), extraintestinal, and systemic manifestations.
   a. **Local symptoms** include diarrhea, abdominal cramping, and emesis.
   b. **Extraintestinal manifestations** may include signs of vulvovaginitis, conjunctivitis, endocarditis, osteomyelitis, or meningitis.
   c. **Systemic manifestations** may include fever and malaise, rash, arthritis, or seizures.

3. **Differential diagnoses**
   a. **Feeding difficulty** with reflux or dumping due to overfeeding
   b. **Anatomic gastrointestinal defects**
      (1) Malrotation
      (2) Hirschsprung's disease
      (3) Volvulus
      (4) Intussusception
   c. **Malabsorptive states**
      (1) Monosaccharidase and disaccharidase deficiency
      (2) Immunoglobulin A (IgA) deficiency
      (3) Celiac disease
      (4) Cystic fibrosis with pancreatic insufficiency
   d. **Toxigenic food poisoning**
      (1) Scombroid poisoning
      (2) Ciguatera poisoning
      (3) *Amanita* mushroom poisoning
   e. **Endocrine deficiency states**
      (1) Congenital adrenal insufficiency
      (2) Adrenogenital syndrome
   f. **Inflammatory bowel disease**
      (1) Crohn's disease
      (2) Ulcerative colitis
      (3) Acrodermatitis enteropathica

4. **Evaluation**
   a. **Laboratory studies**
      (1) A **serum electrolyte panel** is necessary for children with significant dehydration.
      (2) A **CBC** is usually not helpful.
      (3) **Fecal analysis.** Stool specimens should be analyzed for blood, mucus, and leukocytes. Blood and leukocytes detected in a stool sample merit culture of the stool for bacterial agents.
      (4) **Serology.** Antigen-detection methods for rotavirus may be helpful for infants with vomiting and diarrhea during the winter months. Nonspecific serologic markers of infection (e.g., febrile precipitins, acute-phase reactants) are not helpful and do not aid in the specific diagnosis.
      (5) **Blood cultures** are beneficial in children with fever and studies that may suggest *Salmonella* gastroenteritis.

(6) **Aspiration of vasculitic lesions** may yield evidence of the organism on Gram stain or culture.

(7) **Urinalysis** is not helpful unless extraintestinal spread is suggested.

b. **Radiographic studies** usually are not warranted unless a secondary pneumonia or osteomyelitis is suspected.

5. Therapy

   a. **Management of dehydration** is the cornerstone of therapy for diarrhea, regardless of the cause. If symptoms do not resolve in 2–3 days with conservative replacement of fluid and electrolytes, cultures or antigen detection may be necessary to determine the cause of the diarrhea.

      (1) **Oral rehydration** is the treatment of choice for all but the most severely affected infants.

         (a) **Commercially available rehydration solutions** usually have a carbohydrate source that is easily digestible and aids in electrolyte absorption. Ongoing losses should be replaced with oral electrolyte solution.

            (i) The **sodium concentration** is usually at least 90–140 mmol/L.

            (ii) The **carbohydrate:sodium concentration** should be approximately 1:8 to 1:2.

            (iii) The **osmolality** is 300–350 mOsm/L.

         (b) **Home remedies** (e.g., fruit juices, gelatin, tea, decarbonated soda, sports drinks) should not be used because of their unsuitable low-sodium concentrations and excessive carbohydrates.

      (2) **Intravenous rehydration.** Severely dehydrated children should receive 20 mL/kg of lactated Ringer's solution or normal saline to improve perfusion. After the initial resuscitative bolus is administered, further fluid therapy should be guided by serum electrolyte determinations and the clinical response to the infusion. Additional boluses (20 mL/kg) of the previously used fluid administered over 1 hour may be necessary to establish urine flow.

   b. **Serum electrolyte disturbances** (e.g., hyponatremia, hypernatremia) should be corrected in the hospital within 16–24 hours.

   c. **Feeding.** Once rehydration is complete, **introduction of bland foods** such as bananas, apples, rice cereal, or a high-protein source (e.g., chicken) is helpful.

      (1) **Dairy products should be withheld** for 3–5 days because of the induced disaccharidase deficiency.

      (2) **Breast-fed infants** should resume their feedings as soon as possible.

   d. **Antidiarrheal compounds** generally are not warranted for most cases of childhood diarrhea.

   e. **Antibiotic therapy** is indicated when certain bacterial pathogens have been implicated, primarily to shorten the clinical course or to decrease excretion of the organism to prevent secondary spread.

   f. **Antiviral therapy** (including fractionated albumin, high-titer breast milk, or egg white) is not useful in otherwise healthy children.

   g. **Vaccination** is not warranted in most cases of gastroenteritis in the United States but may be helpful for *Salmonella typhi* or *Vibrio cholerae* infection in other countries.

6. Disposition

   a. Most children may be easily managed by oral rehydration at home with a commercially available electrolyte solution and lactose avoidance followed by a bland but protein-rich diet.

   b. Children who are isotonically dehydrated may be discharged to home after appropriate oral or intravenous rehydration, and after a trial of oral hydration is effective.

   c. Children with hypernatremic or hyponatremic dehydration usually require admission to the hospital for rehydration and correction of deficits over an 18- to 24-hour period.

B Intestinal obstruction

1. Discussion

   a. **Incidence.** Intestinal obstruction is not common in pediatrics but occurs with a frequency of approximately 1:2000 live births.

    b. Etiology. In adults, intestinal obstruction is usually a complication of fibrotic bands that have formed after surgery. In children, intestinal obstruction usually is the result of maldevelopment of the embryonic intestine or mechanical factors that have allowed the intestine to slide or move.

    c. Types. Intestinal obstruction can be partial or complete but the distinction is often difficult.

2. Clinical features vary with the cause of the obstruction, the level and completeness of the obstruction, and the time between the obstruction and the presentation for care.

    a. Symptoms

      (1) Nausea and **vomiting.** Obstruction is associated with accumulation of intestinal secretions, ingested food, and gas from fermentation of contents of the intestine. This results in dilatation proximal to the obstruction. Because of the osmolality of the obstructed contents, intraluminal fluid shifts occur that result in fluid and electrolyte depletion. The resultant electrolyte depletion, intraluminal fluid accumulation, and decreased intestinal motility lead to nausea and eventually to vomiting.

        (a) Nausea, vomiting, and abdominal distention are classic signs, with **bilious emesis** found only when the site of obstruction is high in the intestinal tract but below the pylorus.

        (b) Lower intestinal obstruction in adults often results in **feculent vomiting** but is seldom seen in children with similar obstruction.

      (2) Pain and **cramping** are intermittent and often positional. Vomiting often provides relief.

      (3) Obstipation (intractable constipation) is common but not diagnostic by itself or exclusive of obstruction in children.

    b. Physical examination findings

      (1) Fever usually is not seen unless the blood supply to the obstructed bowel becomes compromised, resulting in bacterial proliferation and the development of sepsis.

      (2) Peritoneal signs (i.e., an increasingly tender, distended abdomen with rebound tenderness; involuntary guarding; and rigidity) develop as the obstruction progresses and peritonitis ensues.

      (3) Profound dehydration (evidenced by **poor capillary refill, hypotension,** and **shock**) may be seen in children who present late in the course of their illness as a result of increasing loss of fluid into the bowel lumen.

3. Differential diagnoses

    a. Hypertrophic pyloric stenosis

    b. Congenital gastric outlet obstruction

    c. Gastric duplication syndromes

    d. Duodenal atresia, which is associated with the "double bubble" sign of intestinal obstruction and often with other congenital anomalies

    e. Duodenal bands and webs

    f. Annular pancreas

    g. Jejunal and ileal atresia

    h. Malrotation, which is usually associated with bilious vomiting and, later, small bowel volvulus

    i. Intestinal duplication syndromes

    j. Meckel's diverticulum

    k. Appendicitis

    l. Intussusception

    m. Sepsis

    n. Incarcerated hernia

4. Evaluation. Often, the obstructive process is complete when the patient presents, and little diagnostic skill or laboratory evaluation is required to make the initial diagnosis. Obstructive processes that are incomplete offer a diagnostic challenge of episodic pain and vomiting that have often resolved by the time care is sought.

a. **Physical examination** and **history findings** are usually suggestive of obstruction.

b. **Laboratory studies** are supportive of the diagnosis but not diagnostic. They often reveal hypochloremic alkalosis with hemoconcentration. A CBC often reveals only leukocytosis; a shift to more immature forms is suggestive of impending peritonitis.

c. **Diagnostic imaging studies**

(1) **Ultrasonography** may be useful but only for the diagnosis of pyloric stenosis and rarely for other forms of obstruction.

(2) **Radiographic studies**

(a) **Plain radiographs.** Flat and upright radiographs of the abdomen reveal distention of the bowel at and above the obstruction and the presence of multiple air–fluid levels in various locations in the abdomen. If perforation is present, free air is noticeable in the subdiaphragmatic region, but small amounts are not visible unless lateral decubitus radiographs are performed with air layering over the liver edge.

(b) **Contrast studies** are indicated only when an obstructive pattern exists on plain radiographs but no obvious source of obstruction is apparent despite ultrasonography.

(i) **Water-soluble oral contrast** is useful for recognizing atresia, volvulus, and congenital web or band syndromes, as well as some presentations of malrotation. These contrast agents should be used carefully, particularly in ill patients in whom the risk of perforation is high.

(ii) **Water-soluble enemas** are useful for the diagnosis of malrotation, intussusception, or colonic duplications.

(3) **CT examination** of the abdomen is seldom useful in localizing the site of the obstruction, even with contrast.

5. **Therapy**

a. **Stabilization.** Initial treatment involves **fluid** and **electrolyte resuscitation** to compensate for intraluminal losses.

b. **Nasogastric decompression** is beneficial for the relief of pain and vomiting. This conservative therapy is indicated only for children with postoperative bands, strictures, or adhesions; these patients must be frequently re-evaluated.

c. **Prompt surgical consultation** must be obtained, and additional diagnostic maneuvers should be directed by the surgeon in charge of the case. **Immediate surgical consultation and operation** are imperative for any child who has signs of **peritonitis.**

d. **Hydrostatic reduction of suspected intussusception** is usually not performed by the emergency physician because perforation may result.

e. **Antibiotic therapy** may be instituted after appropriate cultures are obtained for an ill child with signs of peritonitis. The antibiotic regimen should provide broad coverage against anaerobic as well as fecal aerobic organisms.

6. **Disposition.** Most patients are hospitalized for stabilization and gastrointestinal decompression via nasogastric suction.

a. Most patients with intestinal obstruction but no evidence of peritonitis can be managed conservatively. If there is no response while the patient is hospitalized, the condition requires surgical intervention.

b. **No child with suspected intestinal obstruction is ever discharged home without surgical consultation.**

C Volvulus

1. **Discussion.** The most common type of volvulus is gastric, but small bowel volvulus can also occur with intestinal malrotation. A volvulus occurs when the gastrocolic, gastrohepatic, or gastrosplenic ligament is absent, resulting in rotation of the stomach upon itself, which compromises blood flow.

2. Clinical features
   a. History suggests **early satiety** and, in small infants, **failure to thrive.**
   b. Symptoms. Volvulus is characterized by the **acute onset of severe epigastric pain** and **intractable, nonbilious vomiting.**
   c. Physical examination findings. Failure to pass a nasogastric tube is characteristic and diagnostic. **Peritoneal findings** are usually not present in patients with unrecognized volvulus; however, unrecognized volvulus can progress rapidly to strangulation and perforation.

3. Differential diagnoses
   a. Hypertrophic pyloric stenosis
   b. Congenital gastric outlet obstruction
   c. Gastric duplication syndromes
   d. Duodenal atresia
   e. Malrotation
   f. Intussusception
   g. Sepsis
   h. Appendicitis
   i. Incarcerated hernia

4. Evaluation
   a. Careful physical examination often reveals signs of acute obstruction but no peritoneal findings unless it is late in the course.
   b. Laboratory studies. A **CBC** and **electrolyte determination** are essential.
   c. Radiographic studies
      (1) Plain abdominal radiographs reveal a dilated stomach, and upright films reveal the characteristic proximal beak appearance of the lower esophageal junction.
      (2) Contrast radiographic studies usually are not indicated except when small bowel volvulus is suspected. In this case, a barium enema may be helpful.

5. Therapy
   a. Stabilization
      (1) Intravenous electrolyte solution should be administered to stabilize the patient's blood pressure and re-establish urine flow.
      (2) Emergent referral for surgery is necessary to prevent progression of volvulus to perforation and frank peritonitis. All patients with suspected volvulus must have a surgical consultation.
   b. Antibiotic therapy usually is not warranted. However, in critically ill infants with perforation and peritonitis, coverage for aerobic Gram-negative organisms as well as anaerobic infection is justified.

6. Disposition. Patients at **high risk for volvulus** must be emergently taken to surgery or transferred to a center where such care is available.

D Incarcerated hernia

1. Discussion. An incarcerated hernia occurs when the contents of a hernia sac cannot be reduced back into the abdominal cavity. The incarcerated organ is usually an intestine but may be any abdominal organ—most commonly the mesentery or the ovary.

2. Clinical features. This condition usually is associated with signs and symptoms of intestinal obstruction, such as bilious vomiting, abdominal distention, and constipation.
   a. Symptoms. Children are irritable, are inconsolable, and often refuse most or all feedings. They have vomiting that may or may not be bilious in character.
   b. Physical examination findings
      (1) The abdomen is often distended and tympanitic, and peritoneal signs of rigidity or erythema may be noted. A tender, edematous, slightly discolored to pale mass is noted in the inguinal area.

    (2) A swollen erythematous mass that becomes erythematous to violaceous and is exquisitely tender is usually a sign of a strangulated hernia.

    (3) Fever and toxicity suggest frank necrosis of the incarcerated organ and impending or completed perforation.

3. **Differential diagnoses** are the same as for volvulus (see X C 3). Testicular torsion must be considered as well.

4. **Evaluation.** Incarcerated hernia must be considered in all children with intestinal obstruction who have no other obvious reason for obstruction, such as antecedent surgery.

    a. Careful physical examination is the most useful diagnostic test that can be performed.

    b. Laboratory studies

        (1) CBC may confirm the presence of impending strangulation.

        (2) A **serum biochemistry profile** guides therapy for replacement of fluid and electrolytes but is not helpful diagnostically.

    c. Radiographic studies. Air–fluid levels are visible on plain radiographs; however, radiographs do not localize the source any better than a careful physical examination. Contrast studies are usually not indicated and add nothing to the diagnosis.

5. **Therapy**

    a. Stabilization. Electrolyte solution is administered intravenously to stabilize blood pressure and re-establish urine flow.

    b. Reduction of a nonstrangulated hernia can be accomplished in approximately 95%–98% of cases.

        (1) The patient is usually best aided by sedation and placement in mild Trendelenburg position.

        (2) Gentle traction on the hernia and the contents of the sac are usually sufficient to allow for loss of volume and rapid retraction of the contents of the sac into the abdominal cavity.

        (3) After reduction of the hernia, elective repair may be accomplished 24–48 hours after edema subsides.

    c. Emergent referral for surgery to prevent progression of incarceration to perforation and frank peritonitis is mandatory for those patients with hernias that cannot be reduced and for those patients with strangulation. Absolutely **no delay** should occur from the time of diagnosis of an unreduced incarcerated hernia to surgical consultation, because the need for surgery increases the morbidity 25-fold.

    d. Antibiotic therapy usually is not warranted. However, in critically ill infants with perforation and peritonitis, coverage for aerobic Gram-negative organisms as well as anaerobic infection is justified.

6. **Disposition**

    a. Discharge. Children with an incarcerated hernia that is promptly reduced in the ED may be sent home if they are not dehydrated, provided that close surgical care is arranged.

    b. Admission

        (1) Patients at **high risk for strangulation** must be emergently taken to surgery or transferred to a center where such care is available.

        (2) Dehydrated children should be hospitalized and scheduled for surgery in the next 48–72 hours to allow time to correct fluid and electrolyte imbalances.

E Pyloric stenosis

1. **Discussion.** Pyloric stenosis is the most commonly considered diagnosis in a small infant who is vomiting.

    a. Incidence. Pyloric stenosis occurs at a rate of 3–5/1000 live births in the United States. Boys, particularly firstborns, are affected four to six times more frequently than girls. A positive family history of pyloric stenosis increases the probability of the diagnosis in an infant by a factor of 40.

   b. **Etiology.** The cause of pyloric stenosis is unknown, and no direct evidence is available to suggest a preventive strategy. There is an association of other congenital anomalies, particularly tracheoesophageal fistula and trisomy 18.

   c. **Pathogenesis.** Vomiting causes **contraction of the intravascular space** and the development of a marked **hypochloremic alkalosis** with **hypokalemia** and **dehydration.**

2. **Clinical features**

   a. **Symptoms** usually begin after the second or third week of life but have occurred as early as the first week.

   (1) The initial manifestation is most often **nonbilious vomiting** that is **nonprojectile** and often confused with feeding intolerance or gastroenteritis. Vomiting is often intermittent and not associated with an ill appearance. Affected infants appear well after an episode of vomiting and are usually hungry and ready to feed again. The development of **projectile vomiting** appears to be related to the degree of obstruction at the pylorus.

   (2) As the disease progresses and the **infant loses weight,** a **visible peristaltic wave is often seen across the abdomen** that parents may notice.

   b. **Physical examination findings**

   (1) A **pyloric mass** (pyloric olive) that is often firm, movable, and nontender is often palpated immediately under the edge of the liver. Palpating the mass is diagnostic in 60%–90% of affected infants.

   (2) **Dehydration.** In the past, infants presented late in their disease course and were often misdiagnosed, which made them more likely to finally present with signs of significant dehydration. Increased awareness of the entity has decreased the incidence of dehydration dramatically.

3. **Differential diagnoses** include poor maternal–infant bonding or poor feeding technique, congenital gastric outlet obstruction, gastric duplication syndromes, duodenal atresia, malrotation, intussusception, and sepsis.

4. **Evaluation**

   a. **Laboratory studies.** A CBC and serum electrolyte panel are usually not indicated, except in infants who are dehydrated or who have evidence of hemodynamic instability. Blood cultures are usually not warranted.

   b. **Diagnostic imaging studies**

   (1) **Radiography**

   (a) **Plain radiographs** are obtained to exclude other causes in the differential diagnosis but are not diagnostic of pyloric stenosis.

   (b) **Contrast radiographs** are seldom used to make the diagnosis and are associated with a risk of aspiration.

   (2) **Ultrasonography** is safe and has a sensitivity that exceeds 95% when performed by an experienced radiologist. An ultrasonogram can establish the diagnosis on the basis of pyloric thickness and length.

5. **Therapy.** The infant must not be given anything by mouth. Vomiting usually subsides with the last bout of emesis after the stomach is empty.

   a. **Stabilization.** Initially, treatment is directed at **correcting fluid** and **electrolyte disturbances** and **replenishing intravascular volume.** Fluid therapy should be instituted concurrent with obtaining surgical consultation and should be continued until the patient is clinically rehydrated and the serum bicarbonate concentration is near normal.

   b. **Nasogastric suction** is rarely needed.

   c. **Prompt surgical consultation is mandatory,** and most children require hospitalization to correct any electrolyte abnormalities.

6. **Disposition.** Most children who undergo **ultrasound examination** of the pylorus and have **no evidence of stenosis** may be discharged home with appropriate follow-up care.

F **Intussusception**

1. **Discussion.** Intussusception is the most common cause of intestinal obstruction in infants and children between the ages of 3 months and 6 years. This condition occurs when a portion of the intestine telescopes into itself at one or more locations. Intussusceptions are most commonly located in the ileocolic junction but can also occur as a triple ileoileocolic or cecocolic process and may extend for great lengths, involving the vascular supply for the bowel.

   a. **Incidence.** As is the case with pyloric stenosis, intussusception is more common in boys than in girls by 4:1 or 5:1.

   b. **Etiology.** The cause is unknown, but a viral etiology is suspected because of a seasonal predisposition for spring and autumn months. One postulation suggests that intercurrent gastroenteritis or allergic stimuli cause intestinal lymphatic tissue to swell and become a lead point to pull the mass into the adjacent proximal intestine. Only 8%–10% of children who require surgery for reduction have a recognized lead point, usually Meckel's diverticulum, a polyp, duplication, or lymphosarcoma in older children.

   c. **Pathogenesis.** Most intussusceptions cause incarcerations immediately and strangulation within 24 hours, with progression to shock and, if untreated, death.

2. **Clinical features**

   a. **Symptoms**

      (1) In typical cases, there is a sudden onset of **severe abdominal pain** that is colicky in nature and often so profound that the child drops to the floor in agony with crying and pain. Children who are so affected appear to be normal between paroxysms of pain.

      (2) As the intussusception progresses, the child becomes progressively more **irritable and lethargic** until **shock** develops.

      (3) **Vomiting** initially occurs with the early phase of the illness and is bilious in 30% of cases.

      (4) Stools are initially normal early in the course of the disease, but rapidly become bloody and mucoid within the first 12 hours (**currant jelly stool**).

   b. **Physical examination findings.** Palpation of the abdomen usually reveals a **tender, sausage-shaped mass** that is variable in size and firmness with spasms of pain.

3. **Differential diagnoses** include hypertrophic pyloric stenosis, congenital gastric outlet obstruction, gastric duplication syndromes, duodenal atresia, malrotation, appendicitis, sepsis, testicular torsion, incarcerated or strangulated hernia, gastroenteritis with enterocolitis, Henoch-Schönlein purpura, and diabetic ketoacidosis.

4. **Evaluation.** Typically, the **clinical history** and **physical findings** are sufficient for diagnosis.

   a. **Laboratory studies**

      (1) A **CBC** and **serum biochemistry profile** are not indicated and are nondiagnostic in the first 12 hours of the illness but may be warranted in children with hypotension and symptoms of greater than 16 hours' duration.

      (2) **Urinalysis** is not helpful, although it may give some idea of fluid status.

   b. **Diagnostic imaging studies**

      (1) **Radiography**

         (a) **Plain abdominal radiographs** may show areas of increased soft tissue density or scattered air–fluid levels that suggest an ileus or partial obstruction.

         (b) **Contrast radiographs.** A barium enema is therapeutic as well as diagnostic, revealing a **filling defect.** A "coil spring," caused by the tracking of barium around the lumen of the edematous intestine, is a classic sign.

      (2) **Ultrasonography** is useful in some cases and may have a sensitivity as high as 75% when the diagnostic criteria of concentric areas of wall thickness are used.

5. **Therapy**

   a. **Stabilization** is the same as for pyloric stenosis (see X E 5 a). The child should not be given anything by mouth.

    b. Nasogastric suction should be instituted to attempt to decompress the obstruction from above.

    c. Barium or air reduction is appropriate after surgical consultation if symptoms have been present for fewer than 12 hours and there are no signs of peritonitis. Children who have had symptoms longer than 12 hours or who have signs of peritonitis should not be considered candidates for barium or air reduction. These children should be stabilized and taken expeditiously to the operating room because untreated intussusception is almost always fatal.

    d. Partial or complete regression of the invaginating segment may be curative in 75% of cases and is also diagnostic.

6. Disposition

    a. Discharge. Most children who undergo ultrasound examination of the abdomen and have no evidence of intussusception must undergo a barium enema if suspicion is high. They may be discharged home to await appropriate surgical consultation.

    b. Admission. Prompt surgical consultation is mandatory, and most children require hospitalization to correct any electrolyte abnormalities prior to surgery.

G Meckel's diverticulum

1. Discussion

    a. Cause. Meckel's diverticulum is a remnant of the embryonic yolk sac that failed to involute. This results in the presence in the mesenteric or antimesenteric border of a blind pouch that is usually 50–75 cm from the ileocolic junction. Meckel's diverticulum usually becomes clinically apparent during the first 2 years of life but is equally common in the first 10–15 years of life.

    b. Pathogenesis

      (1) Diverticula become symptomatic when ectopic mucosae secrete acid, causing intermittent painless rectal bleeding following ulceration of the adjacent mucosa.

      (2) Occasionally Meckel's diverticulum may be associated with partial or complete bowel obstruction when the diverticulum becomes edematous and acts as a lead point for an intussusception. Such diverticula may become inflamed and mimic appendicitis or result in perforation and peritonitis.

2. Clinical features

    a. Symptoms. Many diverticula remain clinically silent and are found in approximately 3%–5% of autopsy cases as an incidental finding.

      (1) Chronic or **acute abdominal pain** may precede frank bleeding and may be difficult to distinguish from appendicitis or another intestinal obstructive event.

      (2) Melenic stools are intermittent and may correlate with clinical symptoms. Symptoms characteristic of intussusception may occur; currant jelly stools can lead to misdiagnosis.

      (3) Nausea, vomiting, and **abdominal distention** may mirror appendicitis.

    b. Physical examination findings

      (1) Signs of intestinal obstruction are often present and are associated with bands that may result from inflammation of the diverticula.

      (2) Signs of shock or **dehydration** are rarely seen and are not usual unless perforation and peritonitis are present from ulceration.

3. Differential diagnoses include peptic ulcer disease, caustic ingestions, gastric duplication syndromes, annular pancreas, malrotation, appendicitis, colonic diverticulitis, testicular torsion, incarcerated or strangulated hernia, gastroenteritis with enterocolitis, Henoch-Schönlein purpura, diabetic ketoacidosis, and intussusception.

4. Evaluation

    a. Laboratory studies

      (1) A **CBC** usually reveals anemia from chronic blood loss and may show a leukocytosis if inflammation of the diverticulum is present or if there is impending peritonitis.

(2) A **serum biochemical profile** is not useful unless protracted vomiting or signs of peritonitis are evident.

(3) **Blood** and **urine cultures** are warranted in ill-appearing children with signs of peritonitis.

b. **Diagnostic imaging studies**

(1) **Radiography**

(a) **Plain radiographs of the abdomen** usually show evidence of ileus or may show obvious free air with perforation.

(b) **Contrast radiographic studies** rarely demonstrate the diverticula and almost never fill the sac.

(2) A **Meckel radionuclide scan** reveals acid-secreting mucosa and can be enhanced with glucagon, gastrin, or cimetidine; this study is sensitive in 85%–90% of cases.

(3) **Ultrasonography** is of no value and is not warranted unless the purpose is to exclude other causes.

5. **Therapy** entails **stabilization, nasogastric suction,** and **barium reduction** as described for intussusception (see X F 5 a–c). The child should not be given anything by mouth. **Broad-spectrum antibiotic therapy** is indicated for children with peritonitis or diverticulitis.

6. **Disposition.** Children at risk for Meckel's diverticulum must be hospitalized following surgical consultation for antibiotic therapy and exploration. **Prompt surgical consultation is mandatory,** and most children require hospitalization to correct any electrolyte abnormalities prior to surgery and to treat peritonitis.

H Appendicitis

1. **Discussion.** Appendicitis is the most common condition requiring emergency abdominal surgery in childhood.

a. **Etiology.** Appendicitis is inversely related to the amount of fiber in the diet and is uncommon in third-world countries. The cause of appendicitis is unknown but may be due to luminal obstruction with fecal material, inflammation, enteric bacteria, viruses, or tumor mass.

b. **Pathogenesis.** Perforation rates are two to five times higher in children when compared with adults because of nonspecific symptoms and delays in presentation. Approximately 50%–60% of children with perforation were seen by a physician in the preceding 24 hours. Perforation risk is inversely related to age, with the highest risk of perforation being 70%–80% in the 1- to 4-year-old group and lowest in adolescents (30%–40%).

2. **Clinical features**

a. **Classic symptoms** consist of anorexia, fever, vomiting, and pain that initially begins as vague periumbilical discomfort. Progression of symptoms is usually subacute and occurs over 36–48 hours, with perforation rates that exceed 75% at 48 hours.

(1) **Fever** is usually not reported or is low grade but may be elevated with perforation.

(2) **Pain** always precedes the development of vomiting and fever and is an important point in differentiating from infectious gastroenteritis. As inflammation progresses, pain becomes more localized to the site of inflammation in the right lower quadrant. A large retrocecal appendicitis may frequently produce pain in the right upper quadrant that resembles cholecystitis in adults and is usually misdiagnosed in children as nonspecific abdominal pain.

(3) **Diarrhea** is very rare and is often small, pasty, and mucoid and resembles the stool pattern of *Shigella* but without blood.

b. **Physical examination findings** are inconsistent. During the physical examination, pertinent differential diagnostic points (e.g., recent constipation, cough, urinary symptoms, headache, myalgias) should be noted as well.

(1) **Rebound tenderness,** particularly percussion tenderness, is suggestive of impending peritonitis.

(2) An **inflammatory mass** palpated on rectal examination suggests the diagnosis, particularly if the mass is painful.

3. **Differential diagnoses** include peptic ulcer disease, caustic ingestions, gastric duplication syndromes, annular pancreas, malrotation, foreign body obstruction, colonic diverticulitis, testicular torsion, incarcerated or strangulated hernia, gastroenteritis with enterocolitis, Henoch-Schönlein purpura, diabetic ketoacidosis, intussusception, lower lobe pneumonia, tubal ectopic pregnancy (in adolescents), pelvic inflammatory disease (PID), and inflammatory bowel disease.

4. **Evaluation**
   a. **Laboratory studies**
      (1) A **CBC** usually reveals a leukocytosis if inflammation of the appendix is present or if there is impending peritonitis.
      (2) A **serum electrolyte determination** is not useful unless protracted vomiting or signs of peritonitis are evident.
      (3) **Blood** and **urine cultures** are warranted in ill-appearing children with signs of peritonitis.
      (4) **Urinalysis.** Sterile pyuria is occasionally noted because of irritation of the inflamed appendix on the right ureter or bladder.
   b. **Diagnostic imaging studies**
      (1) **Radiography**
         (a) **Plain radiographs of the abdomen** usually show evidence of ileus or may show obvious free air with perforation and, in 15%–20% of cases, may reveal a calcified appendicolith.
         (b) **Contrast radiographic studies** rarely demonstrate the appendicitis—they may show indentation of the cecum with the inflammatory mass but almost never fill the sac.
      (2) **Ultrasonography.** A useful study is an **appendiceal compression ultrasound,** which has a false-negative rate of 8%–10%.
      (3) **CT** is usually helpful and diagnostic. CT is also useful for percutaneous drainage if an abscess is found.

5. **Therapy** entails **stabilization, nasogastric suction,** and a **barium enema** (if intussusception or Meckel's diverticulitis cannot be excluded) as described in X E 5. Children who have had symptoms longer than 36–48 hours or who have signs of peritonitis should not be considered candidates for immediate **surgical exploration.** Children with peritonitis should receive **broad-spectrum antibiotic therapy** and should be hospitalized following surgical consultation.

6. **Disposition**
   a. All children **at risk for appendicitis** must have an intravenous access established and be promptly fluid resuscitated if signs of peritonitis or perforation are present. After surgical consultation, they should be hospitalized for antibiotic therapy and exploration.
   b. Children in whom the **diagnosis is unclear** merit a period of hospital admission and observation or re-examination 6–12 hours later, preferably by the same physician.

XI SEIZURES

A **Discussion**   Seizures represent abnormal neural discharges in the cerebral cortex or brain stem that are paroxysmal in nature and may be either physically silent or expressed motorically in the form of repetitive movements and actions.

1. **Etiology.** Seizures are most often caused by birth trauma, congenital infection, or congenital anatomic defects in young infants. In infants and older children, there may be no apparent cause (idiopathic), or seizures may be the sequela of an acute infectious process.

2. **Classification.** Seizures may be classified according to many schemes, depending on anatomic site of seizure, duration and type of movement disorder (if any), or recurrence patterns.
   a. **Acute nonrecurring seizures**
      (1) **Febrile convulsions** are seizures that accompany febrile disorders but are not directly caused by CNS infections. Febrile convulsions usually occur between the ages of 6 months

and 3 years, sometimes to 5 years of age. Febrile convulsions are the most common type of acute nonrecurring seizures.

(2) **Seizures secondary to toxic ingestions** (e.g., isoniazid or clonidine toxicity)

(3) **Metabolic disturbances** (e.g., hypoglycemia, hypocalcemia, hyponatremia)

(4) **Intracranial disorders** (e.g., cerebral tumor, meningitis, tumor)

b. **Chronic recurring seizures**

(1) **Partial simple seizures** start focally and do not cause loss of consciousness. They usually are motor and nongeneralized and often result in deviation of the eyes and head.

(2) **Partial complex seizures** were previously known as psychomotor or temporal lobe seizures. These seizures usually start focally and classically are associated with a loss of awareness or consciousness but not with loss of motor control.

    (a) Minor changes in behavior or affect may be the only visible manifestation.

    (b) However, these changes may be dramatic, with repetitive purposeless activity. Some patients may perform acts of which they are unaware for minutes or hours. Often, these activities involve walking or running distances, which may put them in great jeopardy.

(3) **Generalized seizures**

    (a) **Generalized tonic–clonic seizures** are the prototype, alternating between the brief tonic phase of generalized muscle contraction and a longer period of rhythmic spasms.

        (i) Classically, children old enough to describe their symptoms report a **prodrome** or **aura** that may be characterized by muscular discomfort, gastrointestinal upset, scotomata, or noxious gustatory stimuli.

        (ii) **Postseizure somnolence** followed by confusion and ataxia is common and may last for several hours.

    (b) **Myoclonic seizures** are a variant that consists of sudden movements of the trunk and extremities, causing the patient to fall. Myoclonic seizures are a common presentation of metabolic or neurodegenerative diseases in infancy (infantile spasms).

(4) **Absence seizures** consist of staring and eye-blinking episodes that usually last 10–20 seconds. These seizures represent brief interruptions of consciousness without overt loss of motor control. Episodes happen many times per day and are usually precipitated by exertion or emotional upset, with resulting subsequent hyperventilation, or by photic stimulation described by blinking lights. Absence seizures usually are not overtly associated with generalized motor manifestations.

(5) **Akinetic seizures** are central seizures that cause a sudden loss of muscle tone. Previously called **"drop attacks,"** these seizures put children in danger of falling at inappropriate times.

(6) **Status epilepticus** or **serial status**

    (a) **Status epilepticus** is a continuous seizure (i.e., the patient does not regain consciousness or function without intervention).

    (b) **Serial status** usually represents bursts of status epilepticus that last for variable periods of time only to recur after an interstatus interval.

(7) **Neonatal seizures** are a special form of seizures because of the lack of stereotypic repetitive behavior. They require a high index of suspicion for subtle symptoms of pedaling movements of legs, stiffening, or lip smacking.

B **Clinical features** depend on the type of seizure. Most seizures are composed of a brief tonic phase of generalized contraction of all or partial muscle groups followed by a more prolonged clonic phase of rhythmic repetitive spasms of the same muscle groups or recruitment of others.

1. **Partial complex seizures** are usually focal and do not generalize but usually are associated with a loss of awareness of surroundings.

2. **Absence seizures** are associated with staring or blinking episodes that last for seconds and with brief interruptions in consciousness but no loss of motor tone. These seizures usually are precipitated by an emotional event or photic stimulation.

3. **Myoclonic seizures** or infantile spasms are associated with sudden flexion of the trunk at the waist with extension or flexion of the arms or legs, resulting in the child falling to the ground.

4. **Akinetic seizures** are similar to myoclonic seizures in that the child falls to the ground, but these seizures are caused by loss of muscle tone, not flexion or muscle spasms.

5. **Neonatal seizures** may be the most difficult to characterize because of the variable presentation of symptoms. A high index of suspicion must be maintained, particularly with infants who present with stiffening episodes or repetitive movements of the eyes, mouth, or tongue. A hospitalized careful observation period is warranted, with video recording to characterize such movements.

C **Differential diagnoses**

1. **Anatomic and structural defects**
   a. Hydranencephaly
   b. Absent corpus callosum
   c. Dandy-Walker cyst

2. **Metabolic and storage diseases**

3. **Phycomycoses**
   a. Tuberous sclerosis
   b. Neurofibromatosis

4. **CNS tumor**

5. **Infection**
   a. Meningitis
   b. Encephalitis
   c. Brain abscess
   d. Cerebral cysticercosis

6. **Trauma**
   a. Subdural effusion
   b. Intracerebral hemorrhage
   c. Cortical infarct

D **Evaluation**

1. A careful **physical examination** should be performed, including growth and development parameters and analysis of perinatal factors and family history.

2. **Laboratory studies.** Appropriate studies include:
   a. Serum biochemistry profile
   b. Liver tests
   c. ABG analysis
   d. Urinalysis and urine amino acid analysis
   e. Serologic screens [e.g., for cytomegalovirus (CMV), toxoplasmosis, HIV, varicella zoster virus]
   f. CSF analysis
   g. Determination of serum anticonvulsant concentrations is important in children with established seizure disorder.

3. **Diagnostic imaging studies**
   a. **Electroencephalography** should be performed alone, with hyperventilation, and with photic stimulation. **Continuous electroencephalogram (EEG) recordings** may provide helpful information.
   b. **Computed axial tomography (CAT) scanning** or **magnetic resonance imaging (MRI)** may be necessary.

E **Therapy**

1. **Simple febrile convulsions** require no further evaluation if patients have no focal neurologic deficits, convulsions lasting fewer than 5 minutes, a short postictal period, and no neurologic disorders following the seizure.

2. **Recurrent febrile seizures** may be treated with oral valproic acid, phenobarbital, or diazepam, but these must be given continuously to avoid prolonged subtherapeutic dosing.

3. **Seizures** as a result of **toxic ingestions** or **metabolic disorders** require no specific treatment except correction of the underlying cause.

4. **Chronic seizures** are treated in consultation with a neurologist based on the EEG findings and the seizure type.

5. **Status epilepticus** requires emergent treatment with either lorazepam or diazepam intravenously. **Benzodiazepines** given rectally are not useful because of erratic absorption.
    a. **Careful monitoring** of pulse oximetry and vital signs is imperative.
    b. If benzodiazepines are ineffective, parenteral loading and maintenance with **phenytoin** are indicated. Children requiring further therapy should be transferred to a regional pediatric center and to the care of a pediatric neurologist.

F **Disposition**

1. **Discharge. Children with febrile seizures** who are normal on examination and to parents do not merit further evaluation and may be discharged home.

2. **Admission** is indicated for:
    a. Children who have **prolonged febrile seizures, focal deficits,** a **prolonged postictal time,** or **neurologic deficits** after a seizure
    b. Children with **new-onset seizure** that is not associated with fever, who should be hospitalized for further evaluation with definitive treatment at that time
    c. **Children with status epilepticus** or **serial status**

XII CHILD ABUSE

A **Discussion**   Child abuse is one of the leading causes of death in children between the ages of 1 and 12 months. With first episodes of child abuse, the mortality rate is approximately 5%–8%, but repeated cases of child abuse are associated with a mortality rate higher than 50%.

1. **Types of abuse**
    a. **Physical abuse** is the intentional injury of a child (e.g., beating, shaking).
    b. **Sexual abuse** is any sexual activity between an adult and a permissive or nonpermissive child.
    c. **Physical neglect** is the failure of caregivers to provide the necessities of life such as nourishment, shelter, clothing, supervision, medical care, cleanliness, education, or monetary support.
    d. **Emotional neglect** is failure of caregivers to provide the necessities of emotional support for self-esteem and normal development.
    e. **By-proxy neglect (Münchhausen syndrome)** is a condition in which the parents induce or fabricate illness, causing the child to undergo unnecessary diagnostic and therapeutic interventions.

2. **Incidence.** Approximately 30% of instances of child abuse occur in children younger than 12 months of age, 33% in children 1–6 years of age, and 37% in children older than 6 years. When the child or family has a life of poverty, crises, or limited access to social resources, the incidence of child abuse is increased.

3. **Characteristics of the abuser.** In 90%–95% of cases, the abuser is a related adult (average age, 25 years), who does not have serious psychiatric illness. The most common perpetrators are the father (21%), mother (21%), mother's boyfriend (9%), babysitter (8%), and stepfather (5%).

Most abusing adults tend to be unhappy, lonely, angry single parents who have no knowledge of child development and unrealistic expectations of child development for age.

B **Clinical features** Physical abuse should be suspected when an injury is **unexplained** by caregivers, is unexplainable by mechanism, or is **implausible,** or when a **significant delay in seeking medical care** is noted. **Bilateral, symmetric,** or **geometric injuries** increase clinical suspicion for child abuse. **Unexplained falls** from heights, **electrocutions,** or **drowning** is always suspicious for child abuse or neglect.

1. **Bruises** are the most common manifestation of child abuse and may be found on any body surface area. Usually, bruises are localized over bony prominences and in areas that cannot be reached or would be unusual in a fall. Bruising may take the shape of the inflicting instrument in the case of a belt buckle, belt, looped electrical cord, flyswatter, coat hanger, or hand.

2. **Fractures** are usually caused by wrenching or pulling injuries that damage the bone metaphysis. Spiral fractures are also seen.

3. **Damaged hair.** At first, tinea capitis may be suspected, but this diagnosis can be eliminated on the basis of lack of skin involvement, broken hairs of varying lengths, and no evidence of fungal elements on the surface of the hair.

4. **Burns** account for 10%–15% of all cases of abuse and usually take on characteristics of the burning object. Cigarette burns result in circular punched-out burns, immersion burns result in a linear pattern on the outer body, and steam-iron burns result in V-shaped burns, particularly if they cross joint spaces.

5. **Head trauma** is the most common cause of death and usually presents as coma, convulsions, apnea, signs of intracranial hypertension, or protracted vomiting.
   a. **Subdural hematomas** are the most frequently seen injury.
   b. **Skull** and **rib fractures** are common together and indicate slamming of the body and head against a wall or mattress.
   c. **Head** and **neck petechiae** associated with subconjunctival hemorrhage are commonly caused by choking.
   d. **Retinal hemorrhages** occur with shaking, are often found in association with subdural hematomas, and rarely result from CPR or from infectious processes.

6. **Intra-abdominal injuries** are the second most common cause of death and usually result in shock if the liver or spleen ruptures.

C **Differential diagnoses** include accidental orthopedic trauma (e.g., nursemaid's elbow, shoulder dislocation, humerus fractures, forearm fractures, wrist fractures, cervical spinal injuries), soft tissue trauma, osteochondrosis of the capitellum (Panner's disease), epicondylitis of the lateral humeral condyle, septic arthritis of the elbow, hemarthroses secondary to hereditary coagulopathy, accidental burns or immersions, metabolic abnormalities (e.g., osteogenesis imperfecta), accidental trauma to sexual organs, and underlying medical conditions leading to failure to thrive.

D **Evaluation**
1. A properly performed **physical examination with careful attention to the historical facts of the injury** is perhaps the most important part of the evaluation process.
   a. In girls, when sexual abuse is suspected, **standard rape testing protocols** should be followed (see Chapter 14 X C 3). In addition, a **culdoscopic examination** should be performed. Photographic evidence may be necessary for later forensic examination.
   b. Suspicious traumatic lesions should be **photographed;** appropriate color correction is necessary.

2. **Laboratory studies**
   a. **Screening tests** for a bleeding diathesis should be obtained in all cases of bruising, along with a **CBC.**

    b. Urine and **stool samples** should be screened for blood in cases of abdominal trauma.

    c. **Cultures of rectal, vaginal, urethral,** and **pharyngeal smears** may be indicated in suspected cases of sexual abuse.

3. Diagnostic imaging studies

    a. A **radiographic bone survey,** including the skull, thorax, long bones, and pelvis, is warranted in all cases of physical abuse. Other bones should be scanned as clinically indicated.

    b. A **CT scan** of the head and abdomen may be indicated in severely traumatized children.

E **Therapy** Life-threatening conditions such as seizures, apnea, or respiratory arrest should be treated promptly. All surgically remediable injuries should be quickly evaluated in consultation with a surgeon.

F **Disposition**

1. Admission is indicated when the medical condition requires inpatient management, when the diagnosis is unclear, when no alternative for the safety or well-being of the child can be assured, or when custody is unavailable.

2. In all cases of physical or sexual abuse, the proper **authorities should be notified,** and the case should be reported as mandated in almost all states. The child should not be released until his or her safety can be assured. The perpetrator should have no access to the child or should be in custody pending evaluation.

3. Children suspected of being abused or neglected should receive adequate **psychological support** and **evaluation.**

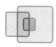

Study Questions

Directions: *Each of the numbered items or incomplete statements in this section is followed by answers or by completions of the statement. Select the ONE lettered answer or completion that is BEST in each case.*

1. Which one of the following signs and symptoms may be associated with foreign body aspiration syndrome in children?

- (A) Cyanosis
- (B) Wheezing
- (C) Absent breath sounds on the affected side
- (D) Decreased chest excursion on the side of the obstruction
- (E) All of the above

2. Which one of the following statements regarding sudden infant death syndrome (SIDS) is correct?

- (A) SIDS is the most common cause of postnatal deaths in developed countries.
- (B) Most cases of SIDS are seen almost exclusively in children younger than 2–3 weeks of age.
- (C) Autopsy findings are diagnostic of SIDS.
- (D) Almost all children are normal prior to the event that results in SIDS.
- (E) The incidence of SIDS is equal in full-term infants and in preterm infants.

3. A previously healthy 15-year-old boy develops a mild pneumonia with nonproductive cough and no evidence of effusion. He does not appear extremely ill, although some mild exertional dyspnea is noted. Pulse oximetry results are normal. The most appropriate therapy is

- (A) amoxicillin sodium
- (B) erythromycin base
- (C) trimethoprim–sulfamethoxazole
- (D) cephalexin
- (E) penicillin sodium

4. A 2-month-old infant with moderately severe bronchopulmonary dysplasia who is on home oxygen therapy is admitted to the hospital with fever, wheezing, and moderate to severe respiratory distress. No obvious cyanosis is seen, but nasal flaring and retractions are noted. A chest radiograph shows hyperinflation and bilateral, interstitial infiltrates with no alveolar process. The complete blood count (CBC) is unremarkable, and pulse oximetry is 96% on supplemental oxygen by nasal cannula at 2 L/min. A nasal washing for respiratory syncytial virus (RSV) is positive. The most appropriate therapy is

- (A) oral amoxicillin sodium
- (B) intravenous ampicillin
- (C) intravenous ceftriaxone
- (D) oral erythromycin
- (E) ribavirin by aerosolization

5. A 3-year-old crying child is brought to the emergency department (ED). He is rubbing both ears and is somewhat inconsolable. Physical examination reveals an erythematous, bulging right tympanic membrane with no light reflex. The two most likely bacterial causes of this illness are

- (A) *Streptococcus pyogenes* and *Staphylococcus aureus*
- (B) *Haemophilus influenzae* and *S. aureus*
- (C) *H. influenzae* and *Streptococcus pneumoniae*
- (D) *S. pneumoniae* and *S. aureus*
- (E) *Moraxella catarrhalis* and *S. pyogenes*

6. A 3-year-old white boy presents to the emergency department (ED) with a sore throat, dysphagia of solids but not liquids, and tender anterior chain adenopathy that measures 3 × 3 cm. The most appropriate initial therapy in this child is

    (A) penicillin sodium
    (B) cephalexin
    (C) amoxicillin
    (D) trimethoprim–sulfamethoxazole
    (E) ampicillin

QUESTIONS 7–8

A 15-month-old girl is brought by her parents to the emergency department (ED) with a history of subjective fever, listlessness, and a rash. Physical examination reveals an ill-appearing infant with a normal temperature, but an obvious petechial rash on the extremities and the trunk. The fontanelle is not palpated, but positive Kernig and Brudzinski signs are present. The capillary refill is delayed at 4 seconds.

7. The most appropriate next step in the management of this patient is

    (A) establishment of an intravenous line with administration of a resuscitative bolus and administration of antibiotics
    (B) complete blood count (CBC) and blood culture
    (C) lumbar puncture with cerebrospinal fluid (CSF) analysis
    (D) Gram stain and culture of an aspirate of petechiae
    (E) securing the airway with endotracheal intubation

8. What is the most likely causative organism?

    (A) *Haemophilus influenzae* type b
    (B) *Streptococcus pneumoniae*
    (C) *Neisseria meningitidis*
    (D) group B β-hemolytic streptococci
    (E) *Staphylococcus aureus*

9. Which one of the following statements is true regarding intussusception in children?

    (A) Most intussusceptions are ileocolic and may be confused with appendicitis, except that there are symptom-free intervals.
    (B) Bouts of abdominal pain are colicky to continuous, may last hours to days, and are usually not associated with vomiting.
    (C) Most children are alert during the painful episode and appear playful and active.
    (D) Masses representing the intussusception are not usually palpated.
    (E) A barium enema may reveal a classic "coil spring" appearance but usually does not aid in the treatment of the disease.

10. Which one of the following statements regarding appendicitis is true?

    (A) Appendicitis occurs more frequently in children younger than 5 years of age.
    (B) Appendicitis is often easy to diagnose; anorexia, pain, and vomiting usually point to the diagnosis.
    (C) The incidence of perforation is high and exceeds the incidence in adult cases because of delay in presentation of symptoms and misdiagnosis.
    (D) Laboratory studies are often helpful in the diagnosis and are useful in differentiating appendicitis from other causes of abdominal pain.
    (E) Definitive diagnosis can usually be established by a period of observation; surgery is not necessary.

Answers and Explanations

1. The answer is E Cyanosis, aphonia, absent breath sounds, and wheezing all may be associated with foreign body aspiration syndrome. The actual symptoms are determined by the location of the obstructing object. In general, cyanosis and aphonia are associated with obstruction at or just below the glottis, and are often accompanied by stridor. Absent breath sounds on the affected side, decreased chest excursion on the side of the obstruction, and wheezing all point to an obstructive process that is in the central trachea or a mainstem bronchus and is caused by obstruction of a lobar segment or the entire lobe of the lung. Unilateral or bilateral wheezing implies partial obstruction below the level of the mainstem bronchus that results in turbulent flow air trapping and wheezing produced around the obstruction point.

2. The answer is A SIDS is the most common cause of infant mortality in developed countries (e.g., the United States). Most cases are seen in infants older than 6 weeks, and the syndrome is decidedly rare before 4 weeks of age. The autopsy findings are inconsistent and nondiagnostic and, in most cases, give no clue to parents, physicians, or the police as to the exact events that resulted in the death. No evidence for prevention is noted. Most children have feeding difficulties in the day prior to the event and many are felt by parents to be more subdued and lethargic. The incidence of SIDS is greater in premature infants and in families with smokers and single parents.

3. The answer is B The most common nonviral causes of pneumonia in children older than 5 years, and in particular those who have been immunized fully, are *Mycoplasma pneumoniae* and *Streptococcus pneumoniae*. Pneumonia caused by *Mycoplasma* is usually milder and not associated with the toxicity of other bacterial agents. It is usually characterized by a nonproductive cough and mild exertional dyspnea. The clinical picture is more consistent with *M. pneumoniae*, because pneumonia caused by *S. pneumoniae* is characterized by a septic appearance and the production of rusty sputum. The treatment of choice for pneumonia caused by *Mycoplasma* is erythromycin. Amoxicillin sodium, trimethoprim–sulfamethoxazole, cephalexin, and penicillin sodium are treatment for *S. pneumoniae*. Trimethoprim–sulfamethoxazole has some activity against *M. pneumoniae*, but is associated with more side effects than erythromycin.

4. The answer is E This infant has evidence of severe bronchiolitis. The positive nasal washing would indicate that the cause is RSV. The moderate to severe respiratory distress associated with significant oxygen-requiring bronchopulmonary dysplasia is a relative indication for institution of aerosolized ribavirin therapy in a monitored intensive care unit. Severe infection is more common in children with severe underlying pulmonary disease and is usually not associated with secondary bacterial infection. Therefore, antibiotic therapy is usually not warranted. Hospitalization is always warranted in such compromised infants because of the increased incidence of apnea. Therapy includes supplemental oxygen, fluids, and possibly intubation, if deterioration of pulmonary function occurs.

5. The answer is C This child is presenting with the signs of classic acute otitis media (i.e., the characteristic features of severe otalgia and a bulging and highly erythematous tympanic membrane with impaired mobility). Bacterial and, to some extent, respiratory viruses are the primary agents of otitis media. The most common causes in all age groups are *S. pneumoniae* and nontypable, unencapsulated *H. influenzae*. Less common causes include *M. catarrhalis*. In chronic otitis media, *S. aureus* is a common causative organism.

6. The answer is A In a child younger than 5 years who has tender adenopathy, exudates, and dysphagia, the most likely diagnosis is streptococcal pharyngitis. Penicillin is clearly the drug of choice because of its relatively inexpensive cost and safety. Cephalexin and amoxicillin would also be efficacious but at the expense of increased cost and possible adverse reactions. Trimethoprim–sulfamethoxazole has no activity against streptococci and should not be used. The side effect profile and lack of efficacy are such that they clearly outweigh any benefit gained from the relatively inexpensive cost.

7. The answer is A This case represents a classic presentation of meningitis caused by an unknown organism. The initial step should be to suspect septic shock and to attempt to augment circulating intravascular volume with intravenous fluids. The absence of temperature elevation but the presence of petechiae should suggest a bacterial process that merits administration of high-dose antibiotic therapy. All other laboratory studies may be processed while an intravenous line is established and antibiotics are started, which should not be delayed pending laboratory results. Securing the airway to control cerebral edema secondary to inflammation may be necessary but not before the administration of antibiotics in this particular clinical situation

8. The answer is C This case represents probable meningococcal sepsis and meningitis, which must be substantiated by culture and chemical analysis of the cerebrospinal fluid (CSF) and blood. *H. influenzae* and group B β-hemolytic streptococci can cause an identical clinical picture. The age of the patient (15 months) precludes group B β-hemolytic streptococci but does not exclude *H. influenzae*. Antibiotic coverage must be directed at the most likely organism, and no assumption about the specific cause should be made until culture results are available.

9. The answer is A Most intussusceptions are ileocolic and may be confused with appendicitis during a painful interval. However, with resolution of the pain, the child appears normal and may have no anorexia. The intervals usually decrease in frequency and usually do not persist longer than 48 hours without obstruction with bilious vomiting or the appearance of a bloody stool. Typically, the child is profoundly lethargic during an acute attack but may appear normal afterwards. A painful sausage-shaped mass may be palpable in 50% of patients, particularly during a painful episode. The barium enema (rarely used nowadays) or air-contrast enema (more commonly used) is both diagnostic and therapeutic and is successful in 80% of cases.

10. The answer is C Appendicitis is more common in children between the ages of 10 and 15 years; it is unusual in children younger than 5 years. The presentation in children is usually atypical and is misdiagnosed 50% of the time because of delay in presentation and poorly localizing signs. Because of these difficulties, the incidence of perforation is many times higher in children than in adults. Laboratory studies are helpful only in the context of the physical examination and are never of such specificity to exclude the diagnosis. Periods of observation in the hospital usually are sufficient to establish the diagnosis in approximately 70% of patients with questionable physical findings; 30% of patients may require surgery for definitive diagnosis. Appendicitis is not found in 5% of patients who undergo diagnostic laparotomy.

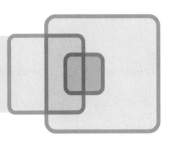

chapter **16**

Hematologic and Oncologic Emergencies

STEPHEN THOMAS

I APPROACH TO THE BLEEDING PATIENT

A Discussion

1. Patients with spontaneous bleeding or multisite hemorrhage should be suspected of having bleeding diathesis.

2. Delay of bleeding for several hours after trauma, persistent hemorrhage, or bleeding into deep tissues or joints may be harbingers of hematologic abnormality.

B Clinical features

1. Patients may present with normal-appearing bleeding, which is abnormal only when delayed or persistent.

2. Bleeding may be visually worrisome, such as appearance of hemarthrosis or petechiae, but not hemodynamically threatening.

3. The most dangerous clinical presentation of bleeding disorders is hemorrhage into potential spaces (e.g., retroperitoneum), which may be life-threatening.

C Differential diagnosis of patients with bleeding disorders primarily involves determination of which one of the multitudes of congenital and hematologic abnormalities is responsible for the patient's presentation.

D Evaluation

1. **Patient history.** Details regarding the patient's current problem, past disease, and family medical history are particularly important in patients who present to the emergency department (ED) with abnormal bleeding.
   a. Most patients with hematologic disease are aware of their diagnosis and are knowledgeable about manifestations and therapy of their disease process. Patients with bleeding abnormalities who may have been unaware of their own diagnosis may be able to provide important aspects of family history.
   b. Past medical history, including such items as postdental extraction bleeding, may also provide useful information about a patient's hemostatic disease. Similarly, chronic liver disease affects hemostasis in many cases, and should therefore be investigated.
   c. A medication history is useful because certain drugs [e.g., nonsteroidal anti-inflammatory drugs (NSAIDs), ethanol] may have deleterious effects on clotting.

2. **Physical examination** includes searches for sites of bleeding and other findings to provide clues to the nature of hemostatic disruption.
   a. **Mucocutaneous bleeding** (petechiae, ecchymoses, respiratory or gastrointestinal tract hemorrhage) is characteristic of platelet disorders.

    b. Delayed bleeding after trauma and **deep tissue or joint hemorrhage** are characteristic of hemophilia.

    c. Postural hypotension and other signs of **volume loss** may be present on examination of patients with significant blood loss.

3. Laboratory evaluation begins with a complete blood count (CBC), platelet count, prothrombin time (PT), and partial thromboplastin time (PTT). Other specialized hematologic tests (e.g., coagulation factors, fibrin degeneration products, inhibitor screens) are ordered as indicated by the differential diagnosis, and results are not usually obtained in the ED.

E **Therapy**   Treatment priorities and initial therapy (e.g., normal saline administration to correct hypotension) are the same as those for any other patient in the ED.

1. Stabilization

    a. Airway compromise may be threatened by blood in the upper airway. When indicated, **intubation** should be performed with an endotracheal tube large enough (preferably 8.0) to allow subsequent bronchoscopy.

    b. Hemodynamic instability should be first treated with **crystalloid replacement,** with progression to blood component therapy as indicated by the situation.

2. Pharmacologic adjuncts [e.g., steroids for idiopathic thrombocytopenic purpura (ITP)] may be indicated.

3. Blood component therapy is indicated for some patients with abnormal bleeding in the ED. Blood component therapy is commonly administered in many EDs, necessitating familiarity with infusion indications, methods, and complications.

    a. Blood type. Type AB patients may receive any blood type; all patients may receive type O. Type A and B patients may also receive blood types A and B, respectively.

        (1) ED patients who may not require immediate transfusion may still require **type and cross match in preparation** for impending blood product therapy. Patients with the following disease processes should be typed and crossed: shock, gastrointestinal bleeding, anemia (hemoglobin less than 10 g/dL), significant or continuing blood loss, or impending surgical procedures that pose a risk of hemorrhage.

        (2) Incompletely matched blood may be transfused in some emergency situations. These emergency transfusions may be life-saving, but they also carry significantly increased risks of transfusion reactions. **Type O blood** (Rh negative in patients of childbearing age) may be used when there is insufficient time to obtain type- and Rh-specific blood. Because type-matching and Rh-matching require only 10–15 minutes in the laboratory (compared with up to 60 minutes for fully cross-matched blood), use of type O blood is becoming less common.

    b. Blood components. Whole blood is essentially unavailable in civilian hospitals, because units of donated blood are separated into components to allow optimal storage and directed therapy.

        (1) Packed red blood cells (PRBCs) represent the most commonly transfused blood component. This component consists of red blood cells (RBCs) and 10%–20% of the plasma from 1 U (450 mL) of donated blood.

            (a) Administration of PRBCs results in **increased oxygen-carrying capacity** in patients with significant blood loss.

            (b) There is no specific threshold for PRBC transfusion, and the risks of blood-borne viral disease have resulted in expectant management of levels of anemia that would have prompted transfusion in past decades. The most important variable, besides the actual hematocrit or hemoglobin level, is whether blood loss is acute or chronic.

                (i) **Acute blood loss** can be replaced with crystalloid until the lost volume approaches 25%–30% of circulating volume.

        (ii) Chronic blood loss. Patients with chronic blood loss may tolerate decrements in hemoglobin to 8 g/dL or lower without requiring a transfusion. Symptomatic patients require PRBCs, and patients with very low hemoglobin levels (e.g., below 7) may be considered candidates for PRBCs depending on the physician's recommendations.

(2) Other formulations of RBCs are transfused in special circumstances.

    (a) Leukocyte-poor RBCs are administered to patients who have undergone transplants or who have had febrile nonhemolytic transfusion reactions.

    (b) Frozen RBCs represent an expensive method of providing reduced antigen exposure or keeping rare blood types stored for longer periods of time than the usual 42-day shelf life of PRBCs.

    (c) Washed RBCs have had plasma proteins and some leukocytes and platelets removed, preventing the precipitation of hemolysis.

(3) Platelets represent another blood component commonly administered in the ED. Usually given in 6-U packs, platelets may also be prepared specially (with HLA matching or radiation) to minimize reactions. Indications for platelet transfusion depend on both the platelet count and the cause of thrombocytopenia. Normally functioning platelets are not associated with bleeding at levels higher than 50,000/μL, so transfusion is aimed at maintaining this minimum level.

    (a) Thrombocytopenia caused by antiplatelet antibodies is **generally refractory** to platelet transfusion.

    (b) Platelet counts of 10,000–50,000/mm³ may be associated with spontaneous bleeding, especially in patients with concurrent hepatorenal disease. Bleeding patients with platelet counts at this level should be treated with platelet transfusion.

    (c) Prophylactic platelet transfusion (to prevent spontaneous hemorrhage) is indicated in patients with platelet counts below 10,000/mm³.

(4) Fresh frozen plasma (FFP) units are 200–250 mL in volume and are used for replacement of coagulation factors and fibrinogen. Indications for FFP transfusion include factor deficiency or other coagulopathy in patients who are bleeding or who will undergo procedures that may induce hemorrhage.

    (a) Patients taking warfarin and those with coagulopathy from liver disease or disseminated intravascular coagulation (DIC) may require treatment with FFP.

    (b) Patients with acquired or congenital factor deficiency, or antithrombin III deficiency, may be treated with FFP when specific therapy is unavailable.

    (c) FFP may be administered to patients with coagulopathy related to massive transfusion therapy.

(5) Cryoprecipitate is derived from FFP and is used for replacement of fibrinogen and von Willebrand's factor (vWF).

    (a) Cryoprecipitate may be infused when factor VIII therapy is unavailable to treat von Willebrand's disease patients whose bleeding is uncontrolled with desmopressin.

    (b) Patients with fibrinogen levels below 100 mg/dL, as may occur with DIC, may be treated with cryoprecipitate.

(6) Albumin infusion is controversial, with efficacy of the protein for traditional indications (colloid replacement in volume depletion, patients undergoing large volume paracentesis, and burns) increasingly being questioned.

(7) Immunoglobulins have been demonstrated to enhance immune response in certain impaired hosts (e.g., transplant patients, patients with leukemia, patients with immune disorders), and also to aid treatment of certain inflammatory conditions (e.g., Kawasaki disease).

(8) Antithrombin III has inhibitory effects on many coagulation factors, and levels may be low because of congenital or acquired disorders. Antithrombin III infusion is currently indicated for patients with hereditary deficiency of this protein.

(9) Specific factor replacement therapy is the optimal choice for replacement of coagulation factors (see II B). Specific factor replacement therapy minimizes the risks associated with pooled blood component therapy.

c. **Administration protocols**

(1) **General considerations**

(a) The **first step** is to **identify the patient's needs** and choose the correct product.

(b) Blood products are infused through **large-bore catheters** to minimize the risks of hemolysis and to allow rapid infusion of blood products when necessary. **Micropore filters** should be used when administering blood products to remove aggregates of platelet, fibrin, and leukocytes.

(2) **PRBCs.** Transfusion of 1 U of PRBCs is expected to raise the hemoglobin level by 1 g/dL and the hematocrit by 3%.

(a) **Normal saline,** the only crystalloid compatible with blood, is usually given along with PRBCs for dilution and infusion facilitation. The saline may be heated to 39°C–43°C in an electric blood warmer (not in a microwave) to prevent hypothermia when multiple units are transfused.

(b) **Transfusion rate.** When the clinical situation allows, blood product infusion should proceed slowly for the first half hour, when transfusion reactions are most likely. Patients without a history of congestive heart failure (CHF) may be administered 1 U of PRBCs over 1–2 hours. The rate is halved for patients with CHF.

(3) **Platelets** are administered in 6-U infusions with a volume of 300 mL. Infusion of one "six-pack" of platelets is expected to result in a platelet count increment of 50,000–60,000/mm^3 as assessed 1 hour after infusion. Some patients (e.g., those with fever, DIC, excessive hemorrhage, hypersplenism, antiplatelet antibodies) may be refractory to platelet transfusion.

(a) **ABO blood type compatibility is recommended** for platelet transfusions to minimize the risks of transfusion reaction from accompanying plasma.

(b) **Rh-negative females of childbearing age** should receive platelets from Rh-negative donors.

(4) **FFP units** should also be transfused from ABO-compatible donors. The initial dose is 8–10 mL/kg (2 bags). In some clinical circumstances, the desired FFP dose is calculated by determining the magnitude of desired increment in factor activity. Patients should be re-evaluated for bleeding after transfusion of the first two FFP bags, with further therapy indicated if coagulation studies remain abnormal in the setting of continued hemorrhage.

(5) **Cryoprecipitate** is infused in initial doses of 2–4 bags/10 kg body weight. ABO compatibility is required only if large amounts of cryoprecipitate are administered.

(6) **Specific factor therapy** is guided by the patient's factor levels and desired magnitudes of increment.

d. **Transfusion complications**

(1) **Acute intravascular hemolysis,** usually resulting from ABO blood group incompatibility, represents the most dangerous acute transfusion reaction. Advanced hemolytic reactions may progress to cardiovascular, pulmonary, and renal failure.

(a) Clinical presentation of a hemolytic transfusion reaction includes fever, chills, back pain, dyspnea, or localized burning at the infusion site. Laboratory tests in patients with acute hemolytic reactions reveal elevated free plasma hemoglobin, haptoglobin, and bilirubin; hemoglobinuria is also found. Coombs' testing should be performed on pre- and posttransfusion blood samples.

(b) Therapy of hemolytic reactions should begin before confirmative testing, and includes cessation of transfusion and institution of aggressive hydration.

(2) **Rh incompatibility hemolysis.** A less acute hemolysis, caused by Rh incompatibility, may occur in the extravascular space of the spleen. These patients often are asymptomatic and do not require specific therapy.

(3) **Febrile nonhemolytic transfusion reactions** occur relatively commonly, especially in patients undergoing multiple transfusions. These nonthreatening reactions are caused by antigen–antibody reactions involving donor plasma, platelets, or leukocytes.

   (a) Clinically, nonhemolytic reactions begin within the first few hours after transfusion and manifest as temperature elevation and chills.

   (b) Because these reactions cannot be differentiated clinically between early acute hemolytic reactions, transfusions must be discontinued when reactions are first suspected and repeat cross matching and Coombs' testing of blood are indicated.

   (c) Patients with previous nonhemolytic reactions may be pretreated with acetaminophen and opioids or may be administered leukocyte-depleted components.

(4) **Allergic reactions** to transfused blood components occur in 1 of 100 transfusions. True anaphylaxis is rare. Symptoms are classic for allergic reactions.

   (a) Patients with history of allergic transfusion reactions should be premedicated with diphenhydramine (50 mg intravenously) before blood product administration.

   (b) In patients who develop allergic symptoms, the transfusion should be interrupted and diphenhydramine should be administered. If symptoms improve with diphenhydramine, transfusion may be restarted and can be completed in some cases.

(5) **Hypervolemia** may result from PRBC or FFP transfusion. Headaches or dyspnea should alert the clinician to the possibility of too-rapid intravascular volume enlargement. Diuresis with furosemide (40 mg intravenously) and reduction in infusion rate are therapeutic.

(6) **Hypothermia** resulting from transfusion of multiple PRBC units can be ameliorated by using warmed saline to dilute the packed cells.

(7) **Infection.** The risk of contracting **HIV** is estimated at 1 in 150,000 U. **Hepatitis B** and **hepatitis C** transmission risks are 1 in 50,000 U and 3 in 10,000 U, respectively.

(8) **Graft-versus-host disease,** which is usually fatal, occurs when nonirradiated (i.e., immunocompetent) leukocytes are administered to, and attack host tissue in, patients without functioning immune systems.

(9) **Electrolyte abnormalities** secondary to transfusion are unusual. Hypokalemia or hyperkalemia may occur, necessitating monitoring of potassium in all transfusions.

(10) **Noncardiogenic pulmonary edema (NCPE)** develops within 4 hours of transfusion, and presents as respiratory distress in the setting of fever, chills, and tachycardia. Usually, hospitalization and supportive care are sufficient, although the entity may be life-threatening in patients with significant comorbidity.

(11) **Asymptomatic anemia,** caused by a delayed hemolytic transfusion reaction, may occur more than 1 week after transfusion. A previously negative Coombs' test is positive.

(12) **Complications of massive transfusion** (i.e., transfusion of a volume of blood equal to the patient's normal circulating blood volume over a 24-hour period)

   (a) **Bleeding,** related to platelet and coagulation factor deficiencies, is the most frequent complication of massive transfusion. Routine replacement of platelets and coagulation factors is not recommended but should be guided by clinical situations.

      (i) **DIC** may occur in the setting of massive transfusion.

      (ii) **Platelet dysfunction.** Platelet levels often are not below 100,000/mm³, but dysfunction occurs because of coexistent hepatorenal disease or DIC. Platelet transfusion is not indicated unless documented thrombocytopenia exists in the setting of bleeding.

      (iii) **Coagulopathy** may be exacerbated by the fact that stored blood loses much of its factor activity, especially for factors V and VIII. FFP should be given only when significant bleeding exists with documented coagulopathy.

   (b) **Citrate toxicity** is primarily a historical problem occurring with transfusion of large amounts of whole blood.

(c) **Hypothermia** may be a significant component of disease states (e.g., major trauma, burns) that require massive transfusion, and particular attention must be paid to preventing the exacerbation of hypothermia when large-volume transfusions are performed.

F **Disposition** Most patients with significant bleeding require admission; however, some may receive treatment and be discharged. All patients should have disposition arranged in conjunction with a hematology consultation.

II HEMATOLOGIC EMERGENCIES

A Von Willebrand's disease

1. **Discussion.** von Willebrand's disease is the most common hereditary bleeding disorder. Genetic transmission is heterogenous because of multiple disease subtypes. von Willebrand's disease is caused by quantitative and/or functional deficiency of vWF, which is necessary for normal bleeding times.
   a. **Type I von Willebrand's disease.** The **amount** of vWF is low.
   b. **Type II von Willebrand's disease.** The **structure** of vWF is abnormal.
   c. **Type III von Willebrand's disease.** Patients have **little or no functioning vWF.**

2. **Clinical features**
   a. **Bleeding** involves primarily the skin and mucosal surfaces.
      (1) More than half of patients with von Willebrand's disease have a history of **epistaxis;** 40% report **easy bruising** and **hematoma formation.**
      (2) One third of patients with von Willebrand's disease have chronic **gingival bleeding;** an equal proportion of females with von Willebrand's have **menorrhagia.**
      (3) **Gastrointestinal bleeding** is less common (10% of patients).
   b. **Hemarthrosis** occurs primarily in patients with severe disease.
   c. A **severe bleeding diathesis,** similar to that seen in patients with severe hemophilia, is seen in patients with type III disease.

3. **Differential diagnosis.** Mild von Willebrand's disease can be difficult to differentiate from mild hemophilia. Severe bleeding in patients with types II and III von Willebrand's disease may present similarly to that in patients with hemophilia, but laboratory tests (see II A 4) usually provide the correct diagnosis in these cases.

4. **Evaluation.** Laboratory evaluation of von Willebrand's disease can be difficult, because variable results may cause the clinician to confuse vWF deficiency with hemophilia, especially in mild cases.
   a. The PT is normal, and the activated PTT is normal except in cases of severe deficiency.
   b. The bleeding time is prolonged, and the vWF activity is low.
   c. The vWF antigen and factor VIII activity are low or normal.

5. **Therapy**
   a. **Desmopressin.** Primary therapy for patients with bleeding due to von Willebrand's disease is desmopressin (0.3 µg/kg every 12 hours) subcutaneously or intravenously. For patients with type I von Willebrand's disease, no therapy besides desmopressin is necessary.
   b. **Aminocaproic acid** administration may be necessary for patients with oral bleeding.
   c. **Blood component transfusion.** For patients with type II or III von Willebrand's disease, **vWF replacement with cryoprecipitate** (2 bags/10 kg) or **factor VIII concentrate** (10 IU/kg) is usually indicated.

6. **Disposition.** Most patients with von Willebrand's disease, and all patients with significant bleeding, require hospital admission.

B **Hemophilias A and B**

1. **Discussion.** Hemophilias A and B are X-linked recessive disorders that may occur in patients without family history of bleeding disorders. Females are generally asymptomatic carriers of hemophilia with 50% of normal factor activity.

   a. **Types**
      (1) **Hemophilia A** is caused by **factor VIII deficiency;** 85% of patients with hemophilia have hemophilia A.
      (2) **Hemophilia B** is caused by **factor IX deficiency.**

   b. **Severity** depends on the level of factor deficiency.
      (1) Patients with mild or moderate disease have 6%–60% and 1%–5% of normal factor activity, respectively.
      (2) Severe disease is manifested as less than 1% factor activity.

   c. **Pathogenesis.** Minor lacerations rarely cause bleeding problems; however, deep hematomas or hemarthroses may occur with minimal or no trauma and may be delayed for hours.
      (1) **Hemarthroses** may lead to chronic arthropathy.
      (2) **Soft tissue** or **muscular hematomas** may cause problems such as obstruction, mass effect (e.g., airway composite compartment syndrome), or volume depletion.
      (3) **Intracranial bleeding** is a major cause of death in people with hemophilia.

2. **Clinical features.** Mucocutaneous bleeding may occur in the respiratory or gastrointestinal tracts. Hematuria is common but rarely severe. Symptoms of compartment syndrome (i.e., pain, paresthesias, neurovascular findings) may accompany intramuscular bleeding in the extremities.

3. **Differential diagnoses.** Hemophilias cause prolongation of the intrinsic pathway, so the initial differential consists primarily of other diseases that result in prolonged activated PTT.

4. **Evaluation**
   a. **History** should focus on bleeding disorders in the patient or family, including previous requirements for factor replacement.

   b. **Physical examination** should begin with assessment for volume depletion and should include a thorough search for bleeding sites.

   c. **Laboratory tests**
      (1) **Blood work** should begin with a **CBC** (with special attention paid to the hematocrit) and coagulation screening, which reveals prolongation of the **activated PTT** and a normal **PT.** In patients with more than 30% factor activity, the activated PTT may be normal, and definitive diagnosis may be difficult.
      (2) **Lumbar puncture.** With the increased frequency of HIV infection in patients with hemophilia, these patients often require diagnostic lumbar puncture to rule out meningeal infection. Factor levels should be raised to 30% 30–45 minutes prior to the procedure.
      (3) **Other tests** important in the hemophilia work-up (factor assays, inhibitor testing) may be ordered after the initial evaluation in the ED.

   d. **Diagnostic imaging studies.** A cranial **computed tomography (CT) scan** should be performed in hemophiliacs with headache or neurologic signs. Patients with abdominal, back, groin, or thigh pain may have retroperitoneal bleeding and should undergo an urgent abdominal CT scan.

5. **Therapy** for hemophilia depends on the type of hemophilia, the severity of disease, the presence of factor inhibitors, and the location and severity of the acute bleeding episode.
   a. **General measures**
      (1) **Stabilization**
         (a) Primary (e.g., volume loss) and secondary (e.g., airway compromise) effects of bleeding must be assessed. Early endotracheal intubation is indicated for patients with impending airway compromise. Oral intubation is preferable to nasal intubation because of the risk of epistaxis associated with the latter approach.

(b) The placement of central venous lines, intramuscular injections, and arterial puncture should be avoided in patients with hemophilia.

(2) FFP contains all clotting factors and is therefore useful for initial therapy for patients with hemophilia A or B when specific factor therapy is delayed or unavailable. Because of decreased risk of blood-borne disease transmission, patients with mild or moderate hemophilia B may be treated with FFP monotherapy.

(3) Factor concentrates, created from large numbers of pooled donors, represent effective hemophilia therapy but are associated with some risk of blood-borne disease transmission. Intermediate-purity factor concentrates have lower factor activity and more non-factor proteins. They are less desirable than high-purity factor concentrates.

  (a) Types

   (i) Factor VIII (1 IU/kg) raises the factor activity approximately 2%. The amount of **factor VIII required** for therapy is determined by the following equation: **patient's weight (kg) × 0.5 × % increase in factor activity required.**

   (ii) Factor IX (1 IU/kg) raises the factor level approximately 1%. The amount of **factor IX required** for therapy is determined by the following equation: **patient's weight (kg) × % increase in factor activity required.**

  (b) Assessment of compartment pressures and fasciotomy (if necessary) should occur after factor replacement to minimize the risk of further bleeding.

(4) Prothrombin complex concentrations may be indicated for factor therapy in some patients with factor VIII inhibition.

(5) DDAVP (1-deamino-8-D-ARGININE VASOPRESSIN; DESMOPRESSIN) is useful for patients with hemophilia A but not hemophilia B. The dose is 0.3 µg/kg intravenously every 12 hours. Response should be seen within 1 hour.

(6) e-Aminocaproic acid (100 mg/kg four times daily) and **tranexamic acid** (25 mg/kg three to four times daily) are plasminogen inhibitors, which prevent clot lysis. These agents are used primarily for mucosal bleeding (e.g., after dental procedures) because prevention of clot resorption in other areas (e.g., joints) may lead to chronic complications.

(7) Cryoprecipitate. With the advent of factor VIII concentrates, the administration of cryoprecipitate is rarely indicated for patients with hemophilia A. Cryoprecipitate contains no factor IX and is not indicated for treatment of hemophilia B.

b. Therapy for specific conditions in hemophilia

  (1) Lacerations. Patients with lacerations requiring suturing usually require factor replacement at the time of suturing and also at the time of suture removal.

  (2) Intra-articular and intramuscular bleeds. Most bleeding in hemophiliacs occurs into the joints and muscles.

   (a) Intra-articular bleeds. Ice, splinting, and **elastic bandages** often provide symptomatic relief to patients with intra-articular bleeds. **Factor replacement** should strive to achieve a level of at least 30%–40% initially.

   (b) Intramuscular bleeds. Immobilization is also indicated in patients with intramuscular hematomas, and **factor replacement** often is required in these patients as well.

  (3) Fractures. Factor replacement to a level of 50% is necessary.

  (4) Dental procedures. Oozing can usually be controlled with ε-aminocaproic acid.

  (5) Hematuria. Patients with persistent hematuria that does not respond to intravenous fluids usually require factor replacement to 50%.

  (6) Intracranial bleeding was, before the advent of AIDS, the major cause of mortality in patients with hemophilia. It may occur without prior history of trauma. In the case of patients with severe disease who suffer any potentially significant cranial trauma, factor replacement to 100% should proceed even before diagnostic imaging is obtained.

  (7) Epistaxis can usually be controlled by direct pressure or packing with microfibrillar collagen. Cautery and traditional petroleum packing can lead to rebleeding upon removal of packing or sloughing of cauterized area. In patients who do require factor replacement, levels should be increased to 50%.

(8) **Gastrointestinal** or **retropharyngeal bleeding.** Patients should receive factor replacement to a level of 50%–100%.

(9) **Retroperitoneal bleeding** is an additional life risk for hemophiliacs. Therapy is with cryoprecipitate (6 bags/10 kg) and factor replacement to 75%–100% (factor VIII) or at least 50% (factor IX).

6. **Disposition.** Patients with significant bleeding (e.g., retroperitoneal) or those at risk for potentially serious sequelae (e.g., compartment syndrome, airway obstruction) should be admitted for observation and specialist consultation when appropriate.

C **Anemia**

1. **Discussion.** Causes of anemia include:

   a. **Blood loss,** which can be occult, is the most common cause of anemia.

   b. **Autoimmune hemolysis** may present as disease occurring in the absence of obvious precipitating factors (warm antibodies) or in the setting of hypothermia (cold antibodies) or drug ingestion (drug-induced hemolysis).

      (1) **Warm autoimmune hemolysis** is often idiopathic, but there may be underlying leukemia, lymphoma, or lupus.

      (2) **Cold autoimmune hemolysis** occurs when RBCs interact with abnormal antibodies in the cooler peripheral circulation, resulting in hemolysis on entering the central circulation.

   c. **Glucose-6-phosphate dehydrogenase (G6PD) deficiency** is seen in up to 10% of the world population. Resultant weakness in the RBC membrane predisposes these patients to hemolysis in the presence of oxidant stress (e.g., fava bean ingestion, antimalarial medication).

   d. **Hereditary spherocytosis** with splenic RBC destruction is the most common hemolytic disease found in individuals of northern European descent.

   e. **Aplastic anemia,** manifested as pancytopenia, results from bone marrow failure, usually after exposure to a drug or toxin.

   f. **Red cell aplasia** is caused by immunologic disease (e.g., thymoma) and is characterized by decreased numbers of RBCs and other cells derived from erythroid precursors.

   g. **Hypochromic disease** is present when RBCs are being produced but are poorly hemoglobinated.

      (1) **Iron deficiency** is the most common cause of hypochromic disease, and it is usually caused by a precipitating disease process.

      (2) **Anemia of chronic disease** may be seen in almost any chronic disease state. These patients suffer from **poor iron utilization.**

      (3) **Defective heme or porphyrin synthesis,** as is seen with **porphyrias,** is a common cause of hypochromic anemia.

      (4) **Impaired globin synthesis,** as is seen in **thalassemias,** may also present as hypochromic anemia.

   h. **Megaloblastic anemia,** resulting from disruption in DNA synthesis, is primarily caused by folate or vitamin B_{12} deficiency.

      (1) Because all stem cell lines in the marrow divide rapidly, patients with significant folate or vitamin B_{12} deficiency can present with profound pancytopenia.

      (2) Other rapidly dividing cell lines are affected, and the patient with folate or B_{12} deficiency may present with disease in the skin, gastrointestinal tract, or mucosae.

   i. **Alcoholism.** The direct bone marrow suppressive effects of ethanol and the presence of concomitant hepatic dysfunction, combined with chronic nutritional deficiencies, make anemia an entity commonly seen in alcoholics.

    j. Mechanical disruption of RBCs may result in anemia.

        (1) Following valvuloplasty or **vascular surgery.** The incidence is decreasing with today's implant technology. Patients with implants and increasing anemia should be evaluated for implant dysfunction.

        (2) Microangiopathic hemolytic anemias involve fragmentation of morphologically normal RBCs by microvascular fibrin strands; examples of this may be seen in DIC, thrombotic thrombocytopenic purpura (TTP), hemolytic–uremic syndrome (HUS), hypertension, renal graft rejection, and mitomycin C toxicity.

2. Clinical features

    a. Chronic blood loss anemia. Patients may be asymptomatic from the gradually developing anemia, but may present with fatigue, exercise intolerance, anginal exacerbation, or syncope when hemoglobin levels drop to critical values.

    b. Autoimmune hemolysis

        (1) Cold agglutinin disease is usually acute and transient, with rare development of severe anemia or chronic disease. In **paroxysmal cold hemoglobinuria,** patients present with urinary discoloration, chills, fever, and abdominal or back pain. The disease is usually transient, but may result in severe anemia.

        (2) Drug-induced hemolytic anemia may be significant but is usually of moderate severity. Hemolysis may develop weeks after institution of drug therapy, and positive Coombs' tests may persist for up to 1 year after drug discontinuation.

    c. Anemia attributed to G6PD deficiency may present as hemolytic crisis in patients who have ingested oxidant drugs (e.g., sulfa drugs) or who have intercurrent infection or acidosis. Hemolysis may occur up to 3 days after the precipitating insult. Laboratory testing reveals a hemolytic state with hemoglobinuria.

    d. Hereditary spherocytosis may also present as an acute hemolytic state, although the anemia is usually relatively mild. Hematologic findings expected in hereditary spherocytosis include a normal mean corpuscular volume (MCV) and an elevated mean corpuscular hemoglobin (MCH).

    e. Aplastic anemia presents with a marked pancytopenia, which is easily recognized upon ED laboratory testing.

    f. Pure red cell aplasia presents with severe anemia and absence of reticulocytosis in patients with normal WBC and platelet counts.

    g. Hypochromic anemia. The presentation is similar to that of other patients with decreased RBC counts. Fatigue and generalized malaise are the most common presenting complaints. Iron deficiency anemia may be characterized by **koilonychia, pallor,** or **cheilosis.**

    h. Megaloblastic anemia. Patients may be folate- or vitamin B_{12}-deficient from underlying disease processes.

        (1) The most noteworthy findings associated with vitamin B_{12} deficiency are peripheral neurologic abnormalities, which are not seen with folate deficiency.

        (2) Inpatient testing (e.g., Schilling test for vitamin B_{12} absorption) is required to determine the nature of the vitamin deficiency in these patients.

3. Evaluation. Although the history may be diagnostic in patients with anemia, physical examination (e.g., jaundice from hemolytic anemia) and laboratory testing (e.g., peripheral RBC smear) often provide diagnostic direction.

    a. Physical examination findings

        (1) Adenopathy, hepatomegaly, splenomegaly, neuropathy, or **bony tenderness** may be present in patients with anemia of various causes.

        (2) Patients with significant volume loss may be **orthostatic** and have other signs of **hypovolemia.**

    b. Laboratory studies

        (1) Stool guaiac. All patients with anemia should undergo stool guaiac for blood. Other findings depend on the degree of blood loss and the specific cause of anemia.

(2) Blood work

- **(a)** A **CBC** quantifies the anemia and assesses the WBC and platelet counts. The **MCV** is an important part of the CBC, because its results direct further work-up. **Other tests** are indicated as directed by the clinical situation. Much of the subsequent evaluation, such as iron-binding capacity, haptoglobin levels, and bone marrow evaluation, takes place outside the ED.

    - **(i)** In patients with a **normal MCV,** serum iron levels, total iron-binding capacity, reticulocyte counts, haptoglobin levels, a Coombs' test, and a peripheral smear should be obtained. Further testing is directed by results of these analyses.

    - **(ii)** Patients with a **low MCV** require assessment of serum iron and iron-binding capacity, with ferritin levels and bone marrow analysis indicated if these tests are below normal. Normal iron testing in patients with a low MCV should prompt hemoglobin electrophoresis.

    - **(iii)** Patients with a **high MCV** should undergo reticulocyte count and assessment of folate and vitamin B_{12} levels.

- **(b)** The **reticulocyte count** allows assessment of the hematopoietic response to anemia.

- **(c)** A **peripheral smear** provides morphologic information on the presence of abnormal cells, such as spherocytes or schistocytes, which are RBC fragments indicating mechanical hemolysis.

    - **(i)** **Heinz bodies,** intra-RBC hemoglobin precipitates, may be seen in **G6PD-deficient patients** with acute hemolysis.

    - **(ii)** Patients with **hereditary spherocytosis** may have splenomegaly and jaundice in addition to characteristic **spherocytosis** on peripheral RBC smear.

- **(d)** **Plasma free hemoglobin, lactic dehydrogenase (LDH),** and **unconjugated bilirubin levels** are elevated in patients with hemolysis.

- **(e)** **Haptoglobin levels** are decreased in patients with hemolytic anemia, although the acute phase character of haptoglobin may cause a rise initially.

- **(f)** **Plasma iron levels, ferritin levels,** and **transferrin saturation** are low and **iron-binding capacity** is high in patients with iron deficiency.

- **(g)** **Direct Coombs' test.** This test evaluates RBC surface immunoglobulin or complement and is positive in cases of autoimmune hemolysis. (An indirect Coombs' test assesses for free antibodies and is used in the setting of transfusion screening.)

(3) Urinalysis may reveal a source of occult bleeding.

(4) Enzyme assay. In patients without previously known disease, the diagnosis of G6PD deficiency is made with an enzymatic assay.

(5) Osmotic fragility test. An osmotic fragility test is necessary to definitively diagnose hereditary spherocytosis.

c. Diagnostic imaging studies (e.g., CT scan, radionuclide imaging) may be required to delineate occult hemorrhage.

4. Therapy

a. Blood loss or **anemia of chronic disease.** In the ED, therapy may include transfusion or vitamin and iron supplementation.

b. Autoimmune hemolysis

(1) Patients with severe autoimmune hemolysis may require **oral prednisone** (1 mg/kg/day) or **transfusion therapy.** Because cross matching is difficult, transfusion therapy in these patients is complicated and should be undertaken only after hematologic consultation. **Splenectomy** or **immunosuppressive drugs** are sometimes required for long-term disease management.

(2) Treatment of underlying disease (e.g., leukemia, syphilis) and **avoidance of precipitating factors** often result in improvement or cure of autoimmune hemolysis.

- **(a)** Therapy for drug-induced autoimmune hemolysis is discontinuation of the offending agent.

(b) Patients with cold antibody hemolytic anemia should avoid cold temperatures to prevent hemolysis.

c. **G6PD deficiency anemia.** There is no specific therapy for this disorder. Optimal therapy for these individuals consists of prevention of hemolytic episodes by avoidance of oxidant drugs and other precipitating factors.

d. **Hereditary spherocytosis.** Therapy is splenectomy, which results in discontinued RBC destruction and prevents anemia.

e. **Aplastic anemia.** Therapy involves expectant management (when marrow function is expected to recover) or possible marrow transplant.

f. **Pure red cell aplasia.** Patients may respond to immunosuppressive therapy, bone marrow transplantation, or antithymocyte globulin.

g. **Iron deficiency anemia** is treated by addressing the underlying disease and attempting to restore body iron levels to normal. Subjective improvement may be seen within days of institution of iron therapy. The determination of nonresponse (and need for parenteral iron) should be made by hematologists.

    (1) **Salts of iron** provide effective oral replacement therapy and are best given in divided doses. Because these medications irritate the gastrointestinal tract, doses should increase gradually to the recommended 325 mg of ferrous sulfate three times daily.

    (2) **Ascorbic acid** may increase absorption of oral iron preparations.

h. **Megaloblastic anemia.** Folate (200 μg orally) or **vitamin B_{12}** (1–5 μg intramuscularly) may be useful. Long-term therapy is generally indicated.

5. **Disposition.** All patients with significant hemorrhage require hospital admission. In cases where outpatient management is judged to be reasonable, follow-up is important for continuation of work-up and potential definitive therapy (e.g., splenectomy).

D **Platelet abnormalities**

1. **Discussion.** Platelet abnormalities may be classified as disorders of quantity (for which transfusion is effective) or disorders of dysfunction (for which transfusion therapy may be futile).

a. **Decreased platelet production** may be seen in patients with marrow dysfunction caused by infiltration, infection, drugs, or radiation.

b. **Increased platelet destruction** is seen in patients with ITP or TTP, HUS, DIC, or viral infections. Thrombocytopenia is also associated with commonly used drugs: NSAIDs, heparin, some antibiotics, dextran, and many others.

c. **Splenic sequestration of platelets** can occur in hypothermic patients or in those with hypersplenism (e.g., with portal hypertension).

d. **Platelet loss** can be seen with hemorrhage or hemodialysis.

e. **Thrombocytosis,** seen in patients with polycythemia vera, splenectomy, or malignancy, may result in coagulopathy when platelet counts exceed 1 million/mm³.

2. **Clinical findings**

a. **Asymptomatic.** Incidental thrombocytopenia may be found by laboratory testing in asymptomatic patients.

b. **Hemorrhage.** Patients with significant platelet dysfunction may have some form of mucocutaneous hemorrhage, and extreme platelet disease may result in catastrophic cerebrovascular hemorrhage.

    (1) The presence of **petechiae, ecchymosis, or purpura** may provide clues to the presence of thrombocytopenia.

    (2) **Mucocutaneous bleeding** is suspicious for platelet abnormality.

c. **Splenomegaly.** The finding of splenomegaly on abdominal examination may help define the cause.

3. **Evaluation.** Laboratory assessment includes a **hematocrit, platelet count,** and **coagulation profile.** Measurement of the **bleeding time** to assess platelet function is usually performed in a spe-

cialized laboratory. The bleeding time usually becomes abnormal with platelet counts lower than 50,000/mm^3 (normal counts range from 150,000–450,000/mm^3). Pseudothrombocytopenia may be associated with laboratory error introduced by agglutination or platelet adherence to other cells.

4. **Therapy**

   a. **Platelet administration** is indicated for all patients with platelet levels below 10,000/mm^3 and for many patients with platelet levels below 50,000/mm^3. Administration of platelets may be counterproductive in some patients with hematologic disease (e.g., TTP). Consultation should be obtained before transfusing platelets in such patients.

   b. **Other therapies** are necessary when thrombocytopenia is caused by platelet destruction. **Prednisone** is often indicated for patients with TTP, ITP, or HUS. **NSAIDs** can supplement steroids in patients with TTP and HUS.

E Sickle cell anemia

1. **Discussion**

   a. **Incidence.** Approximately 8% of the black population of the United States carries the sickle hemoglobin gene. Most of these patients do not have homozygous disease (i.e., Hb SS, seen in 0.15% of blacks born in this country) but are asymptomatic carriers of sickle cell trait (i.e., Hb SA). Others, although not homozygous for sickle disease, have mixed hemoglobinopathies (e.g., Sβ thalassemia, SC) with phenotypic manifestations varying from nearly asymptomatic to severe sickle disease. Patients with heterozygous disease (Hb Sβ$_{thal}$ or Hb SC) may present to the ED with unknown disease states, because these individuals often sickle only under certain circumstances (e.g., high altitude).

   b. **Pathogenesis**

      (1) The **hallmark of sickle cell disease** is **substitution of valine for glutamic acid** on the β-hemoglobin chain. This substitution results in distortion of reduced RBCs into a characteristic sickle shape.

      (2) The sickle-shaped RBCs obstruct capillary blood flow, resulting in a cycle of increased **hypoxia** and worsening RBC sickling. Recurrent episodes of hypoxia may cause **chronic tissue ischemia** and **resultant organ failure.**

      (3) Sickled RBCs are subject to **hemolysis,** and patients with sickle disease suffer **chronic anemia.** Hematopoiesis accelerates in an attempt to maintain RBC numbers.

      (4) One of the most important features of sickle cell disease is the **increased risk of infection.** Hyposplenism (due to repeated ischemic insults) and other immunologic dysfunctions render sickle cell patients especially susceptible to attack from encapsulated organisms (e.g., *Streptococcus pneumoniae, Haemophilus influenzae, Salmonella* species).

2. **Clinical features**

   a. **Vaso-occlusive pain crisis.** RBC sickling and the resultant microvascular occlusion with tissue ischemia are a source of potentially severe pain. The location and type of pain may differ between presentations. Patients with pain crisis typically have low-grade fever, mild leukocytosis, and reticulocytosis, as well as the chronic anemia expected for those with sickle cell anemia. There are different types of vaso-occlusive crises, depending on location.

      (1) **Chest crisis,** most commonly seen in children with sickle cell anemia, is characterized by chest pain with dyspnea, hyperventilation, or both. Although chest crisis may be caused by microvascular occlusion in the thorax, pulmonary infarction and other intrapulmonary disease must be considered.

      (2) **Bone crisis** usually involves extremities, but back pain can occur.

      (3) **Joint crisis** may present as monoarticular or oligoarticular pain.

      (4) **Abdominal crisis** usually is manifest by acute and constant abdominal pain without localized tenderness or peritonitis.

   b. **Aplastic crisis.** In these patients, there is failure of hematopoiesis to keep pace with ongoing hemolysis.

    c. Sequestration crisis. Heterozygous patients may develop sequestration, presenting with acute anemia. The anemia is caused by the sudden sequestration of a large portion of circulating RBCs, usually in the spleen, but the liver may also be involved.

    d. Other acute conditions seen in patients with sickle disease are either more likely to occur or are associated with increased morbidity in these patients.

      (1) Approximately 10% of sickle cell patients have a **cerebrovascular accident.** Cerebrovascular accident often occurs in patients younger than 10 years.

      (2) Pulmonary infarction is much more common in patients with sickle cell anemia than in the general population. In addition, there is increased incidence of venous thromboembolism and fat embolism (from bone infarction).

      (3) Those with sickle cell anemia are no more likely to develop **hyphema** than the general population, but complications are potentially worse in patients with sickle trait or disease.

      (4) Priapism occurs relatively more frequently among those displaying sickle cell anemia and may result in erectile dysfunction if not addressed.

    e. Chronic conditions

      (1) Symptomatic anemia may result from the chronicity of sickle cell disease.

      (2) Sickle lung disease, resulting from chronic hypoxia and recurrent infection and infarction, may cause **cor pulmonale** in those older than 30 years of age.

      (3) Leg ulcers, resulting from chronic tissue hypoxia and venous stasis, also occur commonly.

      (4) Cholelithiasis, due to chronic hemolysis, is also seen frequently.

3. Differential diagnosis

    a. The primary differential in patients with acute sickle crisis is investigation for presence of **precipitating infectious disease.** Noninfectious precipitating factors, including hypoxia, stress, dehydration, hemorrhage, fever, acidosis, alcohol intoxication, and pregnancy, should also be considered.

    b. Patients with bony pain may have **fractures** or **osteomyelitis.**

    c. Sickle cell patients with chest crisis should be evaluated for other **cardiopulmonary disease,** including pneumonia, pulmonary embolus, and pulmonary or myocardial infarction (MI).

    d. Though sickle crisis presenting as abdominal pain may mimic **surgical abdominal disease,** diagnoses of pyelonephritis, biliary tract disease, hepatitis, appendicitis, gynecologic disease, and hepatic or splenic infarction should also be considered in sickle cell patients with abdominal complaints.

    e. Joint pain in the setting of sickle cell disease may be due to joint crisis, but may also be due to **infection, gout,** or **trauma.**

4. Evaluation

    a. History. Pain crises may be precipitated by acute infection, and crisis patients should be thoroughly evaluated for the presence of encapsulated organisms or other infectious agents. The history should address possible precipitating factors, including potential sites of infection, and whether the patient is taking prophylactic penicillin.

    b. Physical examination of patients with sickle cell disease should be thorough to differentiate types of crises and to rule out concurrent disease states.

      (1) Orthopedic examination. Patients with bone crisis may be expected to have slight local bony tenderness, but presence of warmth or erythema should increase suspicion of skin or deep tissue infection. Significant bony tenderness may signal fractures. Identification of **joint effusions** is important in patients with sickle cell who display arthralgias. Such effusions require diagnostic drainage.

      (2) Pulmonary examination, for respiratory rate and auscultation, is particularly important in patients with chest symptoms and possible pneumonia.

      (3) Neurologic examination. Because microvascular deficiencies in sickle cell disease usually involve the central nervous system (CNS), careful neurologic examination may unmask the presence of acute stroke caused by sickle cell disease.

(4) **Abdominal examination**

(a) Sickle cell patients with abdominal crisis must be examined carefully for significant abdominal tenderness and signs of peritonitis, which are usually absent in vaso-occlusive abdominal sickle crisis. Bowel sounds should be normal in patients with abdominal crisis, even in patients with significant pain.

(b) Identification of an enlarged, painful, and tender liver or spleen is critical to making the diagnosis of acute syndromes of sequestration in these organs.

(5) **Extremities.** Nonpitting edema in the extremities is a clue to the presence of dactylitis ("hand-foot syndrome"), which can be the first manifestation of sickle disease.

(6) **Vision.** Evaluation of visual acuity is important in sickle cell patients with visual complaints, because they may have proliferative or nonproliferative retinopathy.

c. **Laboratory studies.** For adult patients with acute crisis, ancillary studies have traditionally included a CBC and reticulocyte count, with other tests performed only if indicated. For pediatric patients, most authorities recommend performing routine urinalysis and chest radiograph, as well as the CBC and reticulocyte count.

(1) **Blood work**

(a) The **CBC** is always important in evaluating sickle cell patients in the ED. Hematocrit can drop to 30% below baseline low levels in acute sequestration syndromes, and can also be low in aplastic crisis. Comparison to known baseline levels is desirable. A leukocyte count of 12,000–17,000 cells/mm^3 is consistent with uncomplicated sickle pain crisis, but WBC counts exceeding this number should increase suspicion of underlying infection.

(b) The **reticulocyte count** is important in ruling out aplastic crisis (in which the reticulocyte count is low) and in differentiation of aplastic from sequestration crises (normal to high reticulocyte count).

(2) **Urinalysis** for identification of urinary tract infection (UTI) is indicated for all children with sickle crisis, as well as for adults with abdominal pain.

(3) **Arterial blood gas (ABG) determination.** The threshold for obtaining an ABG analysis is relatively low in sickle cell patients with chest complaints.

(4) **Blood cultures** should be obtained from those sickle cell patients with identified or strongly suspected infection.

(5) **Blood chemistries** and **liver enzyme tests** are indicated for crisis patients with abdominal pain. Other tests may be indicated as directed by the clinical situation.

(6) **Arthrocentesis** and **laboratory evaluation of joint fluid** are necessary to rule out infection in patients with joint effusions.

(7) **CSF analysis.** In the setting of neurologic deficit and negative cranial CT, **lumbar puncture** should be performed to exclude subarachnoid hemorrhage or infection.

d. **Diagnostic imaging studies**

(1) **Radiography.** The presence of any chest symptoms mandates a **chest radiograph.** Bony pain from sickle crisis, if located in a specific area, is an indication for **plain radiography of the involved region** to search for fracture or osteomyelitis.

(2) **Ultrasonography** may help identify biliary disease and sequestration.

(3) **Emergent cranial CT scan** to rule out cerebrovascular accident should be performed on sickle cell patients with neurologic symptoms. Subsequent **magnetic resonance imaging (MRI)** or **arteriography** may be required. Arteriography should be performed on patients with sickle cell anemia only after adequate hydration and transfusion to maintain an Hb S level of less than 30% to avoid cerebral vasospasm from hyperosmolar contrast exposure.

5. **Therapy.** For the majority of sickle cell anemia patients visiting the ED for vaso-occlusive crisis, therapy is based on hydration and analgesia, usually intravenous opioids. Administration of supplemental oxygen has not been demonstrated to be of aid in vaso-occlusive crisis.

a. **Analgesia.** The chronicity of sickle disease and the inability to confirm crisis pain with bedside or laboratory testing have resulted in an unfortunate pattern of crisis pain undertreatment. Studies have found that although those with sickle cell anemia are not particularly likely to become addicted to opioids, patients with sickle crises receive substantially less analgesia than other chronic pain sufferers who present to the ED.

   (1) **Meperidine should not be administered** to patients with sickle crisis pain. Repeated dosing, which is almost always required in patients with sickle cell anemia, leads to accumulation of the epileptogenic metabolite normeperidine.

   (2) **Oral and injectable NSAIDs** are an option for pain control in patients with sickle cell disease, but precautions for renal effects of these agents should be particularly heeded. Individuals in whom oral agents have failed at home are unlikely to respond to enteral therapy in the ED.

b. **Transfusion** may be required for refractory pain or pain associated with **aplastic crisis.** Given the difficulty of diagnosing pulmonary infarction and the fact that ventilation–perfusion (V/Q) scans are often unreliable in patients with chronic pulmonary abnormalities, some hematologists advocate transfusion for all patients with **chest crisis.**

c. **Antibiotic therapy**

   (1) For patients with infectious complications requiring admission, a reasonable choice for initial empiric therapy is **intravenous ceftriaxone** (1 g in adults, 50–75 mg/kg up to 1 g in children). Other agents may be more appropriate depending on the site of infection (e.g., antistaphylococcal agents for osteomyelitis) and other clinical variables. Prompt administration of antibiotics is important.

   (2) Pediatric patients with localized infectious processes not requiring admission should be prescribed antibiotics reliably covering pneumococcus and *H. influenzae* (e.g., **amoxicillin–clavulanate**). These patients should receive conservative ED return precautions as well as close follow-up.

   (3) Some practitioners believe that the prevalence of pneumonia in sickle cell patients with chest crisis is sufficiently high to warrant **empiric antibiotic coverage** in these patients. The emergency physician is advised to consult a hematologist for aid in guiding therapy of patients with chest crisis.

d. **Management of specific disorders in sickle cell disease**

   (1) **Cerebrovascular accident.** Therapy for patients with cerebral infarction includes **standard management** and **simple** or **partial exchange transfusion** with a goal of reducing the overall burden of Hb S to lower than 30%. Similar therapy is used for sickle cell patients with hemorrhagic cerebrovascular accident. The duty of the emergency physician is to rapidly obtain cranial imaging and contact consultants for aid in guiding appropriate therapy of sickle cell patients with cerebrovascular accidents.

   (2) **Increased intracranial pressure (ICP).** Therapy is similar to the standard therapy, except that special care must be made to **avoid extreme hypocarbia** (i.e., an arterial carbon dioxide tension of less than 24 mm Hg), which can worsen vasospasm, hypoxia, and RBC sickling.

   (3) **Priapism.** Therapy in patients with sickle cell anemia includes hydration and analgesia. Urologic consultation (for corpora aspiration or a shunting procedure) is indicated for patients whose priapism persists beyond 4–6 hours.

   (4) **Hyphema.** Early **ophthalmologic consultation** is indicated for sickle cell patients with hyphema, because surgical management is often indicated. **Acetazolamide,** used to decrease intraocular pressures, is **contraindicated** in sickle cell patients because its pH effects promote sickling.

   (5) **Acute sequestration syndromes.** Therapy includes **transfusion** and **vigorous hydration** to mobilize RBCs.

e. **Management of sickle cell disease in pregnant women.** Other than **lowering the transfusion threshold,** treatment of sickle crisis in pregnancy does not differ from that in other patients.

6. **Disposition.** Patients with refractory pain, infection, dactylitis, priapism, transfusion requirement, neurologic deficit, pulmonary complications, or sequestration syndromes require admission. Thresholds for both prophylactic antibiotics and admission of pediatric sickle cell patients are lower than those for adults.

F **DIC**

1. **Discussion.** DIC is a syndrome of consumptive coagulopathy that occurs in the presence of another disease. Widespread activation of the coagulation pathway results in secondary activation of fibrinolysis, with resultant thrombosis, hemorrhage, or both.
   a. **Mechanisms.** Intravascular coagulation is prompted by one of three mechanisms:
      (1) Extrinsic procoagulant (e.g., amniotic fluid, snake venom)
      (2) Blood contact with a foreign surface (e.g., grafts, burns)
      (3) Intrinsic procoagulant (e.g., promyelocytic leukemia)
   b. **Pathogenesis.** After diffuse microcirculatory clot formation, fibrinolysis occurs with a subsequent release of **fibrin degradation products (FDPs),** and the body's homeostasis between clot and lysis becomes disrupted.
      (1) Circulating plasmin cleaves fibrinogen and further decreases levels of factors V and VIII.
      (2) FDPs add to the overall disruption of hemostasis, delaying fibrin polymerization and impairing platelet function.

2. **Clinical features.** In many cases, the most striking clinical feature of DIC is the comorbid disease that prompts its development. Most commonly, DIC is seen in ED patients who are pregnant, burned, septic, or severely traumatized, or who have severe hepatic disease.
   a. **Primary hematologic complications** of DIC are bleeding and clotting, which may occur concurrently.
      (1) **Bleeding** occurs in up to 75% of patients with DIC, and usually occurs from **skin and mucous membrane sites.** Oozing venipuncture or surgical wound sites, epistaxis, petechiae, and ecchymoses are common manifestations of DIC.
      (2) **Hematuria** or **gastrointestinal** or **intracerebral bleeding** may also be seen. The presence of intracerebral blood is associated with a particularly poor prognosis.
      (3) **Thrombosis** in DIC may be manifest as end-organ damage to involved structures (e.g., mental status change, renal failure, extremity gangrene).
      (4) **Purpura fulminans,** resulting from widespread vascular thrombi, may be seen in patients with DIC caused by *N. meningitidis* or *S. pneumoniae.*
   b. **Microangiopathic hemolytic anemia,** resulting from shear damage to RBCs passing intravascular fibrin strands, is characteristic of chronic DIC.
   c. **Localized DIC** may occur in the kidney or liver in patients with malignant hypertension and cirrhosis, respectively.
   d. Patients with **chronic DIC** may have compensated levels of clotting factor production, as well as laboratory abnormalities without significant clinical disease.

3. **Differential diagnosis.** Because an extremely wide range of disease states can produce DIC, the investigation for underlying pathology in DIC patients in the ED must be comprehensive. Differentiation of DIC from other hematologic abnormalities is based on **laboratory evaluation.** A panel of hematologic abnormalities (see II E 4), rather than one specific test, makes the diagnosis of DIC.

4. **Evaluation.** Despite the relatively loose definition of DIC, evaluation for its presence is relatively straightforward and is primarily based on clinical presentation and laboratory analysis. The CBC—particularly platelet count, PT, PTT, fibrinogen, and fibrin split products—are the main tests used in the ED to identify DIC.
   a. PT and PTT are prolonged.
   b. Fibrin split product levels are increased.

   c. Fibrinogen levels and platelet counts are low.

   d. Levels of factors V and VIII are decreased.

   e. Increased levels of FDPs may be the primary clue to presence of chronic DIC, in which patients may have compensated for lower levels of other clotting factors.

   f. CBC and electrolyte analysis are necessary for determination of overall patient status (e.g., level of anemia, volume deficit).

5. **Therapy.** Although DIC sometimes resolves with treatment of the underlying disease process leading to its development, specific therapy is often indicated.

   a. **Basic life support** (oxygen and fluids for hemodynamic support) is indicated for patients with stable laboratory results and no significant clinical problems.

   b. **Replacement of depleted clotting factors** may be accomplished with FFP, cryoprecipitate, and platelets. Replacement therapy is indicated if the PT is prolonged two to three times normal in a bleeding patient. Factor levels, which should be maintained higher than 50% of normal, can also be used to guide therapy if they are obtainable.

      (1) **FFP** (200–250 U of each factor per unit of FFP) is used to replace clotting factors, and should be administered 2 U at a time. Attention should be paid to pulmonary status during FFP therapy, which involves significant volume infusion.

      (2) **Cryoprecipitate** (10 bags at a time) is administered to maintain fibrinogen levels greater than 100–150 mg/kg.

      (3) **Platelets** should be administered (6 U at a time) in bleeding patients with a platelet count below 50,000/mm^3 and in all patients with a platelet count below 25,000/mm^3.

   c. **Vitamin K** and **folate** should be given to all patients with DIC.

   d. **Heparin.** Though its use is generally reserved for patients not responding to more conservative therapy, heparin may be used to treat patients with thrombosis as the primary manifestation of DIC.

      (1) The ability of heparinization to help patients with DIC is still somewhat controversial, and heparin should be avoided in some circumstances.

         (a) **Contraindications.** Patients who have had recent surgery, and those with active CNS or gastrointestinal bleeding, should not receive heparin.

         (b) **Precaution.** Hypertensive patients should have blood pressure controlled prior to heparinization to reduce risk of precipitating CVA.

      (2) Heparin may be particularly useful in DIC patients with meningococcemia, acute promyelocytic leukemia, or Trousseau's syndrome (i.e., migrating superficial thrombophlebitis in the setting of visceral malignancy). Suggested doses of heparin range from low-dose to full-dose heparinization, depending on the clinical situation.

6. **Disposition.** Almost all patients with DIC require admission to address both the DIC and the underlying medical conditions.

III   ONCOLOGIC EMERGENCIES

A **Discussion**   Emergencies attributed to cancer can be classified as biochemical, immunologic, or mechanical.

1. **Biochemical derangements** from cancer may involve electrolyte, endocrine, or rheologic vascular dysfunction.

   a. **Hypercalcemia** occurs with renal cell carcinoma; multiple myeloma; bone metastases from breast, prostate, or lung primaries; and lymphoma.

   b. **Syndrome of inappropriate antidiuretic hormone (SIADH) secretion** may be seen in patients with intracerebral, intrathoracic, and certain abdominal–pelvic tumors.

   c. **Hyperviscosity syndrome** occurs in patients with Waldenström macroglobulinemia, chronic myelocytic leukemia, and multiple myeloma.

   d. Adrenal insufficiency and **shock** may be seen in patients in whom chronic steroid replacement is withdrawn, or in those with lung or breast carcinomas, malignant melanoma, or retroperitoneal malignancy.

   e. Tumor lysis syndrome is usually anticipated and treated prophylactically by oncologists, but may be seen in patients presenting to the ED. This entity is most commonly seen in patients with leukemia or lymphoma and is characteristically seen 1–5 days after chemotherapy or radiotherapy of sensitive and fast-growing tumors. Acute cell lysis occurs, with release of potassium, nucleic acids, and phosphates. Multiple organ failure and death can result.

2. **Immunologic complications** of cancer are partially caused by cancer-mediated immunosuppression, but they primarily result from chemotherapy or radiation therapy.

   a. Myelosuppression, with resultant granulocytopenia and sepsis, is a primary concern in cancer patients. Opportunistic infection is also a significant risk in the immunosuppressed patient.

   b. Immune-mediated thrombocytopenia can be seen.

   c. Suppression of marrow function can result in anemia.

   d. Overwhelming infection, which may occur with opportunistic microbes, is a major cause of death in patients with cancer.

3. **Mechanical complications of tumor growth** may be the first manifestations of cancer, and they often threaten life or limb.

   a. Airway obstruction may be seen in patients with tumors of the ears, nose, or throat; lymphoma; and metastatic lung carcinoma. Tumor impingement may occur at all levels of the respiratory tract, with upper respiratory tract, ear, nose, and throat tumors causing proximal obstruction and endobronchial lesions restricting airflow distally.

   b. Malignant pericardial effusion and **tamponade** may be seen after radiation therapy or in patients with breast, ovary, or lung carcinoma. In addition, acute leukemia, Hodgkin's lymphoma, or melanoma may present with pericardial disease.

   c. Superior vena cava syndrome is seen in patients with lymphoma or with oat-cell or squamous-cell lung carcinomas.

   d. Spinal cord compression may be the first sign of neoplasm, and it is seen in patients with multiple myeloma, lymphomas, and carcinoma of the lung, breast, or prostate.

B **Clinical features**

1. **Biochemical derangements**

   a. Hypercalcemia, occurring in up to 40% of patients with multiple myeloma, may cause **back pain, constipation,** or **altered mental status.**

   b. SIADH is **primarily a laboratory diagnosis** in patients presenting with **inappropriate free water retention.**

   c. Hyperviscosity syndromes occur when the serum viscosity is greater than five times that of water, and it may be seen when the hematocrit increases beyond 50%–60%. A leukocrit exceeding 10% may also be associated with significant hyperviscosity.

   (1) **Fatigue, headache, anorexia,** and **somnolence** are early nonspecific symptoms of hyperviscosity.

   (2) **Localized neurologic deficits,** with possible progression to coma, may develop as microthromboses develop in the CNS.

   d. Adrenal insufficiency, like hyperviscosity, can manifest as **altered mental status.** There is an added component of potentially life-threatening cardiovascular involvement with adrenal shock.

   e. Tumor lysis syndrome can be characterized by **multiple organ failure** and death.

2. **Immunologic complications.** Features of **thrombocytopenia** (from immune-mediated platelet destruction) and **anemia** in cancer patients are similar to presenting signs and symptoms of these disorders in other patients.

3. **Mechanical complications**
   a. **Airway obstruction** may be indicated by dyspnea, stridor, nasal flaring, or wheezing.
   b. **Malignant effusions** accumulate over long periods of time and, therefore, may reach significant size (sometimes greater than 500 mL) before causing **symptoms characteristic of pericardial fluid accumulation.**
   c. **Superior vena cava syndrome** is frequently diagnosed first in the ED, and it may be the presenting sign of cancer. The syndrome results from tumor restriction of blood flow in the superior vena cava. **Blood flow obstruction** results in elevated venous pressures in the areas drained by the superior vena cava (i.e., arms, neck, face, cerebrum). **Symptoms** reflect the anatomic distribution of the vein's drainage, and include **headache, facial** or **arm edema,** and **fullness in the neck and face.** As the disease progresses, an increase in ICP and syncope may be noted.
   d. **Spinal cord compression** may present as **paraparesis, hypoesthesia,** or **gait disturbance.** Paraplegia, marked sensory deficits, urinary incontinence or retention, and loss of rectal sphincter tone usually indicate a more advanced process.

4. **Signs and symptoms of other, concurrent, diseases.** Concurrent disorders occur in cancer patients with increased frequency because of the malignancy, cancer therapy, or the patient's generalized debilitated state.
   a. **Coronary artery disease** can coexist with cancer and may be exacerbated by anemia. In addition, many chemotherapeutic agents have cardiotoxicity.
   b. **Hypercoagulability** and **thrombosis** (e.g., Trousseau's syndrome of visceral malignancy) are prominent features of many neoplasms.
   c. **Intravascular volume depletion,** common in cachectic cancer patients, may result in prerenal azotemia.
   d. **Rapidly progressive renal failure** from glomerular amyloid deposition may be seen in patients with multiple myeloma or lymphoma.
   e. **Gastrointestinal bleeding** in cancer patients may be caused by tumor therapy.
      (1) **Intra-arterial chemotherapy** may result in upper gastrointestinal tract bleeding.
      (2) **Vomiting,** a well-known complication of tumor therapy, may result in **Mallory-Weiss tears,** causing esophageal bleeding.

C **Differential diagnosis**   The long list of tumor-related emergencies implies a similarly extensive list of differential diagnoses.

1. Because oncologic emergencies may affect blood chemistries, organ function, airway patency, and perfusion, the potential of cancer-related illness should be considered in any cancer patient who presents to the ED.

2. Because many of the oncologic emergencies discussed in this section may represent the presenting signs of cancer, these entities must also be considered in patients without a known history of neoplasm.

D **Evaluation**

1. **Biochemical derangements**
   a. **Hypercalcemia of malignancy** represents a relatively easy diagnostic entity. Calcium levels are readily measured by the hospital laboratory.
      (1) **Ionized calcium levels** should be interpreted in light of pH and serum albumin.
      (2) An **electrocardiogram (ECG)** may demonstrate a **shortened QT interval** in patients with hypercalcemia.
   b. **SIADH** is evaluated by laboratory analysis of serum and urine sodium and urine-specific gravity. Physical examination clues may point toward intracerebral or intrapulmonary processes in patients with SIADH and no known tumor.
      (1) The **primary abnormalities** in SIADH are hyponatremia and urine that contains a high sodium level (greater than 30 mEq/L) and is not optimally concentrated.

        (2) **Normal renal, adrenal,** and **thyroid function** must be demonstrated before the diagnosis of SIADH is established.

    c. **Hyperviscosity syndromes** may be difficult to diagnose clinically because presenting symptoms can be vague. Laboratory analysis is usually diagnostic.

        (1) **Blood work.** A **CBC** reveals elevated hematocrit and microscopic Rouleau formation. Sometimes the clue to the diagnosis of hyperviscosity comes with laboratory technicians reporting that the **blood is "too thick" to run tests.**

        (2) **Neurologic examination** may reveal focal deficits.

        (3) **Funduscopy** should be performed to search for "sausage-link" retinal vasculature, hemorrhages, or exudates.

    d. **Adrenal insufficiency** is suspected based on either electrolyte analysis or the clinical appearance of a patient with potential adrenal dysfunction. Because treatment is empiric, response to therapy may aid in making the diagnosis.

        (1) **Primary laboratory abnormalities** are hypoglycemia, hyponatremia, hyperkalemia, and eosinophilia.

        (2) **Physical examination** for cardiovascular stability is important in patients with adrenal insufficiency, because hypotension may lead to hemodynamic collapse.

    e. **Tumor lysis syndrome.** The diagnosis may be made based on the history in some cases. Patients presenting to the ED with lysis may relate a history of receiving steroids within the past few days (sometimes for an unrelated illness such as anaphylaxis). Some of these patients may not have a known history of neoplasm. Laboratory analysis helps make the definitive diagnosis.

        (1) **Hyperkalemia** occurring in tumor lysis syndrome may also cause **peaked T-wave ECG changes.**

        (2) **Hyperuricemia** can be found in patients with tumor lysis. Uric acid levels should be checked on all patients who are candidates for this diagnosis.

        (3) **Hyperphosphatemia** may cause dangerous hypocalcemia.

2. **Immunologic complications**

    a. **Infection.** The frequency and severity of infection increase with granulocyte counts lower than 1000/mm^3, emphasizing the importance of the differential WBC count in cancer patients with potential infection. Evaluation of such patients involves radiography, body fluid analysis, and culturing to detect the site of infection.

    b. **Immune-mediated thrombocytopenia** may be suggested by the presence of **petechiae** on physical examination.

    c. **Anemia.** Patients report fatigue, and the physical examination may reveal skin or palpebral conjunctival pallor. The **CBC is diagnostic,** but optimal interpretation requires **comparison with a known hemoglobin baseline.**

3. **Mechanical complications**

    a. **Airway obstruction.** Portable chest radiography is usually performed because of potential patient instability. Fiberoptic laryngoscopy may be used for airway visualization.

    b. **Malignant pericardial effusion** and **tamponade** present with similar physical findings as do other causes of pericardial tamponade. Beck's triad of hypotension, venous distention, and muffled heart tones is a late finding.

        (1) **Echocardiography** is the best tool for evaluation of pericardial fluid but may not be available in the ED.

        (2) **Pericardiocentesis** is indicated in patients with hemodynamic compromise, and is both diagnostic and therapeutic.

    c. **Superior vena cava syndrome,** in its advanced stages, may be associated with papilledema caused by increased ICP.

        (1) **Early findings** are neck and upper thoracic venous distention, facial plethora and telangiectasia, and mild edema of the face and arms.

    (2) A **palpable supraclavicular mass** may be identified.

    (3) A **chest radiograph** often demonstrates mediastinal or lung abnormality.

  d. Spinal cord compression may present as acute urinary retention. Patients with this or any other neurologic complaint suggestive of cord compression (e.g., loss of perirectal sensation) should undergo examination of reflexes, gait, sensorimotor function, and sphincter tone to further evaluate for signs of acute cord compression. A sensory level or distal flaccid paralysis may be seen. Patients with suspected cord compression require further consultation, often including emergent CT scan, MRI, or myelographic imaging.

E **Therapy**

  1. Biochemical derangements

    a. Hypercalcemia associated with cancer usually improves with **saline infusion** (1–2 L) and **intravenous furosemide** (80 mg). Hemodialysis or peritoneal dialysis is reserved for patients who do not respond to more conservative measures. Mithramycin, oral phosphate, and glucocorticoids take 1–2 days to lower calcium levels and are interventions best reserved for after a patient's ED stay.

    b. SIADH. Treatment focuses on **free water restriction** and, in cases of cardiac or neurologic toxicity, includes **infusion of 100–250 mL of 3% saline solution.**

    c. Symptomatic hyperviscosity syndrome in patients with a hematocrit greater than 60% is treated with **hydration** and **phlebotomy** (of 1–2 U) with **saline** and **RBC replacement.**

    d. Adrenal insufficiency and **shock.** Primary therapy is the administration of **intravenous hydrocortisone** (100 mg) along with **volume resuscitation.** This dose may be repeated every 6–8 hours. Occasionally, higher doses or pressors may be necessary. If the diagnosis of adrenal insufficiency is unclear, treatment can proceed using **dexamethasone** (4 mg intravenously) while performing an adrenocorticotropic hormone (ACTH) stimulation test.

    e. Tumor lysis syndrome. Ideally, therapy is preventive, but the ED physician can effectively address many of the abnormalities resulting from lysis.

      (1) Vigorous hydration, with careful attention to renal function, is a cornerstone of tumor lysis syndrome treatment.

      (2) Urinary alkalinization (to pH greater than 7) and **allopurinol** (300 mg orally) are recommended to address increased uric acid levels caused by tumor lysis.

      (3) Careful monitoring of calcium levels is important, especially for patients receiving bicarbonate for urinary alkalinization.

  2. Immunologic complications

    a. Infection. In a patient with **fever** or **rigors** in the setting of malignancy, the emergency physician should assume the presence of a serious infection and begin empiric therapy.

      (1) Antibiotic therapy. One acceptable regimen includes **ceftriaxone** (75 mg/kg up to 1 g intravenously) and **gentamicin** (2 mg/kg), with addition of anaerobic coverage (**metronidazole** or **clindamycin**) in patients with possible abdominal infection. As is usually the case, many antibiotic combinations are acceptable, and other choices may be made after early specialist consultation. The primary goal is to administer appropriate antibiotics as early as possible.

      (2) Support for cancer patients with infection should also include **intravenous fluids,** because volume depletion is almost universally present in this setting.

    b. Immune-mediated thrombocytopenia may require transfusion, but transfused platelets also are likely susceptible to destruction. Hematology consultation is recommended before platelet transfusion in these patients.

    c. Anemia. Indications for transfusion in anemia are not significantly different in cancer patients as compared with other individuals.

3. **Mechanical complications**
   a. **Airway obstruction** is treated by establishment of a secure airway. Those patients with true airway emergencies require intubation in the ED. Other oncologic patients with airway compromise may require surgical tracheostomy.
   b. **Malignant pericardial effusion and tamponade** are treated with **fluid resuscitation** and **pericardiocentesis.**
   c. **Superior vena cava syndrome,** when accompanied by papilledema, should be treated with **furosemide** (40 mg intravenously) and **methylprednisolone** (120 mg intravenously) to reduce the ICP pending definitive mediastinal radiotherapy.
   d. **Spinal cord compression** is a true emergency, and it is amenable to rapid therapy in the ED. Patients should receive **dexamethasone** (10 mg intravenously) while awaiting definitive radiographic, radiotherapeutic, or operative intervention. Emergency surgical decompression or radiotherapy can prevent irreversible neurologic impairment.

4. **Concurrent disorders.** Cancer patients are known to have increased frequency of **thrombotic disease,** but the dangers of anticoagulation in this group may prompt mechanical (i.e., filter placement) rather than pharmacologic therapy.

F **Disposition** Admission is the rule for patients with oncologic emergencies. Early nephrology consultation is indicated in patients with tumor lysis syndrome and potential renal insufficiency, because hemodialysis may be helpful.

Study Questions

Directions: *Each of the numbered items or incomplete statements in this section is followed by answers or by completions of the statement. Select the ONE lettered answer or completion that is BEST in each case.*

1. What is used initially to replace fluid deficits in hypotensive patients with hemorrhage caused by hemophilia or von Willebrand's disease?

- A Whole blood
- B Factor VIII
- C Cryoprecipitate
- D Normal saline
- E Packed red blood cells (PRBCs)

2. Which of the following hematologic test results is most reliably present in a patient with mild von Willebrand's disease?

- A Prolonged prothrombin time (PT)
- B Low von Willebrand factor (vWF) antigen
- C Prolonged bleeding time
- D Prolonged thrombin clotting time
- E Prolonged activated partial thromboplastin time (PTT)

3. In which one of the following cases is splenic immune activity likely related to red blood cell (RBC) destruction?

- A A 22-year-old man who does not show the expected response to packed red blood cell (PRBC) transfusion and is found to have received Rh-incompatible blood
- B A 32-year-old woman with sickle cell anemia
- C A 23-year-old woman with acute hemolysis after taking a sulfa drug to treat a urinary tract infection (UTI)
- D A 50-year-old man with syphilis and paroxysmal cold hemoglobinuria
- E A 21-year-old man with thymoma and decreased levels of blood cells derived from erythroid precursors

4. Which one of the following represents a first-line emergency department (ED) therapy for hypercalcemia associated with neoplastic disease?

- A Hemodialysis and mithramycin
- B Intravenous phosphate and glucocorticoids
- C Peritoneal dialysis and oral phosphate
- D Mithramycin and peritoneal dialysis
- E Saline and furosemide

5. Which one of the following represents an appropriate indication for immediate transfusion of the named blood component?

- A A 58-year-old man with a mechanical valve and a hemoglobin level of 8.0 [packed red blood cells (PRBCs)]
- B A 34-year-old woman with von Willebrand's disease (cryoprecipitate)
- C A 23-year-old man with mucosal bleeding and thrombocytopenia caused by antiplatelet antibodies (platelets)

D A 23-year-old trauma patient with loss of 15% of his blood volume (PRBCs)

E An asymptomatic 45-year-old patient with no known hemorrhage and a platelet count of 9000/mm^3 (platelets)

6. Which one of the following bleeding patterns does NOT usually require factor replacement in hemophiliacs with factor levels lower than 30%?

A Intra-articular hemorrhage

B Intramuscular hemorrhage

C Retroperitoneal blood accumulation

D Traumatic lacerations

E Intracranial hemorrhage with stable neurologic examination

7. A patient is diagnosed with a bleeding disorder. The patient has an X-linked recessive disorder that causes factor VIII deficiency, and so this patient has which of the following?

A Hemophilia A

B von Willebrand's disease

C Disseminated intravascular coagulation (DIC)

D Hemophilia B

E Hereditary spherocytosis

8. An 18-year-old male patient presents with diffuse mucosal hemorrhage, gross coagulation profile abnormalities, and purpura fulminans, and is later found to have sepsis caused by *Neisseria meningitides*. Which of the following is the likely cause of the bleeding abnormalities?

A Hereditary spherocytosis

B von Willebrand's disease

C Disseminated intravascular coagulation (DIC)

D Hemophilia D

E Lupus erythematosus

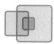

Answers and Explanations

1. The answer is D Although patients with hematologic disease ultimately require specialized replacement therapy, the initial approach to these patients should be the same as for any other patient with acute hemorrhage. Normal saline (or other crystalloid) serves as a temporizing measure while history and laboratory information is obtained.

2. The answer is C Patients with von Willebrand's disease usually have a normal PT and thrombin clotting time. The activated PTT is prolonged only in cases of more severe disease. The vWF antigen and factor VIII activity may be abnormal in patients with von Willebrand's disease, but these findings are variable and are often unavailable in the emergency department (ED).

3. The answer is A The 22-year-old man who received Rh-incompatible blood has extravascular immune hemolysis in the spleen. Such reactions are usually mild and may be asymptomatic. The spleen of the woman with sickle cell anemia has been rendered inactive from repeated infarction long before the age of 32 years. Diseases present in the other patients—such as glucose-6-phosphate dehydrogenase (G6PD) deficiency in the 23-year-old patient who reacted to the sulfa drug, paroxysmal cold hemoglobinuria in the 50-year-old patient, and pure red cell aplasia in the 21-year-old man—are unrelated to splenic activity.

4. The answer is E Saline diuresis represents the first line of therapy in the treatment of patients with oncologic hypercalcemia. Dialysis is reserved for patients in whom saline diuresis fails, and the other therapies (i.e., mithramycin, intravenous phosphate and glucocorticoids, oral phosphate) are effective only after a 1- to 2-day delay.

5. The answer is E Platelet counts below 10,000/mm^3 represent an absolute indication for transfusion to reduce the risk of intracerebral hemorrhage. Platelet administration in the setting of autoimmune disease is unlikely to result in clinical improvement, because transfused platelets are also subject to destruction. Patients with chronic anemia may tolerate hemoglobin levels of 8.0 or lower before requiring transfusion, and trauma patients may lose at least 25%–30% of circulating blood volume before transfusion is mandated to maintain tissue oxygen delivery. Cryoprecipitate therapy is used in patients with von Willebrand's disease only when desmopressin is not sufficient monotherapy, and factor replacement is unavailable.

6. The answer is D Lacerations do not characteristically result in significant bleeding in hemophiliacs, but patients with hemophilia and bleeding in the other regions have potentially serious hemorrhage and require factor replacement to at least 30%–40%.

7. The answer is A Hemophilia A is characterized by factor VIII deficiency. Patients with hereditary spherocytosis have persistent spherocytosis after splenectomy, which simply removes the organ responsible for red blood cell (RBC) destruction in these individuals. Skin and mucosal bleeding (with easy bruising and hematoma formation occurring in up to 40% of patients) characterize von Willebrand's disease, which is treated with desmopressin.

8. The answer is C Purpura fulminans and DIC are characteristic of severe infection with *N. meningitidis.*

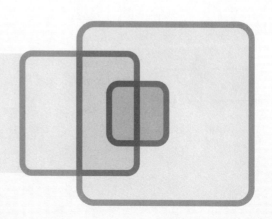

PART **III**

Traumatic Emergencies

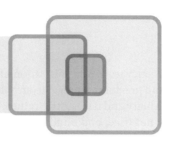

chapter 17

Traumatic Emergencies

JUDITH A. DATTARO

I   **INTRODUCTION**

Trauma is the leading cause of mortality in the first four decades of life. It accounts for approximately 60 million injuries and 9 million disabilities per year. Injuries cost $75–$100 billion annually (including direct healthcare costs as well as indirect costs, such as lost wages).

II   **GENERAL APPROACH TO THE TRAUMA PATIENT**

A **Introduction**   Death from trauma may occur within minutes from injuries such as lacerations of the brain, brain stem, high spinal cord, heart, aorta, or other large vessels. If patients survive the initial minutes after trauma, death may occur within minutes to a few hours of the injury—this is the **"golden hour,"** the time when identification of injuries and resuscitation of patients must take place.

1. Injuries accounting for deaths in this period of time include subdural and epidural hematomas, hemopneumothorax, tension pneumothorax, pericardial tamponade, ruptured spleen, lacerations of the liver, and pelvic fractures.

2. **The goal of immediate trauma care** is to rapidly assess the patient in a systematic fashion, initiate resuscitation and stabilization, establish priorities of care, and begin treatments and diagnostics required in the first hour of emergency care.

B **Patient history**   Whenever possible, an **AMPLE** history (**A**llergies, **M**edications, **P**ast medical history, **L**ast meal, and **E**vents surrounding the injury and its mechanism) should be obtained from the patient and prehospital personnel.

C **Primary survey**   The primary survey—the **"ABCs"** of trauma care—identifies immediately life-threatening conditions. Asking a patient, "How are you?" establishes the patency of the airway, verifies the patient's ability to breathe, and provides information on the patient's neurologic status.

1. **A—airway and cervical spine control.** The patency of the airway is assessed, and the cervical spine is immobilized. The presence of a cervical spine injury should be assumed. A patent airway is established by lifting the patient's chin or thrusting the patient's jaw and by clearing any foreign bodies from the mouth. The patient is intubated, or a cricothyrotomy is performed as indicated.

2. **B—breathing and ventilation.** The chest is inspected, and the quality, depth, and rate of respirations are noted. The patient's chest is auscultated bilaterally for symmetric breath sounds, and the chest is palpated for any deformities. The patient should be placed on a high concentration of oxygen. If identified, a tension pneumothorax requires immediate decompression. Open pneumothoraces should be sealed with a sterile dressing taped on three sides.

3. **C—circulation and hemorrhage control.** Capillary refill, pulses, and the color of the skin should be assessed. Any exsanguinating hemorrhages should be identified. Management includes the placement of two large-bore (14- to 16-gauge) intravenous catheters while blood is obtained for chemistries, hematology, type and cross match, arterial blood gases (ABGs), and possibly

toxicology screens and pregnancy tests. Administration of intravenous fluid (initially, warmed Ringer's lactate) is started, and pressure is applied to any bleeding sites. The patient is connected to a cardiac monitor, and urinary and nasogastric catheters are placed unless contraindicated. Ordinarily, tourniquets are not used, and blind clamping of bleeding sites with hemostats is contraindicated.

4. **D—disability.** A rapid **neurologic assessment** is performed, assessing the **pupils** for size, equality, and reactivity and **level of consciousness** using the **AVPU** scale: **A**lert, response to **V**erbal stimuli, response to **P**ainful stimuli, or **U**nresponsive.

5. **E—exposure.** The patient should be completely undressed.

D **Secondary survey** The secondary survey entails a complete examination of the patient, starting with examination of the head and continuing caudally, examining each region systematically, including assessment of the vital signs. This survey is carried out after completion of the primary survey and after resuscitative measures have been performed.

1. **Head**
   a. The head and face should be inspected for deformities, lacerations, hemorrhages, and other significant injuries. The head is palpated, looking for depressions and abnormal motion.
   b. The eyes are inspected, including reassessment of the pupils. Periorbital ecchymoses (**"raccoon's eyes"**) may indicate a cribriform plate fracture.
   c. The nose is examined for deformity, septal hematoma, rhinorrhea, and bleeding.
   d. The ears should be inspected for the presence of hemotympanum and ecchymosis over the mastoid region of the skull (**Battle's sign**), which may indicate a basal skull fracture.

2. **Cervical spine and neck.** The neck and body should be immobilized as a unit (i.e., with a hard cervical collar and backboard) until the absence of spinal injury has been ensured. The cervical spine should be palpated for tenderness or deformity. The neck should be inspected for injuries, tracheal deviation, distended neck veins, or bruits.

3. **Chest.** The chest should be auscultated again, noting the presence or absence of equal breath sounds and any crepitations. Visual inspection may reveal deformities of the chest wall (e.g., a flail chest, sucking chest wounds, bruising). The ribs, sternum, and clavicles should be palpated, noting tenderness or deformity.
   a. Absence of breath sounds or findings consistent with **tension pneumothorax** (decreased breath sounds, tracheal deviation, distended neck veins, and respiratory distress) require immediate chest decompression.
   b. Beck's triad (decreased blood pressure, decreased heart sounds, and neck vein distention) suggests **pericardial tamponade,** which must be treated with pericardial decompression (e.g., pericardiocentesis, pericardial window, or thoracotomy for open decompression of the pericardial sac).

4. **Abdomen.** The abdomen is inspected for any obvious injuries, distention, and bruising.
   a. The abdomen should be auscultated, then percussed and palpated to search for tenderness and any signs of peritoneal irritation. A repeat evaluation of the abdomen may be required at a later time if the patient's response to pain is altered by alcohol or other drugs, neurologic injury, or pain from a distracting injury.
   b. Focused abdominal sonography is usually indicated at the bedside.
   c. Peritoneal lavage is rarely indicated.

5. **Rectum and perineum**
   a. A rectal examination is performed, noting the presence of blood, sensation, sphincter tone, and the position of the prostate (a high-riding prostate is an indication of urethral disruption).
   b. Perineal examination is performed to search for hematomas or blood at the urinary meatus.
   c. Vaginal examination is performed in women. Blood in the vagina or lacerations should be noted.

6. **Pelvis and extremities**

   a. The pelvis is compressed with both hands in both the anterior-posterior (AP) and lateral directions, assessing for pain, deformity, or instability. The symphysis pubis is palpated. Use of a pneumatic antishock garment should be considered for patients with pelvic fractures.

   b. The extremities are inspected and palpated for deformity, abnormal motion, and any hematomas. Fractures are splinted.

7. **Back.** The patient is log-rolled to maintain spinal immobilization, and the back is inspected and palpated for injuries, bruises, and any deformity, maintaining spinal immobilization as indicated.

8. **Sensory and motor function and level of consciousness.** The neurologic examination is completed, assessing sensory and motor function. The Glasgow coma scale (see Chapter 9, Table 9–1) should be used to assess the level of consciousness. The patient must remain immobilized until spinal cord injury has been ruled out.

E Ongoing care

1. **Re-evaluation.** The patient should be frequently re-evaluated (i.e., by reassessing the ABCs and repeating the secondary survey), particularly if a change in condition is noted.

2. **Oxygenation, perfusion,** and **temperature** must be maintained at all times.

3. **Tetanus prophylaxis** and **antibiotics** are given as indicated.

4. **Arrangement for transfer.** Early contact should be made to arrange for transfer of the patient to a specialized care center (e.g., trauma center, spinal cord center, burn center) as needed.

III TRAUMATIC SHOCK

A Discussion

1. **Definition.** Various definitions of shock exist. Here, shock is defined in terms of its ultimate effect at the cellular level. Shock is the inadequate oxygenation of tissues caused by decreased perfusion (hypoperfusion).

2. **Causes of hypoperfusion.** There are several causes of hypoperfusion, three of which relate to the trauma patient:

   a. **Hypovolemic shock** in the trauma patient is caused by loss of blood volume **secondary to hemorrhage.** In response to a decrease in cardiac output, vasoconstriction occurs, with an initial increase in systemic vascular resistance.

   b. **Cardiogenic shock.** Myocardial dysfunction may be caused by **pericardial tamponade, tension pneumothorax, air embolism, myocardial contusion,** or, in patients with underlying heart disease, **myocardial infarction (MI).**

   c. **Neurogenic shock** may be seen in the patient with **spinal cord injury** with loss of sympathetic tone. Isolated head injuries do not result in neurogenic shock.

B Clinical features

1. **Hypovolemic shock.** In adults, the blood volume is estimated to be 7% of the body weight in kilograms (i.e., approximately 5 L in a 70-kg person), and in children, it is estimated to be approximately 8%–9% of the body weight, or approximately 80 mL/kg. Hemorrhage is classified according to the following Advanced Trauma Life Support (ATLS) guidelines:

   a. **Class I hemorrhage (loss of up to 15% of blood volume).** With this degree of volume loss, minimal tachycardia may occur, and no changes in blood pressure, pulse pressure, or respiratory rate are expected. Capillary refill time is less than 2 seconds.

   b. **Class II hemorrhage (loss of 15%–30% of blood volume; approximately 800–1500 mL of blood in a 70-kg person).** Signs include increased heart rate, tachypnea, anxiety, increased capillary refill time, and a **narrowed pulse pressure** (due to a rise in diastolic pressure). Urine output is maintained at 20–30 mL/hour.

    c. **Class III hemorrhage (loss of 30%–40% of blood volume—approximately 2000 mL in a 70-kg person).** Signs include marked tachycardia and tachypnea, longer than 2-second capillary refill, altered sensorium, and a **decline in systolic blood pressure.**

    d. **Class IV hemorrhage (loss of more than 40% blood volume).** Signs include significant tachycardia; marked decrease in blood pressure; negligible urine output; decreased level of consciousness; cold, clammy skin; and the appearance of **frank shock.** Loss of consciousness, blood pressure, and pulse is seen with losses that exceed 50% of the blood volume.

2. **Cardiogenic shock** should be suspected in patients with chest trauma.

3. **Neurogenic shock.** Signs include hypotension without tachycardia or vasoconstriction of the skin.

C **Differential diagnoses**   The majority of trauma patients in shock are in hypovolemic shock, and fluid resuscitation should be carried out. The patient must be carefully assessed to rule out tension pneumothorax, pericardial tamponade, or neurogenic shock. Emergency department (ED) physicians should consider what may have caused the trauma, especially in a patient in extremis with minimal evidence of injury.

1. **Precipitating factors.** MI, drug overdose, massive stroke, or pulmonary embolism experienced while driving may precipitate a motor vehicle collision that results in trauma.

2. **Medications.** Several medications (e.g., calcium channel blockers, β blockers) may alter the patient's sympathetic response.

3. **Drugs.** Agitation, although it may be an early sign of hypoperfusion, may also be caused by alcohol or other ingested drugs.

4. **Metabolic derangements** (e.g., diabetic ketoacidosis, adrenal crisis) and **hypothermia** may also be factors.

D **Evaluation**

1. **Physical examination.** Early recognition of shock is critical. During the primary and secondary survey, the following should be noted:
    a. Vital signs, including the temperature
    b. Capillary refill time
    c. Sites of obvious hemorrhage
    d. Presence of Beck's triad (hypotension, neck vein distention, and distant heart tones), which is indicative of pericardial tamponade
    e. Urine output (normal is approximately 30 mL/hour in an adult or 1 mL/kg/hour in a pediatric patient)

2. **Laboratory studies.** An ABG determination, to monitor the degree of acidosis as well as the adequacy of ventilation and oxygenation, should be obtained.

E **Treatment**

1. **Initial treatment** in all trauma patients includes establishment of an airway, adequate ventilation, administration of oxygen, and control of hemorrhage with direct pressure to bleeding sites. A pneumatic antishock garment may be applied in the presence of unstable pelvic fractures to control hemorrhage, but is contraindicated in the presence of pulmonary edema and rupture of the diaphragm. Use of a pneumatic antishock garment is relatively contraindicated in the presence of major thoracic injury.

2. **Fluid resuscitation**
    a. **Intravenous fluids.** Initial fluid resuscitation in an adult is with 1–2 L of lactated Ringer's solution. In a child, 20 mL/kg of crystalloid should be infused as a bolus and may be repeated once.

b. **Blood transfusion.** Ideally, blood should be fully typed and cross matched. In a severely hemorrhaging patient, type-specific blood may be given, or O-negative blood may be given if no typed blood is available.

(1) In an adult patient who fails to respond to approximately 2500 mL of crystalloid infusion, blood should be transfused. The amount of blood required is variable and depends on the patient's clinical response.

(2) In a child, the initial transfusion is 10 mL/kg of packed red blood cells (PRBCs).

3. **Early surgical intervention** should be considered for patients who fail to respond to fluid resuscitation.

4. **Frequent re-evaluation** of the patient is required to determine the response to therapy and stability.

F **Disposition**   Patients who present in shock should be admitted to an intensive care unit (ICU), transferred to the operating room, or transferred to a facility that can provide a higher level care if the initial stabilizing facility cannot provide the specialized care required.

IV   HEAD INJURIES

A **Discussion**   Head injuries may involve the scalp, skull, or underlying brain and blood vessels. Injuries may be focal, such as an intracranial bleed, or diffuse.

1. **Mortality rates.** Head injury is associated with **approximately 50% of trauma deaths,** with the mortality rate approaching 35% in patients with severe head injuries. In patients with severe head injuries, the initial score on the Glasgow coma scale and the type of lesion responsible for the neurologic deficits are good indicators of outcome.

2. **Pathology**

a. **Unconsciousness** may be induced by either bilateral cerebral cortical injury or injury to the reticular activating system.

b. **Increased intracranial pressure (ICP)** results from increased intracranial volume either from a mass (such as a hematoma) or edema, and may be the final result of many different head injuries. It can lead to altered level of consciousness, coma, hypertension, bradycardia (Cushing's phenomenon), and, finally, death.

(1) **Herniation syndromes** can result from focal or diffuse increases in ICP.

(a) **Subfalcial herniation** results from one cerebral hemisphere protruding beneath the falx cerebri into the opposite supratentorial space.

(b) **Uncal herniation** occurs when increased ICP causes the uncus of the temporal lobe to protrude through the opening of the tentorium between the cerebral peduncle and the tentorium. This causes compression of the ipsilateral third cranial nerve, the ipsilateral corticospinal tract within the cerebral peduncle, and the brain stem, leading to clinical signs of an ipsilateral fixed, dilated pupil; contralateral hemiparesis; and deteriorating level of consciousness. An uncal herniation is a true neurosurgical emergency.

(c) **Cerebellar tonsillar herniation** through the foramen causes compression of the medulla with bradycardia, slowing of the respirations, and death.

(2) **Cerebral perfusion pressure derangements.** The cerebral perfusion pressure is the mean arterial pressure minus the ICP. Autoregulation of cerebral blood flow may be lost either focally or globally if the ICP remains persistently high.

B **Clinical features**

1. **Diffuse brain injuries** include concussion and diffuse axonal injuries.

a. **Concussion** is defined as a transient loss of consciousness or other neurologic function that lasts for a few seconds or minutes (and occasionally longer) and occurs immediately after blunt head trauma. Concussions are caused by impairment of the reticular activating system, and there are typically no permanent sequelae. However, postconcussive syndrome, consisting of headache, decreased memory and attention, insomnia, and dizziness, may persist.

   b. **Diffuse axonal injury** is secondary to shearing or tearing of nerve fibers and is characterized by coma in the absence of a focal lesion. The mortality rate ranges from 35%–50%, and autonomic dysfunction (i.e., increased blood pressure, increased temperature, sweating) may be seen.

2. **Focal lesions** include subarachnoid hemorrhage, epidural hemorrhage, subdural hematoma, penetrating head injuries (e.g., gunshot wounds, impalement injuries), skull fractures, scalp lacerations, and brain contusions.

   a. **Subarachnoid hemorrhage** (Figure 17–1A) is the most common site of bleeding after head trauma. It results in bloody cerebrospinal fluid (CSF). The patient may complain of headache and photophobia.

   b. **Subdural hematoma** (Figure 17–1B) accounts for approximately 30% of severe head injuries. It is a collection of blood lying between the dura and the arachnoid mater. A subdural hematoma usually results from tearing of the bridging veins traversing the subdural space. There may be neurologic deficit both from mass effect from the hematoma and from contusion to the underlying brain.

   c. **Epidural hemorrhage** (Figure 17–1C) accounts for approximately 1% of head injuries. It results from tearing of a dural artery (usually the middle meningeal artery).

      (1) Epidural hemorrhage should be suspected in patients with skull fractures involving the temporal bone where the middle meningeal artery passes between the dura and the skull.

      (2) It is classically characterized by a brief initial period of unconsciousness, a lucid interval lasting minutes to hours, and subsequent deterioration in neurologic status secondary to increasing ICP.

   d. **Penetrating head injury** is usually obvious in its presentation and is associated with a high mortality rate. Radiographs can help to identify the degree of penetration and path of the object. Any impaled object should be left in place until surgical removal can be accomplished.

   e. **Skull fractures** may be either open or closed. Linear fractures do not displace bone edges. Depressed skull fractures may require surgical elevation.

   f. **Scalp lacerations** may cause significant bleeding and may be a source of shock in children.

C **Differential diagnosis** Causes of altered level of consciousness after head injury that must be ruled out include hypoglycemia, hypoxia, hypotension, hypothermia, alcohol and other drugs, electrolyte abnormalities, and metabolic abnormalities. It is helpful to ascertain the patient's baseline mental status, if possible.

D **Evaluation**

1. **Physical examination**

   a. **Primary survey.** All trauma patients should have their ABCs evaluated initially, as outlined in II C.

      (1) Pupillary size and reactivity should be evaluated, and baseline mental status should be documented.

      (2) An odor of alcohol on the breath should be noted, if present.

      (3) The cervical spine must be evaluated for injury in patients with head injury because approximately 10% of patients with severe head injury have an associated cervical spine injury. If the absence of spinal injury cannot be assured (e.g., because of altered mental status in the patient), the hard cervical collar must remain in place.

   b. **Secondary survey**

      (1) **Head examination.** The head should be examined, noting the presence of depressed skull fractures, open skull fractures, otorrhea, or rhinorrhea (CSF leaking from the ears or nose). The tympanic membranes should be evaluated for hemotympanum, the eyes should be

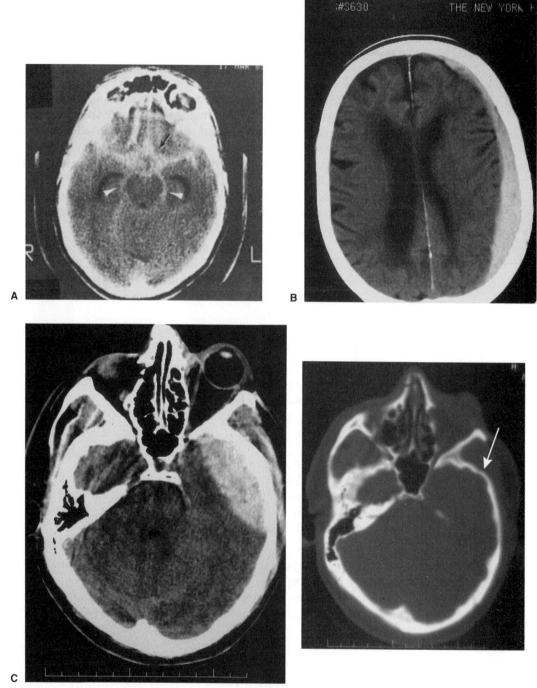

FIGURE 17–1 **(A)** Traumatic subarachnoid hemorrhage at the base (*black arrow*). The *white arrows* outline blood in the ambient cisterns around the brain stem. The patient complained only of headache, and nuchal rigidity was the single abnormality on neurologic examination. **(B)** Left-sided subdural hematoma. **(C)** A left-sided epidural hematoma is seen as a biconvex hyperdensity (*whiteness*) on a computed tomography (CT) scan. The adjacent CT scan shows the bony windows (*arrow*) associated with the fracture causing the underlying epidural hematoma. (Part A is reprinted with permission from Schwartz GR, Bouzarth WF, Goldman HW. Management of head injuries. In: Schwartz GR, Cayten CG, Mangelsen MA, et al. *Principles and Practice of Emergency Medicine.* 3rd Ed. Baltimore: Williams & Wilkins, 1992:948. Parts B and C are compliments of Irina Iordanescu, M.D., and Judith Dattaro, M.D.)

inspected for periorbital hematomas ("raccoon's eyes"), and the mastoid area should be inspected for ecchymosis (Battle's sign), all of which may indicate basilar skull fracture.

(2) **Neurologic examination**

   (a) A complete neurologic examination should be performed, noting lateralizing signs, altered pupils, or deteriorating mental status. After the initial examination, neurologic assessments should be performed at frequent intervals to search for changes from the initial examination.

   (b) The Glasgow coma scale evaluates the level of consciousness in a quantitative manner, noting eye opening response, verbal response, and best motor response. Coma is defined as a Glasgow coma scale score of less than 8, whereby a patient has no word verbal response, no eye opening, and no ability to follow motor commands (see Chapter 9, Table 9–1).

(3) **Vital signs** should be closely assessed, especially noting hypertension in the setting of bradycardia (Cushing's phenomenon).

2. **Diagnostic imaging studies**

   a. **CT.** A head CT scan should be performed on patients who have loss of consciousness or amnesia, altered mental status, abnormal neurologic examination findings, or seizures. A head CT scan should be considered for those with a questionable mechanism of injury who may not be available for a follow-up examination (e.g., patients going to the operating room for treatment of other traumatic injuries).

   b. **Skull radiographs** should be performed on patients with a penetrating head injury or a possible depressed skull fracture (if a head CT scan is not clearly indicated).

3. **Laboratory studies** should include an initial glucose level and oxygen saturation level to rule out these factors contributing to altered mental status. Other laboratory tests to consider, depending on the degree of injury, include ABG determinations, a serum electrolyte panel, an alcohol and toxicology screen, and coagulation studies.

E **Treatment**

1. **Initial stabilization.** The ABCs must be ensured.

   a. **Fluid resuscitation.** If a patient with a head injury is hypotensive, volume resuscitation must be initiated first. Intravenous fluids must be adequate to maintain blood pressure while avoiding overhydration if increased ICP is suspected.

   b. **Adequate oxygen and glucose levels** must be maintained.

2. **Lowering the ICP**

   a. **Hyperventilation.** If the patient's Glasgow coma scale score is lower than 8, intubation should be considered. Hyperventilating a patient to a partial pressure of carbon dioxide (P_{CO_2}) of approximately 25–30 mm Hg causes cerebral vasoconstriction and helps decrease the ICP. Prolonged and aggressive hyperventilation should be avoided if possible because of decreased cerebral perfusion.

   b. **Additional treatments** for increased ICP may include elevation of the head of the bed, sedating the patient, and administration of mannitol (20% solution at 1 g/kg) and furosemide.

3. **Treatment of seizures.** Seizures are usually treated with **phenytoin** (1 g infused at 50 mg/min for adults; approximately 15 mg/kg at 0.5–1 mg/kg/min, not to exceed 50 mg/min for children) **with or without benzodiazepines.**

4. **Treatment of scalp wounds.** Scalp wounds should be copiously irrigated. Pressure should be applied to control bleeding (which can be extensive), and the wound should be closed in a single layer with sutures or staples.

5. **Emergent neurosurgical consultation** should be sought for patients with lateralizing signs, large focal mass lesions, or any signs of herniation. Evacuation of hematomas, placement of bur

holes, or a ventriculostomy may be required. Subarachnoid hemorrhage of traumatic origin does not usually require intervention other than admission for observation.

F Disposition

1. **Discharge.** Patients with minor head injury, defined as a Glasgow coma score of 15, normal mental status, and no loss of consciousness, may be discharged home. Head injury instructions should be reviewed with the patient and a family member, spouse, or friend. The patient and caretaker should be advised to watch for persistent headache, vomiting, dizziness, alterations in mental status, or other signs of deteriorating neurologic function.

2. **Admission.** Patients with loss of consciousness or unreliable follow-up should generally be admitted to the hospital for 24-hour observation. Patients with severe head injury require admission to an ICU.

V SPINAL INJURIES

A Discussion Spinal injuries may be blunt or penetrating and involve either the bony elements of the spinal column or the spinal cord. Bony injuries and cord injuries may exist independently of each other. Motor vehicle collisions account for the largest number of spinal cord injuries, followed by falls, firearm injuries, and recreational injuries. Approximately 10% of patients with head or facial injuries have associated cervical spine injuries.

B Clinical features

1. **Complete cord injuries** involve total loss of motor and sensory function below the lesion. It is important to check for any areas of sparing of cord function (e.g., sacral sensation, rectal tone).

2. **Incomplete cord injuries** carry a better prognosis than complete injuries for some recovery of function. Most can be classified in one of the three following clinical syndromes:
   a. **Anterior cord syndrome** usually follows a cervical flexion injury that compresses the anterior spinal cord or injures the anterior spinal artery. Motor paralysis, decreased sensation (including loss of pain and temperature sensation), and preservation of posterior column function (e.g., position sense, light touch, vibratory sensation) distal to the trauma characterize this lesion.
   b. **Brown-Séquard syndrome,** or hemisection of the cord, is usually the result of penetrating injuries or lateral mass fractures. It presents as paralysis and loss of gross proprioception and vibration on the same side as the lesion and as loss of pain and temperature sense on the contralateral side.
   c. **Central cord syndrome** is most commonly vascular in origin. It may follow a hyperextension injury, most often in patients with degenerative arthritis of the cervical spine. The ligamentum flavum buckles into the cord, resulting in a concussion of the most central portions of the cord (the gray matter and the most central portions of the pyramidal and spinothalamic tracts). Neurologic deficits of the upper extremities are greater than those of the lower extremities, and scattered sensory losses are seen.

3. **Spinal shock** is the immediate neurologic condition seen after spinal cord injury, and it is characterized by flaccidity and areflexia. As spinal shock resolves (days to weeks), function may return or spasticity replaces the flaccidity initially present.

4. **Neurogenic shock** is associated with cervical or high thoracic injuries causing impairment of the descending sympathetic pathways. It is characterized by hypotension (due to loss of vasomotor tone) and bradycardia (secondary to unopposed vagal tone to the heart). Other causes of hypotension must be ruled out in the trauma patient, but the presence of bradycardia and warm, well-perfused skin in the hypotensive patient are clues.

5. **Cervical spine fractures** may result from flexion, axial loading (vertical compression), extension, rotation, or distraction.

   a. **C1 fracture (atlas fracture, Jefferson fracture)** occurs secondary to vertical compression forces directed from the occipital condyles downward toward the superior articular surfaces of the lateral masses of the atlas, resulting in a "blowout" of the ring of C1. C1 fractures are unstable and are often associated with C2 fractures. On a lateral radiograph, they may be seen as widening of the predental space (to greater than 3 mm in an adult or 5 mm in a child). On an odontoid (open mouth) view, the lateral masses of C1 lie lateral to the articular surfaces of C2.

   b. **C2 (axis) injury** may involve dislocation or fractures.

      (1) **Posterior dislocation** of the dens (odontoid) onto the spinal cord may occur if there is injury to the transverse ligament that attaches the dens to C1. Immobilization must be maintained to prevent cord injury.

      (2) **Rotary subluxation injury** of the odontoid may be seen as asymmetry of the lateral masses on the odontoid view.

      (3) **Fractures** at the base of the odontoid are usually unstable. A fracture of the posterior elements of C2 resulting from extension and distraction or extension and axial compression forces (**hangman's fracture**) is unstable.

   c. **C3 through C7 fractures** may occur secondary to flexion, axial loading, extension, rotation, or distraction. The alignment of the vertebral bodies and spinous processes must be assessed radiographically. Increases in the soft tissue spaces of the neck, which suggests hematoma, may also be visible on radiographs.

   d. **Thoracic spine fractures** are usually caused by hyperflexion, leading to wedge compression of the vertebral body. Most of these fractures are stable because of the stabilizing nature of the remainder of the bony thorax. However, because of the narrow space in the thoracic spinal canal, thoracic cord injuries are often complete.

   e. **Thoracolumbar fractures** most often occur secondary to hyperflexion and rotation, in which the lumbar spine is relatively mobile compared to the thoracic spine. These fractures are often unstable. The spinal cord terminates at the level of L2, where the nerve roots of the cauda equina arise. The patient must be assessed for bowel and bladder signs as well as neurologic deficit in the lower extremities.

C **Differential diagnoses**   Spinal shock may mimic a complete cord injury. Assessment of tendon reflexes must be evaluated in light of any local muscle or tendon trauma.

D **Evaluation**

1. **Patient history.** A history of a mechanism of injury involving a fall from a height, high-speed motor vehicle collision, an electrical injury, or a diving accident mandates evaluation for possible spinal injury. No patient who is unconscious, is intoxicated, or has a significant distracting injury can be clinically cleared when a possibility of spinal injury exists.

2. **Physical examination**

   a. **Primary survey.** The ABCs must be evaluated initially in all trauma patients. In patients with lower cervical and upper thoracic spinal cord injuries, hypoventilation may be seen secondary to paralysis of the intercostal muscles. Injury to spinal cord segments C3 through C5 may lead to phrenic nerve damage and subsequent diaphragmatic paralysis.

   b. **Secondary survey**

      (1) **Palpation of the spine.** The spine should be palpated, while the patient is kept immobilized, to assess for tenderness or deformity of the spine. A patient who has a normal mental status and who has no complaint of pain, no neurologic deficit, no tenderness on examination, and no distracting pain may be clinically cleared.

      (2) **Neurologic examination.** A complete assessment of neurologic function, including motor strength and tone, sensory examination, presence of reflexes, and evaluation of autonomic dysfunction (looking for loss of rectal sphincter tone, urinary retention, gastric distention, ileus, or priapism), is required to determine injury and to establish the patient's baseline.

3. **Diagnostic imaging studies**
    a. **Radiography.** A radiographic evaluation of the cervical spine should be completed in patients with suspected cervical spine injury. Radiographs should be evaluated for alignment of contour lines (Figure 17–2); soft tissue swelling, which suggests hematoma; increases in the predental space; abnormal angulation; and subluxation.

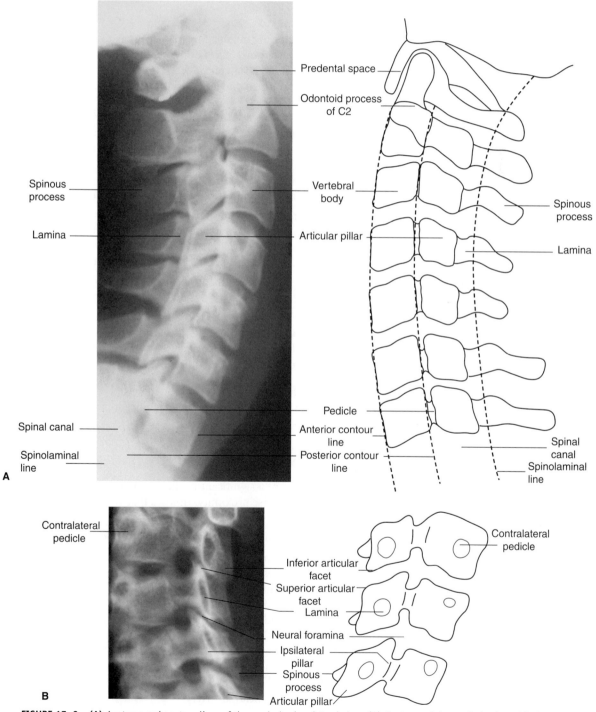

FIGURE 17–2 **(A)** Anatomy and contour lines of the cervical spine, lateral view. **(B)** Anatomy of the cervical spine, oblique view.

(1) A **cross-table lateral radiograph** of the cervical spine should be obtained first. Up to 15% of injuries can be missed if this is the only film obtained. All seven vertebrae must be visualized.

(2) The standard **"three-view" series** consists of:

    (a) A **swimmer's view** (with the arm raised), which may help to visualize the lower cervical vertebrae

    (b) An **open-mouth (odontoid) view,** obtained to evaluate the dens and the lateral masses of the atlas

    (c) An **AP view** of the cervical spine

(3) **Oblique views** of the cervical spine are obtained by many centers to better evaluate the posterior elements, including the laminae, facets, and pedicles. These views should be done to confirm subluxation seen on the lateral view.

(4) **Flexion and extension views,** performed under physician supervision, may be needed to rule out ligamentous injury.

b. **CT.** A CT scan of the cervical spine may be needed to further evaluate any possible fractures to assess the cervical canal, or to visualize vertebrae not seen on a plain film radiograph.

c. **Additional studies** may include **magnetic resonance imaging (MRI)** and **tomography.**

E Treatment

1. **Spinal immobilization** should be maintained until spinal injury has been ruled out.

2. **Airway management** should be accomplished without manipulating the cervical spine. In-line traction should be maintained by an assistant. In a spontaneously breathing patient, nasotracheal intubation can be attempted if there is not significant facial injury. Cricothyrotomy should be performed if an airway cannot be rapidly and safely secured by any other route.

3. **High-dose methylprednisolone** is used in the treatment of spinal cord injury caused by blunt trauma. The patient should receive a loading dose of 30 mg/kg over 15 minutes followed by a continuous infusion of 5.4 mg/kg/hour for the next 23 hours.

4. **Neurosurgical consultation** should be obtained for patients with known or suspected spinal cord injuries, as well as for any unstable spinal fractures. Traction with Gardner-Wells tongs or surgical decompression of a spinal cord injury may be required.

F Disposition Any patient with significant spinal injury should be managed at a regional trauma center or spinal cord center. Patients with unstable spinal injuries, significant pain, or ileus must be admitted to the hospital.

VI PENETRATING AND BLUNT NECK TRAUMA

A Discussion Injuries to the neck can present a significant challenge in emergency management because of the number of vital structures in close proximity. Injuries that violate the platysma are considered penetrating neck injuries.

1. **Zones.** For the purposes of injury management, the neck is divided into zones (Figure 17–3).

2. **Triangles.** The neck is also divided into triangles.

a. The **anterior triangle** is above the clavicles, anterior to the posterior border of the sternocleidomastoid muscle, and is covered by the platysma. It overlies the submandibular gland, part of the thyroid gland, nervous structures (including the cervical branch of the facial nerve, the glossopharyngeal nerve, the vagus nerve, and the sympathetic chain ganglia), vascular structures (including the external and internal carotids and the internal jugular vein), the larynx, the trachea, and the esophagus.

b. The **posterior triangle** is bordered by the sternocleidomastoid muscle, the clavicle, and the trapezius. It overlies vital structures at its base, including the spinal accessory nerve, the brachial plexus, and the proximal portion of the subclavian artery.

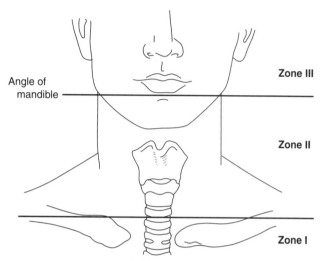

FIGURE 17–3 Zones of the neck. Zone I is the thoracic inlet and lies below the head of the clavicles (or below the cricoid cartilage by some definitions). Zone II extends from above the clavicles to the angle of the mandible. Zone III is the area above the angle of the mandible.

B **Clinical features**   Categories of neck injuries include:

1. **Laryngotracheal (airway) injuries** may be caused by direct blunt trauma, sudden acceleration or deceleration forces, increased intratracheal pressure against a closed glottis, or penetrating injuries. They may include fracture of the thyroid cartilage, disruption of the arytenoid cartilage, dislocation of the cricothyroid joint, and thyrotracheal separation, all of which result in airway compromise. Signs include dyspnea, stridor, hemoptysis, dysphonia, subcutaneous emphysema, and pain.

2. **Pharyngoesophageal injuries** may also be secondary to either penetrating or blunt trauma. Perforation of the esophagus may be particularly devastating, because it can lead rapidly to mediastinitis and high mortality if there is delay in diagnosis. Findings include pain, drooling, bleeding, and crepitus.

3. **Vascular injuries** may result from direct blunt trauma, stretching of the vessels, basilar skull fractures, or penetrating injuries. Hematomas, bruits, or obvious bleeding may be observed. Complications include airway compromise secondary to bleeding or expanding hematoma, hemorrhage, air embolus, and thrombus formation in the carotid arteries, which can lead to cerebral ischemia and neurologic deficits. Vertebral artery injuries are seen less frequently because these vessels are relatively well protected, but they should be suspected with injuries to the posterior neck.

4. **Neurologic injuries** include injuries to the brachial plexus, cervical plexus, and the glossopharyngeal, vagus, spinal accessory, and hypoglossal nerves. Regional motor and sensory deficits may be seen, and Horner's syndrome (i.e., ptosis, miosis, and anhydrosis) is seen with injury to the cervical sympathetic chain.

5. **Soft tissue injuries** include injury to muscle (most commonly), as well as to the thyroid, parathyroid, and salivary glands.

C **Differential diagnosis**   Assessing neurologic injuries may be difficult in patients who are intoxicated or in shock. Arterial bleeding and brisk venous bleeding may appear similar, and sources of respiratory difficulty (e.g., from expanding hematoma or direct tracheal injury) may not be readily known. Controlling the bleeding and maintaining an airway are the key issues in immediate emergency management. The specific diagnosis may not be known until operative or diagnostic procedures are completed.

D **Evaluation**

1. **Primary survey and initial stabilization.** As with all trauma patients, the standard ATLS ABCs must be addressed first, with airway control presenting a particular challenge in patients with neck trauma.

   a. **Airway control.** The patient should be assessed, noting blood in the airway, intraoral penetration, stridor, dysphonia, dysphagia, odynophagia, hemoptysis, hoarseness, drooling, tracheal deviation, crepitus, tenderness, and any thrills or bruits. **Early airway control with intubation needs to be considered** in every patient with neck injury before an elective airway becomes a difficult emergency airway obscured by blood and edema—initially stable airways may quickly become compromised as blood and air accumulate in the neck. Unnecessary manipulation of the airway, however, should be avoided because of the possibility of activating hemorrhage from previously clotted injuries.

   b. **Bleeding control.** Bleeding should be assessed, and bleeding sites should be **controlled with direct pressure.** Expanding hematomas, bruits, and perfusion status (capillary refill and blood pressure) should be evaluated.

   c. **Extent of wound.** It should be determined whether the wound has penetrated the platysma, and the bony structures should be evaluated. Wounds should not be probed, because probing may disrupt a clot and precipitate hemorrhage or air embolus in vascular injuries.

2. **Physical examination.** The cervical spine should be evaluated in patients with a **blunt neck injury.** Patients with blunt trauma to anterior neck structures should be observed for edema, hematomas, and other signs (see VI D 1 a). A **complete neurologic examination** is necessary to assess for brachial plexus, cranial nerve, and cervical sympathetic nerve (Horner's) injury.

3. **Diagnostic imaging studies**

   a. **Radiography**

      (1) **Cervical spine radiographs** should be obtained if a potential for cervical spine injury exists.

      (2) A **soft tissue neck radiograph** is indicated for locating foreign bodies (e.g., bullets, depth of knife blade) and for aiding the evaluation of edema and air in the soft tissues.

      (3) A **chest radiograph** is indicated to evaluate for pneumothorax or hemothorax in patients with zone I injuries.

   b. **Angiography and esophagography**

      (1) **Zone I injuries.** Patients require an emergent angiogram to evaluate the aorta and the innominate, carotid, and subclavian vasculature, as well as to help determine an operative approach. The patient also requires evaluation of the esophagus with esophagography (with Gastrografin, which is less irritating to the tissues if leakage should occur) and esophagoscopy. Diagnostic evaluation of the trachea should be considered.

      (2) **Zone II injuries.** Patients are usually taken to the operating room for exploratory neck surgery. If this is not done, an angiogram and an esophagogram should be obtained, esophagoscopy should be performed, and study of the trachea may be necessary.

      (3) **Zone III injuries.** Patients require an angiogram and careful inspection of the oropharynx.

      (4) **Vertebral artery injuries.** A vertebral artery angiogram should be obtained if penetrating trauma has occurred near these vessels.

   c. **CT.** A CT scan should be performed to evaluate laryngotracheal injuries in stable patients.

E **Treatment**

1. **Airway control.** Blind nasotracheal intubation should be avoided if massive facial trauma exists or if the patient is apneic. Orotracheal intubation should be accomplished without moving the cervical spine if possible spinal injury has occurred. Cricothyrotomy may be the procedure of choice, but caution must be exercised if there is a possibility of laryngotracheal separation. Surgical airway intervention may separate the trachea, causing it to retract into the mediastinum. Supplemental oxygen should always be administered to trauma patients.

2. **Immobilization of the neck.** If a cervical spine injury cannot be ruled out, the neck should be immobilized.

3. **Bleeding control**
   a. **Direct pressure** is used to control bleeding.
   b. **Occlusive dressings** should be maintained over major bleeding sites to avoid **air embolus.** If a stable patient suddenly becomes tachypneic, tachycardic, and hypotensive, an air embolus must be considered. A "machinery murmur" may be auscultated. The patient should be placed in the Trendelenburg position in the left lateral decubitus position and, if there is no improvement, aspiration of the right ventricle to remove air should be accomplished.

4. **Establishing intravenous access.** Placement of central lines in proximity to an injury should be avoided if there is a possibility of vascular disruption. Intravenous access should be accomplished below the diaphragm if injury to the subclavian vessels is suspected.

5. **Treatment of pneumothoraces and hemothoraces.** Pneumothoraces and hemothoraces are treated with **thoracostomy tubes.** If tension pneumothorax exists, emergent needle thoracostomy with a 14-gauge angiocatheter at the second intercostal space, on the side contralateral to tracheal deviation, should be performed (pending chest tube placement).

6. **Wound repair.** Wounds superficial to the platysma should be irrigated and repaired in the standard fashion, with tetanus prophylaxis given as indicated. To avoid increased risk of infection, stab wounds should not be sutured closed.

[F] Disposition Patients with superficial wounds and no evidence of cervical spine injury may be discharged. All other patients should be admitted for diagnostic studies, observation, or operative intervention.

VII THORACIC TRAUMA

[A] Discussion Chest injuries account for 25% of trauma deaths. Approximately 15% of traumatic chest injuries require operative intervention; the remaining 85% can be managed in the ED. Chest injuries may be either penetrating or blunt injuries, and the mechanism of injury determines the work-up and intervention.

1. **Anatomy.** The chest is defined as the area within the rib cage. The chest is further divided into the following compartments:
   a. The **cardiac (anterior) box** has the following borders: the sternomanubrial angle superiorly and the lower ribs inferiorly (including the epigastric area) measured at the midclavicular lines. Penetrating injuries within these margins are at risk of involving the heart.
   b. The **thoracoabdominal area** is bounded superiorly by the nipples anteriorly and the tips of the scapulae posteriorly. The inferior margins are formed by the inferior costal margins. Trauma in this area is at risk of causing injury to the diaphragm, as well as the liver and spleen.
   c. The **posterior box** is formed by the medial borders of the scapulae and the inferior costal margins. Posterior mediastinal structures, including the esophagus, the aorta, and the trachea, are at risk of injury in this area.

2. **Immediate life threats in thoracic injury** include tension pneumothorax, open pneumothorax, flail chest, massive hemothorax, and obstructed airway. Other life-threatening injuries include aortic disruption (80%–90% of patients die immediately at the scene), pulmonary contusion, myocardial contusion, rupture of the diaphragm, esophageal disruption, and tracheobronchial disruption.

3. **Other possible injuries** include chest-wall injuries (e.g., rib fractures, clavicle fractures, sternal fractures, and soft tissue injuries), other great vessel injuries, aspiration of gastric contents, esophageal injuries, and thoracic duct injuries.

B Clinical features

1. **Simple pneumothorax** is a collection of air in the pleural space that does not communicate with the external chest wall. Findings include decreased breath sounds and hyperresonance on the affected side, dyspnea, and chest pain. Chest-wall injury may or may not be present.

2. **Open pneumothorax.** "Sucking chest wounds" are in communication with a defect in the chest wall. If the wound is greater than two thirds of the diameter of the trachea, air may enter the chest through the wound rather than through the normal airway, causing collapse of the ipsilateral lung on inspiration and severe ventilatory defects.

3. **Tension pneumothorax** is an accumulation of air under pressure in the pleural space in which the injury acts like a one-way valve, allowing air to enter the pleural space but not to exit from it, causing collapse of the ipsilateral lung. Increased intrapleural pressure leads to mediastinal shift and compression of the contralateral lung and great vessels, resulting in deceased cardiac filling, decreased cardiac output, and severe respiratory compromise. Findings may include dyspnea, agitation, cyanosis, tachypnea, air hunger, subcutaneous emphysema, hypotension, tachycardia, increased jugular venous pressure, decreased breath sounds, hyperresonance, tracheal shift to the uninvolved side, and increased resistance to ventilation. Tension pneumothorax is a clinical diagnosis that requires immediate decompression (physicians should not wait for a confirmatory radiograph).

4. **Hemothorax** occurs when there is blood found in the chest cavity. It may be secondary to lung injury or bleeding from intercostal or internal mammary vessels. **Massive hemothorax** is defined as blood loss of greater than 1500 mL into the chest cavity. Decreased breath sounds or dullness may be found on the affected side. Blunting of the costophrenic angles generally is not seen on an upright chest radiograph until approximately 250 mL of blood has been lost.

5. **Flail chest** occurs when a segment of the chest wall does not move in continuity with the rest of the chest because of three or more adjacent ribs with fractures at two points. There is paradoxic inward motion of the flail segment with inspiration and outward movement on expiration. Crepitus and abnormal chest-wall motion may be present. If the patient is splinting secondary to pain, a flail chest may not be initially appreciated. Underlying pulmonary contusion is a major cause of respiratory compromise.

6. **Pulmonary contusion** results in parenchymal lung damage with interstitial edema and capillary damage. Patients may present with dyspnea, tachypnea, tachycardia, chest-wall bruising, hypoxia, and an increased arterial–alveolar (A-a) gradient on blood gases. Opacifications may be seen immediately on chest radiograph and always within 6 hours. If opacifications persist on the chest radiograph for longer than 48 hours, **pulmonary laceration** should be suspected.

7. **Tracheobronchial injuries** may be caused by penetrating or blunt injury. Labored or noisy breathing, subcutaneous emphysema, and hemoptysis may be seen. Most injuries from blunt trauma to a major bronchus occur within 2.5 cm of the carina as a result of a deceleration mechanism, leading to tearing of the mainstem bronchus. Persistence of a large air leak or pneumothorax after placement of a chest tube for pneumothorax should raise the suspicion for a major bronchial tear. Tears of the trachea or bronchi outside of the pleura allow air to escape into the mediastinum and soft tissues of the neck. Pneumomediastinum may be seen on the chest radiograph.

8. **Esophageal trauma** is seen most often after penetrating injury. It should also be suspected after blunt trauma to the upper abdomen or lower sternum accompanied by forceful emptying of gastric contents into the esophagus, which can lead to an esophageal tear with mediastinal leak and subsequent mediastinitis. The patient may have severe pain. Pneumomediastinum may be seen on the chest radiograph. Delay in diagnosis can lead to significant morbidity and increased mortality.

9. **Cardiac contusion** should be suspected if a patient has sustained blunt trauma to the chest. The patient may complain of chest-wall or retrosternal pain. Various atrial and ventricular dys-

rhythmias, conduction disturbances, altered cardiac wall motion, and decreased cardiac output may be present. The electrocardiogram (ECG) may be normal, and the most commonly encountered rhythm is sinus tachycardia. There is considerable controversy about the optimal work-up and diagnosis of cardiac contusions. ECGs, cardiac enzyme studies, and cardiac imaging studies (e.g., an echocardiogram) are often not diagnostic. Permanent sequelae are uncommon after cardiac contusion.

10. **Pericardial tamponade** usually follows penetrating trauma to the chest and is rare after blunt trauma. Bleeding into the nondistensible pericardial sac increases intrapericardial volume and pressure, leading to decreased cardiac output. **Beck's triad** may be seen and consists of increased central venous pressure (seen as jugular venous distention if the patient is not hypovolemic), decreased blood pressure, and muffled heart tones. **Pulsus paradoxus** (i.e., a drop in systolic blood pressure of more than 10 mm Hg during inspiration) and **electrical alternans** (alternating morphology and amplitude of the QRS complex on the ECG) may be found. Removal of even small amounts of fluid (10–20 mL) can lead to significant improvement in patients with acute pericardial tamponade.

11. **Myocardial rupture** is nearly always immediately fatal. The ventricles are most often involved, although the right atrium (near the superior vena cava or inferior vena cava) is most often involved in patients who survive to reach the hospital. The septum, chordae, papillary muscles, valves, and pericardium may also be involved. Rupture is most likely to occur following blunt trauma when the cardiac chambers are distended. Shock or evidence of tamponade may be seen.

12. **Traumatic rupture of the aorta** may be caused by bending, shearing, or torsional forces on the aorta or sudden increased intrathoracic pressure. The isthmus of the aorta between the left subclavian artery and the ligamentum arteriosum is the most common site of rupture. The descending aorta is relatively fixed by the ligamentum arteriosum and the intercostal arteries as compared to the relatively mobile ascending aorta. An intact adventitial layer may contain the hematoma and allow the patient to survive until arrival at the hospital. Mechanism alone may be the main reason to pursue this diagnosis.

    a. **Causes.** Traumatic rupture of the aorta should be suspected in patients who have sustained blunt trauma following:
    (1) Deceleration or acceleration of greater than 30 mph
    (2) A fall from greater than a 30-foot height
    (3) Sudden compression of the chest (e.g., car falling onto the chest)

    b. **Symptoms.** The patient may have minimal symptoms and no apparent chest wall injury. A minority of patients may have retrosternal or intrascapular pain. Dyspnea, stridor, or dysphagia (from hematoma compressing the trachea, laryngeal nerve, or esophagus); alteration in perfusion to the extremities; edema to the base of the neck; hypertension; or hypotension may be seen.

    c. **Radiographic findings** may include:
    (1) Widened mediastinum
    (2) Obscured aortic knob
    (3) Obliteration of the aortopulmonary window (the space between the pulmonary artery and the aorta)
    (4) Presence of an apical pleural cap
    (5) Deviation of the trachea or esophagus
    (6) Fracture of the first or second rib
    (7) Elevation and rightward displacement of the right mainstem bronchus
    (8) Depression of the left mainstem bronchus
    (9) Widening of the paravertebral stripe

13. **Diaphragmatic injury** may follow either blunt or penetrating trauma. It must be ruled out in all patients with thoracoabdominal penetrating injuries. The patient may present with respiratory distress, and a chest radiograph may show viscera or a nasogastric tube in the chest. Presence of

peritoneal lavage fluid in a chest tube confirms the diagnosis. These injuries may be difficult to diagnose.

14. **Rib fractures** mandate a search for other injuries and are primarily of concern because of the structures that the ribs cover. Pain with breathing may impair ventilation secondary to splinting.
    a. **Upper rib fractures.** The upper three ribs are more protected. Their fracture may imply greater force of injury to the chest, and intrathoracic injury should be ruled out.
    b. **Lower rib fractures** (ribs 9–12) are at risk of puncturing the liver or spleen. All rib fractures should have associated pneumothorax ruled out.
    c. **Sternal fractures** (often diagnosed on lateral chest radiograph) carry the risk of injury to the underlying heart and lung.

C **Differential diagnoses**

1. Tension pneumothorax may be confused with pericardial tamponade, the former being more common. Hyperresonance and absence of breath sounds in the hemithorax can help to distinguish the two. Hypotension and increased central venous pressure can also be seen in superior vena cava obstruction, right ventricle contusion, rupture of the tricuspid valve, and pulmonary edema.

2. Pneumomediastinum may be seen in esophageal or tracheobronchial tears, as well as in nontraumatic conditions (e.g., asthma).

3. Particulate matter seen in a chest tube can be seen in diaphragmatic rupture or esophageal rupture.

4. Adult respiratory distress syndrome (ARDS) may have a similar appearance to that of pulmonary contusion on the chest radiograph but is generally more diffuse and appears later.

D **Evaluation**

1. **Patient history.** The physician should seek to define the mechanism of injury. Once this is ascertained, information specific to the mechanism of injury should be obtained:
    a. **Motor vehicle collisions**
       (1) Were the passengers wearing seat belts?
       (2) What was the approximate speed of the vehicle?
       (3) Was the patient ejected from the vehicle?
       (4) Was there any deformity of the steering wheel?
       (5) Did any of the other vehicle occupants die?
    b. **Falls.** What was the approximate height from which the fall occurred?
    c. **Gunshot wounds**
       (1) How many shots were heard?
       (2) How many wounds were sustained? (The patient may not know.)
       (3) What type of weapon was used, and what was the range?
       (4) Did the patient fall after being shot?
    d. **Stab wounds**
       (1) How long was the knife?
       (2) In which direction did the stabbing occur?

2. **Primary and secondary survey.** The patient should be completely undressed and a complete primary and secondary survey should be performed, with special attention to inspection, auscultation, and palpation of the chest looking for symmetry of the chest and breath sounds, bruits, murmurs, Hamman's crunch (a crunching sound heard over the heart in systole when pneumomediastinum is present), crepitus, tenderness, bruises, wounds, and impaled objects. **The presence of alcohol or other drugs should be assessed** to determine the reliability of the history and examination.

3. **Specific protocols**
    a. **Blunt chest trauma.** Patients should have a chest radiograph and an evaluation of oxygen saturation or blood gases. Whenever possible, the patient should have an upright chest radio-

graph performed to eliminate a spurious finding of widened mediastinum seen on the supine film. Patients who have sustained a blunt injury to the anterior chest should be evaluated for cardiac contusion. Work-up varies with the age and health of the patient, but generally involves serial cardiac enzymes, an ECG, cardiac monitoring, and cardiac imaging (e.g., an echocardiogram) prior to discharge.

b. **Traumatic rupture of the aorta.** Patients with **rapid acceleration or deceleration injuries** (greater than 30 mph), **falls from a height of 30 feet** (approximately three stories), or **sudden compression** of the chest must be evaluated for traumatic rupture of the aorta. According to the availability of special procedures and the patient's clinical stability, patients can undergo aortic arch angiography, CT scan of the chest with contrast, or transesophageal echocardiography.

c. **Penetrating chest injury.** All patients with penetrating injury to the chest should have a chest radiograph performed. If it is negative, an expiratory film, a posteroanterior film, and a lateral film should be obtained. A pneumothorax may be more evident with the lung in expiration. If all films are negative, the patient should have a repeat chest radiograph in 6 hours.

   (1) **Penetrating wounds in the anterior box.** Patients should have an echocardiogram or chest CT scan to evaluate the heart and mediastinal structures.

   (2) **Penetrating wounds in the posterior box.** Patients are at risk of tracheal, esophageal, and aortic injuries.

      (a) **Stab wounds.** It is necessary to obtain a chest radiograph.

         (i) If there is mediastinal air, then the presence of an esophageal injury should be evaluated using esophagography or esophagoscopy. Any evidence of widened mediastinum mandates further aortic evaluation (chest CT scan or aortography).

         (ii) A patient with a normal chest radiograph should have a repeat chest radiograph in 6 hours.

      (b) **Gunshot wounds.** Patients require a chest radiograph, evaluation of the aorta and esophagus, and, if there is evidence of tracheobronchial injury, bronchoscopy.

E **Treatment**

1. **General measures.** All patients require intravenous access, supplemental oxygen, initial cardiac monitoring, and pulse oximetry measurements.

   a. **Intravenous access and fluid resuscitation.** Central venous cannulation should be on the same side as the pneumothorax to avoid injury to the uninvolved lung. A catheter should not be placed into a potentially injured vessel. If there is a possibility of superior vena cava injury, at least one intravenous line should be placed below the diaphragm. Fluid and blood resuscitation is as outlined in the section on traumatic shock (see III).

   b. **Ventilation.** If the patient is hypoxic despite supplemental oxygen, he or she should be intubated.

2. **Specific measures**

   a. **Pneumothorax and hemopneumothorax.** Pneumothoraces (except very small ones in stable, asymptomatic patients who have sustained blunt trauma) and most hemopneumothoraces are treated with tube thoracostomy. If a chest tube is not placed for a simple pneumothorax, a repeat chest radiograph must be obtained in 6 hours or if there is a change in the patient's clinical condition.

   (1) **Chest tube placement.** The usual placement is at the nipple line (fifth intercostal space), at the mid- to anterior axillary line on the affected side.

   (2) **Chest tube size.** A 24–28 French chest tube is placed for pneumothoraces, and a 32–40 French chest tube is placed for hemothoraces. In children, the appropriate chest tube size depends on the size of the child and the type of injury being treated. An estimate of the size of the intercostal space is useful in determining tube size to avoid kinking of the tube during expiration.

        (3) **Indications for chest tube placement.** All patients with a pneumothorax require a chest tube if they are undergoing:

           (a) Positive-pressure ventilation

           (b) General anesthesia

           (c) Air transport

        (4) **Indications for open thoracotomy**

           (a) Initial blood loss through the chest tube of 1500 mL

           (b) Ongoing blood loss of approximately 300 mL/hour

           (c) Persistent hypotension after adequate blood replacement

           (d) Radiographic evidence of increased hemothorax despite functioning chest tubes

           (e) Worsening of the patient's clinical condition

    b. Tension pneumothorax may be treated initially with insertion of a 14-gauge angiocatheter at the second intercostal space in the midclavicular line to relieve the tension while preparation for a chest tube is under way.

    c. Suspected pericardial tamponade. Pericardiocentesis may be performed while awaiting formal thoracotomy.

    d. Suspected traumatic rupture of the aorta. Care should be taken to avoid agitation or gagging in the patient, which could precipitate hypertension and increase shearing forces on the adventitia of the aorta. Efforts to control the blood pressure may need to include pharmacologic agents if sedation of the patient alone fails to do so. Definitive treatment involves surgical repair.

    e. Penetrating and blunt trauma. Resuscitative thoracotomies for traumatic arrest may be performed in patients with penetrating injuries (except gunshot wounds to the head) if there is known loss of vital signs for fewer than 20 minutes. Patients who have sustained blunt trauma but who arrive in the ED with signs of life (reactive pupils, respiratory effort, cardiac rhythm) may also undergo thoracotomy. (Blunt trauma patients with loss of vital signs in the field usually have injuries from which recovery is not expected.) Open thoracotomy allows for:

        (1) Pericardiotomy to relieve tamponade

        (2) Direct evaluation and stabilization of cardiac injuries

        (3) Clamping of the descending aorta to preserve cardiac output to the coronary and cerebral arteries (Note: clamping the aorta for longer than 30 minutes increases the risk of ischemia to the spinal cord and structures below the chest.)

        (4) Open cardiac massage

  F Disposition Patients with stab wounds who are responsible and who have no evidence of intrathoracic penetration on a repeat chest radiograph after 4–6 hours may be discharged home with instructions (after local wound care and tetanus prophylaxis have been given). Most other patients with thoracic trauma require admission to a monitored bed, ICU, or operating suite for further care.

VIII   ABDOMINAL TRAUMA

  A Discussion Abdominal trauma may follow either penetrating or blunt trauma (direct blows and deceleration injury).

    1. Anatomy

      a. Regions of the abdomen are defined as follows:

        (1) **Anterior abdominal area:** costal margins to the inguinal ligaments, from midaxillary line to midaxillary line

        (2) **Thoracoabdominal area:** above the costal margins, below the nipple line anteriorly and below the tips of the scapulae posteriorly

        (3) **Flank and back:** posterior to the midaxillary line between the inferior tips of the scapulae and the iliac crests

      b. Retroperitoneum. The retroperitoneum contains the aorta, venae cavae, pancreas, kidneys, ureters, and parts of the colon and duodenum.

2. **Management goals**
   a. The primary goal in the emergency management of abdominal trauma is determining whether the patient requires emergent operative intervention, not identifying the specific abdominal injury. **Indications for emergent operative management** include:
      (1) Shock or hemodynamic instability with ongoing blood loss
      (2) Peritoneal irritation
      (3) Retained instrument (e.g., knife blade, impaled object) causing trauma
      (4) Evisceration
      (5) Transabdominal missile injury
      (6) Free air
      (7) Gross blood on nasogastric or rectal examination
   b. The physician must determine if there has been peritoneal, retroperitoneal, or diaphragmatic penetration. A rapid ultrasound examination is usually effective in determining if the patient is bleeding internally. Less commonly, diagnostic peritoneal lavage involves passage of a catheter into the peritoneum, with sampling of the intraperitoneal fluid. If there is no gross blood obtained (5 mL of blood) on initially entering the peritoneum, 1 L of Ringer's lactate or normal saline (or 15 mL/kg of fluid in children) is instilled into the abdomen, and the lavage fluid is subsequently sampled to assess for hemoperitoneum. Approximately 4 mL of blood in 1 L of saline produces a red blood cell (RBC) count of 20,000/mL. Diagnostic peritoneal lavage does not sample the retroperitoneal area unless there is injury through both the peritoneal and retroperitoneal areas.
      (1) **Preparation.** Prior to the lavage procedure, all patients should have a Foley catheter and nasogastric tube placed to decompress the bladder and stomach.
      (2) **Position.** Diagnostic peritoneal lavage is usually performed in the **infraumbilical** position. The **supraumbilical** position is indicated if the patient meets any of the following criteria:
          (a) Has undergone previous abdominal surgery
          (b) Is pregnant (use **suprafundal position**)
          (c) Has a pelvic fracture

B **Clinical features** The mechanism of injury raises the index of suspicion for certain types of organ injuries.

1. **Diaphragmatic injuries** should be suspected in patients who have sustained a sudden compressive injury to the abdomen or a thoracoabdominal penetrating injury. Injuries to the posterolateral aspect of the left hemidiaphragm are most often diagnosed.

2. **Hollow organ injuries** may be suspected if there is sudden compression by a lap belt. CT scans poorly evaluate hollow organ injury. Hollow organs are more often involved in penetrating injuries.
   a. The **duodenum** can be injured following frontal impact or penetrating injuries. Duodenal injury may be suspected if there is blood on nasogastric aspirate, retroperitoneal air, or elevated lavage enzymes.
   b. The **stomach** is relatively resistant to blunt injury unless it is distended, because it is relatively well protected by the rib cage and is mobile.
   c. The **transverse colon** is most often involved in penetrating injuries, whereas the cecum, ascending, and sigmoid colon are more susceptible to blunt, compressive forces because they are relatively immobile.
   d. The **rectum** is an extraperitoneal structure. It is important to identify injury here prior to any operative intervention because these injuries are difficult to diagnose on standard laparotomy approach. Pelvic fractures should raise the index of suspicion for rectal injuries, and rectal examination should be performed.

3. **Pancreatic injuries** should be suspected after a direct epigastric blow (e.g., handlebar injury) that compresses the organ against the vertebral bodies. The pancreas may also be involved in penetrating injuries.

4. **Hepatic injuries.** The liver is commonly injured following penetrating and blunt trauma because it is the largest solid organ and it is relatively immobile. Liver injury should be suspected in patients with right lower rib fractures or right upper-quadrant tenderness, or in patients who are hypotensive after abdominal trauma. Although many liver injuries can be managed nonoperatively, liver injuries may involve major venous or arterial damage with massive bleeding and high mortality.

5. **Splenic injuries.** The spleen is the most commonly injured organ in blunt abdominal trauma. Symptoms of splenic injury are those findings consistent with blood loss (e.g., hypotension, tachycardia, peritoneal signs) and should be suspected with left lower rib fractures. Kehr's sign, pain referred to the left shoulder, may be seen with injury to the spleen.

C **Differential diagnoses** Abdominal injuries, especially in the retroperitoneum, may reveal very few findings on initial evaluation, rendering an essentially normal examination. Diaphragmatic injuries may be missed despite work-up; difficulty breathing may be attributed to concomitant thoracic injury.

D **Evaluation** of the patient is determined by the type and mechanism of injury.

1. **General protocol**
   a. **Primary survey.** The first priority is the evaluation and treatment of the ABCs. A **nasogastric tube** should be placed both for decompression of the stomach and for diagnostic purposes.
   b. **Patient history.** Information that may need to be obtained should include the type of injury, the use of restraints, the type of weapon, the gun caliber, the number of gunshot wounds and at what distance, and the number of stab wounds sustained.
   c. **Secondary survey.** The entire abdomen, back, and flank should be evaluated. Bruises, wounds, retained implements, and their location should be noted.
      (1) **Abdominal examination.** The abdomen should be auscultated for bowel sounds and bruits. Percussion and palpation should identify any tenderness, distention, or peritoneal signs (e.g., rebound tenderness, involuntary guarding). A **repeat abdominal examination** by the same examiner should be done regularly if there is possibility of intra-abdominal injury or if there is change in the patient's status.
      (2) **Rectal examination.** In patients with suspected pelvic fracture, a rectal examination should be performed, noting blood, position of the prostate, and any bony fragments.
   d. **Laboratory studies** should include a complete blood count (CBC); electrolyte, blood urea nitrogen (BUN), creatinine, amylase, and coagulation studies; urinalysis; blood type (if significant blood loss is suspected); and a toxicology screen.
   e. **Diagnostic imaging studies.** Increasingly, **ultrasonography** has been used to identify free fluid (e.g., blood) in the abdomen allowing noninvasive monitoring of the patient's abdomen. **Laparoscopy** may also play an increasing role in evaluation of abdominal trauma.

2. **Specific protocols**
   a. **Patients with indications for operative intervention** (see VIII A 2 a) need no further diagnostic work-up of their abdomen in the ED except for a rectal examination.
   b. **Blunt abdominal trauma**
      (1) The abdomen needs **further work-up** if:
         (a) There is an unreliable examination, such as patients with spinal cord injury or patients with altered mental status (e.g., intoxication, head injury)
         (b) There are equivocal findings on examination
         (c) The patient's examination cannot be followed (e.g., the patient is going to the operating room for treatment of other injuries)
      (2) The patient should have a **diagnostic peritoneal lavage** performed to evaluate for solid organ injury. The diagnostic peritoneal lavage is considered positive if the RBC count is greater than 100,000/mL; the white blood cell (WBC) count is greater than 500/mL; or bile, bacteria, or fecal or vegetable matter is detected. Alternatively, an abdominal CT scan with intravenous and oral contrast can be used to evaluate for solid organ injury.

   c. **Penetrating injury.** Evaluation depends on the mechanism (e.g., stab wound or gunshot wound), the location of the injury, and the possible pathway of the implement.

     (1) **Stab wounds**

       (a) **Stab wounds of the anterior abdomen** penetrate the peritoneum in approximately 50% of cases. Of the wounds that penetrate, approximately 50% require operative intervention. Local wound exploration may be considered to help rule out peritoneal penetration. Some physicians perform diagnostic peritoneal lavage on patients with anterior abdominal stab wounds if there is any question of intra-abdominal extension. If the RBC count is greater than 100,000/mL, the lavage is considered positive.

       (b) Patients with **stab wounds in the thoracoabdominal area** should have diagnostic peritoneal lavage performed. It is considered positive if the RBC count is greater than 10,000/mL (presumptive evidence of diaphragmatic penetration). There is some controversy as to the optimal RBC count to discern peritoneal penetration or diaphragmatic injury without having too many false-positive tests. Some centers use an RBC count of 5000/mL to avoid missing any diaphragmatic injuries.

       (c) Patients with **stab wounds of the back and flank** should have diagnostic peritoneal lavage performed to evaluate for peritoneal penetration. The lavage is considered positive if the RBC count is greater than 10,000/mL. If the lavage is negative, CT scan with oral, intravenous, and rectal contrast is recommended. Alternatively, if the patient is stable, CT scan alone may be used if it is probable that the stab wound is tangential to the skin.

     (2) **Gunshot wounds** that penetrate the abdomen require operative intervention, because more than 98% of these injuries cause damage that requires surgical repair.

E **Treatment**

   1. **Resuscitation.** Patients with abdominal trauma require the standard trauma-resuscitative measures, including fluid resuscitation and oxygen therapy.

   2. **Antibiotic therapy.** Patients with suspected bowel injury require preoperative antibiotics to cover aerobes and anaerobes, pending operative findings.

   3. **Thoracotomy.** Patients with continued hemorrhage and hypotension despite fluid and blood resuscitation may require thoracotomy with cross-clamping of the aorta pending operative intervention.

   4. **Surgery.** Treatment of surgical patients is dictated by operative findings and ongoing blood loss.

F **Disposition** of the patient depends on the extent of the injury sustained. Patients with nonpenetrating stab wounds may be safely discharged home after local wound care. Patients with a minor mechanism of blunt trauma, reliable examinations, and no evidence of injury may also be discharged home with instructions to return if there is any abdominal pain. Most other patients require admission for observation and treatment as dictated by their injuries.

IX   PELVIC TRAUMA

A **Discussion**   Pelvic trauma most commonly results from motor vehicle collisions (especially those involving pedestrians) or falls from heights.

   1. **Anatomy** (Figure 17–4A)

     a. The **bony pelvis** provides support for the body and is the point of attachment for major muscle groups. The **pelvis** consists of the two innominate bones (consisting of the ilium, the ischium, and the pubis, which fuse at the acetabulum), the sacrum, and the coccyx. The **pelvic ring** consists of the two innominate bones and the sacrum.

     b. **Soft tissue structures.** The pelvis contains the lower urinary tract and portions of the lower gastrointestinal tract, including part of the descending colon, the sigmoid colon, the rectum,

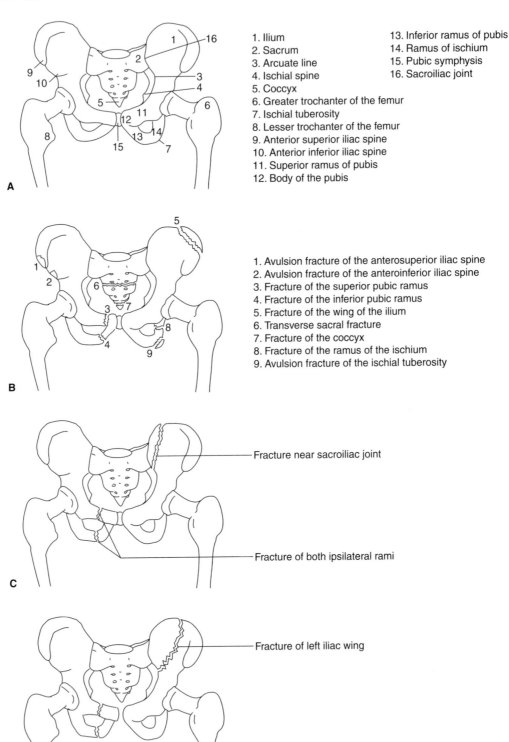

1. Ilium
2. Sacrum
3. Arcuate line
4. Ischial spine
5. Coccyx
6. Greater trochanter of the femur
7. Ischial tuberosity
8. Lesser trochanter of the femur
9. Anterior superior iliac spine
10. Anterior inferior iliac spine
11. Superior ramus of pubis
12. Body of the pubis
13. Inferior ramus of pubis
14. Ramus of ischium
15. Pubic symphysis
16. Sacroiliac joint

1. Avulsion fracture of the anterosuperior iliac spine
2. Avulsion fracture of the anteroinferior iliac spine
3. Fracture of the superior pubic ramus
4. Fracture of the inferior pubic ramus
5. Fracture of the wing of the ilium
6. Transverse sacral fracture
7. Fracture of the coccyx
8. Fracture of the ramus of the ischium
9. Avulsion fracture of the ischial tuberosity

Fracture near sacroiliac joint

Fracture of both ipsilateral rami

Fracture of left iliac wing

FIGURE 17–4 **(A)** Normal pelvis. **(B)** Type I pelvic fractures. **(C)** Type II pelvic fractures. **(D)** Type III pelvic fractures.

and the anus. The normal width of the symphysis pubis is no greater than 5 mm. The sacroiliac joint is 2 to 4 mm wide.

c. **Major arteries and veins** pass through the pelvis. There can be significant hemorrhage in pelvic trauma from pelvic vessels, the pelvic bones, and the pelvic muscles. The majority of the blood supply to the pelvis is from the internal iliac (or hypogastric) arteries. Most pelvic hematomas are venous in origin; an intact peritoneum may tamponade the hematoma in the retroperitoneum.

2. **Major mechanisms of pelvic fracture** include lateral compression (e.g., pedestrian struck from the side), anteroposterior compression (e.g., head-on motor vehicle collision), and vertical shear forces (e.g., fall from a height).

B **Clinical features**   There are several classifications of pelvic fractures.

1. **Type I fractures** are fractures of **individual bones not involving a break in the continuity of the ring** (Figure 17–4B).

2. **Type II fractures** are **single breaks in the pelvic ring** (Figure 17–4C). Fractures involving single breaks in the ring are stable, whereas two or more breaks in the ring are unstable. Type II fractures include:
   a. Fractures of both ipsilateral rami
   b. Subluxation or fracture near the symphysis pubis
   c. Subluxation or fracture near the sacroiliac joint

3. **Type III fractures** are **double breaks in the pelvic ring** (Figure 17–4D). These fractures are unstable, but the degree of instability varies with the individual fracture patterns. A significant amount of force is required to produce these fractures, and there is a high degree of association with intraperitoneal and retroperitoneal injuries. Type III fractures include:
   a. **Straddle fractures** (fractures of both rami on both sides of the symphysis pubis or of both ipsilateral rami in association with separation of the symphysis pubis)
   b. **Fractures involving double vertical pelvic fractures,** anterior and posterior to the acetabulum (**Malgaigne fractures**)
   c. **Multiple severe fractures**

4. **Type IV fractures** are **fractures of the acetabulum.** These may be displaced or nondisplaced.

C **Differential diagnoses**   Multiple trauma patients may have hypotension from numerous sources, but significant hemorrhage should be anticipated with severe pelvic fractures. It may be difficult to diagnose specific fractures on initial radiography, and further studies based on patient stability may be required.

D **Evaluation**

1. **Primary survey.** As with all trauma patients, the patient should have initial evaluation of the trauma ABCs.

2. **Secondary survey**
   a. **Pelvic examination.** AP and lateral compression of the pelvis should be performed, as well as palpation over the symphysis pubis.
   b. **Genitourinary examination.** The presence of blood at the urinary meatus and any scrotal or perineal hematomas should be noted. Female patients should have a vaginal examination and a pregnancy test.
   c. **Rectal examination.** On rectal examination, the physician should note the presence of gross blood, the position of the prostate, sphincter tone, and any bony abnormality.
   d. **Extremities** should be examined for distal pulses, sensation, dislocation, and any leg-length discrepancy.

3. **Diagnostic imaging studies**
   a. **Radiography.** A standard AP view of the pelvis is necessary. Additional views may also be needed, such as:
      (1) Inlet view to visualize AP displacement of the ring
      (2) Outlet views to visualize inferior-superior displacement
      (3) Internal and external oblique views (Judet views) to better visualize the acetabulum
   b. **CT.** A CT scan of the pelvis can better demonstrate acetabular disruption, the sacroiliac joint, and the amount of rotation of the pelvis, as well as nonbony injuries.
   c. **Angiography** may be performed in patients who continue to bleed despite efforts to terminate hemorrhaging. Angiography allows localization of arterial bleeding sites and, possibly, transcatheter embolization of smaller arteries.

4. **Additional studies** (e.g., abdominal or genitourinary procedures) should be performed as indicated. For example:
   a. **Diagnostic peritoneal lavage** should be employed in the patient with pelvic trauma and hypotension to rule out an intra-abdominal source of bleeding. In cases of pelvic fracture, the supraumbilical open or semi-open technique should be employed to avoid entering a pelvic hematoma that may have dissected anteriorly up the abdominal wall.
   b. **Retrograde urethrography and cystography** are indicated for patients with **penetrating pelvic trauma.** These patients should also undergo **rigid proctosigmoidoscopy,** and, in women, **vaginal speculum examination.** Diagnostic peritoneal lavage should be performed to rule out intraperitoneal injury, and **triple-contrast** (oral, intravenous, and rectal) **CT scans** should be obtained.

E **Treatment**   The major life threat with pelvic fractures is hemorrhage.

1. **Resuscitation.** Patients with pelvic trauma should have all the standard resuscitative measures initiated. Intravenous catheters should not be placed in the lower extremities if there is possible proximal venous disruption.

2. A **pelvic compression belt,** a **pneumatic antishock garment,** or **military antishock trousers (MAST)** should be considered in hypotensive patients with pelvic fractures. The pneumatic antishock garment may help compress the pelvic area and tamponade venous bleeding, stabilize pelvic fractures, and improve bony alignment. Pulmonary edema and rupture of the diaphragm are absolute contraindications to placement of a pneumatic antishock garment.

3. **Early orthopedic consultation** should be sought, and an external fixator may be placed to stabilize pelvic fracture.

4. **Operative intervention** may be required but entails the risk of increased bleeding from disruption of the tamponade effect of the peritoneum on pelvic bleeding.

5. **Conservative therapy** (i.e., **analgesia, rest**) is indicated for patients with isolated type I avulsion injuries, isolated ramus fractures, coccygeal fractures, and isolated transverse sacral fractures without associated injuries. Treatment of coccygeal fractures consists of **stool softeners** and **sitting on a doughnut-shaped cushion.**

F **Disposition**   Patients with fractures that can be treated with analgesia and rest may be discharged home or admitted for pain control as needed. Patients with more severe pelvic fractures require admission for associated injuries, ongoing resuscitation, and treatment of individual fractures.

X   **GENITOURINARY TRAUMA**

A **Discussion**   Genitourinary trauma should be suspected in patients who have sustained high-speed deceleration injuries, those who have sustained direct blunt trauma to the back or flank with lower rib fractures, those who have sustained a fall from a height, and those who have sustained penetrating injuries.

B **Clinical features**   Signs include flank tenderness, flank hematoma, fractures of the transverse processes of the vertebrae, and hematuria. The degree of hematuria does not correlate well with the severity of the injury.

1. **Kidneys.** The kidneys are retroperitoneal structures. They receive approximately 1200 mL/min of blood flow (approximately 20%–25% of the cardiac output). The renal pedicle is composed of the major renal vessels and the ureter. Renal injury is the most common form of genitourinary injury. Blunt trauma accounts for more than 90% of renal trauma. Patients with pre-existing renal disease are predisposed to additional renal damage.

   a. **Renal contusion** (Figure 17–5A) involves parenchymal ecchymoses, subcapsular hematomas, and small lacerations. Hematuria is usually present, and the intravenous pyelogram shows normal function. Contusions account for approximately 90% of renal injuries.

   b. **Renal lacerations** may involve either the cortex or the pelvicaliceal system (Figure 17–5B).

   c. **Renal fracture** ("**shattered kidney**") involves complete disruption of the parenchyma from the collecting system (Figure 17–5C). The patient appears hemodynamically unstable secondary to blood loss.

   d. **Renal pedicle injury** (Figure 17–5D) may result from penetrating trauma or deceleration from high speed. Injuries include lacerations and thromboses of the renal arteries and veins. Patients with penetrating renal pedicle trauma and renal vascular thrombosis secondary to

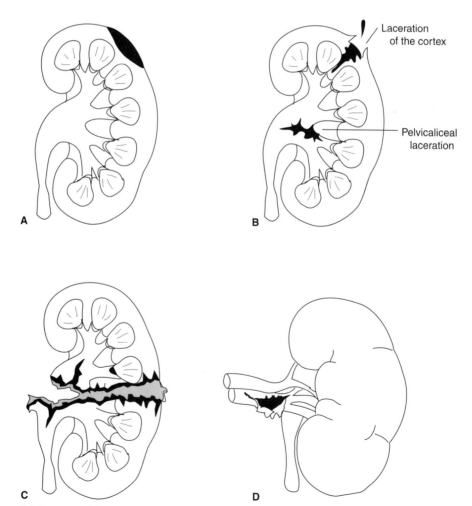

FIGURE 17–5   **(A)** Renal contusion. **(B)** Renal lacerations. **(C)** Renal fracture. **(D)** Renal pedicle injury.

blunt trauma may not have hematuria. The most common renal pedicle injury after blunt trauma is renal artery thrombosis.

2. **Ureters.** Traumatic injury to the ureters is rare. Most penetrating ureteral injuries are in the upper third of the ureter. Blunt trauma can cause avulsion of the ureter at the ureteropelvic junction, where it is in close proximity to the bony pelvic brim. Hematuria may be seen with partial tears but is usually not seen with complete ureteral disruption.

3. **Bladder** injuries are the second most common traumatic genitourinary injuries. They are most commonly seen after blunt trauma and pelvic fractures and usually are associated with a distended bladder (which elevates the bladder from its relatively protected position in the pelvis).
   a. **A bladder contusion** is a bruising of the wall of the bladder; the amount of hematuria is not well correlated with the severity of the injury. The bladder wall is intact.
   b. **An intraperitoneal bladder rupture** is a tear typically found in the fundus or posterior wall of the bladder. (The peritoneal surface of the bladder is the weakest area of the bladder wall and therefore most likely to rupture.) The tear allows opening into the peritoneum and spillage of urine into the peritoneal cavity.
   c. **An extraperitoneal bladder rupture** is a tear outside of the peritoneum that allows urine to spill into the perivesicular space but not into the peritoneum.

4. **Urethra.** Urethral injuries are uncommon.
   a. **Men.** In men, the urethra is divided by the urogenital diaphragm into the anterior and posterior urethra.
      (1) The **anterior urethra** consists of the bulbous and penile urethra. Anterior urethral injuries are associated with direct trauma to the urethra, such as with straddle injuries or fractured penis. Blood at the urinary meatus and perineal hematoma are usually seen.
      (2) The **posterior urethra** consists of the membranous and prostatic urethra. Posterior urethral injuries are typically associated with pelvic fractures. Examination reveals perineal hematoma, a high-riding prostate with a boggy consistency, and blood at the urinary meatus.
   b. **Women.** In women, urethral injuries are not common and are associated with pelvic fracture and perineal injury. These injuries should be sought in patients with vaginal lacerations.

5. **Penis.** Penile injuries range from simple lacerations to amputation. Penile fracture occurs when an erect penis is subjected to a direct blow, with tearing of the tunica albuginea. Reimplantation of an amputated penis may be attempted within approximately 6 hours of dismemberment.

6. **Testicles.** Testicular injuries include contusions, lacerations, rupture, and dislocation, usually as a result of a fall or direct blow.

C **Differential diagnoses** Hypotension, as seen with severe renal lacerations and renal pedicle injuries, may be ascribed to other injuries in the multiply traumatized patient. A high index of suspicion needs to be maintained to diagnose genitourinary trauma, especially in patients with ureteral injuries, who may initially have few symptoms.

D **Evaluation**
1. **Primary survey.** Standard trauma assessment of ABCs is necessary.
2. **Secondary survey.** The **perineum** should be carefully inspected for hematomas or lacerations. The **rectum** should be examined, noting sensation, tone, position, and quality of the **prostate** (a high-riding prostate may signify urethral disruption, whereas a boggy-feeling prostate may indicate hematoma). The **scrotum** should be inspected for hematoma and tenderness. The **penis** should be examined, noting any blood at the urethral meatus. A **vaginal examination,** noting blood or lacerations, should be performed in women.
3. **Diagnostic imaging studies.** The work-up of patients with blunt trauma and microscopic hematuria is controversial. If hematuria fails to clear or is associated with shock, further work-up is undertaken. Patients with penetrating trauma also require further work-up.

a. **Radiography.** Radiologic studies generally proceed in a caudad to cephalad direction.
   (1) Radiographs of the **pelvis** should be obtained, noting any pelvic fractures. Radiographs of the **abdomen** should be evaluated for fractures of the transverse processes as well as other pathology.
   (2) When blood is noted at the urinary meatus, a **retrograde urethrogram** is performed by instilling radiopaque material into the distal urethra and obtaining a radiograph to visualize the urethra. This should be performed before urinary catheterization is attempted to avoid converting a partial urethral disruption into a complete disruption.
   (3) **Cystography** should be performed next in patients with pelvic fracture by instilling approximately 350 mL of contrast into the bladder through a Foley catheter by gravity. An additional 50 mL is then instilled, and radiographs are obtained. The contrast is drained from the bladder, and a "washout film" is obtained, which helps to visualize any extravasation of contrast behind the bladder that may have been obscured when the bladder was full of contrast.
b. **CT.** An abdominal CT scan should be performed in cases of suspected renal trauma. An abdominal CT scan can show the retroperitoneal space, hematomas, renal disruption, and vascular injuries.
c. **Arteriography.** A renal arteriogram may be indicated in cases of renal nonfunction.
d. **"One-shot" intravenous pyelography (IVP)** should be performed when patients are too unstable to undergo CT scan or when assessment of contralateral renal function is necessary (i.e., if a nephrectomy is anticipated on the affected side). Caution should be taken in hypotensive patients (who may not be able to adequately concentrate contrast material in the kidney). Also, care must be taken to avoid precipitating renal failure, especially if multiple contrast studies are anticipated.

E Treatment
1. **General care**
   a. **Resuscitation.** All patients should be resuscitated in the standard fashion for associated injuries. Many patients with genitourinary injuries have sustained multiple injuries, and maintenance of airway and hemodynamics, including urinary output, is key.
   b. **Consultation.** Early urologic and orthopedic consultations should be sought.
   c. **Antibiotic therapy.** Patients with rectal or vaginal lacerations should receive intravenous antibiotics. Use of antibiotics in other genitourinary injuries depends on:
      (1) The location of the injury
      (2) Whether operative intervention is required
      (3) Whether urinary extravasation has occurred
      (4) Associated injuries (e.g., an associated pelvic fracture)
      (5) Whether a penetrating bladder injury has occurred
2. **Specific care**
   a. **Renal injuries**
      (1) **Renal contusions** are treated conservatively following serial hematocrits and urinalyses.
      (2) **Renal laceration, rupture, and pedicle injury.** Minor renal lacerations generally heal without sequelae. Hemodynamic instability of the patient secondary to a serious renal laceration may prompt surgical exploration. Severe renal lacerations, renal rupture, and some renal pedicle injuries may need to be resolved by nephrectomy. Some renal pedicle vascular injuries may be repaired by primary anastomosis or vascular grafting.
   b. **Ureteral injuries** require surgical repair.
   c. **Bladder contusions** resolve with conservative treatment. Bladder ruptures require surgical repair.
   d. **Urethral injuries.** Partial anterior and posterior urethral lacerations may be managed with an indwelling urinary catheter (fluoroscopically placed) or suprapubic cystostomy. Complete anterior and posterior urethral injuries require surgical repair.
   e. **Testicular injuries** associated with clot or rupture may benefit from early surgical exploration.
   f. **Penile ruptures or lacerations** require surgical intervention.

F **Disposition**   Most patients, except those with very superficial external genitourinary injuries (who have no difficulty urinating), should be admitted to the hospital for observation or surgical intervention.

XI PEDIATRIC TRAUMA (see also Chapter 15)

A **Discussion**   Trauma accounts for approximately one half of deaths in the pediatric age group. The initial assessment of children proceeds as with the adult, first completing a primary survey, the ABCs, and then the secondary survey. Children may cry from fear as well as pain, and they may be less able to localize their pain than adults. Other differences include:

1. A child's **head occupies a relatively larger proportion of body surface area than an adult's.** Bony sutures fuse by 18–24 months. A child's brain has a larger proportion of unmyelinated fibers, making it more susceptible to shear injury.

2. Children have **shorter necks with less muscle support and more cartilage.**

3. The **larynx is more cephalad and anterior,** located at approximately C3–C4 in the infant (C4–C5 in the adult). In children younger than 8 years, the subglottic area at the cricoid ring is the narrowest part of the upper airway (in adults, it is at the level of the vocal cords). It is this area that is the limiting factor in determining endotracheal tube size.

4. The **chest is much more compliant** in the child, with less bony structure in the chest wall, more cartilage, less overlying protective muscle mass, and a more horizontally placed and more distensible diaphragm. The child is more dependent on movement of the diaphragm for breathing.

5. The **mediastinum is more mobile** in the child and more susceptible to greater shift in tension pneumothorax.

6. The **abdominal wall is thinner with less protective muscle and fat** overlying it. The liver, spleen, and bladder (which is an intraperitoneal structure in children) are all more subject to injury in the child than in the adult.

7. **Vascular access may be more difficult** in the child, and **intraosseous infusion,** with placement of a needle into the marrow space, should be considered early if other peripheral access cannot be obtained. Intraosseous infusion needles, 18- to 20-gauge spinal needles, or 14- to 20-gauge needles can be used. The anterior tibial area, 1–2 cm distal and medial to the tibial tuberosity, is readily accessible (avoiding the epiphysis). Intraosseous infusions should not be employed in a fractured extremity.

8. Children have a **higher proportion of body surface area to body mass** and are more subject to heat loss and hypothermia.

9. The **anterior fontanelle** closes by approximately 18 months of age, and the **posterior fontanelle** closes by approximately 2 months of age.

10. **Children's bones contain growth centers** at the physes, and the epiphyseal–metaphyseal junction is an area of relative weakness. Growth centers may be confused with fractures on radiographic studies.

11. There may be **radiographic variations** seen on pediatric radiographs that are not seen on adult films. These include:
    a. **Pseudosubluxation,** anterior displacement of one vertebra on another, may be seen at C2 or C3. It is less commonly seen on C3–C4. There may be 3 mm of movement seen at these areas on flexion–extension films.
    b. The **predental space** (space between the anterior arch of C1 and the dens) may be greater than that seen in the adult.

B Clinical features

1. **Shock** can be rapidly fatal to a child. Children have extensive compensatory capabilities, and a drop in blood pressure is a late and ominous sign, not occurring until there has been 25%–30% of blood volume loss. **Early recognition of hypovolemia to prevent shock cannot be overly stressed.**

   a. **Tachycardia** is the primary response to hypovolemia in children. Tachycardia may also be associated with pain and anxiety in children.

   b. **Tachypnea.** Respiratory rate may also be increased to compensate for metabolic acidosis secondary to decreased tissue perfusion.

   c. **Delayed capillary refill.** Capillary refill may be delayed (longer than 2 seconds) if there is decreased perfusion or if the extremities have been exposed to cold.

2. **Head injury** is very common in the pediatric population and accounts for approximately 50% of accidental deaths. Children younger than 5 years are more likely to be injured secondary to a fall and are more likely to be injured at home. Nonaccidental injury, such as shaken baby syndrome, must be ruled out. In the older age groups, bicycle injuries and injuries outside the home are more common. Motor vehicle collisions account for the largest number of deaths. Skull fractures, concussions, contusions, lacerations, vascular injuries, and neuronal injuries may be seen. Children with isolated head injury may be hypotensive. Vomiting is commonly seen after head injury and is usually not a sign of increased ICP. Children with head injury may also be transiently pale and lethargic. Persistent or worsening vomiting should prompt further investigation.

   a. **Scalp lacerations** may cause extensive blood loss in children, and pressure should be applied to control bleeding.

   b. **Subgaleal hematoma** may be seen as fluctuant swelling in the scalp. It is caused by blood and tissue fluid accumulating between the galea and the periosteum. Large blood losses can occur in this area.

   c. **Subgaleal hygroma** is uncommon and is usually caused by a laceration of the dura and arachnoid membranes from a skull fracture causing CSF to accumulate in the subgaleal space.

   d. **Skull fractures** are concerning because of possible injury to the underlying brain. Most skull fractures in children are **linear** and may have no associated symptoms except local tenderness. **Depressed skull fractures** usually result from direct blunt trauma and may be open. **Basilar skull fractures** include fractures in the basal portion of the frontal, temporal, and occipital bones, and ethmoid and sphenoid fractures. Findings are the same as those seen in the adult.

   e. **Concussions, contusions,** and **cerebral lacerations** are defined as in the adult.

   f. **Epidural hematomas** are relatively uncommon and occur more frequently in older children.

      (1) Most epidural hematomas are caused by hemorrhage from the middle meningeal artery. However, in children, a significant number of epidural bleeds may be secondary to meningeal and diploic vein hemorrhage. Posterior cranial fossa bleeds secondary to a deep venous sinus bleed may also be seen.

      (2) Intervening periods of lucency between concussion and further neurologic deterioration are seen less often than in adults. Fractures are seen in only approximately 50% of pediatric patients with epidural hemorrhages.

   g. **Subdural hematomas** are seen much more often than epidural bleeds and are more common in infants than older children. They usually occur secondary to a venous bleed. Nonspecific symptoms may be seen, such as irritability and vomiting. Seizures are usually seen. There is greater morbidity associated with subdural hematoma than epidural hematoma secondary to underlying brain injury.

   h. **Subarachnoid bleed** may be seen commonly on head CT scans in children with severe head trauma and may be caused by disruption of major cranial vessels or smaller leptomeningeal vessels. Headache and nuchal rigidity may be seen.

    i. Increased ICP may be seen after acute brain swelling. Findings may include headache, altered sensorium, vomiting, and (in infants) fullness of the fontanelles. Herniation syndromes are similar to those seen in the adult.

    j. Seizures. Approximately 10% of children hospitalized for head trauma develop seizures.

      (1) Immediate. Seizures may be seen immediately and may be caused by depolarization of the cortex secondary to trauma and usually have no prognostic impact.

      (2) Early seizures (within 1 week) are usually secondary to local injury and may be focal or generalized; approximately 25% of these children develop posttraumatic epilepsy.

      (3) Late posttraumatic seizures may be caused by cortical scarring; approximately 75% of these children continue to have seizures.

3. Spinal cord injury is uncommon in the pediatric age group, accounting for approximately 5% of all spinal cord injuries seen. More children than adults, though, may have spinal cord injury without radiographic abnormality (SCIWORA).

4. Chest injuries may be seen without any evidence of external chest-wall injury. Children are less tolerant of a flail chest, given the increased compliance of their chest walls. Signs of respiratory distress include tachypnea, nasal flaring, grunting, and use of accessory muscles (seen as retractions).

    a. Pulmonary contusions and hemorrhages may be seen more often in children secondary to the elasticity of the chest. Patients may show minimal radiographic or physical signs. Tachypnea, rales, hemoptysis, and decreased arterial oxygen tension (PaO_2) may be seen.

    b. Pneumothoraces, tension pneumothoraces, and **hemothoraces** may occur in children as well as in adults. Displacement of the mediastinum may occur more readily in the child because the mediastinum is less rigidly fixed than in the adult. Less major vascular injuries are seen in the child as compared with the adult.

    c. Pericardial tamponade may occur after penetrating or crush injury. The presentation is similar to that in adult patients.

5. Abdominal injuries may occur after blunt or penetrating trauma. Abdominal distention can compromise ventilation more in children than adults because of their greater reliance on excursion of the diaphragm for breathing.

    a. Hepatic and splenic injuries. The liver and spleen are commonly injured. Early symptoms are caused by blood loss.

    b. Pancreatic injuries are caused by rapid deceleration injuries or following direct blows to the upper abdominal area (e.g., handlebar injuries), causing compression of the midportion of the pancreas against the lumbar spine.

    c. Duodenal injuries should also be suspected in a patient with a history of a direct blow to the upper abdomen. Injury may lead to retroperitoneal leak, duodenal disruption, or intramural hematoma. Symptoms of intestinal obstruction may be seen with duodenal hematoma.

    d. Renal injuries are similar to those seen in the adult. Microscopic hematuria after blunt trauma is more aggressively evaluated in the child. Bruising, bleeding, or pain in the vaginal, perineal, or rectal areas in children should raise the question of possible sexual abuse.

C Differential diagnosis of traumatic injuries in the child is similar to that in the adult except that hypotension may be seen in isolated head injury. Child abuse must always be ruled out as a possible cause of trauma.

D Evaluation

1. Primary and secondary survey. The evaluation of the pediatric trauma patient should proceed in a systematic fashion, as in adults, with completion of a primary and secondary survey.

    a. Monitoring. Children should be closely monitored with **frequent evaluation of heart rate, capillary refill, mental status,** and **urinary output.**

    b. Assessment of the fontanelles should be done in infants, noting fullness or depression.

  2. Diagnostic imaging studies

    a. CT. In children with abdominal trauma, a CT scan is preferred to diagnostic peritoneal lavage. If there is any evidence of significant head injury, a CT scan with bone windows should be performed to evaluate for fractures as well as underlying brain injury.

    b. Radiography. Skull radiographs may be considered as a screening tool in young children to rule out fracture.

    c. Ultrasonography. Ultrasound may be used to evaluate for free fluid in the abdomen.

  3. Diagnostic peritoneal lavage. If diagnostic peritoneal lavage is performed, care should be taken because of the thinner abdominal wall in children. Between 10 mL/kg and 15 mL/kg of lavage fluid is instilled, up to 1 L total.

  4. Early surgical or neurosurgical consultation should be sought in patients with evidence of any significant trauma.

E Treatment

  1. Initial stabilization proceeds as with the adult patient (i.e., providing oxygen, fluid resuscitation, and ongoing monitoring). The urine output should be maintained at 1 mL/kg/hour.

    a. Fluid resuscitation. Hypothermic patients may be refractory to fluid resuscitation; therefore, warming lights, blankets, and warmed intravenous fluids should be available.

      (1) Fluid resuscitation is initially accomplished with normal saline or Ringer's lactate (20 mL/kg administered as a bolus over 5–10 minutes). If the patient is stable after initial fluid resuscitation, Ringer's lactate or normal saline may be given at 5 mL/kg/hour for several hours. Fluids are adjusted to maintenance levels if the patient remains stable.

      (2) If the patient fails to respond, a repeat bolus of 20 mL/kg may be administered.

      (3) If the patient requires additional fluid resuscitation, PRBCs, 10 mL/kg, are given.

      (4) If ongoing resuscitation is required, surgical intervention must be considered.

    b. Establishment of a patent airway

      (1) Rapid sequence induction (RSI; see Chapter 1 III B 3) may facilitate intubation in some patients.

        (a) Atropine should be given (0.02 mg/kg, minimum dose 0.1 mg, up to 1 mg total) to prevent bradycardia secondary to vagal stimulation.

        (b) Neuromuscular blockade

          (i) A defasciculating dose of **pancuronium is not needed in young children.**

          (ii) The dose of **succinylcholine** is higher in children: 2 mg/kg, as opposed to 1.5 mg/kg for adults and children older than 10–12 years.

      (2) Endotracheal intubation. Endotracheal tube size may be estimated using the following formula: (16 + age in years) ÷ 4. Uncuffed endotracheal tubes are used in patients younger than 6–8 years (Table 17–1).

      (3) Nasotracheal intubation may be considered in **adolescents** but should be avoided in children.

      (4) Cricothyrotomy is not recommended in children. The cricothyroid membrane may be difficult to locate and is easily damaged, and accidental puncture of the cricothyroid artery (which runs horizontally over the superior portion of the cricothyroid membrane) can be associated with significant bleeding. If an orotracheal airway cannot be obtained, needle cricothyrotomy with a 14-gauge angiocatheter connected to a Y adaptor and a high-flow oxygen source may be used as a temporizing measure.

  2. Management of pneumothorax or **hemothorax. Chest tube placement** or **needle thoracostomy** is carried out as for an adult, with age-appropriate tubes. An 18-gauge needle may be used for needle decompression of tension pneumothorax.

  3. Management of increased ICP is with hyperventilation. Administration of mannitol and furosemide is considered. Seizures are treated acutely with benzodiazepines. Phenytoin (15 mg/kg, to a maximum dose of 1 g) is administered at a rate of 1 mg/kg/min or 25–50 mg/min, whichever is slower.

TABLE 17–1 Pediatric Equipment

Age, Weight (kg)	Airway/Breathing				
	O₂ MASK	ORAL AIRWAYS	BAG-VALVE MASK	LARYNGOSCOPE BLADES	ENDOTRACHEAL TUBES
Premature, 3 kg	Premature infant Newborn	Infant	Infant	0—Straight	2.5–3.0 Uncuffed
Newborn 0–6 months, 3.5 kg	NB	Infant Small	Infant	1—Straight	3.0–3.5 Uncuffed
6–12 months, 7 kg	PED	Small	PED	1—Straight	3.5–4.5 Uncuffed
1–3 years, 10–12 kg	PED	Small	PED	1—Straight	4.0–4.5 Uncuffed
4–7 years, 16–18 kg	PED	Medium	PED	2—Straight or curved	5.0–5.5 Uncuffed
8–10 years, 24–30 kg	Adult	Medium Large	PED Adult	2–3—Straight or curved	5.5–6.5 Cuffed

Reprinted with permission from American College of Surgeons. *Advanced Trauma Life Support (ATLS) Core Course Student Manual.* Chicago: American College of Surgeons, 1988:231.

4. **Management of abdominal injuries.** Abdominal injuries are more frequently managed nonoperatively in the child than in the adult, with close ongoing monitoring and operative intervention if the patient deteriorates. **Nasogastric decompression of the stomach** should be accomplished if there is gastric distention to prevent diaphragmatic elevation.

F **Disposition**   Children with minor head injury and no loss of consciousness, normal neurologic examination, and a reliable caretaker may be discharged. Many children with isolated orthopedic injuries may also be treated and discharged home. Patients with any other significant injury require admission to a general pediatric floor or to an ICU; some patients may require transfer to a pediatric trauma center.

XII TRAUMA IN PREGNANCY

A **Discussion**   Treatment of the pregnant trauma patient proceeds along the same line as treatment of the nonpregnant patient, with some additional significant differences based on anatomic and physiologic changes during pregnancy. The most important factor in determining fetal outcome is the status of the mother; optimally treating the mother provides the best treatment for the fetus. Some of the **important changes that need to be considered in evaluating and treating the pregnant patient** include the following:

1. Cardiovascular changes
   a. **Cardiac output increases** by the 10th week of pregnancy by 1–1.5 L/min.
   b. **Heart rate increases** by approximately 20 beats.
   c. **Systolic and diastolic blood pressure are lower** in the first and second trimesters, reaching approximately normal levels by term. **Profound hypotension,** secondary to the gravid uterus compressing the inferior vena cava and decreasing preload, may be seen when the pregnant patient is in the supine position.
   d. A **leftward axis with a flipped T wave** may be seen on an ECG in leads III and F.
2. Hematologic changes
   a. **Physiologic anemia.** Pregnant patients have a greater increase in plasma volume than in RBC mass, resulting in a physiologic anemia of pregnancy.
   b. The **WBC count is increased.**
   c. Pregnancy results in a **hypercoagulable state** secondary to increased clotting factors and venous stasis.

		Circulation			Supplemental Equipment		
STYLET	SUCTION	BLOOD PRESSURE CUFF	INTRAVENOUS CATHETER	NASOGASTRIC TUBES	CHEST TUBES	FOLEY URINE COLLECTOR	CERVICAL COLLAR
6 Fr	6–8 Fr	Premature infant Newborn	22 Gauge	12 Fr Anderson	10–14 Fr	5 Fr Feeding	—
6 Fr	8 Fr	Newborn Infant	22 Gauge	12 Fr Anderson	12–18 Fr	5–8 Fr Feeding	—
6 Fr	8–10 Fr	Infant Child	22 Gauge	12 Fr Anderson	14–20 Fr	8 Fr	Small
6 Fr	10 Fr	Child	20–22 Gauge	12 Fr Anderson	14–24 Fr	10 Fr	Small
14 Fr	14 Fr	Child	20 Gauge	12 Fr Anderson	20–32 Fr	10–12 Fr	Small
14 Fr	14 Fr	Child Adult	18–20 Gauge	12 Fr Anderson	28–38 Fr	12 Fr	Medium

3. **Pulmonary changes**
    a. The pregnant patient has **decreased oxygen reserve** secondary to decreased functional residual capacity and increased oxygen consumption. The diaphragm is elevated as uterine size increases.
    b. **Increased risk of aspiration.** Decreased gastric motility and gastric emptying times place the pregnant patient at greater risk of aspiration.

4. **Renal changes. BUN and creatinine are decreased** by approximately 50% secondary to increased glomerular filtration rate. Dilatation of the collecting system may be seen.

5. **Orthopedic changes.** There is **widening of the symphysis pubis** from approximately 4 mm to approximately 7–8 mm because cartilages are softened in preparation for childbirth. Blood flow to the pelvis is increased by 20%–35%.

6. **Endocrine changes.** The **pituitary gland increases in size** and is at increased risk of ischemia, necrosis, and decreased pituitary function (Sheehan's syndrome) if blood flow to it is diminished.

B **Clinical features**

1. **Abruptio placentae,** separation of the placenta from the uterine wall, is the most common cause of fetal death after trauma. There may be little evidence of external abdominal trauma. It should be suspected in patients who have sustained deceleration injuries as well as direct trauma to the abdomen. Disseminated intravascular coagulation (DIC) may develop after abruption secondary to release of placental thromboplastin or myometrial plasminogen activator. Findings may include:
    a. Abdominal pain
    b. Uterine tenderness
    c. Tetanic contractions
    d. Amniotic fluid leak
    e. Enlarging uterus
    f. Evidence of fetal distress (noted on fetal heart monitoring)
    g. Vaginal bleeding

2. **Uterine rupture** is not commonly seen and results from significant forces causing increases in intrauterine pressure. It may follow direct abdominal trauma, rapid deceleration injuries, or pelvic trauma. Maternal shock, abdominal pain, peritoneal signs, and fetal parts outside of the uterus may be found.

3. **Fetomaternal hemorrhage,** or passage of fetal RBCs into the normally separate maternal circulation, can occur after relatively minor trauma. In Rh-negative mothers, it can lead to development of maternal antibodies against Rh-positive fetal RBCs and to subsequent hemolysis of fetal RBCs.

   a. **Rh$_o$(D) immune globulin (RhoGAM)** can prevent this isoimmunization if administered within 72 hours of maternal exposure to fetal cells. The usual dose is 300 µg for every 30 mL of fetal blood found in the maternal circulation.

   b. The **Kleihauer-Betke test** can measure the amount of fetal–maternal hemorrhage in milliliters and should be used in suspected cases of massive fetomaternal hemorrhage. In pregnancies of less than 16 weeks' duration, the fetal blood volume, and therefore fetomaternal hemorrhage, would not be expected to exceed 30 mL.

C **Differential diagnosis**

1. **Seizures** may be seen after head injury or in eclampsia (i.e., third-trimester hypertension, hyper-reflexia, confusion, headache, epigastric pain, seizures, or coma).

2. **Peritoneal signs** may be seen with uterine rupture or with other sources of hemoperitoneum (e.g., ruptured spleen or liver).

3. **Decreased blood pressure and increased heart rate** may reflect normal physiologic changes of pregnancy.

D **Evaluation**

1. **Primary and secondary surveys** should be carried out.

   a. **Fetal monitoring** should be performed for at least 4 hours after significant injury or mechanism. **Evidence of fetal distress** (fetal heart monitoring showing late decelerations or loss of beat-to-beat variability) may be an **early sign of maternal distress.** As blood is shunted away from nonessential organs in the mother, uterine blood flow decreases, affecting the fetus before signs of maternal hypotension are seen.

   b. **Pelvic examination** should assess for the presence of blood, amniotic fluid, cervical dilatation and effacement, presenting part, and station.

   c. **Abdominal examination** should assess for uterine size (with estimate of gestational age/viability), uterine tenderness, and contractions.

2. **Patient history.** The patient should be asked about her prenatal history, any problems with the pregnancy (e.g., pre-eclampsia), the presence of abdominal pain or known contractions, known rupture of membranes, the presence of fetal movements, and vaginal bleeding.

3. **Laboratory studies.** The **Kleihauer-Betke test** should be performed if the pregnancy is 16 weeks or longer in gestational age in an Rh-negative mother.

4. **Diagnostic imaging studies.** Indicated **radiographic studies** should be obtained as mandated by the condition of the mother, shielding the abdomen when possible.

5. **Early obstetric consultation** should be sought.

E **Treatment**   The pregnant patient is treated as the nonpregnant patient is, with the following additions:

1. Unless spinal injury is suspected, the pregnant patient with a fetus of greater than 20 weeks' gestational age should be **positioned on her left side.** Alternatively, the backboard can be tilted, or the gravid uterus can be manually displaced off the vena cava.

2. Given the greater circulating blood volume of the pregnant patient, a **greater volume of fluid resuscitation is required,** especially if there is any evidence of fetal distress or maternal hypovolemia.

3. **Tetanus prophylaxis** with either tetanus–diphtheria toxoid or tetanus immunoglobulin may be given as indicated.

F **Disposition**   Pregnant patients should undergo fetal heart monitoring for at least 4 hours. Patients should go to the operating room or ICU as dictated by their injuries.

XIII   **BURNS**

A **Discussion**   Approximately 2 million patients per year present to EDs with burns. Of these, roughly 100,000 patients require hospitalization. There are approximately 20,000 deaths per year related to immediate or delayed complications of burns. Death rates are higher in children younger than 4 years of age and in adults older than 65 years of age.

1. **Classification of burns**
   a. **First-degree burn** involves only the epidermis and is characterized by erythema, edema, pain, and the absence of blistering. Sunburn is an example of first-degree burn.
   b. **Second-degree burn** involves the dermis and is a partial-thickness burn. It may be further classified as a superficial or deep partial-thickness burn. In superficial burns, deeper layers of the dermis, including hair follicles and sweat glands, are not involved. These burns are characterized by blisters and pain.
   c. **Third-degree burns** are full-thickness burns and involve the epidermis, dermis, and subcutaneous fat. The skin is charred and leathery, and thrombosed blood vessels may be seen. These burns are insensate.
   d. **Fourth-degree burns** are those involving structures underlying the skin, including fascia, bone, and muscle.

2. **Size of the burn** is expressed as a percentage of body surface area. Estimating the percentage of burn area is important in determining the amount of fluid resuscitation the patient needs.
   a. The **"rule of nines"** divides the body surface area into areas of approximately 9% each. In children, the head accounts for a larger percentage of body surface area, whereas the legs account for a smaller percentage (Figure 17–6).
   b. The **"rule of palms"** approximates that the palm size of the patient estimates 1% of the patient's body surface area. Adding up the number of palm areas gives the approximate percentage of body surface area burned.
   c. A **Lund-Browder burn diagram** provides for burn estimates adjusted for age.

3. **Inhalation burns,** which may be associated with carbon monoxide poisoning, poisoning by other noxious gases, or thermal injury to the airways, may be suspected if burns occurred in an enclosed space, involved the face, singed nasal hairs, or caused carbonaceous sputum. The **half-life of carbon monoxide** is approximately 4–5 hours at room air, 90 minutes on 100% oxygen, and 20 minutes on hyperbaric oxygen at three atmospheres.

B **Differential diagnosis**

1. **Deep partial-thickness burns** may sometimes be confused with full-thickness burns. Absence of pain may not be diagnostic if there is significant edema present in a partial-thickness burn.
2. Signs of possible **inhalation injury** may overestimate the actual presence of smoke inhalation.
3. **Hypotension** may be secondary to a major burn, but other causes of hypotension secondary to trauma must be ruled out, especially if the burn is associated with explosions, motor vehicle collisions, or falls.
4. **Altered mental status** may be caused by inhalation injury, but other causes of altered sensorium must be ruled out, including head trauma, ingestions, hypoglycemia and other metabolic causes, and decreased perfusion.
5. **Abuse or neglect.** All **pediatric patients** presenting with burns need to be assessed for the possibility of abuse or neglect.

C **Evaluation**   Burn patients should be evaluated as trauma patients until the presence of other injuries has been fully assessed. Efforts should be made to **avoid contamination** of the burn.

1. **Primary and secondary surveys** should be completed on patients with major burns.
   a. Burns should be evaluated for depth and size.

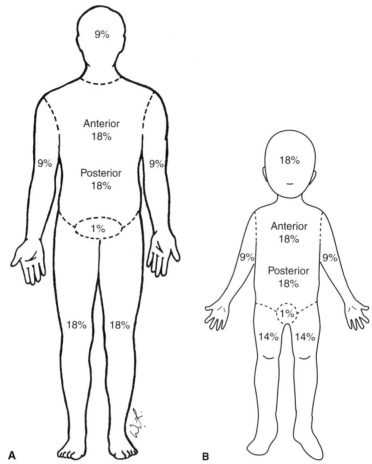

FIGURE 17–6 Approximate burn surface area: **(A)** adult; **(B)** child. (Part A reprinted with permission from Jarrell BE, Carabasi RA III. *NMS Surgery.* 3rd Ed. Baltimore: Williams & Wilkins, 1996:404.)

    b. The **eyes** should be closely examined for presence of any corneal burns.

    c. Peripheral pulses, perfusion, and **sensation** should be carefully evaluated, especially at points distal to circumferential burns.

  2. Patient history. A history of the burn should include where the burn occurred, the time of the burn, possible exposure to gases and chemicals, falls or jumps associated with the burn, and any explosions or other trauma.

  3. Laboratory studies may include a CBC; serum electrolyte panel; BUN, creatinine, and glucose levels; ABG determinations; carbon monoxide level; creatine phosphokinase level; urinalysis; urinary myoglobin; toxicology screen; and ethanol level. Laboratory work is determined by the extent and circumstances of the burn.

  4. Diagnostic imaging studies. A **chest radiograph** should be obtained but may initially appear normal.

  5. Other studies. Fiberoptic bronchoscopy can evaluate the larger airways in patients with suspected inhalation injury.

D **Treatment**

  1. Transport. The burn should be covered with sterile sheets, except for small burns, which may be covered with cool cloths.

2. **Initial burn treatment**
   a. The burning process should be terminated by removing the patient from the burn environment and removing all burning clothing.
   b. The patient should be appropriately immobilized pending assessment of other injuries, and the ABCs of trauma care should be provided.
   c. Patients with possibility of inhalation injury should have **100% oxygen administered** and their airway should be assessed. **Early intubation** should be considered for patients with possible airway compromise.
   d. Hypothermia should be avoided.

3. **Fluid resuscitation** should be undertaken for adult patients with burns that exceed approximately 20% of the body surface area. Lactated Ringer's solution or normal saline is administered at a rate of 2–4 mL/kg/% total body surface area burned. The first half of required fluids should be administered in the first 8 hours from the time of the burn, with the remainder of fluids given over the following 16 hours. Children generally require this amount of fluid in addition to normal maintenance fluids. To assess for adequacy of fluid resuscitation, urinary output should be monitored (30–50 mL/hour in adults or 1 mL/kg/hour in children).

4. **Cleansing, debridement,** and **application of topical antibiotics.** Burn wounds are gently cleansed, and devitalized tissue is débrided. Once evaluated at the definitive treatment center, the burn may be covered with a topical antibiotic ointment (e.g., silver sulfadiazine). Some centers prefer bacitracin for facial burns.

5. **Tetanus immunization** may be indicated, depending on the extent of the burn and the patient's immunization history.

6. Patients with greater than approximately 20% body surface area burn are prone to **ileus** and should have a **nasogastric tube** inserted.

7. **Escharotomy** may be required for circumferential burns to the extremities or chest.

8. **Intravenous antibiotics** are generally not employed initially.

9. **Analgesia** should be administered carefully, monitoring cardiovascular response.

E **Disposition** of the burn patient depends on the extent of the burn, age of the patient, location of the burn, comorbid factors, and associated injuries, as well as factors such as patient's ability to care for the wound, safety for the patient, and capabilities of the hospital to which the patient initially presents.

1. **Admission.** Patients who meet any of the following criteria should be admitted:
   a. Healthy adults with partial-thickness burns affecting more than 15% of the body surface area or full-thickness burns affecting more than 5% of the total body surface area
   b. Young children and older adults with partial-thickness burns affecting more than 10% of the body surface area or full-thickness burns affecting more than 3% of the body surface area
   c. Patients with burns involving the face, hands, perineum, or feet
   d. Patients with circumferential burns or those covering major joints
   e. Patients with electrical or chemical burns
   f. Patients with burns associated with inhalation injury or trauma
   g. Immunocompromised patients
   h. Patients with burns associated with child abuse

2. **Burn center treatment.** Burns for which treatment at a burn center is recommended include burns of greater than 25% in healthy patients aged 10–50 years, burns involving greater than 20% in patients younger than 10 years or older than 50 years, or full-thickness burns involving greater than 10% of the total body surface area.

3. **Discharge.** Patients with burns covering less than 15% of the total body surface area in healthy adults or less than 10% in children and older adults, and those not meeting any other criteria for admission may be treated locally and referred for close follow-up.

Study Questions

Directions: Each of the numbered items or incomplete statements in this section is followed by answers or by completions of the statement. Select the ONE lettered answer or completion that is BEST in each case.

1. A patient presents to the emergency department (ED) with a near-complete amputation of his left lower extremity. The initial intervention for this patient is to

   (A) apply a tourniquet to stop the bleeding
   (B) apply direct pressure to control the bleeding
   (C) clamp off any obvious bleeding vessels
   (D) assess the distal extremity for any pulses
   (E) assess the patient's airway and breathing

2. A patient presents after a motor vehicle collision at which he was found ambulatory at the scene. He is anxious, smells of alcohol, and has a heart rate of 110 beats/min, a blood pressure of 110/90 mm Hg, a normal capillary refill, and normal urinary output. This patient is assessed in which one of the following ways?

   (A) He is intoxicated and an early head computed tomography (CT) scan should be planned to rule out head injury.
   (B) He may be in class I hemorrhage (up to 15% of blood volume loss).
   (C) He may be in class II hemorrhage (15%–30% of blood volume loss).
   (D) He may be in class III hemorrhage (30%–40% of blood volume loss).
   (E) He may be in class IV hemorrhage (40% of blood volume loss).

3. The estimated blood volume in an average adult is

   (A) 7% of body weight (in kilograms)
   (B) 8% of body weight (in kilograms)
   (C) a greater percentage of body weight than that of a child
   (D) approximately 7 L

4. Zone I neck injuries are those in the region including which one of the following anatomic sites?

   (A) The thoracic inlet
   (B) The area between the clavicular heads and the angle of the mandible
   (C) The area above the angle of the mandible
   (D) The area posterior to the sternocleidomastoid muscle

5. A patient presents to the emergency department (ED) after blunt head trauma with unknown loss of consciousness. His family reports that he was initially confused, became alert, but again appears less awake. He has bruising over the left temporal area. Which of the following is the most likely cause of his symptoms?

   (A) Epidural hematoma
   (B) Subarachnoid hemorrhage
   (C) Subdural hematoma
   (D) Diffuse axonal injury
   (E) Concussion

6. A patient with a known history of alcohol abuse is brought to the emergency department (ED) after a fall in which he struck his head. A head computed tomography (CT) scan reveals a crescent-shaped hyperdense lesion. The correct diagnosis is

    A epidural hematoma
    B subarachnoid hemorrhage
    C subdural hematoma
    D diffuse axonal injury
    E concussion

7. A 50-year-old man presents to the emergency department (ED) after a high-speed motor vehicle collision. He has bruises on his head and is comatose. The head computed tomography (CT) scan reveals no focal lesion. Which is the likely cause of his symptoms?

    A Epidural hematoma
    B Subarachnoid hemorrhage
    C Subdural hematoma
    D Diffuse axonal injury
    E Concussion

8. A 16-year-old girl is involved in a 55-mph collision in her car and remembers flexing her neck hard. She sustains multiple injuries, and her neurologic examination reveals motor paralysis, loss of pain and temperature sensation, and preserved posterior column function (position sense, light touch, and vibration). Her diagnosis is

    A anterior cord syndrome
    B central cord syndrome
    C Brown-Séquard syndrome
    D spinal shock
    E neurogenic shock

9. A young male gang member is stabbed in the neck and suffers paralysis, loss of gross proprioception and vibration on the same side as the lesion, and contralateral loss of pain and temperature sensation. His diagnosis is

    A anterior cord syndrome
    B central cord syndrome
    C Brown-Séquard syndrome
    D spinal shock
    E neurogenic shock

10. A 15-year-old male is brought to the emergency room after tackling a large football player. He remembers being knocked backwards hard, and then had a burning sensation and weakness of his arms. His neurologic deficit of the upper extremities is more pronounced than that in the lower extremities with scattered sensory losses. His diagnosis is

    A anterior cord syndrome
    B central cord syndrome
    C Brown-Séquard syndrome
    D spinal shock
    E neurogenic shock

Answers and Explanations

1. The answer is E Although several interventions may occur simultaneously in the trauma patient, the initial assessment in a systematic fashion must always start with the primary survey to identify the immediate life threats. Trauma patients often present with incomplete histories of their injuries, and the obvious injury may not be the only injury (e.g., the patient may have sustained significant head or chest injury at the same time as the extremity injury). The mistake of missing the critical injury while treating the more evident injury should be avoided. Direct pressure to control bleeding is preferred to tourniquets, and blindly clamping open wounds may injure nerves and vessels. Distal pulses should be assessed after airway and breathing are evaluated.

2. The answer is C Narrowed pulse pressure, normal capillary refill, anxiety or mild agitation, and near-normal urine output may be seen in patients with up to 800–1500 mL blood loss (class II hemorrhage). The intoxicated patient always presents a challenge in the evaluation of his injuries, because mental status changes are seen secondary to the amount of alcohol ingested, the examination is unreliable, and details of the mechanism of injury are often unknown. Although evaluating for head injury is mandated in this case, early signs of hypoperfusion should not be prematurely ascribed to an intoxicated state.

3. The answer is A Blood volume is estimated to be approximately 7% of body weight (in kilograms) in the adult, or 5 L in a 70-kg person. In children, blood volume represents a greater percentage of body weight, estimated at 8%–9% of body weight, or approximately 80 mL/kg.

4. The answer is A The neck is divided into zones to aid in injury management. Zone I is the thoracic inlet and lies below the head of the clavicles (or below the cricoid cartilage by some definitions). Zone II is above the clavicles to the angle of the mandible, and zone III is above the angle of the mandible. The neck is also divided into triangles. The anterior triangle is above the clavicles, anterior to the posterior border of the sternocleidomastoid muscle, and is covered by the platysma. The posterior triangle is bordered by the sternocleidomastoid muscle, the clavicle, and the trapezius.

5. The answer is A The first patient has evidence of head trauma in the temporal area and a history of a lucid interval. Epidural hemorrhage should be suspected in patients with head trauma involving the temporal area, where the middle meningeal artery passes between the dura and the skull. A brief initial period of unconsciousness is followed by a lucid interval with subsequent deterioration in neurologic status secondary to increased intracranial pressure (ICP).

6. The answer is C This patient has a subdural hematoma, which usually results from tearing of the bridging veins traversing the subdural space. It is seen as a crescent-shaped density on the head CT scan.

7. The answer is D This patient presents with diffuse axonal injury due to shearing or tearing of nerve fibers. Diffuse axonal injury is characterized by coma in the absence of a focal lesion, and often the CT scan appears normal or with nonspecific findings. Later, magnetic resonance imaging (MRI) studies will reveal significant diffuse edema and swelling, followed by some degree of healing.

8. The answer is A The anterior cord syndrome usually follows a cervical flexion injury that causes compression of the anterior spinal cord. Injury to the anterior spinal artery can also cause the deficits that characterize anterior cord syndrome (i.e., motor paralysis and loss of pain and temperature sensation seen in the presence of preserved posterior column function).

9. **The answer is C** The Brown-Séquard syndrome, or hemisection of the cord, is usually the result of penetrating injuries or lateral mass fractures. It is characterized by paralysis, loss of gross proprioception and vibration on the same side of the lesion, and contralateral loss of pain and temperature sensation.

10. **The answer is B** The central cord syndrome typically follows a hyperextension injury, and is seen most often in patients with degenerative arthritis of the cervical spine. The ligamentum flavum buckles into the cord, resulting in a concussion of the most central portions of the cord (the gray matter and the most central portions of the pyramidal and spinothalamic tracts). Neurologic findings include neurologic deficit of the upper extremities that is more pronounced than that in the lower extremities and scattered sensory losses. Spinal shock is the immediate neurologic condition seen after spinal cord injury. It is characterized by flaccidity and areflexia. Neurogenic shock is associated with cervical or high thoracic injuries, causing impairment of the descending sympathetic pathways. It is characterized by hypotension and bradycardia.

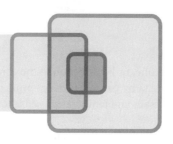

chapter 18

Orthopedic Emergencies

DAVID L. MORGAN

I INTRODUCTION

Orthopedic emergencies are acute medical problems involving the abnormal form or function of the extremities, spine, or associated structures. Orthopedic emergencies are common in the emergency department (ED) and can be a threat to long-term limb function.

A Types of orthopedic emergencies

1. **Muscle contusion (bruise).** A muscle contusion is an extravasation of blood into the muscle tissue. Initially, the bruised muscle will be swollen and tender, and the overlying skin will appear red or blue (ecchymosis). As the blood is resorbed, the skin changes in color from purple to greenish yellow.

2. **Strain.** Muscle strains are classified by the amount of muscle fiber injury that results when the muscle is excessively stretched or when the muscle is forcibly contracted against resistance.
   a. **First-degree muscle strain** is a minor stretching injury of the muscle fibers that is characterized by muscle spasm, mild swelling, local tenderness, and a slight decrease in function.
   b. **Second-degree muscle strain** is a partial tearing of the muscle fibers that is characterized by moderate swelling, ecchymosis, and decreased strength.
   c. **Third-degree muscle strain** is a complete disruption of the muscle that is characterized by swelling, ecchymosis, decreased strength, and a palpable "bulge" caused by the retracted muscle belly. Third-degree muscle strains can lead to significant long-term disability, but fortunately, are not as common as first- and second-degree strains. Third-degree strains require immobilization and early follow-up for potential surgical repair.

3. **Sprain.** Sprains are injuries to joint ligaments that result from a forced abnormal motion of the joint.
   a. **First-degree sprains** are characterized by mild hemorrhage and swelling, minimal point tenderness, and no abnormal joint motion (i.e., the joint is stable).
   b. **Second-degree sprains,** which occur when the ligaments are partially torn, result in moderate hemorrhage and swelling, tenderness, painful motion, loss of function, and minor joint laxity.
   c. **Third-degree sprains** occur when the joint ligaments are completely disrupted. Third-degree sprains may initially appear similar to second-degree sprains, but the patient will have severely abnormal joint motion after the swelling subsides.

4. **Dislocation.** A joint is dislocated when the articular surfaces of the bones are no longer in contact with each other. **Subluxation** is an incomplete dislocation (i.e., the articular surfaces are in partial contact). In order for a dislocation or subluxation to occur, the joint ligaments must be disrupted; therefore, dislocations and subluxations are characterized by swelling, pain, and tenderness around the joint.

5. **Fracture.** A fracture is the disruption of the bony cortex. The broken bone bleeds into the surrounding tissue, resulting in pain, swelling, and deformity.

a. Descriptive terms. The fracture must be fully described for the medical record and for the initial discussion with the orthopedic consultant. Important details include the following: whether the fracture is open or closed, the affected bone and the location of the fracture on the bone, whether intra-articular extension has occurred, the type of fracture line, whether the fracture is complete or incomplete, and the position or alignment of the bone segments.

(1) An **open fracture** occurs when the bone pierces the skin. An open fracture can occur when a bone fragment pierces the skin and then withdraws, leaving only a small puncture wound. Therefore, any fracture with an overlying skin wound should be suspected of being open. A **closed fracture** occurs when the skin and soft tissue overlying the fracture are intact.

(2) An **intra-articular fracture** is a fracture that extends into the joint.

(3) The fracture line may be **spiral, oblique, transverse,** or **butterfly** (Figure 18–1). Fractures in children are often described as **bend, buckle (torus), greenstick,** or **complete** fractures (Figure 18–2). A fracture can also be described as a **compression, avulsion (chip),** or **comminuted (shattered)** fracture.

(4) The bone segments may be in contact with each other or separated by a measurable distance (usually stated in millimeters). The bone segments may be completely **displaced** (i.e., lying next to each other instead of end to end), **partially displaced** (i.e., offset from each other by a measured amount), or **nondisplaced.**

(5) The **angulation** of the two bone segments is described by both the **direction of the angle** (e.g., radial, dorsal, anterior, lateral) and by the **degree of the angle** formed by the two bone segments.

b. Special fractures

(1) Pathologic fractures occur when relatively minor force is applied to diseased or otherwise weakened bone.

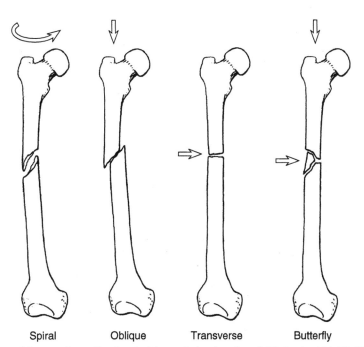

| Spiral | Oblique | Transverse | Butterfly |

FIGURE 18–1 Types of fracture lines. (Reprinted with permission from Jarrell BE, Carabasi RA III. *NMS Surgery.* 3rd Ed. Baltimore: Williams & Wilkins, 1996:528.)

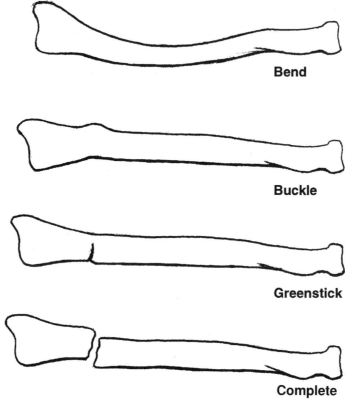

Bend

Buckle

Greenstick

Complete

FIGURE 18–2 Children's fractures. (Reprinted with permission from Jarrell BE, Carabasi RA III. *NMS Surgery*. 3rd Ed. Baltimore: Williams & Wilkins, 1996:529.)

    (2) **Stress fractures** are caused by the repetitive application of minor force to a bone, usually a long bone in the lower extremities. Stress fractures are commonly seen in military personnel and athletes (e.g., joggers, dancers).

    (3) **Salter-Harris fractures** (Figure 18–3) involve the epiphyseal plate (i.e., the growth plate) and are common in children. Damage to the epiphyseal plate may destroy its ability to form new bone, resulting in malformations as the child grows.

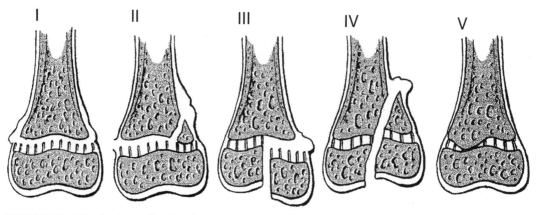

I   II   III   IV   V

FIGURE 18–3 Salter-Harris classification of epiphyseal fractures. Note that type III and IV injuries are intra-articular fractures. Type V injuries are crush injuries. (Reprinted with permission from Jarrell BE, Carabasi RA III. *NMS Surgery*. 3rd Ed. Baltimore: Williams & Wilkins, 1996:533.)

B **Diagnosis of orthopedic emergencies** Most orthopedic emergencies can be diagnosed by a careful patient history and a thorough physical examination. The emergency physician uses the history and physical examination to discern the type and degree of injury and to choose the specific radiographic view that will verify the diagnosis.

1. **Patient history**
   a. **Patient age.** The patient's age may give some indication of the type of injury (e.g., Salter-Harris fractures only occur in young patients, whereas hip fractures are more common in the elderly).
   b. **Chief complaint.** Patients with orthopedic emergencies usually present with one or more of the following extremity complaints: **pain, swelling, redness, deformity,** or an **inability to use the extremity.** Patients with sprains may describe hearing a "pop" at the time of the injury. The location of the chief complaint may or may not reflect the location of the injury (e.g., knee pain may occur with a hip fracture).
   c. **Mechanism of injury**
      (1) The mechanism of injury (i.e., how the injury occurred) is important for predicting the type of injury. For example, if the physician does not know the mechanism of injury, it may be difficult for him or her to reach a diagnosis in a young child with normal radiographs who refuses to use his or her right arm. However, if the physician knows that the child had been recently pulled by that arm, the probable diagnosis (subluxation of the radial head) becomes readily apparent.
      (2) The mechanism of injury also aids in determining which radiographic views to obtain, especially when the patient is unable to cooperate, has referred pain, or has a distracting injury. For example, a patient who complains of acute shoulder pain after an injury may have a normal routine shoulder radiograph. However, if the mechanism of injury suggests posterior dislocation, then an additional view of the shoulder can be obtained to confirm this diagnosis.
   d. **Pre-existing illnesses or conditions.** The physician should inquire about illnesses and conditions that may affect healing (e.g., diabetes, heart disease, steroid therapy, cancer chemotherapy).

2. **Physical examination**
   a. **Inspection.** The entire extremity should be inspected for swelling, discoloration, deformity, abrasions, puncture wounds, and lacerations.
      (1) Orthopedic injuries (including fractures) may have few or no obvious visible abnormalities, especially in children.
      (2) Muscle contusions and severe sprains may result in localized swelling that is similar to the swelling seen with fractures. Sometimes radiographs are needed to differentiate sprains and fractures.
   b. **Palpation** of the entire extremity may reveal point tenderness, subtle deformities (e.g., a "step off"), or bony crepitus. The area distal and proximal to the pain location should be systematically palpated. For example, in a patient who complains of hip pain, the hip, thigh, knee, ankle, and foot should be meticulously palpated. Complete palpation is important for two reasons:
      (1) The patient may be unaware of a second injury because of the pain of the primary injury.
      (2) If radiographs are ordered prior to complete palpation, radiographs of the specific bone may not be obtained.
   c. **Range of motion assessment.** Each joint proximal and distal to the injury should be assessed for both passive and active range of motion. The degree of flexion, extension, and pain should be noted. This examination of the function of the joint may need to be repeated on the contralateral (unaffected) joint to discern slight abnormalities.
   d. **Neurologic examination.** Nerve injury can result in either sensory or motor deficits. Sensation distal to the injury should be identified before any manipulation of the extremity takes place. Muscles that are innervated by the major nerves of the extremity should be examined for motor function.

e. **Arterial blood flow assessment.** Some orthopedic emergencies (e.g., knee dislocation, fracture or dislocation of the ankle, supracondylar fracture of the elbow in children) are commonly associated with vascular (arterial) injuries. The earlier circulatory compromise is identified and addressed, the less likely it is that permanent injury will result.

3. **Radiography**
   a. **Views**
      (1) **Standard.** The area to be examined radiographically should be based on the history and physical examination findings. The joint above and the joint below a fracture should be included on films to detect associated fractures or dislocations. Most extremity radiographs include an **anterior-posterior (AP) view,** a **lateral view,** and, sometimes, an **oblique view.**
      (2) **Special.** Some fractures are only visible using special radiographic views. Some common orthopedic emergencies that require special views include acromioclavicular separation, fracture of the carpal navicular, posterior shoulder dislocation, and sternoclavicular dislocation. Children may need comparison views of the unaffected extremity to detect epiphyseal plate injuries.
   b. **Findings**
      (1) In the case of **stress fractures,** the initial radiographs may be normal. However, the presence of new bone growth or bone resorption (which causes the fracture line to become visible) on radiographs taken 2–3 weeks later may suggest the fracture. If a fracture is highly suspected but the radiograph is normal, treatment for the fracture should be initiated.
      (2) The normal growth plate appears as a transverse, radiolucent line at the end of the bone. The growth plate can be easily confused with a transverse fracture. Frequently, comparison radiographic views of the unaffected extremity are obtained to differentiate a normal growth plate from an injured one.

C **Basic management of orthopedic emergencies**

1. **Sprains.** Because ligaments are relatively avascular, a sprain may require up to 8 weeks to heal. Physicians should take care to avoid dismissing the injury as "only a sprain"; statements like this can give the patient the unrealistic expectation of a rapid and complete recovery.
   a. **First-** and **second-degree sprains.** Initial treatment entails **RICE**—rest, immobilization, compression and cold packs, and elevation—and **analgesics** or **anti-inflammatory agents.** First- and second-degree sprains usually do not result in long-term sequelae.
   b. **Third-degree sprains.** Urgent orthopedic consultation should be obtained for patients with third-degree sprains, which can lead to permanently decreased joint function. These sprains are sometimes immobilized in circumferential casts for several weeks and **may require surgical repair.**

2. **Fractures and dislocations**
   a. **Stabilization of the patient.** Although orthopedic emergencies are seldom life-threatening, concurrent life-threatening injuries may be present. Therefore, **airway, breathing,** and **circulation** (the **ABCs**) should be assessed first, and appropriate measures taken. In multiple trauma patients, airway, head, thorax, and abdominal injuries are treated before orthopedic injuries.
   b. **Reduction of swelling.** Swelling occurs early after a fracture or dislocation and can increase the patient's pain and delay the application of definitive immobilization.
      (1) Elevation of the extremity and application of cold compresses are effective measures for preventing the progression of swelling.
      (2) Jewelry on the affected extremity should be removed.
   c. **Temporary immobilization.** The suspected fracture or dislocation should be immobilized at the beginning of the ED visit. Immobilization reduces the patient's pain, minimizes the potential for damage to the neurovascular bundle, reduces swelling and bleeding, facilitates patient transport, expedites the radiographic examination, and, in the case of fractures, reduces the

chance of a sharp bone fragment puncturing the skin and converting a closed fracture to an open fracture.

(1) For **fractures,** temporary immobilization is accomplished by **splinting** across the fracture and the joints proximal and distal to the fracture.

(2) For **dislocations,** the joint may be immobilized using a **splint** or **sling.**

d. **Pain control.** Most patients with fractures or dislocations will be relatively comfortable at rest when the extremity is sufficiently immobilized and there is only minimal swelling. For those patients who may require general anesthesia at a later time, only parenteral analgesics should be given in the ED.

e. **Reduction** is the process of restoring the bone or joint to its original shape. Early reduction decreases pain, may restore circulatory or nerve function, and prevents the progression of swelling. Not all fractures require reduction—the decision to reduce a fracture depends on the age of the patient, the involved bone, the location of the fracture, and the amount of deformity.

(1) Generally, a radiograph of the bone or joint is obtained prior to the reduction of the fracture or dislocation. However, when there is gross deformity and no palpable distal pulse, emergent reduction is indicated to restore circulation to the limb.

(2) Analgesics and sedatives are usually required for most reductions, which are generally accomplished by applying slow, steady, longitudinal traction.

(3) A postreduction radiograph is always needed to document the success of the procedure, to determine if additional injuries are present, and to assess the need for additional treatment. A neurovascular examination should also be performed following reduction.

f. **Postreduction immobilization.** Reduced fractures, nonreduced fractures, and reduced dislocations must be immobilized before the patient is released from the ED.

(1) **Splints** or **circumferential casts** are usually used to immobilize **fractures.** Splinting is less likely than circumferential casting to lead to pressure sores, circulatory compromise, and neurapraxia. After the swelling has decreased, a circumferential cast can be applied.

(a) Patients with fractures who are not prone to complications and have only minimal swelling may be treated in the ED with circumferential casting.

(b) Splints are usually made from plaster of Paris or fiberglass. Water causes an exothermic chemical reaction, which causes the material to harden over several minutes. During this process, the splint is molded along one side of the extremity, which is held in the appropriate position. Padding is placed between the skin and splint, and the splint is secured to the extremity with an elastic bandage wrapped circumferentially around the extremity and splint.

(2) **Immobilization dressings.** In addition to splints, several dressings are commonly used in the ED. Examples include the **shoulder sling, sling and swath, knee immobilizer,** and **figure-of-eight bandage.**

g. **Disposition**

(1) **Hospital admission.** Patients at high risk for serious complications (see VII) and those with open fractures, fractures that require open reduction or internal fixation, hip fractures, or severe hand infections may require admission to the hospital or to the operating room.

(2) **Discharge.** Most patients with orthopedic emergencies can be treated in the ED and then discharged with follow-up plans. Prior to discharging the patient, the physician should see that the following general measures have been taken:

(a) The patient should be provided with **discharge instructions.** The patient should be advised to:

(i) Keep the extremity elevated at all times

(ii) Alert a physician if excessive swelling, decreased sensation, discoloration, or increased pain in the digits is observed following the application of a splint

(b) If the patient cannot walk or if the patient should not bear weight on a lower extremity, then arrangements for **crutches** or a **walker** (and instructions for their use) should be provided.

(c) **Pain medication** should be addressed for patients with moderate or severe injuries.

(d) Every patient with a dislocation or a fracture requires **follow-up with an orthopedist or a physician skilled in fracture care.** For most orthopedic emergencies, the emergency physician should contact the follow-up physician to arrange an appointment and discuss a discharge plan appropriate to the injury. For simple fractures and reduced dislocations, the patient should usually be seen within 10 days. For a patient with a more complex injury that may require surgical repair, the patient should be seen sooner.

II HAND AND WRIST INJURIES

Injuries and infections of the wrist and hand result in over 6 million visits to the ED each year.

A Descriptive terms

1. **Location.** The terms **radial, ulnar, palmar (volar),** and **dorsal** are used to describe the location of the hand injury.

2. **Digits.** The digits can be numbered or named: **I (thumb), II (index finger), III (long finger), IV (ring finger),** and **V (little finger).**

3. **Joints.** The joints are the **distal interphalangeal (DIP), proximal interphalangeal (PIP), metacarpophalangeal (MCP),** and **carpometacarpal (CM).**

B Diagnosis

1. **Patient history.** Important aspects of the history include hand dominance (right-handed versus left-handed), details of the mechanism of injury, the position of the hand at the time of injury (e.g., fist, fingers extended), the timing and nature of all symptoms, the patient's occupation, previous hand deficits, and the patient's medical history.

2. **Physical examination**

   a. **Inspection.** Abnormal flexion or extension of individual digits when the hand is at rest should be noted, as should swelling, scars, amputations, and discolorations. When inspecting a tendon for injury through an open wound, the position of the hand and fingers must be the same as they were at the time of injury.

   b. **Palpation** of the entire hand and wrist should be performed to determine deformity or point tenderness. The navicular bone lies in the anatomist's snuff-box; palpation for tenderness is necessary to detect fractures of the navicular bone, which are often occult and not visible radiographically.

   c. **Tendon function assessment.** Each muscle–tendon group is tested individually by determining strength against resistance and pain with motion. When the tendon is completely ruptured, there is no movement; with partial ruptures, pain and decreased strength are seen.

      (1) The deep flexor tendons are assessed by having the patient flex each finger at the DIP joint while the examiner keeps the PIP and MCP joints of all the patient's fingers in extension.

      (2) The superficial flexor tendons are assessed in a similar fashion by having the patient flex each PIP joint while the examiner keeps the patient's other fingers in extension.

      (3) The individual extensor tendons are assessed by having the patient extend all digits. The thumb should be extended and abducted (away from the palm) against resistance.

   d. **Wrist function assessment.** Wrist function is examined by having the patient flex the wrist, extend the wrist, and laterally deviate the wrist to the radial and ulnar side against resistance.

  e. **Neurologic examination**
   (1) **Motor function**
    (a) Because the median nerve innervates the abductor pollicis brevis, this nerve can be tested by having the patient abduct the thumb against resistance.
    (b) The ulnar nerve innervates the hypothenar muscles, the thumb adductor, and the intrinsic interosseous muscles of the hand. This nerve can be tested by determining the strength of the index and little fingers when the patient is instructed to abduct the fingers against resistance.
    (c) The radial nerve is injured if the patient cannot extend the wrist against resistance (wristdrop). The radial nerve innervates no muscles in the hand.
   (2) **Sensation**
    (a) Both the radial and ulnar aspect of each digit (digital nerves) should be tested using 5-mm two-point touch.
    (b) All three nerves to the hand should be assessed by determining sensation at the dorsal web space between the thumb and index finger (radial nerve), the tip of the long finger (median nerve), and the tip of the little finger (ulnar nerve). Light touch should be used to test sensation in the dorsal aspect of the fingers and hand because this area is less sensitive than the palmar aspect.
  f. **Arterial blood flow assessment.** The color, warmth, and nail bed capillary refill time should be examined in each finger. Both radial and ulnar pulses should be palpated.

C **Treatment**

 1. **Wounds** that penetrate the skin frequently damage tendons, nerves, vessels, and joint capsules. Deep sutures should never be placed in the hand by ED personnel (except to repair extensor tendons). Elevation, splinting, and close follow-up are important components in the care of hand wounds.

 2. **Tendon injuries.** Although some complete extensor tendon ruptures can be repaired in the ED, flexor tendon injuries should never be repaired in the ED and always require orthopedic consultation. Partial tendon tears can be treated by splinting the finger (possibly for as long as 6 weeks) and close follow-up.

D **Specific injuries**

 1. **Hand**
  a. **Infections**
   (1) **Paronychia** is the most common hand infection and presents as swelling, erythema, pain, and tenderness around the base of the nail. The causative organism is usually *Staphylococcus* or *Streptococcus.* Drainage is performed by inserting a scalpel blade between the nail and the nail fold. Antibiotics are controversial.
   (2) **Felon** is an extremely painful infection of the pulp tissue in the tip of a digit. The causative organism is usually *Staphylococcus,* and the major symptom is pain and swelling of the fingertip. Felons should be drained by making an incision along one lateral aspect of the fingertip; close follow-up is necessary.
   (3) **Tenosynovitis** usually occurs along a flexor tendon and is characterized by tenderness over the tendon, swelling of one finger, pain on passive extension, and a flexed resting position of the finger. If detected early, tenosynovitis can be cured with high-dose intravenous antibiotics, but usually surgical drainage is required.
   (4) **Cellulitis** of the hand typically requires hospital admission, intravenous antibiotics (cephalosporin unless the cellulitis is the result of a bite wound), immobilization, and elevation.
   (5) **Septic arthritis** of any digital joint or of the CM joint can occur. Treatment entails irrigation and drainage in the operating room.

b. Tendon injuries

(1) **Mallet finger** is caused by detachment of the extensor tendon from the distal phalanx. The patient usually complains of pain at the DIP joint and is unable to fully extend the affected finger. The radiograph of the finger may appear normal, or there may be a small avulsion fracture at the base of the distal phalanx. Unless accompanied by a fracture, mallet finger is treated with a dorsal splint that prevents flexion of the PIP for 6 weeks. If it is accompanied by a large avulsion fracture, surgical pinning may be required.

(2) **Boutonniere deformity,** a disruption of the extensor hood apparatus near the PIP, can be easily overlooked. In the ED, it is treated with a dorsal splint with the PIP in full extension or slight flexion. This injury requires close follow-up.

c. Trauma

(1) **Fingertip amputations** are common injuries that require copious irrigation and careful debridement in the ED. If the distal phalanx is not exposed, the digit can be dressed and the patient referred to a hand surgeon for definitive care within a few days.

(2) **Finger sprains**

    (a) Collateral ligament sprains of the MCP, PIP, and DIP are common. Lateral stress should be applied to the extended joint to determine the amount of laxity and the degree of sprain. All sprains should be splinted for several weeks or until the follow-up examination.

    (b) Third-degree sprains that cannot be reduced in the ED frequently require surgical repair. "Gamekeeper's thumb" ("skier's thumb") is a serious injury that is caused by disruption of the ulnar collateral ligament of the MCP joint of the thumb. The patient is unable to grasp items between the thumb and index finger. These injuries require splinting and close follow-up.

    (c) The most significant CM joint sprain involves the first metacarpal joint. These sprains are caused by hyperextension and the joint may be dislocated. Severe sprains require operative treatment.

(3) **Finger dislocations.** Dislocations of the DIP and PIP joints are usually easily reduced using longitudinal traction following digital block anesthesia. Reductions of MCP dislocations can be extremely difficult and may require surgery. All reduced dislocations should be splinted for several weeks or until the follow-up examination.

(4) **Finger fractures**

    (a) **Phalanx fractures**

        (i) **Distal phalanx** fractures are usually treated with a protective splint, leaving all joints free. Subungual hematomas are common and should be drained to alleviate pain. Associated nail bed injuries should be repaired. As discussed in II D 1 b (1), some fractures associated with mallet finger require surgery.

        (ii) **Middle** and **proximal phalanx** fractures that are not displaced can be splinted and the patient referred to an orthopedist. Fractures that are displaced may require surgical pinning after reduction.

    (b) **Metacarpal fractures** usually occur at the distal neck rather than at the head, shaft, or proximal base. All metacarpal fractures can be treated with an ulnar gutter splint in the ED prior to referral.

        (i) **Distal neck fractures.** The most common distal neck fracture is "boxer's fracture" (i.e., fracture of the neck of the fifth metacarpal). Distal fractures of the fourth or fifth metacarpal require reduction if the angulation is greater than 30 degrees. Distal fractures of the second or third metacarpal require reduction if the angulation is greater than 15 degrees.

        (ii) **Head, shaft,** or **base fractures** require early follow-up.

(5) **High-pressure injection injuries** occur when the hand is inadvertently placed over the nozzle of a paint gun, grease gun, hydraulic line, or other high-pressure injector, resulting

in the injection of a large amount of liquid into the hand or finger through a small puncture wound. These injuries can be devastating, depending on the material injected. Initially, there may be only mild swelling and tingling, but these injuries (despite their initial near-normal appearance) require immediate consultation by a hand surgeon.

2. **Wrist injuries**
   a. **Carpal dislocations**
      (1) **Anterior (volar) lunate dislocation** is the most common carpal dislocation. The lunate appears rotated on the lateral radiograph.
      (2) **Posterior perilunate dislocation** is also common. The capitate is dorsally dislocated in relation to the lunate.
   b. **Carpal fractures** may occur when a patient falls on an outstretched hand. Because carpal fractures can be radiographically occult, any patient with significant signs or symptoms of a wrist fracture should be treated with a thumb spica splint and referred to an orthopedic surgeon.
      (1) The **scaphoid (navicular), triquetrum,** and **lunate** are the most commonly fractured carpal bones.
      (2) **Distal radius** fractures with significant displacement are usually reduced in the ED.
         (a) **Colles' fracture** is a fracture of the distal radius in which the distal radius is dorsally displaced, producing a characteristic "dinner fork" deformity.
         (b) **Smith's fracture** is a fracture of the distal radius characterized by volar displacement (i.e., it is a reversed Colles' fracture).
   c. **Carpal tunnel syndrome** is caused by inflammation of the carpal canal, resulting in compression of the median nerve.
      (1) **Etiology.** Carpal tunnel syndrome is usually a result of repetitive wrist flexion.
      (2) **Clinical signs.** Patients usually complain of paresthesia ("pins and needles") in the index finger, long finger, and radial aspect of the ring finger. The paresthesia is exacerbated by tapping the volar wrist (Tinel's sign) or by holding the wrist in the flexed position (Phalen's sign).
      (3) **Treatment.** Emergency treatment consists of a volar wrist splint, nonsteroidal anti-inflammatory drugs (NSAIDs), and referral to a hand specialist.

III   FOREARM, ELBOW, UPPER ARM, AND SHOULDER INJURIES

A **Forearm**   Forearm shaft fractures of the ulna or radius frequently occur together and are usually displaced; therefore, after finding a fracture in one forearm bone, the other bone should be closely scrutinized. Careful examination for swelling, deformity, and point tenderness is required; however, most closed forearm fractures do not result in nerve or vascular injury.

1. **"Nightstick" fractures** are nondisplaced fractures of the ulna often caused by a direct blow to the forearm. These fractures are treated with a long arm splint and close follow-up.

2. **Monteggia fracture–dislocation** is a fracture of the proximal ulna and a dislocation of the radial head at the elbow. Adults with this injury are treated with open reduction and internal fixation. Children are treated with closed reduction and immobilization.

3. **Galeazzi's fracture** (fracture of the distal radial shaft) is often associated with a distal radioulnar joint dislocation near the wrist; it is often thought of as **reverse Monteggia fracture.** The AP radiograph may show only slight widening of radioulnar space. On the lateral view, the ulna is displaced dorsally. This injury is treated with open reduction and internal fixation.

4. **Radial shaft fractures.** In adults, displaced fractures of the radial shaft typically require open reduction and internal (or external) fixation. In children, displaced fractures can sometimes be treated with closed reduction.

B Elbow

1. **Subluxation of the radial head (nursemaids' elbow)** is seen only in children younger than 7 years and is caused by the application of sudden traction to a pronated hand (i.e., by pulling the child by the hand). The child presents in apparently no pain, but keeps the affected arm pronated and in slight flexion. Treatment is by either passive supination or extension of the forearm; a "click" can be felt over the radial head as the subluxation is reduced. Within a few minutes of successful reduction, the child will use the affected arm normally. Immobilization after reduction is usually not required.

2. **Elbow dislocations** are usually posterior and occur following a fall on an outstretched arm.

   a. Because **neurovascular complications** (most commonly, ulnar nerve and brachial artery injuries) are associated with up to 21% of elbow dislocations, the function of the ulnar, radial, and median nerves and the presence of the radial and ulnar pulses should be assessed. Associated fractures should be sought.

   b. **Treatment.** Reduction is accomplished by traction and countertraction after adequate sedation. After reduction, the neurovascular examination is performed again and the arm splinted in 90-degree flexion. Cylindrical casts should not be used.

C Upper arm

1. **Distal humerus fractures** are usually supracondylar in children and intercondylar (intra-articular) in adults. Hemarthrosis, characterized by a posterior "fat pad" sign on the lateral radiograph, may be the only evidence of a nondisplaced fracture.

   a. **Complications.** These fractures often cause severe swelling; injuries to the median, ulnar, and radial nerves; transection of the brachial artery; and Volkmann's ischemic contracture (compartment syndrome; see VII).

   b. **Treatment** for displaced fractures normally consists of open reduction and internal fixation and hospital admission for neurovascular observation.

2. **Proximal humerus fractures** can occur at the anatomic neck, surgical neck, greater tuberosity, lesser tuberosity, or shaft.

   a. **Complications.** Anatomic neck fractures can result in vascular compromise to the humeral head, leading to necrosis of the articular segment. Significantly displaced surgical neck fractures and shaft fractures may have associated brachial plexus and vascular injuries. A significant displaced fracture of the greater tuberosity implies concomitant rotator cuff injury.

   b. **Treatment.** If neurovascular injuries are not present, these fractures are immobilized in the ED with a sling and swath, and the patient is referred for follow-up.

D Shoulder

1. **Acromioclavicular joint injuries (shoulder separations)** are common.

   a. **Classification.** Shoulder separations are classified according to the amount of ligament disruption.

      (1) **Type I** injuries are characterized by a minor ligament sprain. Patients have joint tenderness, but no disruption of the joint.

      (2) **Type II** injuries consist of one ruptured ligament and slight widening of the acromioclavicular joint. There may be a slight step-off deformity that becomes apparent following comparison with the opposite acromioclavicular joint.

      (3) **Type III** injuries are characterized by rupture of all acromioclavicular ligaments and significant widening of the joint.

   b. **Treatment** of all three grades of injury consists of rest, ice, analgesics, and immobilization with a simple sling. In addition, some type III injuries may require open reduction and repair.

2. **Glenohumeral dislocations**

   a. **Anterior dislocations,** in which the humeral head is displaced anterior to the glenoid and inferior to the coracoid, are the most common type of glenohumeral dislocation. A flattening deformity of the lateral aspect of the shoulder can be seen, and the humeral head can usually be palpated anteriorly.

(1) **Complications.** Anterior dislocation is frequently associated with a greater tuberosity fracture, humeral head fracture, rotator cuff tear, disruption of the axillary artery, and transient axillary nerve injury.

(2) **Treatment.** Many reduction techniques have been described and are used in the ED. Because this injury has a recurrence rate of up to 90%, patients are treated with a sling following reduction and referred to an orthopedist for follow-up care.

b. **Posterior dislocations** often occur as a result of a fall or during an epileptic seizure. Posterior dislocations are frequently not clinically recognized, and a lateral shoulder or "scapula Y" radiograph may be required to make the diagnosis.

3. **Clavicle fractures** are the most common fractures of childhood. The mechanism of injury is usually a blow to the shoulder, and most fractures occur in the middle third. Therefore, the clavicle should be inspected and palpated along its entire length in every patient with a suspected shoulder injury. Most clavicle fractures heal within 6 weeks without complications.

a. Nondisplaced fractures require only immobilization with a sling.

b. Displaced fractures do not need immediate reduction and only require treatment with a figure-of-eight brace.

IV   PELVIS, HIP, AND FEMUR INJURIES

A **Pelvis**   Pelvic **fractures** are common and commonly result from blunt trauma sustained during motor vehicle collisions. All multiple trauma patients should be initially suspected of having a pelvic fracture, and a pelvis radiograph should be obtained. Fractures that result in a widened pubic symphysis are unstable.

1. **Diagnosis.** Most pelvic fractures are suggested by mechanism of injury and physical examination findings (e.g., pain on palpation).

2. **Associated injuries and complications**

a. Common associated injuries include intra-abdominal organ injuries, femur fractures, bladder and urethral injuries, nerve root injuries, and vaginal injuries. Rectal examination occasionally reveals superior displacement of the prostate (indicative of urologic injury) or blood in the rectum (indicative of intra-abdominal injury).

b. The pelvis is extremely vascular; therefore, hemorrhage is a major cause of death in patients with pelvic trauma. Retroperitoneal bleeding is very common, and up to 6 L of blood can be accommodated in the retroperitoneal space.

3. **Treatment** consists of resuscitation with intravenous fluids and blood products, immobilization of the pelvis, and a careful search for concomitant injuries. Orthopedic consultation is required. Stable, nondisplaced fractures require only bed rest. Other pelvic fractures may require open reduction and fixation.

B **Hip**

1. **Hip dislocations** are posterior in 90% of patients and occur when force is applied to the anterior of the flexed knee. The leg is shortened, internally rotated, and adducted.

a. **Complications.** Acetabulum fractures and femur fractures often occur with hip dislocations. Dislocation of the hip can disrupt the blood vessels between the acetabulum and the femur, causing avascular necrosis of the femoral head. Sciatic nerve injury is also a common complication.

b. **Treatment** consists of closed reduction under general anesthesia. Ideally, hip dislocations are treated within 6 hours of the injury.

2. **Slipped capital femoral epiphysis** may occur bilaterally and is seen most often in boys between the ages of 10 and 16 years. The cause is unknown; symptoms include the gradual onset of groin

discomfort following activity, knee pain, hip stiffness, and limping. The slightly posterior displaced epiphyseal plate is visible on a lateral radiograph. Treatment entails weight-bearing restrictions and referral to an orthopedist for definitive diagnosis and treatment.

3. **Septic arthritis** usually occurs in children younger than 4 years and is the most common cause of a painful hip in infants. The most commonly implicated organisms are *Staphylococcus, Streptococcus,* and *Haemophilus influenzae.* Patients have severely limited range of motion in the hip, which is held in a flexed, abducted, and externally rotated position. Diagnosis is by needle aspiration of the hip using fluoroscopic guidance. Treatment includes hospitalization, intravenous antibiotics, and, possibly, surgical drainage.

C Femur

1. **Intertrochanteric fractures** are most often seen in elderly patients following a fall or motor vehicle collision. The leg is shortened, adducted, and externally rotated. Movement of the hip or weight bearing produces severe pain. Surgical fixation by an orthopedic surgeon is required.

2. **Subtrochanteric fractures** are usually caused by a fall or motor vehicle collision. Signs and symptoms are similar to those seen with intertrochanteric fractures, but these fractures can cause severe hemorrhage and large amounts of blood can accumulate in the thigh. Orthopedic consultation should be obtained for definitive treatment.

3. **Femoral shaft fractures** usually occur in young adults following a fall or motor vehicle collision. The leg should be splinted in the ED using a traction device that applies a sling to the ankle and foot. The patient requires hospitalization, fracture reduction, and surgical insertion of an intramedullary rod.

V KNEE INJURIES

A Diagnosis
The injured knee should always be compared with the noninjured knee. The patient's gait, degree of active flexion, and degree of active extension should be noted, along with the presence of skin trauma or swelling. The knee is systematically palpated for point tenderness, effusion, hemarthrosis, and increased temperature.

1. **Abduction and adduction stress testing** should be performed by applying lateral stress to the knee while the patient holds it in 30-degree flexion. By comparing the degree of laxity of the injured knee to the noninjured knee, the degree of injury (if any) to the medial and lateral collateral ligaments can be measured. In patients with an acute knee injury, it may be difficult to appreciate joint laxity as a result of hemarthrosis and pain.

2. **Lachman's test.** To perform Lachman's test, the examiner stabilizes the femur in his or her left hand and uses his or her right hand to grasp the posterior aspect of the lower leg below the knee. While the knee is flexed to 20 degrees, the examiner applies anterior force with his or her right hand to pull the lower leg forward. A displacement of greater than 5 mm when compared with the noninjured leg is evidence of a partial or complete tear of the anterior cruciate ligament.

B Specific injuries

1. **Meniscus injuries** usually produce hemarthrosis, a clicking sound with movement, or locking of joint on partial flexion. If a meniscus injury is suspected, orthopedic follow-up should be obtained.

2. **Sprains.** Ligament injuries typically produce hemarthrosis unless the knee capsule is completely disrupted. Minimal ligament injuries that appear stable can be treated with a knee splint, ice packs, elevation, and ambulation as tolerated. More severe injuries require an orthopedic consultation for definitive management.

3. **Dislocations**
   a. **Tibia–femur dislocations** are common, and spontaneous reductions occur frequently. Suspicion of this injury is important because of the associated risk of injury to the ligaments,

popliteal artery, and peroneal nerve. Early reduction and orthopedic consultation are required, and an arteriogram is customarily obtained.

    b. Lateral dislocation of the patella is usually evident on physical examination. Reduction is performed by keeping the hip flexed and then extending the knee while sliding the patella back into place.

  4. Fractures can result from a direct blow to the patella. Nondisplaced, simple patella fractures are treated by immobilization. A comminuted or displaced fracture may require open reduction and fixation.

VI   LOWER LEG, ANKLE, AND FOOT INJURIES

A **Lower leg**

  1. Tibial plateau fractures most commonly occur through the superior aspect of the lateral condyles, but may also affect the medial tibia condyles. These fractures can be difficult to detect by physical examination and radiography.

    a. Nondepressed fractures can be treated with immobilization and restricted weight bearing.

    b. Depressed fractures require open reduction and elevation of the bony segment.

  2. Tibial shaft fractures are common in children and usually result from the application of a twisting force. The fibula is usually fractured also. These fractures require reduction, immobilization, and follow-up with an orthopedist. Compartment syndrome of the anterior compartment of the lower leg is a common complication of tibial shaft fractures (see VII A).

B **Ankle**

  1. Sprains. Ankle sprains most often involve the lateral collateral ligaments and result from the application of an inversion force. The sprain can be graded using the clinical impression of the amount of ligament injury as a basis.

    a. First- and **second-degree sprains** are treated with compression, ice, elevation, and immobilization.

    b. Third-degree sprains require orthopedic consultation and may require surgical repair.

  2. Dislocations. Ankle dislocations usually have concomitant malleolar fractures. The ankle should be reduced with in-line traction and immobilized. Orthopedic consultation is required.

  3. Fractures. Malleolar fractures usually occur when the ankle is forcibly adducted and may be accompanied by avulsion fractures of both the medial and lateral malleolus (i.e., the tibia and fibula, respectively). A malleolar fracture is treated by either closed reduction and immobilization or by open reduction and fixation, depending on the type and severity of the fracture. Severe ligament injuries are commonly associated with malleolar fractures.

C **Foot**

  1. Calcaneal fractures are the most common type of tarsal bone fracture. The mechanism of injury is usually a fall from a height. These fractures are often associated with other injuries to the lower extremity or to the spine. Orthopedic consultation is usually required to reduce these difficult fractures.

  2. Metatarsal fractures. Avulsion fractures of the base of the fifth metatarsal are the most common type of metatarsal fracture. The mechanism of injury is plantar flexion and inversion; patients often say they "slipped while walking." These fractures are often misdiagnosed when local tenderness is attributed to an ankle sprain. Treatment consists of restriction of weight bearing and follow-up.

  3. Phalanx fractures are common and usually result from a direct blow to the toe. Treatment consists of reduction of the fracture by traction following digital anesthesia. The digit is then immobilized by "buddy taping" the broken toe to the adjacent toe or applying a walking cast.

VII COMPLICATIONS OF ORTHOPEDIC INJURIES

A Compartment syndromes are extremely serious complications of orthopedic injuries that, without early recognition and treatment, can result in permanent disability.

1. **Pathogenesis.** Compartment syndromes occur when tissue pressures greater than 20 mm Hg in closed compartments compromise the capillary blood flow, leading to muscle and nerve ischemia and necrosis. Compartment syndromes are caused by either a decrease in compartment size (usually due to constrictive casts or burn eschars) or an increase in compartment contents (usually due to hemorrhage or edema). Palpation of the compartment may not reveal swelling.

2. **Clinical features** include muscle pain at rest that is exacerbated by movement and muscle tenderness. Later, hypesthesia of the area innervated by the ischemic nerve may occur. A diminished distal pulse is a late finding that occurs after muscle necrosis.

3. **Diagnosis.** Compartment syndromes can be difficult to diagnose early. Suspicion of the compartment syndrome must be based on pain location and knowledge of the recent injury. Commonly affected areas include the forearm (usually from supracondylar humerus fractures), hand and thigh (usually from crush injuries), and the lower leg (usually from tibial fractures).

   a. **Differential diagnoses** for a painful extremity include compartment syndrome, fracture, muscle strain, muscle contusion, venous thrombosis, and cellulitis.

   b. **Definitive diagnosis** is provided by inserting an 18-gauge needle into the compartment tissue and measuring the pressure using an electronic monitor or mercury manometer.

4. **Treatment.** A pressure greater than 30 mm Hg usually requires **emergency fasciotomy** in the operating room. This procedure is performed by making longitudinal skin and fascia incisions to free the contents of the compartment and to decrease the pressure.

B Osteomyelitis may occur in a patient with an open fracture or following surgery to repair the fracture. The following precautions are usually taken to prevent osteomyelitis in patients with open fractures:

1. **Prophylactic antibiotics** (e.g., a parenteral cephalosporin and an aminoglycoside) are administered in the ED.

2. **Careful irrigation** and **debridement** are performed in the operating room.

C Pulmonary fat embolus results when a bone marrow fat particle reaches the venous circulation, leading to respiratory compromise. When it occurs, this complication usually develops within a few days of fracturing a long bone.

D Avascular necrosis of the bone segment can occur and may necessitate prosthetic replacement.

E Nonunion occurs when a fracture does not heal.

F Malunion occurs when a fracture heals with a deformity.

G Joint stiffness or **traumatic arthritis** may occur following a fracture.

Study Questions

Directions: *Each of the numbered items or incomplete statements in this section is followed by answers or by completions of the statement. Select the ONE lettered answer or completion that is BEST in each case.*

QUESTIONS 1–3

A 32-year-old man comes to the emergency department (ED) complaining of wrist pain. He tripped over his son's tricycle in the driveway and fell forward, landing on his outstretched left hand. The patient is right-handed. Physical examination reveals significant swelling of the left wrist. The anterior-posterior (AP) and lateral wrist radiographs show a thin, radiolucent, transverse line across the distal radius. There is no displacement, angulation, or deformity.

1. What is the most likely diagnosis?
   - A Type I Salter-Harris fracture
   - B Second-degree wrist sprain
   - C Monteggia fracture
   - D Nondisplaced radius fracture
   - E Colles' fracture

2. How should this patient's injury be immobilized?
   - A No immobilization is necessary
   - B Compression dressing
   - C Splint
   - D Circumferential cast
   - E Surgical fixation

3. What should the patient be told at the time of discharge from the ED?
   - A "Your wrist will be back to normal in a few weeks."
   - B "You should expect severe pain and increased numbness for the next few days."
   - C "You can continue your usual activities, but keep your wrist immobilized at night."
   - D "Use ice as directed, elevate your hand, and do not use your hand for a few weeks."

4. What is the most common hand infection?
   - A Felon
   - B Paronychia
   - C Tenosynovitis
   - D Cellulitis
   - E Septic arthritis

5. The mother of a 4-year-old girl brings her daughter to the emergency department (ED) because she has noticed that the child has been avoiding using her right arm for the last 3 hours. The emergency physician diagnoses subluxation of the radial head. Which of the following statements is consistent with this diagnosis?
   - A The mother states that earlier, she "yanked" her daughter out of the street while the two of them were walking to the bus stop.
   - B The patient is crying and appears to be in distress, and the elbow is swollen and tender.
   - C The patient holds her elbow in full supination and extension.
   - D The radiograph reveals a supracondylar fracture of the elbow.
   - E Reduction of the injury requires sedation and traction.

6. Which one of the following statements regarding clavicle fractures is true?

- [A] They are rarely seen in children.
- [B] They usually occur in the lateral third of the clavicle.
- [C] They are typically caused by a blow to the upper chest.
- [D] The only immobilization required for nondisplaced clavicle fractures is a sling.
- [E] Displaced clavicle fractures usually require surgical treatment and are often associated with many complications.

7. An 81-year-old woman presents to the emergency department (ED) after a fall from a standing position. She complains of right knee pain and is unable to bear weight on her right leg. On physical examination, her knee is nontender, her right hip is tender, and her right leg is shortened, externally rotated, and adducted. What is the most likely diagnosis?

- [A] Posterior hip dislocation
- [B] Knee dislocation
- [C] Femoral shaft fracture
- [D] Intertrochanteric fracture
- [E] Slipped capital femoral epiphysis

8. Which one of the following statements regarding glenohumeral dislocation is true?

- [A] It is also called a "shoulder separation."
- [B] It usually cannot be detected by physical examination.
- [C] The most common type is an anterior dislocation.
- [D] Patients are not prone to recurrence of the dislocation.
- [E] It is not associated with humeral fractures.

9. Which type of fracture is rarely overlooked on a radiograph?

- [A] Tibial plateau fracture
- [B] Scaphoid (navicular) fracture
- [C] Fifth metatarsal fracture
- [D] Nondisplaced supracondylar fracture
- [E] Colles' fracture

10. How does one examine the motor function of the hand?

- [A] The motor component of the radial nerve is tested by having the patient abduct his or her thumb against resistance.
- [B] The motor component of the median nerve is tested by having the patient extend his or her wrist against resistance.
- [C] The motor component of the ulnar nerve is tested by having the patient spread his or her fingers against resistance.
- [D] The deep flexor tendon is assessed by having the patient flex each proximal interphalangeal (PIP) joint.
- [E] The superficial flexor tendon is assessed by having the patient flex each distal interphalangeal (DIP) joint.

Answers and Explanations

1. The answer is D The 32-year-old man who tripped over the tricycle most likely has a nondisplaced fracture of the radius. Because he is an adult, his epiphyseal plate is closed; therefore, the Salter-Harris classification scheme does not apply. The radiograph reveals a distal radius fracture, not a sprain. A Monteggia fracture involves an angulated fracture of the proximal ulna and dislocation of the radial head at the elbow. A Colles' fracture implies dorsal angulation of the distal radius fracture. Because no deformity is evident on physical examination, a Monteggia or Colles' fracture is unlikely.

2. The answer is C The nondisplaced distal radius fracture requires immobilization. Usually, these fractures are immobilized with a plaster of Paris or fiberglass splint. Splints accommodate the swelling that accompanies most fractures and are less likely to cause pressure sores, circulatory compromise, or neurapraxia. At the follow-up visit, a circumferential cast can be applied. Surgical repair and fixation are usually not required for nondisplaced distal radius fractures.

3. The answer is D The patient should be told to keep the extremity elevated, wear the splint at all times, and apply cold compresses intermittently for 24 hours. Fractures take more than a "few" weeks to heal. Every patient with any type of fracture needs a follow-up appointment within 10 days (sometimes sooner) to ensure that the fracture is healing well and there are no complications. Every patient should be told to seek immediate medical treatment if the pain increases after the extremity has been immobilized. Increased pain can be an early symptom of complications, such as compartment syndrome or infection.

4. The answer is B Paronychia, infection of the nail base, is the most common hand infection.

5. The answer is A Subluxation of the radial head ("nursemaids' elbow") always occurs in young children and most often results when an adult pulls sharply upward on the extended hand of the child. The patient appears to be in no distress but keeps the arm pronated and in slight flexion. The radiograph will be normal. Reduction is quickly and easily performed by first fully extending and then flexing the elbow while holding the hand in pronation, while pressing over the proximal radial head. Past teaching was to hold the hand in supination while flexing the elbow, but a higher success rate is achieved when keeping the hand pronated.

6. The answer is D Clavicle fractures are the most common fracture of childhood. They usually occur in the middle third and are usually caused by a blow to the shoulder. If the fracture is displaced, usually only a figure-of-eight brace is required for immobilization. Most displaced clavicle fractures heal without complications. Nondisplaced clavicle fractures can be immobilized using a sling.

7. The answer is D This woman most likely has an intertrochanteric or subtrochanteric fracture. Posterior hip dislocation causes the leg to be shortened, internally rotated, and adducted. Knee dislocations usually are caused by a more severe force than a simple fall, result in swelling and tenderness of the knee, and do not cause external rotation of the leg. Femoral shaft fractures usually occur in young adults involved in motor vehicle collisions. Slipped capital femoral epiphysis occurs in children younger than 16 years of age.

8. The answer is C The most common glenohumeral dislocation is anterior. Glenohumeral dislocations are frequently associated with greater tuberosity (humerus) and humeral head fractures. There is a 90% recurrence rate. A "shoulder separation" is another term for acromioclavicular joint injury, not glenohumeral dislocation.

9. The answer is E Colles' fracture, an angulated fracture with a characteristic "dinner fork" appearance, is rarely missed radiographically. Tibial plateau fractures may be subtle and are frequently missed.

Scaphoid fractures may not be detected radiographically for as many as 10 days after the injury. Fractures at the base of the fifth metatarsal are frequently missed because the ankle radiograph does not include that bone. A nondisplaced supracondylar fracture may be missed because of the difficulty of detecting a fracture through the epiphyseal plate. The only radiographic sign of a nondisplaced supracondylar fracture may be a posterior "fat pad" sign.

10. The answer is C The motor components of the median and ulnar nerves are assessed by abducting the thumb and spreading the fingers, respectively. The radial nerve has no motor component in the hand. The motor component of the radial nerve is assessed by wrist extension. The deep flexor tendons flex the DIP joint, and the superficial flexor tendons flex the PIP joint.

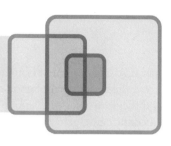

chapter 19

Wound Emergencies

JACK STUMP

I STAGES OF WOUND HEALING

A **Immediate response of tissue to injury**   When an injury exposes tissues, tissue retraction, tissue contraction, and vasoconstriction immediately occur. Platelets begin to aggregate and the clotting cascade is activated, leading to the accumulation of hemostatic coagulum. Once hemostasis is complete, the release of vasoactive amines causes capillary dilatation and an exudate begins to form.

B **Inflammatory phase**   Shortly after the immediate response, granulocytes and lymphocytes accumulate. These cells control the growth of bacteria and prevent infection. Immunoglobulins present in the exudate contribute to the control of infection. Macrophages phagocytize the wound debris, encourage collagen deposition by fibroblasts, and stimulate neovascularization.

C **Epithelialization**   Cells of the stratum germinativum become activated within 12 hours of the injury. Initial epithelialization may be completed in 24 hours, but most wounds require several days. The maturation of this process takes several months.

D **Neovascularization**   This process is critical to wound healing. Without new blood vessels to bring nutrients and oxygen to the healing wound, the cells responsible for healing are unable to remodel the wound. Neovascularization begins at day 3 and peaks at day 7. By day 21 the process is complete and the new blood vessels withdraw as the tissue matures (i.e., regression begins).

E **Collagen synthesis**   The collagen matrix determines the ultimate strength of a wound. Fibrocytes initially lay down a disorganized pattern of collagen. Over the next several months to years this matrix is remodeled to form an organized meshwork of collagen.

F **Wound contraction**   Myofibroblasts are the cells responsible for wound contraction, in which the scar that initially forms contracts to a smaller size.

II PREHOSPITAL CARE OF WOUNDS

A **Care by the public**

1. Most wounds are initially cared for by the injured person or by friends and family. Although wounds evoke an emotional response that may prevent good decision-making in the first few moments, most people recall training that will allow them to provide adequate care. This training is provided by various agencies, such as the American Red Cross, scouting organizations, schools, and summer camps. Emergency medical personnel should recognize this as the first line of medical care, and support such agencies with teaching time and financial support.

2. Immediate care is directed toward stopping bleeding and preventing further injury or contamination. Most bleeding can be controlled by direct pressure and elevation. Any clean covering such

as towels may be used if proper first aid equipment is not available. Thick layers of cloth should be avoided because they prevent the application of good direct pressure and may absorb large amounts of blood, making it difficult to assess the amount of blood loss. If bleeding cannot be controlled, laypersons should contact emergency medical services (EMS).

B **Care by prehospital personnel (EMS)** EMS personnel are expected to provide expert initial care of wounds. They are equipped with proper bandaging and are trained in proper techniques for caring for most wounds. The goals of EMS care are to control bleeding, prevent further injury, limit contamination, perform some decontamination, prevent dehydration of the wound, and collect valuable history and observations.

III EVALUATION OF WOUNDS IN THE EMERGENCY DEPARTMENT (ED)

Emergency physicians treat an estimated 11 million traumatic wounds annually; therefore, they must possess a high level of wound care knowledge. An understanding of anatomy, wound healing, local anesthesia, wound preparation, and suturing guides the physician in the steps needed for successful wound care. The goals of wound care in the ED are to **prevent infection, restore function,** and **restore physical integrity.**

A **Screening examination**

1. **ABCs.** Every patient should have airway, breathing, and circulation (ABCs) evaluated before any other evaluations take place. It is important not to let bleeding wounds distract attention from life-threatening injuries or illnesses. Along with the ABCs, a head-to-toe examination, including vital signs and mental status, should be performed. If abnormalities are encountered, further evaluation and correction of these problems should take place before continuing with wound care.

2. **A brief examination of the wound** allows the physician to assess the level of care the patient may require. Attention to the area of the body injured, and its underlying structures, guides the physician in deciding whether the wound can be treated in the ED or requires a more specialized level of care (e.g., as provided by a plastic surgeon, general surgeon, hand surgeon, or orthopedic surgeon). If other specialties are required, the specialist should be involved in the care of the patient as early as possible.

   a. **Facial wounds** are generally referred to a plastic surgeon, although orofacial surgeons and ear, nose, and throat (ENT) surgeons may elect to repair some facial wounds.

   b. **Hand/forearm wounds** are generally referred to hand surgeons. If a hand surgeon is not available, some plastic surgeons and orthopedic surgeons repair hand injuries.

   c. **Arm and leg injuries** are usually referred to orthopedic surgeons.

   d. **Neck injuries** are treated by trauma/general or ENT surgeons.

   e. **Wounds to the chest and abdomen** should, in most cases, be evaluated by general surgeons because they may involve entry into major body cavities.

B **History** It is tempting to proceed to general inspection of the wound without first obtaining a history from the patient. However, many components of the history guide the examination and determine the course of treatment; therefore, obtaining a history is essential.

1. **History of present injury**

   a. **Mechanism of injury.** Three basic types of mechanisms are involved in producing wounds: shearing, tension, and compression. Although a wound may have components of all three, most wounds are created predominantly by one of these forces. The mechanism of injury affects the amount of tissue involved, risk of infection, method of repair, and amount of scarring.

      (1) **Shearing-type wounds** are lacerations caused by sharp objects (e.g., knife, glass). These wounds usually have a low infection rate, can be closed primarily (see V A), and produce small scars.

    (2) **Tension-type wounds** are caused by blunt objects striking the skin at angles of less than 90 degrees, often producing a flap of injured tissue. They involve larger amounts of tissue, have a high infection rate, and produce larger scars.

    (3) **Compression-type wounds** are caused by direct forces striking the skin at a 90-degree angle, causing crushing of the skin and underlying tissue. These wounds are often irregular in shape (stellate laceration) with maceration of wound margins. Infection rates are high and scarring may be extensive.

  b. Contamination of the wound. The mechanism of injury affects the degree of wound contamination. When ascertaining the mechanism of injury, it is important to obtain information on environmental factors associated with the wound. Wounds with high concentrations of bacterial contamination (e.g., by feces, saliva, or organic matter) need extensive debridement and irrigation. Some of these wounds may have such extensive contamination that they will require delayed closure. Every attempt should be made to rule out foreign bodies.

  c. Exposure to heat or cold. It is important to ascertain whether the injured area or person was exposed to extreme heat or cold. This information helps the physician determine if wound healing will be compromised by cold or if some of the tissue destruction is caused by burns.

  d. Age of injury. The **golden period of wound care** is generally considered to be less than 6–8 hours following injury. Between 8 and 12 hours, some wounds can be closed without significant additional risk of infection. Facial wounds can generally be closed up to 12–24 hours following injury because the higher vascularity of the face leads to lower infection rates than in wounds occurring to the rest of the body. In contrast, in a heavily contaminated wound of the foot, closure may not be safe in as little as 3 hours postinjury.

  e. Extent of injury

    (1) Physicians must be aware of their limitations in caring for wounds. It is inappropriate to attempt to care for an extensive wound in an ED or clinic; doing so puts the patient at risk for infection and future complications.

    (2) When obtaining information regarding the extent of injury, the physician must be on the alert for possible injury to deep structures. Information obtained during the history should guide the physical examination. Patients may be reluctant to discuss other injuries because they think they may be too minor or because of embarrassment due to mechanism or location.

2. Past medical history

  a. Underlying disease processes. Diabetes, immunosuppression (e.g., caused by steroids, AIDS, cancer treatment), and alcoholism are examples of conditions that affect wound healing. These conditions lead to slower healing and higher infection rates. In the presence of such conditions, sutures should be left in longer and prophylactic antibiotics should be considered.

  b. Previous injuries. The patient should be questioned regarding healing of previous wounds. This can give some idea about the patient's rate of healing and severity of scarring. Attention should be paid to the amount of scar formation, especially keloid scar formation. In patients with a history of multiple previous injuries, domestic abuse should be considered (especially in women).

  c. Age of the patient. Patients younger than 2 years and older than 50 years have higher rates of infection. In children and the elderly, the possibility of abuse should be considered.

  d. Smoking status. Tobacco smoking decreases peripheral blood flow and increases the risk of other vascular injury. Wounds in regions supplied by distal circulation (i.e., the extremities) heal more slowly in people who smoke.

  e. Nutritional status. Patients with severe nutritional deprivation have slower wound healing and higher infection rates. Supplemental nutrition may be necessary for these individuals.

  f. Medications. Steroids and immunosuppressive medications may slow healing and increase infection rates. Aspirin may inhibit platelet aggregation and increase bleeding. Patients taking warfarin may experience prolonged bleeding. Both aspirin and warfarin may cause accumulation of blood in wounds that are primarily closed, causing swelling and possible infection.

   g. Allergies. The physician should inquire about allergies to all medications and materials that may be used in treating the patient. Reactions to local skin cleaning solutions, local anesthetics, sutures, tapes, antibiotic ointments, antibiotics, and pain medications should be considered.

   h. Tetanus immunization. Tetanus is a potentially fatal disease that is highly preventable. All patients with wounds should be questioned as to their immunization status.

C **General inspection**

1. Patient comfort and safety

   a. Patients should be safely secured before beginning any inspection or treatment. Rails should be used to protect patients from falling, in case they react to pain by rolling off the gurney or with a vasovagal response.

   b. Patients should be in a comfortable position that will allow examination and repair; the time involved can be anything from a few minutes to many hours.

   c. Pain medication or sedation may be warranted. Pediatric patients may require special sedation or containment (e.g., a papoose for infants).

2. Description of wounds. The general inspection is an appropriate time to begin to describe the wound. Measurements should be taken. The entire wound should be visualized. If the wound is covered by matted blood or hair, it may be necessary to gently clean the wound to allow visualization. Usually, saline-soaked gauze can be used to loosen blood and debris with minimal pain.

3. Functionality of wounded area. The initial general inspection is also the time to evaluate functioning of the area as well as distal functioning. Attention to neurologic function (i.e., sensation, reflexes, strength) prior to the use of local anesthesia is important. Muscle movement and tendon function should be evaluated through the entire range of motion. Vascular integrity should be evaluated (i.e., temperature, color, capillary refill, pulses).

IV   WOUND CARE

The fundamental steps of proper wound care are **inspection, exploration, debridement,** and **irrigation.** These steps are normally preceded by tetanus prophylaxis, cleansing of the wound, and any necessary anesthesia.

A **Tetanus prophylaxis**   Tetanus prophylaxis should be considered part of wound preparation. Tetanus is best prevented by proper wound care (i.e., inspection, exploration, debridement, irrigation) and immunization; the combination of the two is nearly 100% effective in preventing this disease. Tetanus immunizations are safe in pregnancy. Table 19–1 provides guidelines for tetanus immunization.

B **Skin cleansing and wound preparation**   The goals of skin cleansing are to remove debris and decrease the bacterial count of the surrounding skin. The reduction of bacteria and other microbials is necessary before continuing with wound care.

1. The area surrounding the wound must be cleansed to remove blood and other debris. Mild cleansing or scrubbing can usually be accomplished prior to administering local anesthesia. Skin preparation is essential if the anesthesia method involves injecting through the skin (field blocks).

2. Wound care is often based on common practice rather than research. For example, hydrogen peroxide is still used by some medical professionals even though it is a poor antimicrobial solution with significant tissue toxicity. It is incumbent on emergency physicians to know the advantages and disadvantages of the solutions they use and to be able to discuss these with their patients.

3. Several solutions are available for skin cleansing. A skin-cleansing solution should be fast acting and have a broad spectrum of antimicrobial activity. These requirements must be weighed

TABLE 19–1   Guidelines for Tetanus Immunization

	Non–tetanus-prone Wounds	Tetanus-prone Wounds*
Unknown or less than three shots	Td	Td + TIG
Three or more shots; last shot: 0–5 years prior	None	None
Three or more shots; last shot: 5–10 years prior	None	Td

*Tetanus-prone wounds are characterized by one or more of the following: age older than 6 hours; contaminated, infected, nonviable tissue; puncture, missile, or crushing wound; burn; frostbite.

Tetanus immunizations are safe in pregnancy. Td = tetanus and diphtheria toxoid; TIG = tetanus immune globulin.

against the solution's toxicity to wound tissues. Povidone–iodine and chlorhexidine are the two most commonly used skin preparation solutions.

  a. **Povidone–iodine solutions.** Povidone–iodine is a potent germicidal solution. It has broad-spectrum coverage and is fast acting. However, it is toxic to open tissues. Toxicity reduces the immune response, thereby increasing risk of infection. It is an excellent skin cleanser but should not be used inside of wounds.

  b. **Chlorhexidine.** This solution has reasonable bactericidal activity, but its antiviral activity is not well understood. It is toxic to wound tissue, and contact with open wounds should be avoided.

  c. **Hydrogen peroxide.** Because of its poor antimicrobial activity and significant wound toxicity, this solution should not be used for skin preparation or wound irrigation. Hydrogen peroxide may be used to dissolve dried blood and matted hair (e.g., on the scalp). Care should be taken to keep the solution away from wound tissues.

  d. **Alcohols.** These solutions also have poor antimicrobial activity and are toxic to tissues. Alcohols can cause significant pain when used around open wounds, and are not good skin preparation solutions.

  e. **Hexachlorophene.** This solution is damaging to wound tissues. Its use has been dramatically restricted over the past few years.

4. Shaving the area around the wound is no longer recommended because it increases the risk of infection. Furthermore, in many cases, hair lines provide landmarks that should be lined up during repair.

  a. If hair removal is necessary to visualize the wound, the hair should be clipped with scissors.

  b. Eyebrows should never be clipped or shaved. The eyebrows of a small percentage of the population do not regrow.

C Anesthesia   After a neurovascular examination has been completed and documented, it is essential that the area of the wound be adequately anesthetized to allow pain-free examination, cleansing, debridement, irrigation, and closure.

1. **Pain associated with the injection.** For both regional and local anesthesia, several factors affect the level of pain associated with injection of the anesthetic. These factors include the:

  a. **Rate of injection** (a slow injection is less painful)

  b. **Size of the needle** (a smaller needle is less painful)

  c. **Location of the injection** (intradermal is more painful, subdermal is less painful)

  d. **Temperature of the injected agent** (warm is less painful)

  e. **Presence or absence of buffering lidocaine prior to injection**

2. **Regional anesthesia** is the preferred method of anesthesia in most cases when wound treatment is necessary. Regional blocks allow injection of anesthetic agents away from the injury site, which can be quite sensitive, and they allow for longer anesthesia. In addition, more than one wound can be repaired from a single injection site.

   a. Wounds of the fingers, hands, feet, toes, ears, face, and mouth are appropriate for regional blocks. These small areas often have important landmarks. Local anesthesia can distort landmarks and cause tissues to swell, making them more difficult to examine, débride, irrigate, and close.

   b. The injection of anesthesia is usually done with a 27-gauge or 30-gauge needle. The exact location of nerve blocks can be found in various emergency medicine textbooks.

3. **Local anesthesia**

   a. **Injected local anesthesia** is the most commonly used method of local anesthesia; it is the simplest, fastest, and most effective for nearly all wounds. There are two basic approaches:

      (1) **Parallel margin infiltration (field block).** Anesthesia is injected through the **intact skin** next to the wound. If local anesthesia is injected through intact skin, the skin must be cleansed prior to injection to help prevent skin bacteria from being carried subcutaneously.

      (2) Anesthesia may be injected through **exposed subcutaneous tissue** of the wound edge. Injecting through the exposed wound tissue causes less pain, but may carry contaminants in the wound to deeper tissues.

   b. **Topical local anesthesia** is associated with high patient satisfaction because there is no pain associated with injection of anesthesia.

      (1) **Agents**

         (a) **TAC,** a mixture of **tetracaine, adrenaline (epinephrine),** and **cocaine liquid,** has been used for topical wound anesthesia. Results are somewhat mixed, but TAC appears to provide good wound anesthesia for most patients. **Potential risks** of using TAC include increased incidence of infection and wound edge necrosis, although proponents of TAC believe this risk to be minimal. There is also some concern regarding toxic reactions that occur when TAC comes in contact with mucous membranes. In addition, fatal reactions to the cocaine have been reported.

         (b) **LET,** a mixture of **lidocaine, epinephrine,** and **tetracaine,** is a possible alternative to TAC. This compound offers pain control similar to that provided by TAC, but is associated with fewer toxic effects.

      (2) **Administration**

         (a) Both compounds are formulated by the hospital pharmacy and should be applied 20 minutes prior to initiating wound care. Success of anesthesia is made evident by blanching of the area around the wound.

         (b) Neither TAC nor LET should be used on wounds involving areas of distal vascularity (e.g., ears, tip of nose, penis, or digits) because of the constrictive properties of epinephrine and cocaine.

4. **Anesthetic agents**

   a. **Esters.** Procaine, tetracaine, chloroprocaine, benzocaine, and cocaine (not for injection) are examples of esters. Most of these have fallen from common use except as topical agents. These agents may be used for patients who are allergic to amides.

   b. **Amides.** Lidocaine, bupivacaine, and mepivacaine are all examples of amide-type anesthetics. This is a newer class of anesthetics than the esters and may be an alternative for patients who are allergic to ester-type anesthetics.

      (1) **Lidocaine** and **bupivacaine** are the two most commonly used local anesthetics. Lidocaine has a fast onset of action and a duration of action of 20–60 minutes. Bupivacaine has a slower onset of action than lidocaine, but is effective about four times longer.

      (2) Some allergic reactions may be caused by preservatives present in both amide- and ester-type agents. Lidocaine that is used for intravenous administration does not contain these preservatives and may be used if the patient is allergic only to the preservatives.

(3) Buffering of lidocaine to near-neutral pH can decrease the pain of injection. Lidocaine 1% can be buffered with sodium bicarbonate for injection (1 mEq/mL) at a ratio of 10 mL of lidocaine 1% to 1 mL of sodium bicarbonate for injection (1 mEq/mL).

  c. Antihistamines. Diphenhydramine is an amide antihistamine that provides some local anesthesia when infiltrated near a wound. Diphenhydramine can be used in patients who are allergic to ester-type anesthetics.

  d. Epinephrine. Epinephrine added to an anesthetic agent prolongs the agent's activity. In addition, the vasoconstrictive action of the epinephrine reduces local wound bleeding. Agents with epinephrine should be avoided in areas of distal vascularity [see IV C 3 b (2) (b)]. Because epinephrine may weaken the defenses of the wound, increasing the risk of infection, epinephrine should be avoided in wounds that are contaminated or have a high infection potential.

D Inspection and exploration

1. General comments

  a. The wound must be **adequately anesthetized** before inspection and exploration can take place. A **bloodless field** must be obtained by applying a local tourniquet (i.e., a Penrose drain) around a digit, or by using an extremity pneumatic tourniquet. An extremity tourniquet may be inflated for up to 2 hours without risk of causing tissue injury.

  b. The wound edges should be **pulled apart with instruments so that the entire wound can be adequately examined.** It is very important that the bottom of the wound be visualized. The entire wound should be examined for tracts that may lead to other areas of injury. If necessary, the wound should be extended surgically to allow a complete examination.

2. Location of the wound. Vascularity of the wound, stress on the wound, and the bacterial skin count are related to the location of the wound on the body.

  a. Vascularity is one of the most important factors that determine the likelihood of a wound becoming infected. Areas of high vascularity (e.g., face) generally have lower infection rates. Areas with low vascularity (e.g., hands and feet) have higher infection rates.

  b. Bacterial skin count also contributes to the infection potential. Moist areas (e.g., axillae, perineum) have high bacterial skin counts. Careful preparation of wounds in these areas is imperative.

  c. Stress on the wound is a factor in determining scar size. Wounds that are parallel to the lines of tension in the body leave smaller scars than wounds that are perpendicular to these lines (Figure 19–1).

3. Underlying structures. When examining a wound, the physician should consider the surrounding anatomy and any possible injury to underlying structures, such as tendons, joints, nerves, vascular structures, bone, and organs. It may be necessary to extend the wound surgically to obtain adequate visualization of all underlying structures. If the injury is over a joint or tendon, the underlying structures must be examined through their entire range of motion.

4. Foreign bodies. All foreign bodies must be removed from a wound.

  a. The incidence of infection dramatically increases when foreign bodies are left in a wound. In general, 10^6 bacteria per gram of wound tissue cause infection. If a foreign body is present in a wound, as few as 100 bacteria can cause infection. Occasionally, a wound contains so many foreign bodies that it is necessary to take the patient to the operating room for wound cleansing and foreign body removal.

  b. In some situations, radiographic studies may be necessary to locate foreign objects. Radiographic studies should not be used in place of good wound inspection and exploration, but rather as an adjunct.

    (1) Metal, gravel, and some glass may be visualized using ordinary radiographs.

    (2) Wood, plastic, and other less dense objects may be visualized with computed tomography or ultrasound.

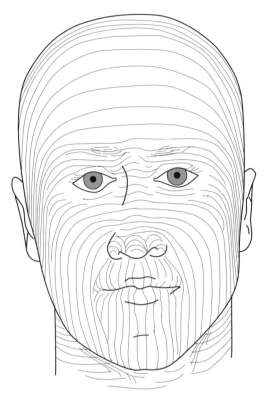

FIGURE 19–1 Skin tension lines of the face. Incisions or lacerations parallel to these lines are less likely to create widened scars than those that are perpendicular to them.

E **Debridement** is the removal of devitalized and heavily contaminated tissue from the wound. Clots from the initial coagulum require removal as well. Devitalized tissue acts much like a foreign body. Any tissue that has lost its blood supply becomes a source of infection. If a wound has significant devitalized or contaminated tissue, surgical consult may be necessary. Upon completion of the debridement process, all tissues in the wound should look healthy and have a good blood supply.

F **Irrigation**   "The solution to pollution is dilution" is an axiom commonly taught in wound care. Irrigation—rather than soaking—is the method used to decrease the bacterial count of a wound.

1. The solutions most commonly used for irrigation are sterile normal saline and nonionic detergents.

2. Irrigation should be high volume (200–2000 mL, depending on the size and contamination of the wound) and high pressure (7 psi). This can usually be accomplished by an 18- or 19-gauge blunt needle on a 35-mL syringe. Most wounds require at least 200–500 mL of irrigating solution. Contaminated wounds require more irrigation.

V   WOUND CLOSURE

A **Categories of wound closure**

1. **Primary closure** is closure using sutures, tapes, staples, or adhesives. It can be performed on wounds with low infection potential.

2. **Secondary closure (intention).** Smaller wounds that have a high infection potential are left open and allowed to heal by granulation and re-epithelialization. This is called secondary closure. These wounds still require proper wound care (i.e., inspection, exploration, debridement, irrigation).

3. **Tertiary closure (delayed primary closure).** Wounds that have a high infection potential and are quite large may be best treated by delayed primary closure. Following proper wound care, the wound may be packed with saline gauze mesh and covered. If the wound does not show any signs of infection after 4 or 5 days of daily dressing changes, it may be closed using percutaneous sutures or tapes. The wound may need to be revised (i.e., trimming of the wound edges until tissue with a good vascular supply is reached). Proper wound care should be repeated prior to closure.

B **Sutures**

1. **General comments**
   a. The purpose of sutures is to restore physical integrity and function. Although the patient may come to the ED to "get stitches," the emergency physician should focus on proper wound care. It does little good to close a wound only to have it become infected later, or to close a wound and leave an underlying structure damaged and nonfunctional.
   b. Sutures need to be placed to adequately close the wound and provide even tension in the wound. Sutures that are too tight may reduce circulation to the wound edge and cause necrosis. Sutures that are too loose may cause the wound to gap open and serve as a portal of entry for infection. The suture itself may invoke an inflammatory response that weakens resistance to infection. As few sutures as possible should be used to adequately close the wound and provide even tension.

2. **Suture types**
   a. **Absorbable.** Sutures that lose their tensile strength in 60 days or less are considered absorbable. Types include synthetic absorbable sutures, plain gut (collagen), chromic gut, and rapidly absorbable gut.
   b. **Nonabsorbable.** These sutures are usually made of polymer. Sutures made from stainless steel, cotton, and silk are rarely used.
      (1) **Monofilament sutures** are used most often.
      (2) **Multifilament sutures,** made of polymers such as nylon, may be used because of their ease of handling. There is some concern that a multifilament suture may wick fluid and contaminants from the surface of the skin into the wound, increasing the risk of infection.

3. **Suture placement**
   a. **Percutaneous suturing** is the most common method of suturing, in which the needle and suture enter through the skin at the edge of the wound. Sutures can be continuous (running) or interrupted. Interrupted sutures are most commonly used. The sutures should be placed evenly and provide even closure and tension on the wound. There are several methods of percutaneous suture placement (Figure 19–2).
   b. **Dermal (subcuticular) suturing.** In this method of wound closure, the sutures are placed just below the surface of the skin. Except at the ends of the wound, the sutures do not enter through the skin. When the wound is closed, only the ends of the suture are visible. If absorbable suture is used, no suture may be visible. Dermal sutures can be used in clean wounds, but should be avoided in contaminated wounds.

C **Staples**   In areas where scars are less likely to show (e.g., the scalp), staples provide a fast and inexpensive method of skin closure. The staple invokes very little inflammatory response. The wound is held securely closed by the strength of the staple, with only a minimal amount of material below the skin surface.

1. Compared with suturing, positioning the wound edges is more difficult using staples, and the staple punctures are larger. Staples should be avoided on the face and other places where scars may be visible.

2. Because of their ease of use, there may be a temptation to rush through proper wound care and proceed directly to stapling. This defeats the purpose of good wound care.

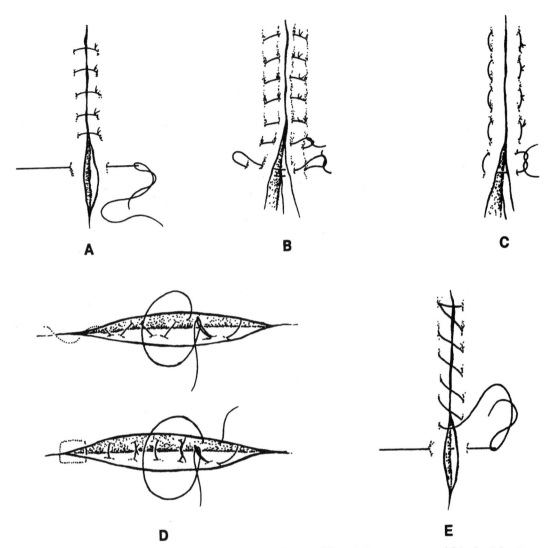

FIGURE 19–2 Types of wound closures: **(A)** simple interrupted suture, **(B)** vertical mattress suture, **(C)** horizontal mattress suture, **(D)** subcuticular suture, **(E)** continuous over-and-over suture. (Reprinted with permission from Jarrell BE, Carabasi RA III. *NMS Surgery.* 3rd Ed. Baltimore: Williams & Wilkins, 1996:479.)

D **Tapes** Tapes (i.e., Steri-Strips) are a fast, painless method of skin closure. They have the lowest rate of infection. As with other methods of closure, proper wound care must be performed prior to their use.

1. The skin must be dry, and tincture of benzoin is generally applied to help the tapes adhere better. Care should be taken to keep tincture of benzoin from coming in contact with the wound because it is quite toxic to wound tissues.

2. Tapes can be used on areas of the skin that have relatively low skin tension and are not over areas of motion (i.e., joints).

E **Adhesives** Several wound adhesives are available. These may prevent some of the problems that occur with sutures and staples, and studies have shown that the wound infection rate and the appearance are as good or better. Some practitioners are concerned that proper wound care may be circumvented if wounds are "glued shut" without inspection, exploration, irrigation, and debridement.

VI **CARE OF SPECIFIC WOUND TYPES**

A **Closed-fist injuries** These wounds are generally associated with young men and alcohol consumption.

1. **Characteristics.** Closed-fist injuries often involve the fist coming in contact with the teeth of another individual. Because the patient is often intoxicated, these wounds may receive delayed care. The laceration is over the metacarpophalangeal (MCP) joint and extends into the joint. These wounds have a high rate of infection.

2. **Therapy.** Inspection, exploration, debridement, and irrigation usually must be done in the operating room. All of these wounds should be radiographed. Intravenous antibiotics that cover Gram-positive and Gram-negative organisms should be administered. Splinting is very important to prevent infection. These wounds are not sutured closed. Most of these patients will need to be admitted for close follow-up and continued antibiotics.

B **Bite wounds**

1. **Characteristics**
   a. From 80%–90% of bite wounds result from dog bites, 5%–10% from cat bites, 2%–3% from human bites, and 2%–3% from other animals (e.g., rats, hamsters).
   b. Cat bites have the highest infection rate, followed by human bites and then dog bites. *Pasteurella multocida* is a common pathogen of cat bites and some dog bites. It is very sensitive to ordinary penicillin, but not sensitive to penicillinase-resistant penicillins. Most bite wounds have mixed-flora inoculum; *Streptococcus* and *Staphylococcus* species are common.

2. **Therapy**
   a. Proper wound inspection, exploration, debridement, and irrigation are necessary. Radiographs may be warranted to evaluate the condition of deep structures and the existence of retained foreign bodies.
   b. Bite wounds on distal extremities should not be sutured closed. Suturing may be considered at other locations. Delayed primary closure may be advisable to reduce the potential for infection.
   c. Although clear evidence of their benefit is still lacking, antibiotics should be prescribed for most bite wounds. Penicillin and a cephalosporin are recommended. If the patient is allergic to penicillin and is not pregnant, erythromycin or tetracycline may be used.
   d. Frequent follow-up visits to watch for infection are a must. Follow-up should take place in 12–24 hours and again in 36–72 hours. The patient may need to be evaluated at 5 and 7 days, as well. Bite wounds should be considered tetanus-prone wounds. Rabies should also be considered in patients with animal bite wounds (see Chapter 6 III D).

C **Puncture wounds**

1. **Characteristics.** Most puncture wounds occur to the feet. If the puncture occurred through a tennis shoe, *Pseudomonas aeruginosa* infections are possible.

2. **Therapy.** Puncture wounds should be opened, inspected, débrided, irrigated, and left open. Soaking puncture wounds is not adequate treatment. Prophylactic antibiotics are usually not required, unless the patient was wearing tennis shoes at the time of injury. In this case, ciprofloxacin may be prescribed. Frequent follow-up visits (on days 1, 3, 5, and 7) to watch for infection are necessary.

D **Fingertip injuries**

1. **Digital tip avulsion**
   a. **Characteristics.** Tip avulsion often occurs as a result of slamming fingers in doors, or by accidentally cutting oneself with a saw or sharp knife. If the bone is not exposed and only skin and soft tissue are missing, these wounds often heal by secondary intention (i.e., secondary closure).

b. **Therapy.** Some hand surgeons may attempt skin grafts. Regardless of the final treatment, these wounds need proper wound care. Digital block with a long-acting anesthetic (e.g., bupivacaine) is indicated. If healing by secondary intention is preferred, these wounds can be covered with antibiotic ointment and petroleum jelly–impregnated gauze and then bandaged. Regular examinations to watch for infection are important.

2. **Digital tip amputation with exposed bone.** Treatment of these injuries depends on the level at which the finger is amputated. If the tip is amputated and bone is exposed, shortening of the bone and movement of a viable flap over the finger may be indicated. If the finger is amputated at the distal interphalangeal (DIP) joint or proximal to the DIP joint, replantation may be indicated. A hand surgery consultation is usually required.

3. **Nail bed injuries**
   a. **Characteristics.** Nail bed injuries are common and usually result from hitting the fingertip with a hammer or slamming the finger in a door.
   b. **Therapy**
      (1) The presence of a subungual hematoma affecting 25% of the nail bed warrants removal of the nail and examination of the nail matrix. Lacerations of the nail bed often require suturing with absorbable suture. Subungual hematomas affecting less than 25% of the nail bed may be drained through the nail.
      (2) When history indicates that enough force may have been present to fracture the distal phalanx, radiographs should be obtained. Approximately 50% of nail bed injuries are associated with distal phalanx fractures. These fractures may require a surgical consultation and stabilization of the fracture with Kirschner wires.

E **High-pressure injection injuries**

1. **Characteristics.** These injuries are often caused by paint guns, grease guns, or air guns. They involve injection of air and other materials under the skin and along vascular and tendon sheaths. The opening to these injuries (i.e., injection site) may be quite small. The patient may not initially complain of pain, but swelling, pain, and severe infection in deep tissues usually develop within a few hours of injury.

2. **Therapy.** Immediate surgical consultation with exploration is nearly always indicated. Pain control, splinting, and intravenous antibiotics are indicated while waiting for consultation.

VII **FOLLOW-UP CARE**

A **Wound care**

1. Most wounds benefit from being covered with antibiotic ointment to prevent them from drying out. Antibiotic ointments have been shown to improve healing and decrease infection. If there is risk of the dressing adhering to the wound, a petroleum jelly–impregnated porous gauze may be indicated. The dressing should then be covered with an absorbent layer to collect exudate from the wound. Bandaging should be firm enough to hold the dressing in place, but not so tight that it restricts circulation.

2. The first dressings are usually left in place for 24–48 hours. After the first dressing change, they should be changed every 24 hours. After 48 hours, the wound is usually sealed and resistant to new infection. A light washing with sterile saline helps to remove accumulated debris from the surface of the wound, allowing for inspection of the wound for infection and reapplication of antibiotic ointment and fresh dressings.

B **Medications**

1. **Pain control** should be considered for all patients. This is easily forgotten while the patient is still in the ED and the wound is still anesthetized. Patients may refuse pain medication at the time of

discharge because pain is reduced from local anesthesia. They may try over-the-counter pain medications, but a prescription for stronger pain medication should be sent with them. Nonsteroidal anti-inflammatory drugs (NSAIDs) and narcotics are often prescribed. It is common for local anesthesia to wear off while the inflammatory response is increasing, causing the patient to wake up in pain in the middle of the night.

2. **Antibiotics.** Patients with wounds that are at high risk of infection (e.g., bites, heavily contaminated wounds) should be given prophylactic antibiotics. Antibiotic therapy is not required for most patients with wounds.

C **Discharge instructions**

1. **Signs of infection** should be explained: redness, increasing pain, swelling, purulent discharge from the wound, red streaks moving up the extremity, and fever.

2. **Care for the wound** should be explained (i.e., dressing changes, pain control, follow-up appointments). Computerized discharge instructions can be a valuable tool for providing all of the following information:

   a. The patient should be told whether he or she is permitted to take a shower or bath. In most cases, showering is permissible, but activities that involve submerging the wound in water (e.g., baths, soaking in a hot tub, swimming) should be avoided for the first 1–3 days.

   b. The patient should also be told how long to keep the wound immobile and elevated, and when to have the sutures or staples removed (Table 19–2).

   c. Patients should know when, where, why, and with whom they should seek follow-up care. The name, address, and phone number of the person the patient is to see should be provided, and if possible, a follow-up appointment should be made prior to the patient leaving the ED.

      (1) Wounds that carry a high risk of infection should be referred for close follow-up. Many of these wounds should be seen in 1, 3, 5, and 7 days.

      (2) Patients should be instructed to return to the ED if their condition worsens acutely.

TABLE 19–2   Guidelines for Suture Removal*

Location	Days Following Closure
Face	3–5
Scalp	7–10
Trunk	7–10
Arms and legs	10–14
Joints	14

*Some sutures may be removed earlier if the wound can be reinforced with tape closure. Patients with conditions causing immunocompromise (e.g., steroid therapy, AIDS) or who have demonstrated slow healing previously may need to have sutures left in place longer.

Study Questions

Directions: *Each of the numbered items or incomplete statements in this section is followed by answers or by completions of the statement. Select the ONE lettered answer or completion that is BEST in each case.*

1. The wound-healing process that involves the accumulation of lymphocytes and granulocytes, and the removal of debris from the wound by macrophages, is called

- (A) epithelialization
- (B) immediate response
- (C) inflammatory response
- (D) neovascularization
- (E) collagen synthesis

2. The history of an injury can help determine treatment required. Which one of the following statements matching history to treatment is correct?

- (A) Age of the wound is important because it can determine scar size after suturing.
- (B) Mechanism of injury has little importance in wound care.
- (C) The extent of injury is of minor importance because emergency physicians repair all wounds.
- (D) The degree of contamination of the wound affects the risk of infection and the amount of wound care required.

3. A 67-year-old diabetic man presents at the emergency department (ED) with a laceration to his hand from a kitchen knife. He is taking aspirin for a heart condition and prednisone for chronic obstructive pulmonary disease (COPD). He is a long-time smoker. Which one of the following statements regarding his history is correct?

- (A) As far as wound care is concerned, the patient is in a young age group.
- (B) If his diabetes is under control, it is not a consideration in treatment.
- (C) His medications could adversely affect healing.
- (D) Because the wound is caused by a kitchen knife, it is a clean wound with little chance of infection.
- (E) The patient's history of smoking is irrelevant.

4. A patient with a forehead wound requires anesthesia. Which one of the following statements is correct?

- (A) Topical local anesthesia may not be effective for this area.
- (B) The pain of injection can be reduced by administering buffered lidocaine prior to infiltration.
- (C) The pain of injection can be reduced by injecting the surrounding tissue with anesthetic quickly.
- (D) An anesthetic agent containing epinephrine is not safe to use in this area.

5. Which one of the following statements regarding irrigation of a wound is correct?

- (A) Antibiotics are more effective than dilution for preventing infection.
- (B) The goal of irrigating a wound is to make the wound sterile.
- (C) Irrigation can be accomplished by slowly dripping saline solution into the wound.
- (D) High-pressure, high-volume irrigation is the preferred method of irrigation.
- (E) Only nonionic detergents should be used as irrigating solution.

6. A 30-year-old man falls out of the back of a pick-up truck, landing on his right knee. His only injury is a severe laceration to the right knee contaminated by several pieces of gravel and dirt. A proximally based flap, 5 cm on each side, is raised from the knee. The wound has irregular, devitalized edges, and there are sections of subcutaneous tissue with poor vascularization. Which of the following statements concerning this wound is true?

- (A) Foreign bodies can be left in the wound if they are small.
- (B) A radiograph may be required because of the risk of foreign bodies in the knee joint and fractures to the underlying tissue.
- (C) The sections of subcutaneous tissue with poor vascularization can be left alone because they are under the skin.
- (D) The devitalized tissue on the edges of this wound does not require removal.
- (E) This type of wound rarely needs to be treated in the operating room.

7. A 25-year-old woman is bitten on the hand by her cat. Which one of the following statements regarding this injury is correct?

- (A) There is little chance of infection because cat bites have a low infection rate.
- (B) Cat bites to the hand can be sutured closed acutely.
- (C) Antibiotics are not required.
- (D) Because the bites wounds are small, they do not need to be opened and irrigated.
- (E) The first follow-up visit should take place in 12–24 hours.

8. A tennis player is swinging back for an overhand shot when he hits the back wall with his right index finger and crushes the fingertip between the wall and the racket handle. Which one of the following statements regarding treatment of this injury is correct?

- (A) If the tip is avulsed, it may be allowed to heal by secondary intention.
- (B) If there is greater than a 25% subungual hematoma, the nail should be left in place.
- (C) If the nail bed is lacerated, radiographs to screen for a distal phalanx fracture are contraindicated.
- (D) The nail bed may be sutured with nylon sutures.

9. Which one of the following statements regarding discharge instructions, medications, and follow-up care for emergency treatment of wounds is correct?

- (A) If the patient is not in pain on discharge from the emergency department (ED), he or she probably will not be in pain later
- (B) The wound should be cleaned daily with saline solution and fresh antibiotic ointment, and dressings should be applied daily.
- (C) Sutures to the face should be removed in 2 weeks.
- (D) All patients with wounds, even minor wounds, should be prescribed antibiotics.
- (E) Follow-up instructions are required only for serious wounds.

Answers and Explanations

1. The answer is C The inflammatory response is characterized by the accumulation of lymphocytes and granulocytes, which are infection-fighting cells. Macrophages phagocytize wound debris.

2. The answer is D The level of contamination of a wound has a direct impact on the risk of infection and the amount of wound care (i.e., debridement and irrigation) required. The age of the wound is important not because it determines scar size, but because the ideal period for closing a wound is generally considered to be within 6–8 hours following the injury. The mechanism of injury helps determine the amount of tissue involved, risk of infection, and method of repair. It is one of the most important components to history. The extent of injury helps determine whether it is appropriate to repair the wound in the emergency department (ED).

3. The answer is C This patient is taking aspirin, which may prevent platelet aggregation and cause blood to accumulate in the wound after it is closed, increasing the risk of infection. He is also taking prednisone, which may suppress the immune system, causing a higher rate of infection and slower healing. His age is of concern because patients who are older than 50 years have an increased potential for infection. His diabetes is a concern whether it is controlled or not. Diabetics often have poor distal vasculature, leading to increased potential for infection. The fact that the wound was caused by a kitchen knife does not mean that it is a clean wound. One needs to ask what he was cutting. The kitchen is a source of bacterial contamination. Smoking affects healing of wounds to the hands and feet because it compromises distal circulation.

4. The answer is B Injecting buffered lidocaine can help decrease the pain of injection. Anesthetic should be injected slowly to decrease the pain associated with injection. Topical anesthetics (e.g., TAC [a mixture of tetracaine, adrenaline (epinephrine), and cocaine liquid] or LET [a mixture of lidocaine, epinephrine, and tetracaine]) are acceptable for anesthetizing forehead wounds. Anesthetics containing epinephrine are safe in highly vascular areas; they are not safe in the fingers, toes, distal nose, or penis.

5. The answer is D High-pressure (7 psi), high-volume (200–2000 mL) irrigation is the most effective treatment against infection. The goal of irrigation is not to make the wound sterile, but to decrease the bacterial count to less than 10^6 per gram of wound tissue (preferably to less than 10^4 bacteria per gram). Effective irrigation cannot be accomplished by slowly dripping saline through a wound or by low-pressure irrigation. Sterile saline and nonionic detergents are both good irrigating solutions. The administration of antibiotics only marginally decreases the infection rate.

6. The answer is B In a patient with a wound that occurs over a joint and is associated with obvious foreign bodies, a radiograph may be required to look for foreign bodies deep in the wound and injury to underlying structures. Foreign bodies increase the infection rate significantly and cannot be left in a wound, even if they are quite small. Devitalized tissue at wound edges acts much like a foreign body in increasing the infection rate. Subcutaneous tissue with poor vascularization may become devitalized, and thus should be removed from the wound. A wound such as this one, with extensive foreign bodies and soft tissue injury, requires exploration. If exploration or radiographic studies indicate that deeper structures are involved, this wound may require treatment in the operating room by an orthopedic surgeon.

7. The answer is E Cat bites have a high infection rate; close follow-up within the first 12–24 hours is important. That this is the patient's pet cat (which implies that she knows the cat is healthy) is irrelevant; the infection rate associated with cat bites is still high. Cat bites to the hand should not be sutured acutely.

They may be closed after 4 days if necessary. Almost all cat bites require prophylactic antibiotics. Even though the bite wound may appear small, the wound should be opened and irrigated.

8. The answer is A Fingertip avulsions that do not involve the bone may be allowed to heal by secondary intention. If a subungual hematoma is greater than 25%, the nail should be removed to inspect the nail bed for lacerations. Nail bed lacerations frequently are associated with distal phalangeal fractures, and radiographs are indicated. Nylon is not a good suture material for nail beds because it requires removal, which is painful.

9. The answer is B Almost all wounds benefit from being cleaned with sterile saline every day and having new antibiotic ointment and dressings applied. Patients who are not in pain on discharge from the ED are probably still feeling the effect of local anesthesia. When the local anesthesia wears off, they may be in considerable pain; thus, some instructions on pain management and/or a prescription for analgesia should be sent with the patient. Sutures to the face generally should be removed in 3–5 days. After 7 days, the risk of scarring from suture marks increases. Very few wounds require prophylactic antibiotics; only wounds with a high risk of infection do. All patients with wounds should be given follow-up instructions.

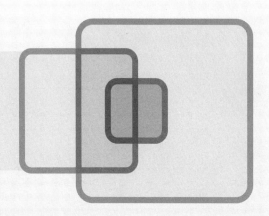

PART **IV**

Toxicologic and Environmental Emergencies

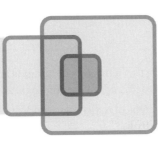

chapter 20

Toxicologic Emergencies

SUSAN E. FARRELL · DAVID C. LEE

I — APPROACH TO THE PATIENT

A Initial stabilization   As with any other patient in the emergency department (ED), initial stabilization of the poisoned patient involves assessment of airway, breathing, and circulation (the ABCs).

1. **Airway.** Check for the presence of a gag reflex, and assess the need for intubation, initially and serially, over the period of observation. Causes of airway compromise include:
   a. Posterior displacement of the tongue [e.g., from central nervous system (CNS) and respiratory depressants]
   b. Oropharyngeal mucosal injury or edema (e.g., from caustic ingestions)
   c. Angioedema [e.g., from angiotensin-converting enzyme (ACE) inhibitors]
   d. Trauma

2. **Breathing.** Assess the adequacy of oxygenation and ventilation with pulse oximetry and arterial blood gas (ABG) determinations. Breathing may be compromised by any of the following:
   a. **Hypoventilation** (e.g., from CNS or respiratory depressants, peripheral muscle toxins)
   b. **Aspiration** (e.g., from CNS or respiratory depressants, peripheral muscle toxins)
   c. **Pulmonary edema** (e.g., from inhalational injuries, heroin, salicylates)

3. **Circulation.** Assess the heart rate and rhythm, the blood pressure, and the adequacy of perfusion. Circulation may be compromised by a multitude of medications and toxins.

B Patient history   The patient may not be cooperative, or may be unable to give an accurate history of ingestion or exposure. Other sources of information include family members, friends, coworkers, rescue personnel, the patient's physician or pharmacist, and old hospital records. Questions to ask include the following:

1. **What?**
   a. What drugs is the patient taking?
   b. What drugs or chemicals are available to the patient?
   c. What chemicals or toxins is the patient exposed to at work?
   d. What (e.g., pill bottles, chemical containers, drug paraphernalia) was present at the scene?
   e. What events have occurred since the ingestion or exposure?

2. **How much?**
   a. How much of the drug or chemical was initially available?
   b. How much of the drug or chemical is remaining in the bottle or container?

3. **When?**
   a. When was the patient last observed to be at his or her baseline?
   b. When did the patient ingest or become exposed to the drug, chemical, or toxin?

C Physical examination
   1. **Vital signs** should be assessed and managed as appropriate.

2. **Neurologic findings.** During the neurologic examination, the level of consciousness, pupil size, and reactivity should be assessed, and focal neurologic abnormalities should be noted.

3. **"Toxidromes"** are physical signs of toxicologic syndromes that may aid in the diagnosis.
   a. **Sympathomimetic "toxidrome"**
      (1) Hyperthermia
      (2) Tachycardia
      (3) Hypertension
      (4) Dilated pupils
      (5) Warm, moist skin
      (6) Altered mental status (e.g., agitation, hallucinations, combativeness) and seizures
   b. **Cholinergic "toxidrome"**
      (1) Profuse salivation
      (2) Bradycardia or tachycardia
      (3) Pinpoint pupils
      (4) Diaphoresis
      (5) Excessive bronchial secretions and bronchospasm
      (6) Hyperactive bowel sounds
      (7) Urinary or fecal incontinence (or both)
      (8) Muscle fasciculations and weakness
      (9) Altered mental status and seizures
   c. **Anticholinergic "toxidrome"**
      (1) Hyperthermia ("hot as Hades")
      (2) Tachycardia
      (3) Hypertension
      (4) Hot, flushed, dry skin ("red as a beet")
      (5) Dilated pupils ("blind as a bat")
      (6) Dry mucous membranes ("dry as a bone")
      (7) Diminished bowel sounds
      (8) Urinary retention
      (9) Altered mental status (e.g., agitation, hallucinations) and seizures ("mad as a hatter")
   d. **Narcotic "toxidrome"**
      (1) Pinpoint pupils
      (2) Respiratory depression
      (3) Altered mental status (e.g., obtundation)

4. **Other findings.** Evidence of trauma (e.g., head trauma) or a medical disorder (e.g., hypo- or hyperglycemia, hypothyroidism) should be sought.

D **Administration of the "coma cocktail"** The "coma cocktail" consists of a group of antidotes that may be of value, both diagnostically and therapeutically, during the initial assessment and treatment of patients with altered mental status.

1. **Thiamine.** Malnutrition or alcoholism predisposes the patient to thiamine deficiency. Patients suspected of having **Wernicke-Korsakoff syndrome** (see Chapter 8 VII) should receive thiamine, 1 g intravenously. To prevent the development of Wernicke-Korsakoff syndrome in alcoholic patients, thiamine (100 mg intravenously) should be administered prior to the administration of dextrose.

2. **Dextrose.** As is the case with any patient with an altered mental status, the serum glucose should be assessed by rapid bedside testing. **Hypoglycemia** is treated with intravenous dextrose.

3. **Naloxone.** If a narcotic toxidrome exists, or the patient's mental status is consistent with **opiate ingestion,** an initial dose of naloxone (0.01 mg/kg intravenously) is administered.

a. Doses as high as 10 mg or more may be required to reverse respiratory depression, and patients who have ingested certain types of synthetic opioids may require large or repeated doses of naloxone.

b. Administration of naloxone may precipitate withdrawal in patients with physiologic dependence to an opiate.

4. **Flumazenil,** a benzodiazepine antagonist, is capable of reversing **benzodiazepine-induced CNS depression.** The dose is 0.5 mg (to a maximum dose of 5.0 mg) administered by slow intravenous push. Flumazenil has a half-life of 57 minutes, so resedation after administration may occur within 1–2 hours and repeat doses may be required.

a. **Adverse effects** include seizures, arrhythmias, induction of benzodiazepine withdrawal, and increased intracranial pressure (ICP) in patients with head trauma.

b. **Contraindications** to the use of flumazenil include:

(1) Previous ingestion of epileptogenic agents, especially cyclic antidepressants

(2) The presence of a seizure disorder that is being therapeutically suppressed with benzodiazepines

(3) A history of chronic benzodiazepine use, suspected benzodiazepine dependence, or potential benzodiazepine withdrawal

(4) Evidence on physical examination of anticholinergic or sympathomimetic "toxidromes"

E **Gastric decontamination procedures**

1. **Activated charcoal** decreases the systemic absorption of many drugs and should be administered once airway patency has been assured. The initial dose is generally 1 g/kg. There are a few substances that are not adsorbed, or are poorly adsorbed, to activated charcoal: alcohols, lithium, iron, lead, hydrocarbons, and caustics. Furthermore, in the case of a caustic ingestion, administration of charcoal will limit endoscopic evaluation of mucosal injury.

2. **Gastric lavage,** in general, has no advantage over activated charcoal in terms of preventing the absorption of toxins. Gastric lavage is appropriate in certain situations and should be considered early in the presentation, but only when the airway is secure. Consider gastric lavage for:

a. Large ingestions of medications or toxins that have high lethality

b. Life-threatening ingestions of medications or toxins for which there is no antidote

c. Life-threatening ingestions of medications or toxins that are not adsorbed to activated charcoal

3. **Whole-bowel irrigation.** Administration of polyethylene glycol solutions at appropriate rates (2 L/hour in adults and 0.5 L/hour in children) speeds the transit of substances through the gastrointestinal tract, thus decreasing their systemic absorption. Unlike cathartics (e.g., magnesium sulfate), whole-bowel irrigation is not associated with any adverse concomitant fluid/electrolyte shifts. Decontamination by whole-bowel irrigation may be of benefit in several cases, once a patent airway has been secured:

a. Life-threatening ingestions of sustained-release drugs

b. Life-threatening ingestions of medications or toxins that are not adsorbed by activated charcoal

c. Ingestion of drug vials, bags, or packets

F **Laboratory and diagnostic studies**   There are several quick studies that can help isolate the toxicologic agent.

1. **Laboratory studies**

a. **Ferric chloride test.** This is a simple qualitative test to assess the presence of **salicylates** in the urine.

(1) **Technique.** Several drops of 10% ferric chloride are added to 1 mL of urine. A purple color change occurs as ferric ion complexes with salicylate, indicating the ingestion of as little as two aspirin in the previous several hours.

    (2) **False-positive results** may occur in the setting of phenothiazine, acetoacetate, phenyl-pyruvic acid, or methyldopa ingestion.

  b. **Urinary fluorescence.** When urine in a plastic container is exposed to ultraviolet light, fluorescence may indicate the presence of fluorescein, a marker for **ethylene glycol,** in the urine. The presence of fluorescence depends on the brand of ethylene glycol ingested, the amount ingested, and the time since ingestion.

  c. **Urinalysis.** The presence of crystals, specifically calcium oxalate, may help confirm **ethylene glycol** ingestion.

  d. **Blood color.** Blood that is chocolate brown in color has at least a 15% **methemoglobin** concentration.

  e. **Toxicology screens.** Screening capabilities vary among laboratories.

    (1) **Urine benzodiazepine screens.** False-negative results may occur with benzodiazepines that are not metabolized to oxazepam (e.g., clonazepam, alprazolam) or in the presence of oxaprozin, a nonsteroidal anti-inflammatory drug (NSAID).

    (2) **Urine opiate screens** assay for morphine and codeine.

      (a) False-positive results may occur if the patient has ingested foods containing a high concentration of poppy seeds.

      (b) Fentanyl and its analogs are not detected on most urine opiate screens, causing false-negative results after their use.

    (3) **Quantitative serum drug levels** are rarely helpful in directing clinical emergency management of the patient except in the following situations:

      (a) Acetaminophen overdose

      (b) Salicylate overdose

      (c) Theophylline overdose

      (d) Lithium overdose

      (e) Lead poisoning

      (f) Carbon monoxide poisoning

      (g) Methemoglobinemia

      (h) Alcohol toxicity

      (i) Digoxin toxicity

2. **Diagnostic studies**

  a. **Electrocardiography.** An electrocardiogram (ECG) is an easy way to evaluate drug-induced rhythm disturbances, conduction abnormalities, and axis changes. It is an especially useful tool in the early diagnosis of **cyclic antidepressant overdose, phenothiazine overdose,** and **antihistamine overdose.**

  b. **Radiography.** The radiopacity of tablets or capsules in the stomach depends on several variables, including the size of the patient, the arrangement of pills (i.e., bezoars), the presence of air around or in the pill, the presence of an enteric coating, and the time since ingestion. The following are often radiopaque:

    (1) Halogenated hydrocarbons

    (2) Iron-containing preparations

    (3) Potassium preparations

    (4) Iodinated compounds

    (5) Heroin or cocaine packets

II   OVER-THE-COUNTER DRUGS

A   Acetaminophen toxicity

1. **Discussion.** Acetaminophen is a commonly used analgesic and antipyretic, available in various formulations, including sustained-release preparations.

    a. Pharmacokinetics. The **recommended maximum dose** is 4 g/day in adults and 90 mg/kg/day in children.

        (1) Absorption and distribution. Acetaminophen is well absorbed and widely distributed. Peak serum levels occur within 4 hours of an overdose.

        (2) Metabolism

            (a) In therapeutic doses, 90% of the dose is conjugated to glucuronide or sulfate. Approximately 5% is metabolized by the **cytochrome P-450 system** to a toxic intermediate, NAPQI, which is detoxified by conjugation to glutathione.

            (b) The **half-life** is 2–3 hours, longer in patients with hepatic dysfunction.

    b. Pathophysiology. The **toxic dose** is 140 mg/kg as a single ingestion.

        (1) Mechanism. In overdose, excess acetaminophen is metabolized via the cytochrome P-450 system to NAPQI. Depletion of glutathione to less than 30% of normal allows the accumulation of NAPQI and other toxic metabolites, leading to hepatic cell death. Renal toxicity and pancreatitis may occur.

        (2) Predisposing factors. If the patient has reduced glutathione stores (such as occurs with malnutrition or chronic alcoholism) or an enhanced ability to form NAPQI through cytochrome P-450 enzyme induction (as occurs with antiepileptic therapy or chronic ethanol abuse), the patient may be at increased risk for toxicity.

2. Clinical features. Acetaminophen toxicity occurs in stages.

    a. Initial stage (0–24 hours). Gastrointestinal symptoms (e.g., nausea, vomiting, anorexia) may be present, but patients at this stage are largely asymptomatic.

    b. Latent stage (24–48 hours). A subclinical increase in hepatic aminotransferases and bilirubin occurs during this stage.

    c. Hepatic stage (3–4 days). This stage is characterized by progressive hepatic failure, manifested as right upper quadrant pain, vomiting, jaundice, encephalopathy, coagulopathy, hypoglycemia, metabolic acidosis, and renal failure.

    d. Recovery stage (4 days–2 weeks). The recovery stage is characterized by resolution of hepatic dysfunction.

3. Differential diagnoses. During the initial stage, acetaminophen toxicity may mimic **gastritis** or **gastroenteritis.** Other hepatotoxic insults (e.g., **iron toxicity, mushroom toxicity**), **pancreatitis, renal failure,** and **sepsis** should also be considered.

4. Evaluation

    a. Serum acetaminophen levels

        (1) Timing. A serum acetaminophen level should be drawn **4 hours postingestion.**

            (a) If the time of ingestion is unknown, a level should be drawn immediately and again in 2–4 hours, and the presence of developing liver dysfunction assessed.

            (b) If a sustained-release preparation has been ingested, a level should be drawn at 4 and 8 hours postingestion, to assess the development of toxic levels.

        (2) Interpretation. The **Rumack-Matthew nomogram** (Figure 20–1) assesses the degree of toxicity. It is based on a single ingestion of regular-release acetaminophen, and a serum level drawn at a known time since ingestion. The level at which treatment is required is approximately 150 μg/mL at 4 hours.

    b. Liver function tests, including the prothrombin time (PT) and bilirubin level, should be ordered. Elevated unconjugated bilirubin is often the first detectable sign of toxicity.

    c. Glucose, blood urea nitrogen (BUN), and **creatinine levels; a serum electrolyte panel; ABG determinations;** and a **pregnancy test** (in women) are indicated.

5. Therapy

    a. Initial stabilization includes airway management and cardiovascular resuscitation, including assessment of hemorrhage.

    b. Gastric decontamination. Activated charcoal should be administered.

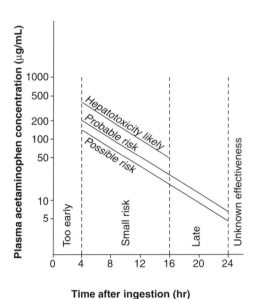

Time after ingestion (hr)

FIGURE 20–1 Rumack-Matthew nomogram. [Adapted with permission from Lewis RK, Paloucek FP. Assessment and treatment of acetaminophen overdose (review). *Clin Pharmacol* 1991;10(10):765–774.]

   c. Antidote treatment. N-Acetylcysteine, a glutathione precursor, repletes glutathione stores and enhances conjugation of toxic NAPQI to glutathione. N-Acetylcysteine should be administered within 8 hours of ingestion for maximum benefit.

     (1) Indications. N-Acetylcysteine is indicated in the following situations:

       (a) Ingestions with potential toxicity (see Figure 20–1)

       (b) Late presentations with potential or ongoing toxicity

       (c) Chronic overdose and evidence of ongoing hepatic damage (e.g., elevated aminotransferases, elevated PT, vomiting)

     (2) Dosage

       (a) Oral. Presently, in the United States, N-acetylcysteine is approved for oral use only. The current protocol is a loading dose of 140 mg/kg, followed by 70 mg/kg every 4 hours for 17 doses.

       (b) Intravenous. The N-acetylcysteine dose is 300 mg/kg intravenously.

6. Disposition

   a. Discharge. Patients with nontoxic levels who present at a known time after a single ingestion of acetaminophen may be safely discharged.

   b. Admission. The following patients should be admitted for N-acetylcysteine therapy:

     (1) Patients with known toxicity or potentially toxic levels

     (2) Patients who have laboratory evidence of ongoing hepatic damage

     (3) Patients with an unknown time of ingestion and symptoms consistent with toxicity

     (4) Patients who present at an unknown time postingestion who still have measurable acetaminophen levels

   c. Referrals. Poor prognostic indicators include a serum pH less than 7.3, grade III encephalopathy, a PT greater than 1.8 times normal, and a creatinine level greater than 3.3 mg/dL. Patients who have these laboratory abnormalities should be referred to a transplant service for consultation.

B **Salicylate toxicity**

   1. Discussion. Acetylsalicylic acid, or aspirin, is contained in analgesics, cold preparations, and topical liniments. Preparations vary in their concentration of salicylate.

a. **Pharmacokinetics**

(1) **Absorption.** Acetylsalicylic acid is a weak acid with a pK_a of 3. Fifty percent is rapidly absorbed from the stomach, and the remainder is absorbed from the small intestine.

(a) Enteric-coated preparations are more slowly absorbed, causing delayed serum levels.

(b) In large ingestions, the dose may precipitate as a bezoar in the stomach that slowly leaches acetylsalicylate, prolonging absorption.

(2) **Distribution.** Most of the drug (50%–80%) is protein-bound. Hypoalbuminemia and serum acidemia increase salicylate penetration of tissues.

(3) **Metabolism and elimination.** In therapeutic doses, 80% of acetylsalicylate is conjugated in the liver. In large doses or chronic dosing, hepatic enzymes become saturated. Renal excretion is dependent on an alkaline urinary pH, adequate serum potassium, normal hepatic and renal function, and the size of the dose.

b. **Pathophysiology.** The **toxic dose** is approximately **160 mg/kg.** The **lethal dose** in adults is approximately **480 mg/kg.**

(1) **Mixed respiratory alkalosis–metabolic acidosis.** Salicylate initially stimulates the respiratory center, causing hyperventilation and respiratory alkalosis.

(a) The serum ionized calcium level decreases. Renal excretion of potassium, sodium, and bicarbonate occurs.

(b) In addition, salicylate interferes with the tricarboxylic acid (TCA) cycle, uncouples oxidative phosphorylation, and limits adenosine triphosphate (ATP) production, causing lactate generation. Fatty acids are metabolized, generating ketone bodies.

(2) **Hypoglycemia.** Oxygen consumption and glucose utilization increase. Heat production increases, and hypoglycemia occurs, especially in the CNS. In children poisoned by salicylate, metabolic acidosis and hypoglycemia predominate.

(3) **Noncardiogenic pulmonary edema (NCPE)** and **direct hepatic toxicity** may also occur.

2. **Clinical features**

a. **Vital signs.** Tachypnea, hyperpnea, tachycardia, and mild to moderate hyperthermia may be seen.

b. **Acid–base status.** Initially, a mixed respiratory alkalosis–metabolic acidosis may be present. A respiratory–metabolic acidosis may indicate coingestion of CNS or respiratory depressants or impending respiratory failure.

c. **Fluid and electrolyte status.** Altered serum glucose is common, and cerebrospinal fluid (CSF) glucose levels may be low despite a normal serum glucose. Serum sodium, potassium, and calcium levels may be low. An anion-gap metabolic acidosis is often present. Mild to moderate dehydration (secondary to vomiting) and insensible losses from tachypnea and perspiration contribute to the fluid and electrolyte derangement.

d. **Gastrointestinal symptoms.** The patient may experience abdominal pain, nausea, vomiting, and blood-tinged emesis.

e. **CNS signs and symptoms.** Tinnitus, hearing loss, lethargy, asterixis, hallucinations, seizures, altered mental status, and coma may occur.

f. **Cardiovascular signs.** NCPE may be seen in older patients, in patients with chronic ingestions, or in conjunction with metabolic acidosis, neurologic symptoms, and serum salicylate levels greater than 40 mg/dL.

3. **Differential diagnoses**

a. Sepsis, pneumonia, pulmonary edema, gastritis, CNS depressant ingestion, and electrolyte abnormalities, especially hypoglycemia in pediatric patients, must be ruled out.

b. Chronic toxicity is most common in geriatric patients and may be misdiagnosed as fever of unknown origin (FUO), pneumonia, pulmonary edema, dehydration, or a change in mental status.

4. **Evaluation**

a. **General laboratory studies**

      (1) **Electrolyte** and **ABG determinations** to assess the acid–base status should be followed frequently to estimate the progression of toxicity and the effectiveness of therapy.

      (2) **Glucose, calcium, BUN,** and **creatinine levels** should be assessed.

      (3) A **complete blood count (CBC)** should be sent.

      (4) **Liver function tests** should be sent and the **PT** assessed.

      (5) The **urinary pH** should be assessed.

      (6) A **pregnancy test** is indicated for women of childbearing age.

  b. Ferric chloride test (see I F 1 a). A purple color change indicates the presence of salicylate. This is only a qualitative test.

  c. Serum salicylate levels. Toxicity occurs at levels exceeding 25 mg/dL. However, toxicity correlates poorly with levels. Evaluation using the **Done nomogram** (Figure 20–2) is based on a single ingestion of regular aspirin and a level drawn at least 6 hours after the known time of ingestion. The Done nomogram underestimates toxicity in cases of severe acidemia or chronic ingestion, and should be evaluated in conjunction with the ABGs. Therapeutic decisions should be based on clinical evaluation, not the Done nomogram.

5. Therapy is directed by the severity of the clinical signs and the progression of toxicity.

  a. Initial stabilization

      (1) Airway management, mechanical ventilation, and cardiovascular resuscitation may be necessary. In patients with respiratory failure, great care should be taken when employing sedation with mechanical ventilation. Sedation-induced respiratory depression may cause a precipitous rise in the carbon dioxide tension (PCO_2), a decrease in the pH, sudden tissue penetration of salicylate, and death.

      (2) Electrolyte imbalances (e.g., hypoglycemia, hypokalemia, hypocalcemia) must be corrected, and acidosis treated aggressively with sodium bicarbonate. The serum pH should be maintained at 7.45–7.50 to maximize protein binding of salicylate and minimize tissue penetration.

  b. Gastric decontamination

      (1) **Gastric lavage** may be indicated for patients who present early after a lethal ingestion, especially if they have ingested a sustained-release preparation.

      (2) **Activated charcoal** binds acetylsalicylate well. It is administered in a 10:1 ratio for maximal adsorption. Multiple-dose activated charcoal should be administered to enhance gastrointestinal elimination of salicylate.

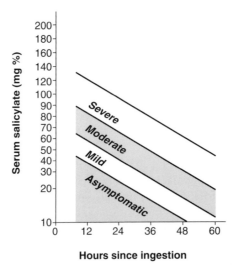

FIGURE 20–2 Done nomogram. (Adapted with permission from Watson WA. Clinical toxicology. In: Young LY, Koda-Kimble MA, Kradjan WA, eds. *Applied Therapeutics: The Clinical Use of Drugs.* Vancouver, WA: Lippincott Williams & Wilkins, 1995:104.1–104.23.)

(3) Whole-bowel irrigation has not been proven to be of benefit in increasing the clearance of salicylate. It may decrease absorption in patients who have large overdoses or who have ingested enteric-coated preparations.

c. **Elimination enhancement**

(1) Urinary alkalinization greatly enhances the renal excretion of salicylate, and should be undertaken when the serum level is greater than 35 mg/dL, or whenever toxicity is suspected. By increasing the urine pH to 8, the amount of ionized salicylate in the tubules increases and is "trapped" (i.e., it cannot be reabsorbed).

(a) Alkalinization may be achieved with an intravenous loading bolus of **sodium bicarbonate** (1–2 mEq/kg), followed by 3 ampules (132 mEq) of sodium bicarbonate in 1 L of 5% dextrose in water (D_5W) to run at 1.5–2 times maintenance.

(b) Hypokalemia must be corrected in order to achieve adequate alkalinization.

(2) Hemodialysis removes salicylate and corrects electrolyte abnormalities. Indications include severe, uncorrectable acidemia, fluid overload and pulmonary edema, cardiac or renal compromise, seizures, and coma. Serum salicylate levels that exceed 100 mg/dL (in acute ingestions) or 60–80 mg/dL (in chronic ingestions) are also an indication for hemodialysis, but the patient's clinical status should always direct treatment, and hemodialysis at lower serum levels should be instituted when appropriate.

(3) Charcoal hemoperfusion provides better salicylate clearance but does not correct the metabolic abnormalities associated with poisoning.

6. **Disposition**

a. **Discharge.** Patients who receive activated charcoal and remain asymptomatic may be safely discharged after 6–8 hours. Patients who have ingested sustained-release preparations may require a more prolonged period of observation.

b. **Admission.** All patients who have toxic levels, are symptomatic, or develop symptoms during observation in the ED should be admitted to a monitored setting.

III PRESCRIPTION DRUGS

A **Drugs used in the treatment of psychiatric disorders**

1. **Benzodiazepine overdose.** Benzodiazepines are used in the treatment of anxiety disorders, insomnia, and pain disorders, and as muscle relaxants.

a. **Discussion**

(1) Toxicity. Benzodiazepines are a common ingestant in overdoses; however, deaths caused by benzodiazepine ingestion alone are very rare. Deaths, when they occur, are usually secondary to benzodiazepines taken in combination with other depressant substances.

(2) Mechanism of action. All benzodiazepines exert varying sedative, hypnotic, amnestic, anxiolytic, anticonvulsant, and muscle relaxant properties, secondary to their potentiation of the inhibitory effect of γ-aminobutyric acid (GABA), the major inhibitory neurotransmitter in the CNS.

(a) The benzodiazepine binds to the CNS benzodiazepine receptor, inducing a conformational change in the receptor. This conformational change facilitates the binding of GABA to the GABA receptor.

(b) GABA binding enhances chloride channel opening in the neuron, and the resultant influx of chloride into the neuron hyperpolarizes the cell. As a result, excitatory activity is inhibited in the hyperpolarized cell.

b. **Clinical features.** CNS depression is the hallmark of overdose. Findings may include:

(1) Dizziness, depression, apathy

(2) Drowsiness, stupor, ataxia

(3) Hypotonia or motor retardation

(4) Low-grade coma

(5) Profound coma, hypotension, respiratory depression, or hypothermia (very rare)

c. **Differential diagnoses** include **head trauma, stroke, hypoglycemia or other metabolic abnormalities,** and **carbon monoxide poisoning.**

d. **Evaluation**

  (1) Physical examination. The ABCs should be assessed and evidence of trauma sought.

  (2) Laboratory studies

    (a) Rapid bedside testing of glucose should be performed.

    (b) A **pregnancy test** is indicated for women of childbearing age.

    (c) An **ethanol level** should be obtained to check for concurrent ethanol ingestion.

    (d) Urine drug screening may help to confirm the diagnosis or suggest other drugs that could be contributing to the patient's altered mental status, but emergency management should not necessarily wait for, or be changed by, these results.

    (e) Quantitative serum levels of benzodiazepines have no usefulness in the emergency management of patients with benzodiazepine overdose.

  (3) Diagnostic studies. An ECG should be obtained.

e. **Therapy.** Most patients require only supportive care and observation.

  (1) Supportive measures. Most patients with benzodiazepine overdose become arousable within 12–36 hours when treated supportively.

    (a) A **patent airway** must be ensured, and aspiration precautions must be in place.

    (b) Activated charcoal and **intravenous fluids** should be administered.

  (2) Antidote treatment is with **flumazenil** (see I D 4), which rapidly reverses the sedative, anxiolytic, anticonvulsant, ataxic, and muscle relaxant effects of benzodiazepines by competitively binding to the benzodiazepine receptor.

    (a) Because flumazenil can have serious adverse effects, it is not indicated for every patient with benzodiazepine overdose. One indication may be for patients with severe CNS depression who may require intubation otherwise.

    (b) Because the half-life of flumazenil is less than that of many benzodiazepines, resedation may occur.

f. **Disposition**

  (1) Discharge from the ED after a period of several hours of observation is appropriate for patients who are awake and who have ingested only benzodiazepines.

  (2) Admission. Indications for inpatient admission include:

    (a) Profound CNS or respiratory depression

    (b) Evidence of concomitant drug ingestion

    (c) The use of flumazenil

2. Lithium toxicity. Lithium's primary use is in the treatment of manic-depressive disorders.

a. **Discussion**

  (1) Toxicity. Lithium has a narrow toxic:therapeutic ratio. Chronic lithium poisoning is associated with higher morbidity and mortality rates than acute lithium poisoning.

  (2) Pathophysiology. Lithium poisoning most often occurs as the result of altered drug pharmacokinetics, leading to chronic toxicity. Many drugs affect lithium metabolism.

b. **Clinical features**

  (1) CNS signs are the most common. Tremors, fasciculations, movement disorders, and a Parkinsonian-like syndrome can be present in mild poisonings. In severe poisonings, stupor, coma, seizures, and a prolonged encephalopathy can be present.

  (2) Renal signs are also common. Lithium compromises the ability of the kidneys to concentrate the urine, leading to transient diuresis, nephrogenic diabetes insipidus, and renal tubular acidosis. Dehydration and high urine output are clinical signs of renal involvement.

  (3) Other signs

(a) **Cardiopulmonary signs** may be present but are rare.

(b) **Gastrointestinal symptoms** (e.g., nausea, vomiting, diarrhea) are common but are usually not life-threatening.

(c) **Endocrine signs** include those of hypothyroidism.

c. **Differential diagnoses** include **head trauma, encephalitis, acute schizophrenia or psychosis, parkinsonism,** and **primary hypothyroidism.**

d. **Evaluation**

(1) **Laboratory studies**

(a) A **serum lithium level, glucose level, serum electrolyte panel, BUN and creatinine level, urinalysis,** and **thyroid function tests** should be obtained for all patients with suspected lithium toxicity.

(b) If diabetes insipidus is suspected, **urinary electrolytes** should be obtained.

(2) **Other studies.** If encephalopathy is suspected, a computed tomography (CT) scan of the head and lumbar puncture should be considered.

e. **Therapy**

(1) **Gastric decontamination. Gastric lavage** and **whole-bowel irrigation** should be considered. Lithium does not bind to charcoal.

(2) **Elimination enhancement**

(a) **Intravenous saline** should be administered to replace and maintain sodium and water balance. Sodium facilitates the elimination of lithium. A Foley catheter should be inserted to monitor fluid status.

(b) **Hemodialysis** is the most effective method of eliminating systemic lithium. Hemodialysis should be considered in patients who meet any of the following criteria:

(i) Chronic poisoning with a lithium level greater than 4.0 mEq/L

(ii) Persistent electrolyte disorders

(iii) Life-threatening neurologic toxicity

f. **Disposition**

(1) **Discharge.** Asymptomatic patients with a serum lithium level of less than 2.0 mEq/L can be discharged.

(2) **Admission** is indicated for:

(a) All symptomatic patients

(b) All patients with a serum lithium level greater than 2.0 mEq/L

(3) **Referral.** Psychiatric consult may be warranted for suicidal patients.

3. **Cyclic antidepressant overdose.** Cyclic antidepressants are the leading cause of death by intentional overdose of a prescription medication.

a. **Discussion**

(1) **Mechanism of action.** Cyclic antidepressants prevent the reuptake of synaptic neurotransmitters (e.g., norepinephrine, serotonin). In addition to improving mood, cyclic antidepressants have class Ia antiarrhythmic effects.

(2) **Pathophysiology.** Death is predominantly caused by dysrhythmias and cardiovascular compromise. Tricyclic antidepressants, the oldest class of cyclic antidepressants, have the greatest potential for cardiac toxicity. The newer agents (e.g., amoxapine, trazodone, clozapine) have less cardiotoxic potential.

b. **Clinical features**

(1) Most cyclic antidepressants have an **anticholinergic effect,** characterized by xerostomia, dry skin, blurred vision, mydriasis, urinary retention, and delirium (see I C 3 c). Agitation and myoclonic jerks are also common findings.

(2) In severe poisonings, hypotension, seizures, respiratory depression, and cardiac dysrhythmias are classic findings.

(3) Findings in advanced poisonings include adult respiratory distress syndrome (ARDS), rhabdomyolysis, and disseminated intravascular coagulation (DIC).

    c. Differential diagnoses include **myocardial infarction (MI), hyperkalemia, sympathomimetic abuse,** and **alcohol withdrawal.**

    d. Evaluation

        (1) Diagnostic studies. Special attention should be paid to the **ECG.** Signs of toxicity include:

            (a) A prolonged QTc (often the first sign)

            (b) Sinus tachycardia and a prolonged QRS interval (longer than 0.1 second)

            (c) An R wave greater than 3 mm in the AVR

        (2) Laboratory studies include an ABG determination, a serum electrolyte panel, and a glucose level.

        (3) Imaging studies. A chest radiograph is indicated if the patient has clinical signs of ARDS.

    e. Therapy

        (1) Initial stabilization. Standard advanced cardiac life support (ACLS) protocols should be employed.

        (2) Treatment of dysrhythmias and hypotension

            (a) Sodium bicarbonate (1–2 mg/kg as an intravenous bolus) should be administered until the dysrhythmias and hypotension resolve. Intravenous sodium bicarbonate (3 ampules in 1 L of D_5W) may then be administered at a rate of 250 mL/hour, titrated until a serum pH of 7.45–7.50 is reached.

            (b) Intravenous saline fluid challenge may also be indicated.

            (c) Hyperventilation. The goal is an arterial pH between 7.45 and 7.50.

            (d) Lidocaine, bretylium, or **phenytoin** can be administered if the dysrhythmias persist. Class Ia antiarrhythmics (e.g., procainamide, quinidine) should be avoided.

            (e) Intravenous norepinephrine or an **intra-aortic balloon pump** may be indicated for patients with life-threatening hypotension.

        (3) Treatment of seizures and agitation. If seizures are present, **diazepam,** a benzodiazepine, is the first-line drug. The dose is 5 mg in adults and 0.1–0.5 mg/kg in children, administered intravenously. Most seizures are short-lived.

        (4) Gastric decontamination. Charcoal (1 mg/kg) should be administered.

    f. Disposition. All patients with known or suspected cyclic antidepressant overdose should undergo cardiac monitoring for at least 6–8 hours.

        (1) Discharge. Asymptomatic patients with a normal cardiac rhythm and normal cardiac conduction intervals at the end of the observation period can be transferred to a psychiatric facility or discharged home.

        (2) Admission. Patients with symptoms or cardiac conduction abnormalities should be admitted to an intensive care unit (ICU).

        (3) Referral. All patients with intentional overdoses should be referred for psychiatric evaluation.

4. Neuroleptic overdose. Neuroleptics are a class of drugs used to modify behavior. Clinically, this category usually includes antipsychotic drugs, specifically phenothiazines, thioxanthenes, and butyrophenone.

    a. Discussion

        (1) Toxicity. Although generally considered to have a high toxic:therapeutic ratio, neuroleptic toxicity varies considerably. Haloperidol is associated with a low rate of life-threatening events, whereas thioridazine is associated with a higher rate of life-threatening events. Death from a pure neuroleptic ingestion is uncommon.

        (2) Pathophysiology. Certain neuroleptics (e.g., thioridazine, mesoridazine) can cause cardiac dysrhythmias and hypotension similar to that caused by cyclic antidepressant overdose.

    b. Clinical features

        (1) Neurologic features of neuroleptic overdose include **sedation** and **depressed mental status, seizures, movement disorders** (including **dystonic reactions** and **tardive dyskinesias), and neuroleptic malignant syndrome (NMS; see Chapter 9 IX). Dystonic reactions**

are a side effect of certain drugs (in particular antipsychotics and antiemetics) thought to be caused by CNS dopamine blockade; they are most commonly associated with haloperidol. Although the signs are often anxiety-provoking (torticollis, tongue protrusion, trismus, and speech impediment), they are rarely life-threatening.

   (2) **Cardiovascular features** include hypotension and cardiac dysrhythmias.

   (3) **Anticholinergic features.** Most neuroleptics have anticholinergic properties (see I C 3 c).

   c. **Differential diagnoses** include an **acute psychotic episode, cyclic antidepressant overdose, sepsis, meningitis,** and **seizures.** In patients exhibiting dystonic reactions, **cerebrovascular accident, psychogenic catatonia, tetanus, parkinsonism,** and **strychnine poisoning** should be considered.

   d. **Evaluation**

   (1) **Glucose, BUN, creatinine,** and **creatinine phosphokinase levels** should be obtained for all patients. A **drug screen** may also be appropriate.

   (2) **Special studies** may be appropriate depending on the patient's clinical presentation:

   (a) **Dystonic reactions.** In patients with prolonged dystonic reactions, **urinalysis** and a **serum electrolyte panel** should also be considered. A **diagnostic challenge with an anticholinergic agent** (e.g., diphenhydramine, 0.5–1 mg intravenously or intramuscularly, or benztropine, 1–2 mg intravenously or intramuscularly) should resolve symptoms within 1 hour.

   (b) **NMS.** In patients with signs of NMS, a septic work-up should be considered.

   (3) A **CT scan** of the head may be warranted.

   e. **Therapy**

   (1) **Initial stabilization.** Standard ACLS protocols should be carried out.

   (2) **Treatment of dysrhythmias and hypotension** is the same as that for dysrhythmias caused by cyclic antidepressant overdose [see III A 3 e (2)].

   (3) **Treatment of seizures** is with intravenous diazepam (5 mg in adults; 0.1–0.5 mg/kg in children).

   (4) **Treatment of dystonic reactions.** Dystonic reactions are treated with diphenhydramine (25–50 mg orally every 6–8 hours in adults, 5 mg/kg/day in children in divided doses) or benztropine (1–2 mg/day) for 24–48 hours to prevent recurrence of the dystonic reaction.

   (5) **Treatment of NMS** entails the administration of a benzodiazepine, bromocriptine (2.5 mg orally twice daily), or dantrolene (0.8 mg/kg orally or intravenously every 6 hours) and vigorous hydration to prevent rhabdomyolysis.

   f. **Disposition**

   (1) **Discharge.** Asymptomatic patients can be discharged.

   (2) **Admission** is indicated for patients who do not show significant improvement within 1–2 hours of therapy.

B **Drugs used in the treatment of cardiovascular disorders**   Medications used for the treatment of hypertension, cardiac dysrhythmias, and angina are a common cause of toxicity and morbidity in overdose.

1. **β-Adrenergic antagonist (β blocker) overdose.** β Blockers are class II antiarrhythmics, used for the treatment of hypertension, angina, dysrhythmias, thyrotoxicosis, migraines, and glaucoma.

   a. **Discussion**

   (1) **Pharmacokinetics.** Most agents are rapidly absorbed from the gastrointestinal tract.

   (2) **Pathophysiology.** In overdose, β blockers cause cardiovascular and CNS effects. Symptoms occur within hours, and the half-life is prolonged. Cardiotoxicity varies, depending on the agent's cardioselectivity (β_1 versus β_2), degree of β agonist activity, membrane depressant effects, and lipid solubility.

   (a) β_1 **Antagonists** decrease the sinus rate, contractility, conduction, and renin release.

   (b) β_2 **Antagonists** increase bronchial smooth muscle contraction and may precipitate bronchoconstriction in patients with asthma. In addition, they alter insulin release and triglyceride metabolism, especially in patients with insulin-dependent diabetes mellitus.

    (c) **Partial agonists** increase the heart rate and smooth muscle tone.

    (d) **Agents that have membrane depressant effects** decrease sodium influx, prolonging depolarization, and calcium release, depressing myocardial contractility and electrical conduction.

    (e) **Lipid-soluble agents** cause more CNS depression, seizures, and apnea.

  b. **Clinical features**

    (1) **Cardiovascular features** include bradycardia, conduction abnormalities, hypotension, and pulmonary edema. Partial agonists may cause hypertension and tachycardia.

    (2) **Neurologic features** include lethargy, dilated pupils, coma, and seizures.

    (3) **Other features** include hypoglycemia and bronchospasm.

  c. **Differential diagnoses** include **calcium channel blocker overdose, digitalis toxicity, primary cardiac disease, sedative-hypnotic overdose, stroke,** and **hypoglycemia.**

  d. **Evaluation.** An ECG and chest radiograph should be obtained. Appropriate laboratory studies include a serum glucose level, serum electrolyte panel, ABG determination, and cardiac enzyme studies.

  e. **Therapy**

    (1) **Initial stabilization** involves airway management, cardiovascular resuscitation, and continuous cardiac monitoring.

      (a) **Hypotension** is treated with intravenous fluid boluses or epinephrine or norepinephrine infusion. These agents have a high lethality in overdose, and some patients may require aortic balloon pump placement to maintain hemodynamic stability sufficient for adequate perfusion during the acute period of toxicity.

      (b) **Bradycardia** is treated with atropine or isoproterenol infusion. Temporary transvenous pacemaker placement should be considered for patients with refractory bradycardia.

      (c) **Seizures** are treated with benzodiazepines.

      (d) **Bronchospasm** is treated with β_2 agonists.

    (2) **Gastric decontamination**

      (a) **Gastric lavage** is indicated if the patient presents early enough in the course of the poisoning.

      (b) **Activated charcoal** should be administered.

      (c) **Whole-bowel irrigation** may be appropriate for patients with massive ingestions or those who have ingested a long-acting preparation.

    (3) **Antidote treatment**

      (a) **Glucagon** is a non–β-adrenergic receptor agonist that increases intracellular cyclic adenosine monophosphate (cAMP) synthesis, enhancing contractility by increasing calcium influx.

        (i) **Indications** include hemodynamic compromise.

        (ii) **Dosage.** The dosage for adults is 5–10 mg administered as an intravenous bolus, followed by an infusion at a rate of 5 mg/hour. Large doses should be mixed in a normal saline diluent.

      (b) **Amrinone** is a phosphodiesterase inhibitor that prevents cAMP breakdown, enhancing calcium influx. A loading dose of 0.75 mg/kg is administered, followed by an infusion at a rate of 5–10 μg/kg/min.

  f. **Disposition**

    (1) **Discharge.** Patients who receive activated charcoal and are observed to be asymptomatic with a normal ECG after 6–8 hours may be discharged.

    (2) **Admission** to a cardiac monitoring unit is indicated for all symptomatic patients and those who have ingested sustained-release or long-acting preparations.

2. Calcium channel antagonist overdose. Calcium channel blockers are class IV antiarrhythmics, used in the treatment of hypertension, dysrhythmias, angina, migraine, and subarachnoid hemorrhage with cerebral vasospasm.

a. Discussion

   (1) Pharmacokinetics. Calcium channel blockers are well absorbed and highly protein bound. With regular-release formulas, the onset of action occurs within 1 hour. Sustained-release preparations have a delayed onset of action.

   (2) Mechanism of action. These agents inhibit calcium influx across voltage-dependent slow channels, decreasing sinoatrial (SA) and atrioventricular (AV) node conduction. They prevent calcium influx across fast channels during the plateau phase of contraction, decreasing contractility, and causing smooth muscle relaxation.

b. Clinical features

   (1) Cardiovascular features include conduction delays and blocks, myocardial depression, reduced cardiac output, vasodilation, and hypotension.

   (2) Neurologic features include dizziness, coma, apnea, and seizures.

   (3) Other features include metabolic acidosis and, possibly, hyperglycemia.

c. Differential diagnoses include β **blocker overdose, digitalis toxicity, primary cardiac abnormalities, sedative-hypnotic overdose,** and **stroke.**

d. Evaluation. Appropriate studies include an ECG, a chest radiograph, ABG determinations, serum electrolyte panel, and cardiac enzyme levels.

e. Therapy

   (1) Initial stabilization involves airway management, cardiovascular resuscitation, and continuous cardiac monitoring. Hypotension and bradycardia often respond to intravenous administration of calcium and glucagon [see III B 2 e (3) (a)–(b)]; other approaches include the following:

   (a) Hypotension can be treated with intravenous fluid boluses or epinephrine or norepinephrine infusion [see III B 1 e (1) (a)].

   (b) Bradycardia can be treated with atropine. Temporary transvenous pacemaker placement may be necessary.

   (2) Gastric decontamination

   (a) Gastric lavage is indicated for early presentations.

   (b) Activated charcoal is effective.

   (c) Whole-bowel irrigation should be considered for patients who have ingested a sustained-release preparation.

   (3) Antidote treatment

   (a) Calcium overcomes the toxicity of calcium channel blockers by entering the cell through other channels, enhancing contractility. It is administered as 10 mL of **10% calcium chloride** or 30 mL of **calcium gluconate.** Repeat boluses are administered every 15–20 minutes, for a total of four to five doses. CaCl should ideally be infused through a central line due to severe vein irritation and pain.

   (b) Glucagon is administered as a 5- to 10-mg bolus intravenously, and then as an infusion at a rate of 5 mg/hour. Large doses should be diluted in normal saline.

   (c) Amrinone may be used in refractory cases to enhance contractility. The dosage is the same as for β blocker toxicity [see III B 1 e (3) (b)].

f. Disposition

   (1) Discharge. Patients who receive activated charcoal and remain asymptomatic with a normal ECG for 6–8 hours (after ingesting a regular-release formula) may be discharged.

   (2) Admission. All symptomatic patients, including those with AV conduction abnormalities, should be admitted to a cardiac care setting. Patients who have ingested sustained-release preparations should be monitored for 24 hours for signs of delayed toxicity.

3. **Digitalis toxicity.** Digoxin is the most common digitalis preparation in the United States. Cardiac glycoside–containing plants include oleander, foxglove, and lily of the valley, and may cause digitalis toxicity if smoked or ingested.

a. **Discussion**

(1) **Pharmacokinetics.** Digoxin is fairly well absorbed from the gastrointestinal tract, and is widely distributed to muscle tissue.

(2) **Pathophysiology.** Ingestion of 0.05 mg/kg of digoxin can produce toxic levels.

(a) **Mechanism.** Digoxin affects the ATPase-dependent sodium–potassium pump, allowing potassium efflux from the cell and sodium and calcium influx into the cell. The result is enhanced excitability and contractility in myocardial muscle, and decreased conduction velocity in conductive tissue.

(b) **Predisposing factors** to enhanced toxicity include advanced age, hepatic or renal disease, electrolyte abnormalities, and pre-existing cardiac disease.

b. **Clinical features**

(1) **Acute toxicity.** The onset of symptoms may be delayed as long as 6 hours.

(a) **Cardiovascular features** include tachydysrhythmias with all grades of AV block, bradycardia, depressed contractility, and decreased cardiac output.

(b) **Gastrointestinal symptoms** include anorexia, nausea, vomiting, and abdominal pain.

(c) **Neurologic symptoms** include confusion, headache, hallucinations, and visual disturbances (e.g., abnormal color perception, yellow halos).

(2) **Chronic toxicity.** Electrolyte abnormalities and renal insufficiency predispose to cardiovascular abnormalities (e.g., dysrhythmias, especially accelerated atrial or junctional tachycardia with all grades of AV block; ventricular automaticity; and extrasystoles) as well as malaise, anorexia, nausea, vomiting, blurred vision, and confusion.

(3) **Acute on chronic toxicity** appears clinically similar to acute toxicity.

c. **Differential diagnoses** include **calcium channel blocker or β blocker overdose, primary cardiac abnormalities, stroke,** and **electrolyte abnormalities.**

d. **Evaluation**

(1) **Laboratory studies**

(a) **Serum digoxin levels** peak within 2 hours of ingestion. Levels drawn 6 hours after ingestion correlate with toxicity, which occurs at serum digoxin levels that exceed 2 ng/mL. Serious toxicity occurs at serum digoxin levels of 10–15 ng/mL, but dysrhythmias may occur at lower levels.

(b) **Serum electrolytes.** Hyperkalemia (a serum potassium level greater than 5.0 mEq/L) indicates serious toxicity. Calcium and magnesium levels should also be assessed.

(c) **BUN, creatinine,** and **cardiac enzyme levels** should also be ordered.

(2) **Diagnostic studies.** An **ECG** and **chest radiograph** should be obtained.

e. **Therapy**

(1) **Initial stabilization** involves airway management, cardiovascular resuscitation, and continuous cardiac monitoring.

(a) **Ventricular ectopy** is treated with lidocaine or phenytoin.

(b) **Symptomatic bradycardia** is treated with atropine. Type Ia antiarrhythmics and calcium boluses should be avoided. Transvenous pacemaker placement may be appropriate.

(c) **Electrolyte imbalances** should be corrected carefully.

(2) **Gastric decontamination.** Gastric lavage (for early presentations) and the administration of activated charcoal are indicated.

(3) **Antidote treatment** is with digoxin-specific antibodies, which consist of Fab fragments that bind digoxin, removing it from cardiac receptors and reversing toxicity.

(a) **Indications** include life-threatening dysrhythmias, a serum potassium level greater than 5.0 mEq/L, a serum digoxin level greater than 10–15 ng/mL, and advanced age.

      (b) Dosing. Fab is administered in an equimolar dose to neutralize the total body load of digoxin (1 mg digoxin = 50–100 mg Fab). The empiric dose for an adult is approximately 10–20 vials.

  f. Disposition

      (1) Discharge. Patients who receive activated charcoal and remain asymptomatic with normal digoxin and potassium levels 6 hours postingestion may be discharged.

      (2) Admission to a cardiac monitoring unit is indicated for symptomatic patients, including those with ECG abnormalities, and patients with chronic toxicity.

4. Clonidine toxicity. Clonidine is used for the treatment of hypertension and as adjunctive therapy in the treatment of opiate withdrawal. It is available in oral and transdermal preparations.

  a. Discussion

      (1) Pharmacokinetics. Clonidine is well absorbed from the gastrointestinal tract and widely distributed in the body. Clonidine is capable of penetrating the blood–brain barrier. The onset of action is within 1 hour.

      (2) Mechanism of action. Clonidine is a centrally acting α_2 agonist that decreases peripheral sympathetic stimulation, decreasing norepinephrine activity and lowering systemic vascular resistance, heart rate, and cardiac output.

      (3) Pathophysiology. In overdose, clonidine may initially exert peripheral α agonist effects, causing hypertension and tachycardia. It also has opiate-like CNS depressant activity. Toxic effects occur 1–3 hours postingestion.

  b. Clinical features

      (1) Cardiovascular features include bradycardia and hypotension. Hypertension and tachycardia may occur transiently.

      (2) Neurologic features include miosis, sedation, coma, hypotonia, hyporeflexia, respiratory depression, and apnea.

  c. Differential diagnoses. Consider **β blocker or calcium channel blocker overdose, narcotic or sedative-hypnotic overdose, stroke, head injury,** and **hypoglycemia.**

  d. Evaluation. An ECG, ABG determination, chest radiograph, glucose level, and serum electrolyte panel should be obtained.

  e. Therapy

      (1) Initial stabilization includes airway management, cardiovascular resuscitation, and continuous cardiac monitoring.

         (a) Early hypertensive symptoms may be treated with nitroprusside infusion.

         (b) Hypotension may be treated with intravenous fluid boluses or dopamine infusion.

         (c) Bradycardia may be treated with atropine.

      (2) Gastric decontamination is with **activated charcoal.**

      (3) Antidote treatment. Naloxone may be of benefit in reversing CNS depression. It has been reported to alleviate respiratory toxicity to a certain degree.

  f. Disposition

      (1) Discharge. Patients who receive activated charcoal and are asymptomatic after 6–8 hours of observation may be discharged.

      (2) Admission. Symptomatic patients must be admitted to a cardiac monitoring setting.

C Theophylline

1. Discussion. Theophylline is used in the treatment of asthma and apnea of prematurity; it improves bronchodilation, diaphragmatic contraction, and oxygen saturation. It is one of the most common causes of drug-induced seizures and status epilepticus.

  a. Pharmacokinetics. The **therapeutic serum range** is **10–20 μg/mL.**

      (1) Absorption. Theophylline is well absorbed from the gastrointestinal tract. Peak levels occur 4 hours after the administration of regular-release preparations, and 12–24 hours after the administration of sustained-release formulas.

    (2) Metabolism and elimination
        (a) Half-life. Congestive heart failure (CHF), hepatic dysfunction, and fever prolong the half-life.
        (b) Clearance. Erythromycin, cimetidine, and ciprofloxacin decrease clearance, and phenobarbital, phenytoin, and cigarette smoking enhance clearance.
  b. Pathophysiology
    (1) Adenosine antagonism and phosphodiesterase inhibition (leading to elevated cAMP levels) cause smooth muscle relaxation.
    (2) Enhanced catecholamine release leads to myocardial stimulation.
    (3) Predisposing factors to enhanced toxicity include advanced age and pre-existing cardiovascular disease.

2. Clinical features
  a. Acute toxicity
    (1) Cardiovascular features include sinus tachycardia, supraventricular tachycardias, and hypotension.
    (2) CNS features include hyperventilation, tremulousness, agitation, seizures, and status epilepticus.
    (3) Gastrointestinal features include nausea and vomiting.
    (4) Metabolic features include hypokalemia, hyperglycemia, hypophosphatemia, and hypercalcemia.
    (5) Other features include leukocytosis and rhabdomyolysis.
  b. Chronic toxicity. Seizures and dysrhythmias occur at lower serum theophylline levels in patients with chronic toxicity.
    (1) Cardiovascular features include sinus tachycardia, supraventricular tachycardias, and atrial fibrillation.
    (2) CNS features include tremulousness and anxiety. Seizures may be the initial sign of toxicity.
  c. Acute on chronic toxicity resembles acute toxicity.

3. Differential diagnoses include **salicylate or stimulant ingestion, sepsis, thyrotoxicosis, primary cardiac dysrhythmias, meningitis,** and **head injury.**

4. Evaluation
  a. Serum theophylline level. In patients with single, acute ingestions, the serum theophylline level correlates roughly with the degree of toxicity: a serum theophylline level of 20–40 μg/mL suggests minimal toxicity, one of 40–100 μg/mL suggests moderate toxicity, and one of 100 μg/mL or more suggests severe toxicity.
  b. A **serum electrolyte panel** (including potassium, glucose, phosphate, calcium, and magnesium), a **CBC,** an **ABG determination,** and **creatine phosphokinase levels** should be ordered. A **PT** and **partial thromboplastin time (PTT)** should be ordered as well (in preparation for invasive elimination procedures). Urine should be assessed for myoglobin.
  c. Diagnostic imaging studies. An **ECG** and **chest radiograph** should be ordered.

5. Therapy
  a. Initial stabilization entails airway management, cardiovascular resuscitation, and continuous cardiac monitoring.
    (1) Arrhythmias. Supraventricular tachycardia may be treated with β blockers or verapamil, and ventricular ectopy or tachycardia is treated with lidocaine.
    (2) Hypotension may be treated with intravenous fluid boluses or epinephrine or norepinephrine infusion.
    (3) Agitation and **seizures** are treated with benzodiazepines.
    (4) Vomiting may be treated with metoclopramide or ondansetron. Electrolyte abnormalities must be corrected carefully.
  b. Gastric decontamination

(1) **Gastric lavage** is indicated if the patient presents early in the course of the poisoning.
(2) **Activated charcoal.** Multiple-dose activated charcoal should be administered to enhance elimination of theophylline.
(3) **Whole-bowel irrigation** with polyethylene glycol solution may be beneficial when the patient has ingested a sustained-release preparation.

c. **Elimination enhancement. Charcoal hemoperfusion** greatly enhances theophylline clearance, and is preferred over hemodialysis, which clears a lesser amount of drug, but also corrects metabolic disturbances. Hemodialysis may be instituted if elimination enhancement is indicated and charcoal hemoperfusion is not readily available. Indications for hemoperfusion include:
(1) Seizures
(2) Hypotension unresponsive to intravenous fluid and pressor administration
(3) Dysrhythmias
(4) Persistent vomiting and the inability to take activated charcoal
(5) A serum theophylline level greater than 90 µg/mL after a single ingestion of a regular-release product
(6) A serum theophylline level greater than 40 µg/mL 4 hours after ingestion of a sustained-release preparation
(7) A serum theophylline level of 40–60 µg/mL in patients with chronic toxicity

6. **Disposition**
a. **Discharge.** The patient may be discharged if the serum level is within normal limits 4 hours after ingestion of a regular-release formula, and the patient has no symptoms of toxicity.
b. **Admission.** All patients with evidence of symptoms, or in whom serum levels are not decreasing or are rising, should be admitted to an intensive care setting. Patients who ingest sustained-release preparations should be monitored for 24 hours for signs of delayed toxicity.

IV DRUGS OF ABUSE

A **Opiate overdose**   Heroin is probably the most commonly abused illicit opiate. Although its popularity has been declining since its height of popularity in the 1970s and 1980s, it has seen a recent resurgence in popularity.

1. **Discussion**
a. Opiates can be ingested, insufflated, smoked, or intravenously injected.
b. **Pathophysiology.** Deaths from opiate abuse usually result from respiratory depression. Newer, synthetic agents can cause other life-threatening events (e.g., meperidine metabolites and dextromethorphan can cause seizures; propoxyphene can cause seizures and cardiac dysrhythmias).

2. **Clinical features**
a. **Symptoms.** Patients usually have depressed mental status.
b. **Physical examination findings** include pinpoint pupils and depressed respiratory drive. Frothy sputum, rhonchi, and rales are suggestive of NCPE, which has been reported in heroin users. Chest wall rigidity is a sign of an idiosyncratic reaction to fentanyl derivatives.

3. **Differential diagnoses** include **organophosphate poisoning, pontine hemorrhage,** and **clonidine overdose.**

4. **Evaluation**
a. **Response to naloxone.** The cornerstone of diagnosis of opiate intoxication is the response to naloxone (an opiate antagonist).
b. A **drug screen** may be helpful but certain opiates (e.g., fentanyl) may not show up on routine drug screens.
c. **ABG determinations** and a **chest radiograph** may be helpful in patients with suspected NCPE.
d. An **ECG** is indicated in patients with propoxyphene overdose.

5. Therapy

    a. Initial stabilization. ACLS protocols should be followed as indicated. Careful attention should be given to maintaining the airway. If the patient does not have an adequate respiratory drive, 100% oxygen should be administered by mechanical or assisted ventilation.

    b. Naloxone should be administered intravenously (1–2 mg every 2–3 minutes) until a total dose of 10 mg is reached or the desired effect is achieved. In patients with a known addiction to opiates, a lower dose of naloxone can be used to avoid withdrawal (0.4 mg every 2–3 minutes until the desired effect is achieved). Soft restraints may be placed before titration of naloxone to help protect the patient and staff members.

    c. Antiarrhythmic agents. Class Ia antiarrhythmic agents should be avoided in patients with propoxyphene-induced dysrhythmias.

    d. Loop diuretics, oxygen, and **vasodilators** should be used for patients with heroin-induced NCPE. Mechanical ventilation and positive end-expiratory pressure (PEEP) should be considered.

    e. Neuromuscular paralysis and **respiratory support** are indicated for patients with fentanyl-induced chest wall rigidity.

6. Disposition

    a. Discharge. Known heroin abusers who respond to naloxone therapy can be discharged after 4–6 hours of observation, when it is certain that respiratory depression will not recur.

    b. Admission

        (1) Patients who abuse or ingest long-acting opiates (e.g., methadone) should be admitted to the ICU.

        (2) Patients who suffered a life-threatening, opiate-induced period of hypoxia should be admitted for a 24-hour period of observation.

    c. Referral. All patients with opium toxicity should receive drug counseling. In addition, referral to a detoxification program should be offered.

B **Amphetamines and cocaine** are sympathomimetic agents that cause stimulation of the CNS. These drugs are among the most popular drugs of abuse.

1. Discussion

    a. Amphetamines and cocaine can be smoked, injected, nasally insufflated, and ingested.

    b. Pathophysiology. Death can be caused by cardiac dysrhythmias, MI, cerebrovascular accident, hyperthermia, and renal failure.

2. Clinical features

    a. Symptoms. Patients may be euphoric, anxious, paranoid, or agitated. They usually present to the ED with more than one complaint, the most common being chest pain.

    b. Physical examination findings. In significant poisonings, various life-threatening presentations can manifest.

        (1) Neurologic findings

            (a) Seizures can occur. These are usually self-limited and brief. Status epilepticus is usually a manifestation of a secondary pathologic process (e.g., intracerebral hemorrhage, coingestion).

            (b) Focal findings on neurologic examination suggest cerebrovascular accident.

            (c) A **"wash-out" syndrome** (i.e., depressed mental status, lethargy, and obtundation) has been described with chronic use or after prolonged binging. Patients usually recover spontaneously with supportive care only.

        (2) Cardiopulmonary findings

            (a) Dysrhythmias, hypotension or **hypertension,** and **signs of MI** are reflective of cardiotoxicity. Approximately 60% of patients who present to the ED with a chief complaint of chest pain shortly after cocaine ingestion have MI.

        (b) **Asthma** or **reactive airway disease** can be precipitated by smoking "crack" (an alkaloidal cocaine) or "crank" (an amphetamine).

     (3) **Profound hyperthermia** (greater than 105°F) can occur.

3. **Differential diagnoses** include **CNS infection, pheochromocytoma, thyroid storm, vasculitis,** and **hypoglycemia.**

4. **Evaluation**

    a. **Laboratory studies** include cardiac enzyme levels, a CBC, a serum electrolyte panel, BUN and creatinine levels, liver function tests, coagulation studies, glucose levels, and an ABG determination.

    b. **Diagnostic studies.** A chest radiograph and head CT scan should be considered. An ECG should be performed.

    c. **Other studies.** A lumbar puncture should be considered if infection or subarachnoid hemorrhage is suspected. If hyperthermia is suspected, a rectal temperature should be obtained.

5. **Therapy**

    a. **Initial stabilization.** ACLS protocols should be implemented if warranted. **Diazepam** (2.5 mg administered intravenously and titrated to effect) is the mainstay of therapy.

    b. **Treatment of cardiotoxicity**

        (1) Patients with evidence of MI should be treated with nitrates, anticoagulants, thrombolytics, and emergency cardiac angioplasty as indicated.

        (2) Patients with malignant hypertension should be treated with a nitroprusside intravenous drip.

        (3) Class Ia antiarrhythmics and β blockers should be avoided.

    c. **Treatment of bronchospasm.** Patients with bronchospasm should be treated with bronchodilators and steroids.

    d. **Treatment of intracranial hemorrhage.** Patients with evidence of intracranial hemorrhage require emergent neurosurgical consultation.

    e. **Treatment of hyperthermia** must be aggressive. The core temperature should be reduced to below 104°F as rapidly as possible.

        (1) Ice baths or constant water misting with intense fanning are used for treating hyperthermia.

        (2) Sedation or neuromuscular paralysis can be employed.

        (3) Phenothiazines should be avoided.

    f. **Treatment of rhabdomyolysis** must also be aggressive (see Chapter 9 VIII B).

6. **Disposition**

    a. **Discharge.** Patients who are asymptomatic and show no evidence of end-organ damage may be discharged.

    b. **Admission.** Patients who are symptomatic and show end-organ toxicity require admission. Patients with cardiac or neurologic toxicity require ICU admission.

    c. **Referral.** All patients should be offered drug counseling and the opportunity to enroll in a detoxification program.

C **Hallucinogens**

1. **Discussion.** Many drugs or compounds have hallucinogenic properties, and certain substances are sought out and consumed for these properties. Synthetic hallucinogens include lysergic acid diethylamide (LSD), 3–4 methylenedioxyamphetamine (MDA), and N,N-dimethyltryptamine. Naturally occurring hallucinogens include psilocybin, peyote, and myristicin.

    a. **Mechanism of action.** The exact mechanism of action has not been elucidated for most hallucinogens. It is thought that hallucinogens interact with serotonin and dopamine mechanisms in the CNS.

    b. **Toxicity.** The effect and toxicity of various hallucinogens are highly variable. Although most drugs of abuse that are consumed primarily for their hallucinogenic properties have low intrinsic toxicity, patients suffer morbidity and mortality from actions that they perform while intoxicated (e.g., driving).

2. **Clinical features**
   a. **Symptoms.** Patients experiencing a "bad trip" will often complain of **anxiety, paranoia,** and **unusual thought processes.** Most patients who are under the influence of hallucinogens have a **"sense of self"** and are therefore oriented and coherent. Phencyclidine (PCP) is one hallucinogenic agent (although usually not consumed primarily for its hallucinogenic properties) in which patients lose this "sense of self."
   b. **Signs.** Certain hallucinogenic agents can have various side effects.
      (1) **Hyperthermia** has been associated with synthetic hallucinogens with amphetamine-like properties (e.g., LSD, MDA).
      (2) **Anticholinergic effects** have been associated with other agents (e.g., psilocybin, myristicin) causing dry mouth, mydriasis, tachycardia, flushed skin, and delirium.

3. **Differential diagnoses** include **acute psychosis, conversion disorder, encephalitis, neurosyphilis,** and **dementia.**

4. **Evaluation.** Most hallucinogenic agents will not be apparent on routine "drugs of abuse" screens performed through the ED. Urinalysis and creatine phosphokinase, BUN, and creatinine levels should be considered in patients with protracted symptoms to rule out rhabdomyolysis.

5. **Therapy**
   a. Most patients have stable vital signs. These patients usually require only reassurance and seclusion in a nonthreatening environment. Anxiolytics (e.g., diazepam, 2.5 mg intravenously or orally, titrated to effect) can also be administered.
   b. Patients with evidence of rhabdomyolysis or hyperthermia require aggressive therapy (see IV B 5 e–f).

6. **Disposition**
   a. **Discharge.** Asymptomatic patients may be discharged after 4–6 hours of observation.
   b. **Admission.** Patients with evidence of hyperthermia, anticholinergic delirium, rhabdomyolysis, or persistent symptoms after a 4- to 6-hour observation period should be admitted.
   c. **Referral.** All patients should be offered drug abuse counseling and the opportunity to enroll in a detoxification program.

V TOXIC ALCOHOLS

The metabolites of toxic alcohols cause morbidity and mortality. A toxic alcohol ingestion should be suspected when an anion gap metabolic acidosis and osmolal gap are present. However, a normal osmolal gap does not exclude a toxic alcohol ingestion.

A **Ethylene glycol** is used as a coolant and in antifreeze solutions. The **lethal ingested dose** is estimated to be **1.0–1.5 mL/kg.**

1. **Discussion.** Ethylene glycol is absorbed rapidly from the gastrointestinal tract. It is sequentially oxidized in the liver to **glycoaldehyde, glycolate,** and **glyoxylate,** producing an elevated reduced nicotinamide adenine dinucleotide (NADH):nicotinamide adenine dinucleotide (NAD) ratio and lactic acidosis.
   a. **CNS euphoria, intoxication,** and **depression** result from ethylene glycol.
   b. **Myocardial depression** is caused by glyoxylate.
   c. **Acute tubular necrosis** results from calcium oxalate crystal deposition and direct toxicity.
   d. An **anion gap acidosis** is caused by glycolate, glyoxylate, and lactate.
   e. **Hypocalcemia** occurs secondary to calcium oxalate crystal formation and deposition.

2. **Clinical features.** Ethylene glycol causes CNS effects that approximate acute ethanol intoxication. There are generally three stages of toxicity from ethylene glycol ingestion:

a. **Stage I** (1–12 hours postingestion) is characterized by CNS depression, cerebral edema, coma, and seizures. Myoclonic jerking, nausea, and vomiting may occur. At this stage, metabolic acidosis is beginning to develop.

b. **Stage II** (12–24 hours postingestion) is characterized by tachycardia, tachypnea, and mild hypertension, followed by the development of CHF and circulatory collapse.

c. **Stage III** (24–72 hours postingestion) is characterized by acute tubular necrosis, oliguria, and acute renal failure.

3. **Differential diagnoses** include **ingestion of another type of toxic alcohol or a CNS depressant, head injury, stroke, pulmonary edema, sepsis,** and **acute renal failure.**

4. **Evaluation**

   a. **Laboratory studies**

      (1) **Ethylene glycol, methanol,** and **ethanol levels** should be ordered.

      (2) An **ABG determination, serum osmolality, serum electrolyte panel, calcium,** and **BUN and creatinine levels** should be obtained.

      (3) **Urine** should be examined for **calcium oxalate crystals** and **fluorescence** when exposed to ultraviolet light. (Fluorescence suggests the excretion of fluorescein, an additive of many antifreezes.) While helpful if present, urinary crystals and fluorescence may be absent despite significant toxicity.

   b. **Diagnostic studies**

      (1) An **ECG** should be evaluated for prolonged QT intervals, suggestive of hypocalcemia.

      (2) A **chest radiograph** should be evaluated for pulmonary edema.

5. **Therapy**

   a. **Initial stabilization** entails airway management, mechanical ventilation, and cardiovascular resuscitation. Acidosis should be corrected by administering intravenous sodium bicarbonate. Electrolyte imbalances should be corrected, and calcium repleted.

   b. **Elimination enhancement. Hemodialysis** is indicated at serum ethylene glycol levels of 25 mg/dL or greater. Hemodialysis should also be initiated under conditions of profound metabolic acidosis, deteriorating vital signs, crystalluria, renal compromise, and pulmonary edema.

   c. **Antidote treatment**

      (1) **Ethanol** competitively inhibits the metabolism of ethylene glycol to its harmful metabolites.

         (a) **Indications.** Ethanol is indicated for patients with anion gap metabolic acidosis, an osmolal gap, and/or a high suspicion of ethylene glycol ingestion.

         (b) **Dosage.** The loading dose is 0.8 g/kg followed by a maintenance dose of 130 mg/kg/hour to obtain a serum ethanol level of 100–150 mg/dL. Ethanol may be administered as a 5%–10% concentration intravenously, or as a 20%–30% concentration orally.

      (2) **Fomepizole** may be given IV and may be more advantageous in some patients as it also slows formation of toxic products of ethylene glycol metabolism.

      (3) **Cofactors** aid in the detoxification of ethylene glycol's metabolites and include:

         (a) **Pyridoxine** (50 mg every 6 hours intravenously)

         (b) **Thiamine** (100 mg every 6 hours intravenously)

B **Methanol (wood alcohol)** is used in solvents, antifreeze, windshield washer fluid, Sterno canned heat, paints, paint removers, and varnishes. The **lethal ingested dose** is approximately **15–30 mL** in adults.

1. **Discussion.** Methanol is rapidly absorbed from the gastrointestinal tract and the skin; it may also be inhaled. It is sequentially oxidized in the liver to **formaldehyde** and **formate,** producing an elevated NADH:NAD ratio and lactic acidosis. These metabolites concentrate in the vitreous humor and optic nerve, causing ocular toxicity.

   a. **CNS depression** and an **osmolal gap** are caused by methanol.

   b. **Ocular toxicity** and an **anion gap acidosis** are caused by formate.

2. **Clinical features.** Methanol causes CNS effects similar to those caused by ethanol. Symptoms occur 40 minutes to 72 hours after ingestion. Serious toxicity is not usually apparent until 12–24 hours postingestion.

   a. **CNS features** include euphoria, intoxication, headache, vertigo, lethargy, confusion, seizures, and coma.

   b. **Ocular features** include blurred vision; decreased visual acuity; classically, a "snowstorm" effect; dilated, minimally responsive pupils; retinal edema; and hyperemia of the optic disk.

   c. **Gastrointestinal features** include nausea, vomiting, abdominal pain, and symptoms of pancreatitis.

   d. **Renal features.** Myoglobinuria and acute renal failure have been reported.

3. **Differential diagnoses** include **ethanol or another toxic alcohol ingestion, CNS depressant ingestion, head injury, stroke,** and **other causes of acute retinopathy.**

4. **Evaluation**

   a. **Ethylene glycol, methanol,** and **ethanol levels** should be obtained.

   b. An **ABG determination, serum osmolality, serum electrolyte panel,** and **BUN and creatinine levels** should be obtained. A **urinalysis** should be ordered to assess myoglobin.

   c. **Visual acuity** should be evaluated.

5. **Therapy**

   a. **Initial stabilization** includes airway management, mechanical ventilation, and cardiovascular resuscitation. Acidosis should be corrected by administering sodium bicarbonate intravenously. Electrolyte imbalances should be corrected, and the patient should be monitored for the development of hypoglycemia and myoglobinuria.

   b. **Elimination enhancement. Hemodialysis** is indicated at serum methanol levels of 20–50 mg/dL or greater. Hemodialysis should also be initiated in patients with profound metabolic acidosis, deteriorating vital signs, visual impairment, or renal failure.

   c. **Antidote treatment**

      (1) **Ethanol** competitively inhibits further metabolism of methanol to its harmful metabolites. The indications and dosage are the same as for ethylene glycol intoxication [see V A 5 c (1) (a)–(b)].

      (2) **Folate,** a cofactor, aids in the detoxification of formate. **Folic** or **folinic acid** (50–77 mg) is administered intravenously every 4 hours.

      (3) **Fomepizole** may be given IV and may be more advantageous in some patients.

C **Isopropyl alcohol (isopropanol)** is used as a solvent and a disinfectant, and is a component of rubbing alcohol, many skin and hair products, antifreeze, and window cleaning solutions. The **toxic dose of a 70% solution** is approximately **1 mL/kg.**

1. **Discussion.** Isopropanol is rapidly absorbed from the gastrointestinal tract. Dermal absorption may also occur. Isopropyl alcohol is metabolized to **acetone.**

   a. **CNS depression** is caused by isopropanol and acetone.

   b. **Cardiovascular collapse** may occur after the ingestion of large quantities of isopropanol.

   c. **Mild acidosis** may occur due to acetate and formate.

2. **Clinical features.** Isopropyl alcohol has twice the CNS depressant effects of ethanol. Acetone may be smelled on the patient's breath.

   a. **CNS features** include euphoria, intoxication, dizziness, incoordination, headache, confusion, and coma.

   b. **Gastrointestinal features** include early abdominal pain, nausea, and vomiting.

   c. **Cardiovascular features** include hypotension, tachycardia, and respiratory depression.

   d. **Other features.** Acute tubular necrosis, hepatic dysfunction, hemolytic anemia, and myoglobinuria have been reported.

3. **Differential diagnoses** include **ethanol or another toxic alcohol ingestion, acetone ingestion, CNS depressant ingestion, head injury, stroke,** and **other causes of ketoacidosis or electrolyte abnormalities.**

4. **Evaluation.** Isopropanol ingestion should be suspected in a patient with ketosis and minimal acidosis. Isopropanol, acetone, and ethanol levels and the serum osmolality should be obtained. ABGs, serum electrolytes, and BUN and creatinine levels should be assessed.

5. **Therapy**
   a. **Initial stabilization** entails airway management, mechanical ventilation (if necessary), cardiovascular resuscitation, intravenous fluid hydration, and supportive care. Most ingestions can be managed successfully with appropriate supportive care.
   b. **Elimination enhancement.** Hemodialysis is recommended for patients with:
      (1) Severe hypotension that is not correctable with fluid resuscitation and pressors
      (2) Deep coma
      (3) Deteriorating vital signs
      (4) Isopropanol levels greater than 400–500 mg/dL

VI CARBON MONOXIDE

A **Discussion** Carbon monoxide is an odorless, colorless, tasteless gas produced during the incomplete combustion of carbon-containing compounds. The leading cause of poisoning deaths in the United States, it is responsible for an estimated 3000 to 4000 deaths annually.

B **Clinical features** Carbon monoxide affects the tissues with the highest oxygen requirements (e.g., CNS tissue, myocardium).

1. With **mild exposures,** headache, nausea, and malaise predominate. The physical examination is often unremarkable.

2. With **significant exposures,** symptoms include chest pain, impaired mental status, syncope, and coma. The examination may reveal a decreased level of consciousness, focal neurologic signs, hypotension, and dysrhythmias. "Cherry red" skin and bright red venous blood are suggestive of carbon monoxide poisoning, but these signs are infrequently noted and are more often a postmortem finding.

C **Differential diagnoses** include **head trauma,** drug or chemical **intoxication** (especially **cyanide** or **hydrogen sulfide exposure**), and **infection** (especially **meningitis** or **encephalitis**).

D **Evaluation**

1. **Carboxyhemoglobin level.** Diagnosis is made by obtaining a carboxyhemoglobin level. The amount of carboxyhemoglobin is measured with a q-wavelength spectrophotometer (co-oximeter). Pulse oximetry and standard ABG testing often will not detect carbon dioxide poisoning.

2. **Pregnancy testing; creatinine phosphokinase, BUN, and creatine levels; urinalysis; a serum electrolyte panel; an ECG;** and a **head CT scan** may be helpful in making the diagnosis and determining treatment protocols.

E **Therapy**

1. **Initial stabilization.** ACLS protocols should be followed as warranted. The administration of **oxygen at the highest possible concentration** is the cornerstone of management (i.e., 100% oxygen via a tight-fitting face mask). Treatment should continue until all symptoms resolve or the carbon monoxide level is reduced to below 5%.

2. **Hyperbaric oxygen therapy** to enhance carbon monoxide elimination is used in the treatment of severe toxicity. Indications for hyperbaric treatment include loss of consciousness, pregnancy, evidence of end-organ damage, and an initial carbon monoxide level of greater than 25%.

F **Disposition**

1. **Discharge.** Patients who are asymptomatic or become asymptomatic within 4–6 hours of observation and treatment, and who have normal examination findings and a normal ECG, may be discharged home.

2. **Admission.** All other patients should be admitted. Patients with ECG changes, a history of chest pain, or depressed mental status should be admitted to the ICU.

VII ANTICHOLINERGICS

A **Discussion**

1. **Causes of anticholinergic poisoning.** Various drugs and plants can cause anticholinergic poisoning.
   a. **Drugs** with anticholinergic properties include antihistamines, benztropine, phenothiazines, cyclic antidepressants, over-the-counter sleep medications, atropine ophthalmic drops, and scopolamine, a drug that has been used to incapacitate and take advantage of unwary victims.
   b. **Plants.** *Datura stramonium* (jimsonweed), ingested to induce a hallucinogenic experience, may also cause a severe anticholinergic reaction. Plant leaves may be used to make tea, dried plant leaves can be smoked, or seeds may be ingested.

2. **Pharmacokinetics.** Most preparations are well absorbed from the gastrointestinal tract, have large volumes of distribution, and are largely protein-bound. Many of these substances delay gastric emptying, prolonging drug absorption and causing delayed onset of symptoms.

3. **Pathophysiology.** These agents inhibit the muscarinic effects of acetylcholine at central and peripheral cholinergic receptors. Hyperthermia, resulting from increased muscle tone and inhibited perspiration, is centrally and peripherally mediated.

B **Clinical features**   The anticholinergic "toxidrome" is described in I C 3 c.

C **Differential diagnoses**   Consider ingestions of **hallucinogens** or **sympathomimetic agents, hypertensive crisis, sepsis, CNS hemorrhage,** or **psychosis.**

D **Evaluation**

1. Quantitative serum levels are of no therapeutic value in the emergency setting. Many over-the-counter preparations of antihistamines contain analgesics and antipyretics, so **acetaminophen** and **salicylate levels** should be obtained.

2. A **glucose level,** a **serum electrolyte panel,** a **CBC,** and an **ABG determination** should be ordered. If rhabdomyolysis is suspected, **creatinine phosphokinase** and **urine myoglobin levels** should be ordered. An **ECG** should be obtained to assess conduction abnormalities.

E **Therapy**

1. **Initial stabilization** involves airway management, cardiovascular resuscitation, and continuous cardiac monitoring.
   a. Hyperthermia must be treated aggressively with rapid cooling measures.
   b. Agitation, hallucinations, and seizures are treated with benzodiazepines.

c. Ventricular dysrhythmias may be treated with lidocaine. Class Ia antiarrhythmics should be avoided. If the ECG reveals a prolonged QRS complex, sodium bicarbonate should be administered to alkalinize the serum to a pH of 7.45–7.55.

d. The bladder should be catheterized.

2. **Gastric decontamination** consists of the administration of **activated charcoal.** The drug may remain in the stomach for as long as 2–4 hours after ingestion. Multiple-dose activated charcoal may be required in some situations.

3. **Antidote treatment. Physostigmine salicylate** is a tertiary amine that reversibly binds cholinesterase enzyme, inactivating it, and enhancing cholinergic tone. It acts at muscarinic and nicotinic receptors and crosses the blood–brain barrier, reversing CNS toxicity.

a. **Adverse effects** of physostigmine include bradycardia, asystole, seizures, and bronchoconstriction.

b. **Indications** include severe agitation, seizures, coma with respiratory depression, and hypotension. Central and peripheral anticholinergic toxicity must be present for physostigmine administration to be warranted. The ECG should reveal a narrow QRS complex and no evidence of conduction abnormalities.

c. **Contraindications**
   (1) **Absolute contraindications** include evidence of ingestion of drugs with class Ia–like cardiotoxic effects, including cyclic antidepressants.
   (2) **Relative contraindications** include bronchospastic disease and intestinal or bladder obstruction.

d. **Dosage and administration**
   (1) Ensure a secure airway. Pretreatment with benzodiazepines may prevent physostigmine-induced seizures.
   (2) The dosage is 0.5 mg administered intravenously over 1 minute, repeated every 5 minutes, up to a total dose of 1–2 mg in adults (0.5 mg in children). The dose may be repeated if necessary in 30–60 minutes.

F **Disposition**

1. **Discharge.** Asymptomatic patients who receive activated charcoal and are observed for 6 hours to have no change in temperature or pulse rate over serial measurements, and no anticholinergic signs, may be safely discharged.

2. **Admission.** Patients with significant toxicity, those who require heavy doses of benzodiazepines for sedation, or those who receive physostigmine should be admitted to a monitored setting.

VIII **INDUSTRIAL CHEMICALS**

A **Organophosphates** and **carbamates** are cholinesterase-inhibiting insecticides, available for use in both industrial and home settings.

1. **Organophosphates**
   a. **Discussion.** Organophosphates are carbon-containing molecules derived from phosphorous acid. The phosphate group is responsible for the molecule's binding and toxicity.
      (1) These agents are absorbed through dermal, conjunctival, gastrointestinal, and pulmonary surfaces. Symptoms occur minutes to hours postexposure. Fat-soluble organophosphates may accumulate in fat, producing delayed or prolonged symptoms.
      (2) The organophosphate forms a complex with acetylcholinesterase. Without treatment, the enzyme is "aged" and destroyed, preventing the breakdown of acetylcholine. There is a wide variability in an individual's "normal" acetylcholinesterase activity. Generally, symptoms occur when the acetylcholinesterase activity is less than 50% of baseline, indicative of acute poisoning. Toxicity is graded according to the percentage of acetylcholinesterase

activity: mild toxicity = 20%–50%, moderate toxicity = 10%–20%, severe toxicity = less than 10%.

    (3) Acetylcholine accumulates, stimulates, and exhausts cholinergic receptors. Cholinergic excess occurs in the parasympathetic system, in the preganglionic synapses of the sympathetic system, and at the neuromuscular junction. Sites of toxicity include:

        (a) Muscarinic sites (i.e., postganglionic parasympathetic synapses)

        (b) Nicotinic sites (i.e., autonomic ganglia, somatic neuromuscular endplates)

        (c) CNS sites

b. Clinical features. Patients often exhibit a garlic-like or petroleum-like odor. NCPE, hyperthermia, and hepatotoxicity may also occur. Other signs and symptoms are classified as:

    (1) Muscarinic (e.g., salivation, lacrimation, urination, defecation, gastrointestinal cramping, emesis, bronchospasm, bronchorrhea, sweating, and miosis)

    (2) Nicotinic (e.g., muscle fasciculations, cramping, weakness, paralysis, areflexia, tachycardia, hypertension, pallor, and hyperglycemia)

    (3) CNS (e.g., restlessness, agitation, headache, drowsiness, confusion, ataxia, delirium, seizures, and coma)

c. Differential diagnoses

    (1) Ingestion of or exposure to carbamates or short-acting cholinesterase inhibitors (e.g., pyridostigmine, and some ophthalmic preparations used to treat glaucoma, such as demecarium and echothiophate) should be considered.

    (2) CNS depressant ingestions, head injury, stroke, pulmonary edema, sepsis, and **severe gastroenteritis** may be ruled out.

d. Evaluation

    (1) General studies. An ABG determination should be made, and the need for mechanical ventilation assessed. A glucose level, CBC, electrolyte panel, BUN and creatinine levels, and liver function tests should be ordered. The ECG should be assessed for dysrhythmias.

    (2) Confirmatory studies

        (a) Erythrocyte (true) cholinesterase is found in nervous tissue and on erythrocytes. This level most accurately reflects cholinesterase activity in nervous tissues.

        (b) Plasma (pseudo) cholinesterase is produced in the liver and circulated in the plasma. This level is more labile and less specific than the true cholinesterase level and is affected by liver disease, cirrhosis, malnutrition, chronic inflammation, and morphine or codeine administration.

        (c) Urine screens. Some metabolites are excreted in the urine. However, this confirmatory analysis may not be available, and treatment should be initiated on clinical suspicion of organophosphate poisoning.

e. Therapy

    (1) Initial stabilization involves airway management (including endotracheal intubation, mechanical ventilation, vigorous suctioning, and the administration of supplemental oxygen as necessary), cardiovascular resuscitation, and treatment of ventricular arrhythmias. Seizures are treated with benzodiazepines.

    (2) Decontamination

        (a) Gastric decontamination. Gastric lavage is indicated if the patient presents early after ingestion. Activated charcoal should be administered.

        (b) Dermal decontamination. Contaminated clothing should be removed and placed in plastic bags for disposal. Skin, hair, and nails should be washed with soap and water, and the conjunctivae should be irrigated.

           (i) Wash water and irrigation fluids must be disposed of separately.

           (ii) Healthcare workers must wear protective clothing, masks, and rubber gloves to prevent secondary exposure and toxicity.

    (3) Antidote treatment

(a) **Atropine** antagonizes the effects of acetylcholine. It reverses muscarinic effects and penetrates the CNS to alleviate effects at central cholinergic receptors.

(i) **Indications.** Atropine should be administered as soon as evidence of cholinergic excess is apparent. Tachycardia is not a contraindication to atropine administration. Heart rate may actually decrease as bronchial secretions dry and oxygenation improves.

(ii) **Dosage.** The initial dose in adults is 2–4 mg intravenously, and in children, 0.05 mg/kg intravenously. This dose may be doubled every 5–10 minutes. The endpoint for atropine administration is the drying of bronchial secretions.

(b) **Pralidoxime (2-PAM)** attacks the phosphorylated acetylcholinesterase, freeing the enzyme. It acts at nicotinic receptors, and may relieve CNS toxicity.

(i) **Indications.** Pralidoxime should be administered as soon as evidence of cholinergic excess is apparent or if organophosphate poisoning is suspected, preferably within 24 hours. Late presentation does not preclude its use.

(ii) **Dosage.** The adult dose is 1 g administered intravenously (20–40 mg/kg, up to a total dose of 1 g in children). This dose may be repeated.

f. **Disposition**

(1) **Discharge.** Patients with inconsequential exposures who have been monitored for 6–8 hours and who have no cholinergic symptoms may be discharged.

(2) **Admission.** Patients who are symptomatic or who have received atropine, pralidoxime, or both should be admitted to an ICU. Patients with ingestions or exposures to fat-soluble organophosphates should be admitted and monitored for delayed onset of toxicity.

2. **Carbamates**

a. **Discussion.** Carbamate insecticides cause cholinergic symptoms, but CNS toxicity is thought to be minimal because these chemicals do not penetrate the blood–brain barrier to a great extent.

(1) Carbamates are readily absorbed after dermal, gastrointestinal, and pulmonary exposure.

(2) Carbamates prevent the normal breakdown of acetylcholine, causing cholinergic excess. However, their bond to acetylcholinesterase spontaneously hydrolyzes, and therefore symptoms are usually less severe and less prolonged (as compared with those of organophosphate toxicity).

b. **Clinical features:** Carbamate-induced cholinergic toxicity consists of muscarinic and nicotinic symptoms, but CNS toxicity is generally less than that of organophosphates.

c. **Differential diagnoses** include **ingestion of organophosphates or other cholinesterase inhibitors** (e.g., physostigmine, pyridostigmine), **CNS depressant ingestion, head injury, stroke, pulmonary edema, cardiogenic shock, sepsis,** and **severe gastroenteritis.**

d. **Evaluation** should proceed as for organophosphates (see VIII A 1 d). True and pseudocholinesterase levels should be obtained.

e. **Therapy** entails airway management, stabilization, and decontamination. Antidote treatment is with atropine. The administration of pralidoxime in cases of carbamate poisoning is controversial, but may improve respiratory function and may also be administered.

f. **Disposition**

(1) **Discharge.** Patients with inconsequential exposures who are monitored for 6 hours and show no signs of cholinergic excess may be discharged.

(2) **Admission.** Symptomatic patients and patients who have been treated with atropine, pralidoxime, or both should be admitted to an ICU.

B **Hydrocarbons** are a diverse group of organic compounds with a wide range of toxicity. In addition, hydrocarbons are often used as a solvent for other chemicals, which can have their own intrinsic toxicity.

1. **Discussion**

a. **Incidence.** Children younger than 5 years have the highest incidence of reported exposure requiring hospital admission.

    b. Pathophysiology. Toxicity occurs mainly in three organ systems:

        (1) Lung toxicity is caused by aspiration and leads to respiratory failure. Aspiration is most likely with hydrocarbons of low viscosity and high volatility. The lungs are the organ most often affected in acute exposures.

        (2) Cardiac toxicity produces dysrhythmias.

        (3) CNS toxicity produces lethargy, stupor, coma, and seizures.

2. Clinical features

    a. Patient history. A history of coughing, grunting, gasping, or vomiting strongly suggests aspiration.

    b. Physical examination findings may include tachypnea, stridor, cyanosis, rales, respiratory distress, irregular heart rate, and CNS depression.

        (1) CNS and cardiac signs usually occur within 1 hour of intoxication.

        (2) Pulmonary signs and symptoms usually become apparent later.

3. Differential diagnoses include **child abuse, salicylate toxicity, caustic ingestion, cardiogenic pulmonary edema,** or **secondary poisonings** (e.g., from pesticides containing hydrocarbons as a solvent).

4. Evaluation is with continuous cardiac monitoring and pulse oximetry. An ABG determination, electrolyte panel, and chest radiograph may also be considered.

5. Therapy. Aggressive supportive care is the mainstay of treatment. There are no specific antidotes.

    a. Initial stabilization is according to ACLS protocols. CPR may be necessary.

        (1) In cases of severe respiratory distress and persistent hypoxia, consider intubation, PEEP, and extracorporeal membrane oxygenation.

        (2) Epinephrine should be avoided because of the theoretical risk of catecholamine sensitization of the heart, leading to ventricular dysrhythmias.

    b. Gastric decontamination is a **relative contraindication** because decontamination procedures may increase the chance of aspiration. Decontamination should be considered in cases of toxic coingestions or when hydrocarbons have been ingested in association with camphor, heavy metals, toluene, benzene, pesticides, carbon tetrachloride, methylene chloride, or other halogenated hydrocarbons.

6. Disposition

    a. Discharge. Patients who are asymptomatic after 4–6 hours of observation and who have normal physical examination findings, normal results on room air ABG determinations or pulse oximetry, and a normal chest radiograph may be discharged home with a responsible party.

    b. Admission. Symptomatic patients must be admitted. Patients who have significant persistent hypoxia should be admitted to an ICU.

IX   IRON TOXICITY

A Discussion   Iron poisoning is one of the most common pediatric poisonings. Most of the poisonings are secondary to the ingestion of ferrous sulfate, the least expensive and most commonly available iron preparation.

1. Pharmacokinetics

    a. Absorption. Iron absorption may occur by aspiration, exposure of nonintact skin, or, most commonly, by ingestion. Iron is absorbed in the duodenum as ferrous (2^+) iron, oxidized to the ferric (3^+) form, and bound either to ferritin for storage or to transferrin for transport in plasma. Delayed absorption may occur with enteric-coated preparations or if bezoars form in the stomach.

    b. Excretion of iron is limited.

2. **Pathophysiology.** Potential toxicity can be estimated based on the dose of ingested elemental iron: 10–20 mg/kg is nontoxic, 20–180 mg/kg is toxic, and 180–300 mg/kg is lethal. Toxicity occurs secondary to free (circulating) iron, which is capable of tissue penetration.

  a. In the gastrointestinal tract, iron has a corrosive effect, causing ulceration, hemorrhage, perforation, and peritonitis.

  b. Vasodilation occurs secondary to direct iron toxicity and is exacerbated by ferritin and the release of serotonin and histamine. Myocardial depression contributes to hypotension.

  c. Disruption of mitochondrial membranes and the TCA cycle enzymes interferes with oxidative metabolism, leading to lactate accumulation and anion gap metabolic acidosis.

  d. Accumulation of iron in Kupffer's cells and hepatocytes causes hepatic toxicity.

  e. Accumulation of iron in the renal capsular space and tubules leads to renal toxicity.

B **Clinical features** Toxicity occurs in several stages:

1. **Initial stage (1–6 hours postingestion).** This stage is characterized by abdominal pain, gastritis, hemorrhage, nausea, vomiting, and diarrhea. Lethargy and tachycardia may occur.

2. **Quiescent stage (12–24 hours postingestion).** Transient improvement and stabilization are noted.

3. **Recurrent stage (12–40 hours postingestion)**

  a. **Gastrointestinal symptoms** include hematemesis and melena.

  b. **Cardiovascular signs** include cyanosis, pulmonary edema, hypotension, and cardiovascular collapse.

  c. **CNS symptoms** include lethargy, seizures, and coma.

  d. **Metabolic signs** include those of an anion gap metabolic acidosis and hyperglycemia.

  e. **Hepatorenal signs** include those of coagulopathy and hepatic and renal failure.

4. **Late stage (2–8 weeks postingestion).** Signs of gastrointestinal scarring and stricture formation may develop if the patient survives the acute episode.

C **Differential diagnoses**

1. The initial presentation may mimic **gastroenteritis.**

2. Late presentations may mimic **gastric hemorrhage, acute abdomen, sepsis,** or **cardiogenic shock.**

3. **CNS depressant ingestion** should be ruled out.

4. **Other causes of hepatic** or **renal failure** must also be considered.

D **Evaluation**

1. **Serum iron levels.** Peak serum iron levels occur 3–5 hours after ingestion.

  a. Correlation of serum iron levels with probable toxicity is shown in Table 20–1.

  b. Toxicity caused by "free" unbound circulating iron is thought to occur when the serum iron level is greater than the total iron binding capacity (TIBC). However, the "measured" TIBC is an unreliable predictor of the actual ability of transferrin to bind iron, and toxicity has

TABLE 20–1 Correlation of Serum Iron Levels and Probable Toxicity	
Serum Iron Level (µg/dL)	**Toxicity**
0–100	Normal (no toxicity)
100–350	Questionable toxicity
350–500	Potentially serious toxicity
500–1000	Serious toxicity
>1000	Fatal toxicity

occurred when measured TIBC levels exceed serum iron levels. Therefore, the TIBC may be of limited value.

2. **Radiologic studies.** Iron is radiopaque and a kidney-ureter-bladder (KUB) view taken within 2 hours of ingestion may show tablets within the stomach or small bowel. False-negatives may occur if the film is taken later than 2 hours postingestion, if there is minimal elemental iron content in the ingested preparation, or if dissolution has already occurred.

3. **Blood work.** Leukocytosis and hyperglycemia are common, but these values are neither sensitive nor specific for toxicity. A CBC, a serum electrolyte panel, BUN and creatinine levels, an ABG determination, a PT and PTT, liver function tests, and blood type and cross match should be ordered.

4. **Other studies.** Stools and vomitus should be tested using a heme test.

E **Therapy**

1. **Initial stabilization** entails airway management and aggressive fluid resuscitation. Gastrointestinal blood loss should be assessed and treated. Coagulopathy should be treated with vitamin K or fresh frozen plasma, depending on the acuity of the bleeding.

2. **Gastric decontamination**
   a. **Gastric lavage** with normal saline is indicated for early presentations.
   b. **Whole-bowel irrigation.** If a KUB view taken after lavage reveals retained iron tablets in the stomach or small bowel, whole-bowel irrigation with polyethylene glycol solution may be instituted to speed the transit of the ingested iron through the gastrointestinal tract and decrease absorption.

3. **Antidote treatment** is with **deferoxamine mesylate,** an avid chelator of ferric ion. It binds free (circulating) and cytoplasmic iron, forming an iron–deferoxamine complex, ferrioxamine, which is then excreted in the urine. Ferrioxamine imparts a "vin-rose" (reddish-brown) tinge to the urine.
   a. **Indications.** Deferoxamine mesylate is indicated for:
      (1) All symptomatic patients (e.g., those exhibiting a change in mental status, hypotension, gastrointestinal hemorrhage, protracted vomiting)
      (2) Patients with a serum iron level greater than 500 µg/dL (however, **antidotal treatment should never be delayed in symptomatic patients while awaiting the serum iron levels**)
   b. **Dosing**
      (1) **Intramuscular.** The dose is 40–90 mg/kg (up to 2 g per injection), given at 4- to 12-hour intervals (up to a maximum dose of 6 g per day).
      (2) **Intravenous.** The dose is 15 mg/kg/hour by continuous infusion. The patient must be monitored for the development of hypotension or a rash.

F **Disposition**

1. **Discharge.** Patients who remain asymptomatic for at least 6 hours and have a negative KUB radiograph may be discharged home.

2. **Admission.** All symptomatic patients, those with retained iron tablets after gastrointestinal decontamination, and those who have received deferoxamine should be admitted.

X **CAUSTIC INGESTIONS**

A **Discussion**

1. **Corrosive injury.** Caustic ingestions cause corrosive injury to the gastrointestinal tract through various mechanisms:
   a. **Acids** cause a **coagulation necrosis** that theoretically forms an immediate scar.
   b. **Alkalis** cause a **liquefaction necrosis** that theoretically allows deeper penetration of the agent.

2. **Secondary toxicity.** Some agents cause secondary toxicity to other organ systems (e.g., paraquat can cause pulmonary fibrosis, hydrofluoric acid can cause hypocalcemia, and certain acids can cause a systemic acidosis).

B **Clinical features**

1. **Symptoms** include chest pain, abdominal pain, odynophagia, and dysphagia.

2. **Physical examination findings** include oral lesions, drooling, stridor, hoarseness, and acute peritoneal irritation. In significant ingestions, the patient may be in shock, evidenced by hypotension and circulatory collapse.

C **Differential diagnoses** include **pancreatitis, gastric perforation, ischemic bowel,** and **Boerhaave's syndrome.**

D **Evaluation**

1. **Laboratory studies** include a CBC, blood type and cross match, a serum electrolyte panel, BUN and creatinine levels, urinalysis, coagulations studies, liver function tests, and ABG determinations.

2. **Diagnostic studies**
   a. An **upright chest radiograph** should be performed to check for an abnormal mediastinum (indicating esophageal perforation) or free air under the diaphragm (indicating gastric or intestinal perforation).
   b. **Endoscopy** should be considered for stable patients; **laparotomy** is preferred for unstable patients.

E **Therapy**

1. **Initial stabilization.** ACLS protocols should be applied as warranted.
   a. Careful attention should be applied to maintaining the airway and preventing aspiration.
   b. Two large-bore intravenous lines should be maintained. Hypotension is treated with isotonic crystalloid solutions.

2. **Decontamination**
   a. The administration of **emetics** and **neutralizing agents** is **contraindicated.**
   b. **Gastric lavage** and **activated charcoal** are **relative contraindications.**

3. **Surgical consultation** is warranted if esophageal, gastric, or intestinal perforation is suspected.

F **Disposition**

1. **Discharge.** Patients who are asymptomatic can be discharged. Patients who were symptomatic but become asymptomatic may require further endoscopic evaluation before being discharged.

2. **Admission.** Patients who are persistently symptomatic require admission and endoscopic evaluation.

Study Questions

Directions: *Each of the numbered items or incomplete statements in this section is followed by answers or by completions of the statement. Select the ONE lettered answer or completion that is BEST in each case.*

1. Activated charcoal would be expected to avidly adsorb which one of the following substances?
   - (A) Lithium
   - (B) Lead
   - (C) Aspirin
   - (D) Iron
   - (E) Hydrocarbons

2. The ocular damage that occurs as a result of methanol poisoning is secondary to the accumulation of which one of the following substances in the vitreous humor and optic nerve?
   - (A) Oxalate
   - (B) Glycolate
   - (C) Lactate
   - (D) Formate
   - (E) Folate

3. The use of flumazenil as an antidote in suspected benzodiazepine overdose may be indicated for which one of the following patients?
   - (A) A patient with significant central nervous system (CNS) depression 2 hours after the ingestion of diazepam
   - (B) A patient with a known seizure disorder who has ingested diazepam
   - (C) A patient with CNS depression 2 hours after the ingestion of a cyclic antidepressant and diazepam
   - (D) A patient with hallucinations, tachycardia, and fever 2 hours after the ingestion of an antihistamine and diazepam
   - (E) A patient on chronic diazepam therapy with potential physiologic tolerance and dependence who develops CNS depression 2 hours after the acute ingestion of an overdose of diazepam

4. Deferoxamine mesylate is an antidote for which one of the following toxins?
   - (A) Acetaminophen
   - (B) Benzodiazepines
   - (C) Methanol
   - (D) Iron
   - (E) Lithium

5. A patient is suspected of having organophosphate poisoning. Which one of the following tests would be most specific for determining the extent of central nervous system (CNS) cholinesterase inhibition?
   - (A) Pralidoxime (2-PAM) level
   - (B) Plasma (pseudo) cholinesterase level
   - (C) Acetylcholine level
   - (D) Urine assay for organophosphate metabolites
   - (E) Erythrocyte (true) cholinesterase level

6. What is the role of urinary alkalinization in the treatment of salicylate poisoning?

   (A) To "trap" ionized salicylate in the renal tubules, preventing reabsorption and enhancing excretion
   (B) To provide adequate diuresis
   (C) To enhance hydrogen ion excretion
   (D) To allow greater reabsorption of potassium from the renal tubules, in exchange for salicylate
   (E) To prevent the precipitation of salicylate-induced myoglobin in the tubules

7. What is the specific antidote for anticholinergic poisoning?

   (A) Flumazenil
   (B) Physostigmine
   (C) Atropine
   (D) Benzodiazepine
   (E) Antihistamine

8. N-Acetylcysteine is an antidote for acetaminophen toxicity. Administration of N-acetylcysteine provides which one of the following detoxifying substances?

   (A) Glutathione
   (B) Glucuronide
   (C) Sulfate
   (D) Folate
   (E) Thiamine

9. What is the most common cause of death in patients with tricyclic antidepressant overdose?

   (A) Cardiac dysrhythmias
   (B) Status epilepticus
   (C) Rhabdomyolysis
   (D) Acute respiratory distress syndrome (ARDS)
   (E) Disseminated intravascular coagulation (DIC)

10. Which one of the following statements regarding carbon monoxide poisoning is true?

   (A) Signs are easily recognizable on physical examination.
   (B) Carbon monoxide poisoning can be detected by calculating the oxygen saturation, using the arterial oxygen tension as a basis for the determination.
   (C) "Cherry red" skin is an early sign of carbon monoxide poisoning.
   (D) Carbon monoxide poisoning affects the central nervous system (CNS) and heart more than the other organs.
   (E) Carbon monoxide is treated by administering an intravenous antidote.

11. Which one of the following medications is indicated in the treatment of cyclic antidepressant overdose?

   (A) Procainamide
   (B) Sodium bicarbonate
   (C) Flumazenil
   (D) Quinidine
   (E) Physostigmine

12. Which one of the following statements regarding dystonic reactions is true?

[A] Antiemetics can cause dystonic reactions.
[B] Dystonic reactions are treated with cholinergic agents.
[C] Dystonic reactions are characterized by muscular flaccidity.
[D] Dystonic reactions are life-threatening.
[E] Dystonic reactions are most commonly caused by over-the-counter medications.

13. Which one of the following statements regarding caustic ingestions is true?

[A] Acids cause a liquefaction necrosis.
[B] Activated charcoal usually facilitates gastric decontamination.
[C] Steroids have been proven to be beneficial.
[D] Theoretically, alkali injuries penetrate deeper than acid injuries.
[E] Neutralization has been proven beneficial.

14. Which one of the following statements regarding hydrocarbon aspiration is true?

[A] Children older than 5 years are most often affected.
[B] Coughing, gasping, and grunting are suggestive of hydrocarbon aspiration.
[C] The onset of symptoms is usually delayed for at least 12 hours.
[D] Hydrocarbons of low volatility and high viscosity are the most likely to cause aspiration.
[E] Hydrocarbon aspiration can be treated with an antidote.

15. A patient is brought to the emergency department (ED) late on a Saturday night after "snorting" a large amount of cocaine at a party. The patient is very anxious. His vital signs are as follows: temperature, 40°C; heart rate, 130 beats/min; respiratory rate, 22 breaths/min; blood pressure, 180/100 mm Hg. What should the emergency physician do next?

[A] Administer activated charcoal.
[B] Administer intravenous propranolol.
[C] Administer oral propranolol.
[D] Administer oral diazepam.
[E] Administer intravenous diazepam.

Answers and Explanations

1. The answer is C Activated charcoal has significant adsorptive capacity for aspirin, as well as many other compounds. Activated charcoal does not adsorb metals (e.g., lead, iron, lithium), hydrocarbons, or alcohols to a significant degree.

2. The answer is D Methanol is metabolized to formate, which causes ocular toxicity. Glycolate and oxalate are intermediate metabolites of ethylene glycol, which does not cause ocular toxicity. Both methanol and ethylene glycol cause elevated lactate levels secondary to the increase in the reduced nicotinamide adenine dinucleotide (NADH):nicotinamide adenine dinucleotide (NAD) ratio, but the elevated lactate level is not responsible for the ocular damage caused by methanol poisoning. Folate is a cofactor used in detoxifying methanol metabolites.

3. The answer is A Flumazenil may be of benefit in a patient with significant CNS depression who has ingested a single dose of a benzodiazepine. Flumazenil is contraindicated in patients who have taken a benzodiazepine along with an epileptogenic agent (e.g., cyclic antidepressants, antihistamines), in patients with known seizure disorders, and in patients who may develop physiologic dependence. Because the chronic use of benzodiazepines is often difficult to rule out, flumazenil is rarely used in the emergency department, but is useful for accidental benzodiazepine ingestion by a normal child.

4. The answer is D Deferoxamine mesylate chelates elemental iron. It is not of use in acetaminophen overdose, benzodiazepine overdose, methanol poisoning, or lithium poisoning.

5. The answer is E Erythrocyte (true) cholinesterase is found in brain tissue, nervous tissue, and red blood cells (RBCs); therefore, the erythrocyte cholinesterase level most specifically reflects cholinesterase activity in nervous tissue. Plasma (pseudo) cholinesterase levels are also adversely affected by organophosphate poisoning, but are a less specific parameter because plasma cholinesterase levels are also affected by liver disease, malnutrition, chronic inflammation, and morphine or codeine administration. Some organophosphate metabolites are excreted in measurable amounts in the urine, but do not give any particular indication of CNS toxicity. 2-PAM is the antidote for organophosphate poisoning.

6. The answer is A Urinary alkalinization "traps" ionized salicylate in the renal tubules, so that it cannot be reabsorbed, leading to its excretion in the urine. Hypokalemia associated with salicylate toxicity must be corrected before alkalinization can be performed effectively.

7. The answer is B Physostigmine is a tertiary amine that reversibly binds cholinesterase to enhance cholinergic activity. It crosses the blood–brain barrier and is effective in reversing central and peripheral anticholinergic symptoms. Atropine and antihistamines are drugs with anticholinergic properties. Flumazenil is an antidote for benzodiazepine-induced central nervous system (CNS) depression.

8. The answer is A N-Acetylcysteine is a precursor for glutathione, which conjugates with NAPQI, the toxic intermediate produced during acetaminophen overdose. In therapeutic doses, 90% of acetaminophen is metabolized by conjugation with glucuronide or sulfate.

9. The answer is A Although tricyclic antidepressants can cause status epilepticus, rhabdomyolysis, ARDS, and DIC, they have the greatest toxic effect on the conduction system of the heart. In patients with tricyclic antidepressant overdose, death is most commonly the result of intractable ventricular tachycardia or fibrillation and hypotension.

10. **The answer is D** Carbon monoxide is the number one toxicologic cause of death. The heart and brain are the two organs most affected by carbon monoxide poisoning. Carbon monoxide poisoning is often difficult to detect on physical examination; a carboxyhemoglobin level is required for diagnosis. The distinctive "cherry red" color of the skin and venous blood in carbon monoxide poisoning is an infrequent finding; when noted, it is usually at autopsy. The mainstay of treatment in carbon monoxide poisoning is the administration of supplemental oxygen; there is no antidote.

11. **The answer is B** Sodium bicarbonate is administered to patients with cyclic antidepressant overdose to treat dysrhythmias and hypotension. Procainamide and quinidine are class Ia antiarrhythmics, which can worsen the effects of cyclic antidepressants on the cardiac conduction system. Flumazenil and physostigmine have been reported to cause seizures when used in patients with cyclic antidepressant overdose.

12. **The answer is A** Dystonic reactions are most commonly caused by agents that cause dopaminergic blockade in the central nervous system (CNS), such as antiemetics and antipsychotics (especially haloperidol). Dystonic reactions, characterized by muscular rigidity, are easily treated with anticholinergic agents and are almost never life-threatening.

13. **The answer is D** Alkali injuries cause a liquefaction necrosis, which, theoretically, allows deeper penetration of the substance into the tissue. Gastric decontamination and neutralization are not indicated, and steroids have not been shown to be beneficial.

14. **The answer is B** Hydrocarbon aspiration is most common in children younger than 5 years who typically swallow low-viscosity, high-volatility hydrocarbons. These children tend to cough, grunt, and gasp. Respiratory symptoms and findings develop within 6 hours and supportive care is the mainstay of treatment.

15. **The answer is E** The next step in the care of this patient would be the intravenous administration of a benzodiazepine, such as diazepam. Benzodiazepines are the pharmacologic mainstay of treatment for cocaine intoxication. Many of the toxic effects of cocaine (e.g., seizures, hypertension, tachycardia, hyperthermia) are centrally mediated. Rapid treatment is necessary to prevent further toxicity. β Blockers (e.g., propranolol) are a relative contraindication in patients with cocaine intoxication.

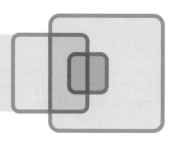

chapter 21

Environmental Emergencies

E. JOHN WIPFLER, III

I   INTRODUCTION

This chapter deals with the diagnosis and treatment of illness and injury related to nature's dangerous forces, including wildlife. Also discussed in this chapter are the special problems encountered when the sick or injured patient is located far from civilization—the subspecialty of **wilderness medicine.**

II   COLD-RELATED ILLNESS AND INJURY

When people interact with cold environments and are unable to protect themselves properly, injuries may result. These injuries may be generalized (e.g., hypothermia) or localized (e.g., frostbite). Both types of injuries may occur at temperatures above and below freezing.

A **Hypothermia**

1. **Discussion**
   a. **Definitions. Hypothermia** is a decrease in core body temperature to 35°C (95°F) or below. Often it is associated with the clinical state of subnormal temperature when the body is unable to generate sufficient heat to function normally.
      (1) **Primary hypothermia (accidental hypothermia)** refers to a spontaneous reduction in core body temperature, usually from exposure to a cold environment without adequate protection. It often occurs in healthy people. (Each year approximately 780 people in the United States die of exposure to cold.)
      (2) **Secondary hypothermia** often occurs as a complication in patients with a systemic disease that compromises the body's thermoregulatory mechanisms (e.g., an endocrine disorder).
   b. **Risk factors** for hypothermia include:
      (1) Increased heat loss owing to extreme cold, insufficient clothing or shelter, infancy (infants have a high surface-to-body ratio), or old age (altered mental status/dementia)
      (2) Decreased heat production (old age, medications, disease)
      (3) Impaired thermoregulation (illness)
      (4) Other factors such as human error, abnormal behavioral responses to cold weather, ethanol abuse, and race (blacks are at higher risk)
   c. **Heat transfer**
      (1) **Mechanisms.** Normal heat loss of the human body occurs through five mechanisms:
         (a) **Radiation** is heat transfer by electromagnetic waves. It accounts for 55%–65% of heat loss in a person at rest in cool climates. The amount of heat lost depends on the temperature gradient between the body surface and the environment.
         (b) **Conduction** is the transfer of heat energy from warmer to cooler objects by direct physical contact. It normally accounts for less than 3% of heat loss; however, if the person is in direct contact with cold surfaces or water, heat loss may increase up to 32 times the normal amount.

617

    (c) Convection is heat transfer to air and water vapor molecules circulating around the body. It accounts for 10% of heat loss; greater heat loss occurs with wind blowing against the skin surface. As ambient temperature rises, the amount of heat dissipated by convection becomes minimal.

    (d) Evaporation is conversion from a liquid to a gas, with a loss of energy of 0.58 kcal/mL of water evaporated. Insensible water loss from the skin and lungs normally accounts for 25% of heat loss. At ambient temperatures above body temperature, evaporative heat loss becomes the primary means of dissipating heat, exceeding radiation.

    (e) Respiration. Warming the inspired air accounts for 2%–9% of heat loss; this percentage varies with the temperature of the ambient air.

  (2) Summary. Considering these mechanisms, it can be said that a person would lose the most heat on a cool, windy, dry, cloudy day in contact with a cool surface while perspiring and wearing few protective items of clothing.

d. Pathophysiology. The pathophysiologic changes that occur in hypothermic patients depend on the severity of the temperature reduction, the underlying cause, and the patient's pre-existing medical condition. The body functions optimally when its core temperature is maintained within 1°C (1.8°F) of its normal value, and any deviation from this narrow range affects all organ systems.

  (1) Cardiovascular responses

    (a) At core body temperatures below 30°C (86°F), **initial tachycardia** is followed by **bradycardia** resulting from decreased spontaneous depolarization of the pacemaker cells. This bradycardia is resistant to treatment with atropine. If tachycardia is present in a significantly hypothermic patient, then hypovolemia, hypoglycemia, drugs, or other conditions must be ruled out.

    (b) Systemic vascular resistance (SVR) increases initially; when the core temperature drops below 24°C (75°F), SVR decreases.

    (c) Most types of **atrial** and **ventricular dysrhythmias** are seen in patients with moderate and severe hypothermia.

      (i) Cardiac cycle prolongation occurs. The QT interval is most prolonged.

      (ii) Atrial fibrillation is seen commonly at core temperatures below 32°C (90°F), and usually converts spontaneously on rewarming.

      (iii) Ventricular fibrillation and **asystole** can occur spontaneously when the core temperature drops below 25°C (77°F), and the patient is often resistant to defibrillation attempts until the body temperature is raised above 30°C (86°F).

  (2) Respiratory responses

    (a) The initial response to hypothermia is an increase in **respiratory rate.** As body temperature declines and the medullary respiratory center becomes depressed, there is a **progressive decrease in minute volume** that is proportional to the decreasing metabolic rate.

    (b) Even though carbon dioxide production is decreased in hypothermia, the patient often develops a **mild respiratory acidosis** due to decreased respiratory ventilation.

    (c) Airway protective reflexes are depressed, resulting in a **cold-induced bronchorrhea.** This leads to atelectasis, bronchopneumonia, aspiration pneumonia, and postwarming pulmonary edema.

    (d) The pH typically rises as body temperature drops. Many studies have shown this mechanism to be protective; therefore, it may be advantageous to allow patients to be **alkalemic.**

  (3) Central nervous system (CNS) responses

    (a) Hypothermia progressively **decreases CNS function.** Significant brain electroencephalogram (EEG) slowing begins below 33.5°C (92°F). Below 20°C (68°F), the EEG demonstrates no brain activity. The alteration in mental status may lead to maladaptive behavior that worsens the patient's condition (e.g., removing the clothes in freezing conditions).

(b) Hypothermia protects the brain from the effects of ischemia. When core body temperatures drop below 20°C (68°F), **total circulatory arrest** may be tolerated for longer than 1 hour with **no neurologic sequelae following rewarming.** Therefore, patients with hypothermia should not be declared brain dead until they have been rewarmed and their brain activity has been re-evaluated.

(c) The reflexes initially are hyperreflexic, but when the core body temperature decreases to below 32°C (90°F), humans become **hyporeflexic,** with the knee-jerk the last reflex to disappear (at temperatures below 26°C, or 79°F).

(4) Renal responses

(a) Exposure to cold induces a **diuresis** despite a decrease in glomerular filtration rate and renal blood flow. The production of a large volume of dilute urine (up to three times normal) results principally from the vasoconstriction and a blunted response to antidiuretic hormone (ADH). As a result, when the hypothermic patient is rewarmed, a relative hypovolemia occurs, contributing to **"rewarming shock."**

(b) Prolonged immobilization and decreased perfusion may lead to **rhabdomyolysis.**

(5) Hematologic responses

(a) Hypothermia impairs coagulation; thus, despite normal prothrombin time (PT) and partial thromboplastin time (PTT) values, **clinical coagulopathy** may be present. Often the coagulopathy resolves when the patient is rewarmed, although rare cases of disseminated intravascular coagulation (DIC) have been reported.

(i) Several factors play a role in impairing coagulation, including hemoconcentration, vasoconstriction, and release of tissue thromboplastin from cold ischemic tissue.

(ii) Cold-precipitated fibrinogen may increase the risk for coronary and cerebral thrombosis.

(b) Hypothermia induces hepatosplenic sequestration and bone marrow suppression, which decreases leukocyte and platelet counts. The **leukopenia** and **thrombocytopenia** reverse with rewarming.

(c) **Blood viscosity increases** by 2% for every 1°C drop in temperature. Hemoconcentration develops, most likely from the cold diuresis.

(d) **The oxyhemoglobin curve shifts to the left,** diminishing the release of oxygen to tissue.

(6) Gastrointestinal responses. Complications of hypothermia may include ileus, pancreatitis, and gastric stress ulcers. Hepatic function is reduced, which can lead to increased levels of lactate, drugs, and toxins in the blood.

e. Classification. Hypothermic patients can be divided into three groups based on core temperature:

(1) Severe hypothermia: core temperature below 24°C (75°F). All endocrinologic and autonomic nervous system mechanisms for heat conservation become inactive. Survival is rare despite aggressive medical treatment.

(2) Moderate hypothermia: core temperature between 32°C and 24°C (90°F and 75°F). Heat loss is minimized by vasoconstriction, but the body is too cold to shiver. (Shivering is synchronized muscle group contractions that produce heat.)

(3) Mild hypothermia: core temperature above 32°C (90°F). Shivering plays a significant role in rewarming, and vasoconstriction, decreased perspiration, and nonshivering basal and endocrinologic heat production help retain body warmth.

2. Clinical features

a. The **history** gathered from bystanders or from an awake patient often enables accurate diagnosis of accidental hypothermia. However, in the case of an unresponsive patient without witnesses, it may be difficult to identify the causative factors.

b. **Signs**
  (1) In wilderness travel, the onset of hypothermia often is slow and subtle; some **early signs** are **mood changes, unusual behavior,** and **impaired judgment.**
  (2) The **core temperature** is **35°C (95°F) or lower.**
  (3) In general, the presenting signs and symptoms of hypothermic patients reflect **decreased function of most organ systems** (see II A 1 d). The patient may demonstrate hypotension with bradycardia, initial tachypnea followed by slowed respirations progressing to hypoventilation, ileus, and a depressed level of consciousness. Shivering may be present or absent. Skin changes may include frostbite, erythema, pallor, cyanosis, edema, and other changes.

3. **Differential diagnoses** include thyroid deficiency, stroke, infection, drugs, and other causes of a depressed body temperature.

4. **Evaluation.** Accurate diagnosis and early treatment are important. The diagnosis of hypothermia can be made once an accurate core temperature is measured. Determining the cause or causes (see II A 1 a–b) can be more difficult, especially if the patient is unable to communicate. Underlying medical problems must be identified and addressed, which may be difficult to do in a comatose hypothermic patient.
  a. **Core temperature** is best determined by measuring the rectal or tympanic temperature. Oral temperatures are an unreliable and often inaccurate indication of core temperature. The tympanic temperature changes most rapidly with core temperature; new infrared tympanic thermometers are proving to be more accurate than the older ones.
  b. **Laboratory studies**
    (1) Specific laboratory tests should be ordered to confirm the diagnosis of hypothermia and to identify any possible underlying cause. A thorough evaluation is required and includes a **complete blood count (CBC), electrolytes, arterial blood gas (ABG) determination, liver function tests, coagulation studies, urinalysis,** and **toxicology screening** if possible. Additional tests useful outside the emergency department (ED) may include endocrine evaluation (cortisol, thyroid) and sputum and blood cultures.
    (2) **Serum pH determination.** The evaluation of arterial and venous blood samples in the hypothermic patient is controversial. Reliable prediction of acid–base status in the clinical setting is not possible; one study showed that 25% of hypothermic patients were alkalotic and 30% were acidotic. Most authors agree that correction of ABG parameters is unnecessary and potentially harmful.
  c. **Diagnostic tests.** Electrocardiogram (ECG) findings in hypothermia may include an Osborn (J) wave if the core temperature is below 33°C (91.4°F). The J wave is seen at the junction of the QRS complex and ST segment, which are upright in the aVL, aVF, and left precordial leads. The size of the J wave increases as the temperature decreases; it is diagnostic but not prognostic.
  d. **Imaging studies.** If a traumatic mechanism is suspected or known, radiologic examination may be appropriate. In a patient with a persistent altered level of consciousness, a brain computed tomography (CT) scan may be appropriate.

5. **Therapy**
  a. **Prehospital management.** The basic prehospital treatment protocol is **rescue, evaluate, insulate, resuscitate,** and **transport.**
    (1) **Rescue.** Make sure the site is safe (e.g., is the patient in an avalanche area?). If the site is unsafe, rescue should proceed only if the benefits outweigh the risks.
    (2) **Evaluate.** Obtain a brief history and perform a physical examination. Assessment, stabilization, and management of airway, breathing, and circulation (ABCs) should be done while handling the patient very carefully. (Hypothermic patients are subject to serious cardiac arrhythmias, which can be precipitated by jostling or otherwise moving the patient. Therefore, unnecessary manipulations should be avoided.)

(3) Insulate. The prime directive in prehospital treatment of the hypothermic patient is the prevention of additional heat loss. However, rescuers at the scene often are hampered by the cold environment, limited supplies, and lack of shelter. If reasonable likelihood of survival exists, the patient's wet clothing should be removed and the patient should be placed in dry, warm clothes or sheets (passive rewarming).

(4) Resuscitation

(a) Cardiopulmonary resuscitation (CPR) should be administered to hypothermic patients in cardiac arrest if survival is considered possible. At core temperatures below 30°C (86°F), the heart may be refractory to pharmacologic interventions and defibrillation.

(b) Warmed, humidified oxygen and **warm intravenous fluids** should be administered as soon as possible to prevent further cooling of the patient. Intravenous access often is difficult to obtain due to peripheral vasoconstriction.

(c) If initial attempts at cardioversion are not successful, continue CPR, warm the patient, and repeat defibrillation attempts with every 2°C–4°C rise in temperature.

(5) Transport. The patient should be transported with care to a medical center.

b. ED management. Resuscitation efforts should be continued as described for prehospital treatment. **Thermal stabilization** should continue, as well as **maintenance of tissue oxygenation** through adequate circulation and ventilation. **ECG monitoring** to detect cardiac arrhythmias and **accurate core temperature evaluation** are required to monitor the severity of hypothermia and the response to treatment.

(1) It is important to determine whether the hypothermia is primary or secondary, and to **treat the underlying medical problems if any are identified.**

(2) Supportive care

(a) Patients with an altered mental status should receive intravenous **naloxone, glucose, and thiamine.**

(b) The hypothermic patient usually is dehydrated and may develop hypovolemia and hypoglycemia as he is rewarmed; therefore, warm (40°C–42°C) **intravenous fluid boluses** of normal saline with 5% dextrose should be administered as needed.

(3) Rewarming methods. The dictum "You are not dead until you are warm and dead" is based on past experience with patients who have been successfully resuscitated despite being unresponsive, stiff, and cold on initial presentation.

(a) Patients with **mild hypothermia** typically have an intact shiver reflex; if shelter and passive external rewarming are provided, endogenous heat production will enable these patients to rewarm gradually on their own.

(b) Patients with **moderate or severe hypothermia** often are unable to rewarm their bodies using passive external rewarming alone. Therefore, the physician may employ **active rewarming techniques** using exogenous heat sources. The active techniques may be external or internal (core), with the choice of technique being controversial.

(i) Active external rewarming directly exposes the body to an exogenous heat source, such as **warm baths, hot water bottles, heat lamps, heating blankets,** or other heat source.

(ii) Active core rewarming may be used in patients with moderate to severe hypothermia, especially in those with unstable cardiac arrhythmias. Techniques include administering **heated, humidified oxygen** by way of a face mask or endotracheal tube; administering **warmed intravenous fluids;** performing **warm fluid lavage** (intragastric, intracolonic, peritoneal or thoracic lavage); and **extracorporeal rewarming** (the most rapid method).

Methods of **extracorporeal rewarming** include **hemodialysis, arteriovenous** or **venovenous extracorporeal rewarming,** and **cardiopulmonary bypass.** The latter is the treatment of choice for the cardiac arrest patient who is severely hypothermic [i.e., with a body temperature less than 30°C (86°F)].

Rapid rewarming has not been shown to improve survival rates among hypothermic patients.

6. **Disposition.** The patient with severe hypothermia may appear clinically dead; however, in the appropriate setting, resuscitative efforts should continue until the patient's core temperature reaches a level (higher than 30°C, or 86°F) that would allow accurate determination of response to resuscitation.

a. **Discharge.** Victims of mild hypothermia who are rewarmed to a normal temperature without complications may be discharged.

b. **Admission.** Survivors of severe or moderate hypothermia should be admitted to a monitored bed in an intensive care unit (ICU) for close observation.

B Frostbite and other localized cold injuries may occur in the absence of generalized hypothermia.

1. **Discussion**

a. The **areas of the body most likely to suffer localized cold injury** are those most exposed to cold and farthest away from the body's core, such as the feet, hands, nose, and earlobes.

b. **Severity.** Several factors influence the severity of localized cold injury, including the conducting surface (wet cold surfaces cool tissue much more quickly than dry cold surfaces), ambient temperature, wind speed, and the physiologic condition of the patient.

c. **Types of localized cold injuries**

(1) **Nonfreezing cold injury** can be divided into two groups, on the basis of exposure to dry or wet cold environments:

(a) **Chilblain (perniosis, "cold sore")** is the term used to describe skin that has been exposed chronically to **cold, dry air** at temperatures above freezing. It is seen most commonly in women and mountain climbers.

(b) **Trench foot (immersion foot)** is caused by several days of exposure to **wet, cold conditions** when the ambient temperature is above freezing. The name is derived from the fact that soldiers exposed to harsh conditions often developed the condition; it is often seen today in homeless patients.

(2) **Freezing cold injury.** Frostbite occurs when a body surface comes in contact with cold, resulting in tissue freezing. The depth of freezing is related to the duration and intensity of the cold exposure. Frostbite has been divided into four pathologic phases:

(a) **Prefreeze phase.** Chilling causes vasospasm and transendothelial plasma leakage. The tissue temperature ranges from 3°C–10°C (37°F–50°F).

(b) **Freeze–thaw phase.** Actual tissue ice crystals form. Owing to underlying radiation of heat energy, the skin must be supercooled to −4°C (24.8°F) to freeze.

(c) **Vascular stasis phase.** Because of the freezing injury to the overlying skin, blood vessels are damaged, and plasma leakage, coagulation, and shunting occur.

(d) **Late ischemic phase.** Arteriovenous shunting, thrombosis, and ischemia lead to gangrene and autonomic dysfunction.

2. **Clinical features**

a. **Chilblain.** The skin has small, erythematous, superficial ulcerations, plaques, nodules, and vesicles over exposed areas, which are pruritic and hypersensitive. The skin lesions appear 12–14 hours after exposure to cold.

b. **Trench foot** resembles superficial burns (hyperemia, pain, edema, vesiculation), and can be very debilitating. Severe cases can progress to liquefaction gangrene.

c. **Frostbite**

(1) **Symptoms** are related to the severity of the injury. True frostbite always results in damaged skin after rewarming. Most patients will report coldness and numbness of the

involved skin initially, but during rewarming will complain of extreme pain. Usually the severity of the injury defines the extent of neuropathologic damage, and a wide variety of symptoms occur.

(2) **Physical examination findings.** Close examination of the skin reveals the degrees of injury. Historically, **four levels of injury** have been described:

   (a) **First-degree injury:** numbness and erythema of skin, with a firm white or yellow plaque in the area of injury

   (b) **Second-degree injury:** superficial skin vesiculation, with clear or milky fluid within the blisters, surrounded by edema and erythema

   (c) **Third-degree injury:** deeper blister formation, with purple, blood-containing fluid, and injury extending into the deep dermis layers

   (d) **Fourth-degree injury:** involves tissue below the dermis, with muscle and bone involvement, causing mummification of the digit or extremity

3. **Differential diagnoses** for localized cold injuries include burns, chemical irritation, tissue damage, infections, trauma, vascular compromise, and cutaneous manifestation of systemic disease. Often the patient's history makes the diagnosis simple.

4. **Evaluation.** If cold injury alone is strongly suspected, no specific tests are necessary. If the diagnosis is uncertain, tests to eliminate differential diagnoses should be obtained.

5. **Therapy**

   a. **Chilblain.** Management is supportive and consists of gentle rewarming, use of local skin moisturizers, and avoidance of cold conditions. Most cases heal well with proper care. The victim is prone to recurrence from similar exposure.

   b. **Trench foot.** Treatment includes local skin care, elevation, rest, and avoidance of wet, cold conditions. Prognosis is better than for frostbite, although these injuries often are clinically indistinguishable initially. Most cases heal well with proper care.

   c. **Frostbite.** The treatment of frostbite is directed at saving as many cells as possible in the skin and underlying tissue.

   (1) **Prehospital management** consists of rapid transportation to a medical center, with the involved extremity wrapped in loose, dry clothing, elevated, and protected from trauma and further freezing. It is very important to prevent refreezing injuries if the patient has been warmed, because refreezing causes more severe cellular damage. For example, any victim who absolutely must walk through snow should do so before the frostbitten feet are thawed.

   (2) **ED management.** Initially, it is difficult to predict the extent of frostbite damage. Only a few patients arrive with tissue still frozen. With rapid rewarming there is almost immediate hyperemia, even in severe injuries. The initial treatment of all four frostbite levels is identical, and so initial distinctions are artificial.

   (a) **Systemic hypothermia should be corrected.** The patient's body temperature should be 34°C (93°F) before frostbite management is attempted.

   (b) **Rapid rewarming** should be started immediately after the patient has been stabilized. Rapid rewarming is accomplished by immersing the affected body part in a gently circulating warm water bath; the water temperature should be 40°C–42°C (104°F–108°F). Adherence to this narrow temperature range is important, because rewarming at higher temperatures produces a burn wound, and lower temperatures are less beneficial for tissue survival.

   (i) Rewarming should continue until the skin is soft, pliable, and erythematous at the affected part's most distal aspect.

   (ii) After rewarming, edema appears within several hours, blisters in 6–24 hours. Over the next several weeks, demarcation, eschar, and mummification occur. Demarcation of viable and nonviable tissue may require several weeks to develop, and this delay allows accurate amputation if indicated.

        (c) Parenteral analgesics are required to manage the significant pain associated with rewarming.

        (d) Other considerations include **tetanus prophylaxis, debridement of white blisters** (hemorrhagic blisters should be left intact), **aloe vera cream, elevation, ibuprofen,** intravenous prophylactic **penicillin G,** and **daily hydrotherapy.**

  6. Disposition. Most patients with frostbite will require **admission to the hospital** for further evaluation and treatment. All patients with potential for significant skin damage should be admitted and observed.

III   HEAT-RELATED ILLNESS

A **Introduction**   Humans have a reasonable ability to tolerate environmental heat stress, but with physical exertion and high temperatures, they may suffer heat illness.

  1. Physiology of temperature regulation. Regulation of human body temperature is complex, involving the thermosensors (located in the skin and centrally in the preoptic anterior hypothalamus), the thermoregulatory effectors (sweating and peripheral vasodilatation), and the brain. The human body is essentially a "furnace" that converts fuel (food) into usable energy while producing by-products and heat from exothermic processes. The basal metabolism consumes 50–60 kcal/hour/m^2; in the absence of cooling mechanisms, this rate of consumption would result in a 1.1°C (2°F)-per-hour increase in body temperature. When the body gains heat faster than it can be eliminated, heat illness may occur.

  2. Factors contributing to increased heat production

    a. Hyperthyroidism

    b. Drugs (e.g., haloperidol, alcohol)

    c. Increased activity level. Heat production may be increased up to 20 times by strenuous exertion.

    d. Hot weather. Environmental heat adds to the heat load, interfering with the dissipation of heat through the four mechanisms of conduction, convection, evaporation, and radiation.

  3. Adaptations to heat

    a. Evaporation is the most effective method of heat loss when environmental temperature is at or above body temperature.

    b. Acclimatization is the physiologic adaptation that occurs in a normal person after 7–14 days of exposure to work in a hot environment. This is characterized by an earlier onset of sweating, increased sweat volume with lowered sweat electrolyte concentrations, and hormonal changes. In trained marathon runners, temperatures as high as 42°C (107.6°F) have been recorded without ill effects.

  4. Predisposing factors to heat illness

    a. Hot environment

    b. Lack of behavior modification (not drinking enough fluids, not seeking shade)

    c. Extremes of age

    d. Drugs

    e. Occupation

    f. Lack of acclimatization

    g. Sweat gland abnormalities

    h. Psychological factors

  5. Categories of heat illness. Heat illness may be divided into four categories: minor heat illness, heat exhaustion, heat stroke, and unusual heat disorders.

B **Minor heat illness**

  1. Discussion. Most cases of minor heat illness occur within the first several days of exposure or work in a hot environment. The person who is not acclimated may develop heat edema, cramps, syncope, and tetany.

2. **Clinical features**
   a. **Heat edema** occurs primarily in nonacclimatized older people who are exposed to climatic stresses of tropical areas. It presents as minor swelling of the feet and ankles, often in people who sit or stand for long periods of time, and results from vasodilation and increased hydrostatic pressure leading to vascular leak and interstitial edema.
   b. **Heat cramps** are brief, often severe muscular cramps that typically affect muscles heavily used by workers or athletes who are sweating profusely in hot environments. The cramps usually occur after the activity has ceased, while the person is relaxing. They result from salt deficiency (sweating heavily but drinking hypotonic fluids) and may be related to hyperventilation.
   c. **Heat syncope** is related to the vasodilation that occurs in people (particularly the elderly) exposed to hot conditions. The vasodilation of cutaneous vessels results in relative hypovolemia of the thoracic blood vessels, decreased central venous return, a drop in cardiac output, and decreased cerebral perfusion. The dehydrated person is at even higher risk for syncope. The syncopal episode may result in injuries from falling; thus, patients should be closely examined for skull, spine, and hip injuries.
   d. **Heat tetany** may be associated with hyperventilation occurring in heat illness, which is caused by central stimulation of respiration. Symptoms include carpopedal spasm and paresthesias of the extremities and perioral area.

3. **Differential diagnoses.** Congestive heart failure (CHF), deep venous thrombosis, and lymphedema must be ruled out in cases of heat edema. Syncope has a wide differential, and other serious causes should be excluded.

4. **Evaluation**
   a. An **accurate history** should be obtained, including the length of exposure to heat, type of work or activity, intake of water or food, salt intake, and events surrounding the onset of symptoms.
   b. **Laboratory studies.** In patients with severe heat cramps or syncope, **analysis of serum electrolytes** and a **CBC** may be required to guide therapy.

5. **Therapy**
   a. **Heat edema** is treated by simple leg elevation. There is no evidence that diuretic therapy is effective. In most patients, the edema will resolve with acclimatization or with the person's return to the home climate.
   b. **Mild heat cramps** are treated with rest and replacement of the deficient salt with an oral salt solution (0.1% sodium chloride). Patients with severe cramps may require intravenous isotonic saline (0.9% sodium chloride). Most patients respond rapidly to treatment.
   c. **Heat syncope** usually resolves when the person faints and assumes a supine position. Because the patient may be dehydrated, intravenous rehydration is often indicated. Persons at risk for heat syncope should be informed of preventive measures such as moving frequently, flexing leg muscles while standing, and sitting or lying down whenever early symptoms (e.g., vertigo, nausea, weakness) appear. Support hose and adequate oral fluid intake are also of benefit.
   d. **Heat tetany** resolves when the hyperventilation is treated with cooling and rehydration.

6. **Disposition.** The minor heat illnesses are easily treated, and most are preventable through patient education and ensuring adequate fluid and salt replacement. Patients with complicating illnesses, unstable vital signs, or abnormal mental status should be admitted and evaluated further.

C Heat exhaustion

1. **Discussion.** Heat exhaustion is a clinical syndrome characterized by volume depletion in patients exposed to heat stress. Most cases of heat exhaustion occur because of mixed salt and water depletion resulting from inadequate fluid and salt replacement in persons working in a hot environment. Heat exhaustion may progress to heat stroke if untreated; the symptoms are similar in the early stages.

2. **Clinical features.** The signs and symptoms of heat exhaustion are variable.
   a. **Symptoms.** Early complaints of fatigue and vague malaise may progress to weakness, vertigo, nausea and vomiting, and headache.
   b. **Physical examination findings.** With significant dehydration, signs may include muscle cramps, orthostatic syncope, tachycardia, hyperventilation, and hypotension. Body temperature often is normal or slightly elevated. Sweating persists and may be profuse. Signs of severe CNS damage are absent, with mental function essentially intact.

3. **Differential diagnoses** include cerebrovascular accident, drug ingestion, exacerbation of pre-existing medical illness, viral syndromes, psychological factors, infection, and heat stroke.

4. **Evaluation**
   a. A **history** and **physical examination** should lead to an accurate diagnosis in most cases.
   b. **Laboratory studies.** In mild cases, no laboratory studies are needed. In moderate to severe cases, a **CBC**, a **serum electrolyte panel**, and **hepatic transaminase values** may be helpful in identifying hypernatremia, hyponatremia, hemoconcentration, or hepatic damage. **Blood urea nitrogen (BUN)** and **urine specific gravity values** aid in determining the level of dehydration.

5. **Therapy.** If any doubt exists about the severity of the heat illness, the patient should be treated aggressively for possible heat stroke (see III D 5).
   a. **Cool environment.** The patient should rest in a cool environment. The patient who has an elevated body temperature should be cooled using a room-temperature water mist spray and a fan to aid in evaporation. Cool packs placed on the neck, axilla, and groin may speed cooling.
   b. **Correction of volume and electrolyte imbalances.** Usually, symptoms resolve rapidly with **intravenous saline rehydration.**
      (1) The type and volume of fluid should be determined by the patient's condition.
      (2) The free water deficit in the hypernatremic patient should be replaced slowly over 48 hours to prevent cerebral edema.

6. **Disposition**
   a. **Discharge.** In young, healthy patients who respond rapidly to treatment, no additional testing is required; these patients may be discharged with education about preventive techniques.
   b. **Admission.** Older patients, particularly those with cardiovascular disease or serious illness, require more careful fluid and electrolyte replacement and should be admitted.

D **Heat stroke**

1. **Discussion.** A true medical emergency, heat stroke is life-threatening and often fatal.
   a. **Definition.** Heat stroke is characterized by hyperpyrexia (core body temperature higher than 40°C or 105°F) and neurologic symptoms.
   b. **Pathophysiology.** In heat stroke, the homeostatic thermoregulatory mechanisms fail to work effectively, and the body is unable to maintain proper temperature. This failure results in elevation of body temperature to extreme levels (over 40°C, or 105°F), which produces multisystem damage, organ dysfunction, and sometimes death.
      (1) **CNS system dysfunction** is a hallmark of heat stroke.
      (2) **Other systemic effects** include **cerebral edema, circulatory/cardiac failure,** and **hepatic damage.**
   c. **Risk factors**
      (1) **Age.** Infants and the elderly are at increased risk. Infants have poorly developed compensatory mechanisms, while the elderly are at increased risk owing to disease, polypharmacy, and a decreased ability to escape hot environments.
      (2) **Occupation** (e.g., roofers, military personnel)
      (3) **Hot, humid environment**
      (4) **Alcohol abuse**
      (5) **Medication side effects**

        (6) Sweat gland abnormalities

        (7) Obesity

        (8) Psychological factors

        (9) Certain diseases (e.g., scleroderma, diabetes)

        (10) Socioeconomic factors (e.g., lack of a fan or air conditioning)

   d. Forms of heat stroke

     (1) Classic heat stroke occurs in conditions of high ambient heat and humidity. The victims are often poor, elderly, and living in poorly ventilated homes. These patients often have poor access to water or cool fluids. Frequently, these patients suffer from psychiatric and medical conditions that predispose them to heat illness, especially if they are taking medications that impair cooling. Sweating is absent in 84%–100% of classic heat stroke patients.

     (2) Exertional heat stroke occurs in previously healthy young people who have exercised or exerted themselves strenuously. In these patients, the endogenous heat production is too high relative to the hot environment and the body's cooling mechanisms are overwhelmed, causing the body temperature to increase to dangerously high levels. Patients are at increased risk for heat stroke, rhabdomyolysis, and acute renal failure, owing to heavy exercise and muscular exertion.

2. Clinical features

   a. Symptoms. Prodromal symptoms are nonspecific and include weakness, nausea, vomiting, vertigo, headache, and anorexia. Later, more serious symptoms include confusion, drowsiness, disorientation, ataxia, and psychiatric symptoms; these CNS symptoms eventually progress to coma and possibly death.

   b. Physical examination findings

     (1) Sweating may persist in early heat stroke, but **is often absent later** owing to failure of compensatory mechanisms.

     (2) Seizures occur in 75% of victims.

     (3) Varied pupil size may be found.

     (4) Cardiovascular findings include tachycardia, an **elevated cardiac index,** and **low peripheral vascular resistance.**

     (5) Coagulation may be aberrant, and **pancreatic** and **hepatic damage** often are present.

     (6) Hypoglycemia may be present in exertional heat stroke.

     (7) The **urine** may be **dark brown** from concentration, myoglobinuria, red blood cells (RBCs), or acute oliguric renal failure.

     (8) Respiratory alkalosis may be severe and may produce **tetany.**

     (9) After exercise, **lactic acidosis** often is present; a high lactate level is associated with increased mortality from heat stroke.

3. Differential diagnoses include meningitis, encephalitis, sepsis, cerebrovascular accident, thyroid storm, drug-induced heat illness (i.e., anticholinergic poisoning), typhus, and delirium tremens.

4. Evaluation

   a. History and physical examination aid in the diagnosis. Information from witnesses or the prehospital medical personnel may be critical if the patient has a severe CNS abnormality. **The initial core temperature does not correlate well with outcome;** often, the patient with heat stroke arrives at the hospital with only a minimally elevated temperature.

   b. Laboratory studies should include a **CBC, serum electrolyte panel, body fluid cultures** if sepsis is suspected, **coagulation studies, liver** and **pancreatic tests,** and **lactate, creatine phosphokinase,** and **myoglobin levels. Lumbar puncture** is required in any uncertain case to rule out meningitis and encephalitis.

   c. Diagnostic tests and **imaging studies.** An **ECG, EEG,** and **radiologic tests** should be considered.

5. **Therapy**
   a. **Prehospital management.** Treatment of heat stroke requires **immediate cooling.** The patient should be removed from the hot environment and, during transport to the hospital, should be unclothed and fanned, and the skin kept wet with tepid water.
   b. **ED management**
      (1) **Stabilization.** Attention must be paid to the patient's ABCs. **Intubation** of the patient with a severely altered mental status is often indicated, and **circulatory support** may require central venous pressure or Swan-Ganz catheter monitoring.
      (2) **Monitoring** of the core temperature, urine output, and cardiac rhythm is important.
      (3) **Supportive care.** Glucose, thiamine, folate, or naloxone may need to be administered to unresponsive patients.
      (4) **Cooling techniques** vary and are controversial. Optimal cooling usually includes disrobing the patient, sponging or misting with room-temperature water, and circulating air over the patient using fans. Other measures include immersion in a tub of ice water, ice packs, cooling blankets, and internal lavage with cool water. When the core temperature reaches 39°C (102°F), the cooling efforts should be slowed to prevent hypothermic overshoot.
      (5) **Antipyretics** (e.g., aspirin, acetaminophen) **are contraindicated.** They are ineffective in heat stroke victims, and may worsen the liver damage and uncouple oxidative phosphorylation.
      (6) **Treatment of complications**
         (a) **Shivering** may be treated with chlorpromazine or diazepam.
         (b) **Myoglobinuria** is treated with mannitol, alkalinization of the urine, and adequate fluid support, with possible dialysis.
         (c) **Acid–base and electrolyte disturbances** should be treated appropriately.

6. **Disposition.** All patients with heat stroke should be hospitalized and closely monitored for complications. Consultation with specialists may be required to deal with organ failure or damage.

7. **Prevention** of heat stroke is very important; people at risk should be educated about preventive measures. A wet bulb globe thermometer should be used by athletes and military units; activity should be restricted in hot, humid conditions. The young and old should receive close supervision and be taken to cooler locations during heat waves.

E **Unusual causes of hyperthermia**

1. **Malignant hyperthermia.** Certain patients with a rare genetic predisposition who undergo general anesthesia may rapidly develop severe hyperthermia, muscular rigidity, and acidosis. Malignant hyperthermia is caused by inappropriate intracellular calcium release. Treatment includes dantrolene (which lowers myoplasmic calcium), cooling, and supportive measures.

2. **Neuroleptic malignant syndrome (NMS).** This rare syndrome is induced by antipsychotic medications, commonly haloperidol, and manifests as muscular rigidity, severe dyskinesia, dystonia, hyperthermia, dyspnea, tachycardia, and urinary incontinence. The mechanism involves dopamine receptor blockade in the brain. Haloperidol also suppresses thirst, which exacerbates the problem. Treatment includes supportive and cooling measures, and administration of dantrolene.

3. **Drug overdose.** Overdose of anticholinergic medications and sympathomimetic agents such as amphetamines may cause fatal hyperpyrexia.

4. **Cerebrovascular accident.** Ischemic strokes involving the thermoregulatory centers in the brain, as well as intracerebral and subarachnoid hemorrhage, can cause elevation of body temperature and should be considered in the differential diagnosis of hyperthermia.

IV **HIGH-ALTITUDE EMERGENCIES**

A **Introduction** In the United States, over 40 million visitors travel to altitudes over 8000 feet annually. These people are at increased risk for hypoxia and related illness, dehydration, hypothermia, frostbite, trauma, delayed access to medical care, lightning injury, and other illnesses. This section focuses on acute mountain sickness (AMS), high-altitude pulmonary edema (HAPE), high-altitude cerebral edema (HACE), and other specific illnesses caused by high altitudes.

1. **Physiologic effects of altitude.** The degree of altitude is defined in three categories based on physiologic effects:
   a. **High altitude, from 1500–3500 meters (4900–11,500 feet):** decreased exercise performance and increased ventilation occur.
   b. **Very high altitude, from 3500–5500 meters (11,500–18,000 feet):** the maximum arterial oxygen saturation falls to less than 90%.
   c. **Extreme altitude, over 5500 meters (18,000 feet):** severe hypoxemia and hypocapnia are present. There is no human habitation above this level.

2. **Acclimatization to high altitude** occurs through increased ventilation, respiratory alkalosis, and an accompanying renal excretion of bicarbonate. These adaptations stabilize after 4–7 days of exposure to high altitude.
   a. Initially, exercise capacity is decreased and sleep disturbance is common.
   b. With continued ascent to higher altitudes, the central chemoreceptors reset to progressively lower $PaCO_2$ values.
      (1) Peripheral vasoconstriction leads to diuresis and hemoconcentration.
      (2) The hematopoietic response includes increased erythropoietin production, leading to an increased RBC mass.
      (3) Pulmonary vasculature constricts secondary to hypoxia, causing increased pulmonary vascular pressures.
      (4) Cerebral blood flow increases.

B **Acute mountain sickness (AMS)**

1. **Discussion.** AMS is found in nonacclimatized persons who ascend rapidly to 2000 meters (6600 feet) or higher. AMS is caused by **hypobaric hypoxia,** and the effects on the body are widespread.
   a. **Pathophysiology.** Varying degrees of cerebral edema result from cytotoxic edema (failure of the sodium–potassium pump) and vasogenic edema (leaky blood–brain barrier). Abnormal water handling by the body is involved, resulting in peripheral edema, mild interstitial pulmonary edema, and fluid retention. Severe AMS may progress to HACE.
   b. **Incidence.** The incidence depends on the rate of ascent, altitude, lung vital capacity, and ventilatory response. Approximately 25% of those going to 2500 meters (8100 feet) and 75% of those going to 4500 meters (14,600 feet) experience AMS.
   c. **Susceptibility.** AMS generally recurs on repeat altitude exposure, and is not related to physical fitness.

2. **Clinical features**
   a. **Symptoms**
      (1) **Mild AMS.** Symptoms include a bifrontal headache, anorexia, nausea, weakness, and fatigue. Sleepiness and malaise are common.
      (2) **More severe AMS** is characterized by vomiting, worsening headache, oliguria, and increased dyspnea; some victims may require help with eating and dressing because of lassitude.
   b. **Physical examination findings** are nonspecific and may include apparent fluid retention, retinal vein dilatation, and variable vital signs.

3. **Differential diagnoses** include viral syndromes, hypothermia, dehydration, exhaustion, carbon monoxide poisoning, infection, and exacerbation of pre-existing illness.

4. **Evaluation.** The early diagnosis is based on the setting, symptoms, and physical examination findings. Often the patient with AMS is in a setting remote from hospital medical care, where most tests are unavailable. Early diagnosis is essential to prevent worsening of symptoms.

5. **Therapy.** Most cases of AMS are self-limited.
   a. **Oxygen** by nasal canula or face mask (although not usually available) will help treat the symptoms in all cases of AMS.
   b. **Aspirin** or **acetaminophen** can be used for headache.
   c. **Intramuscular prochlorperazine** is useful for nausea and vomiting.
   d. **Dexamethasone** (4 mg every 6 hours) is effective treatment, but is best reserved for moderate and severe cases of AMS.
   e. **Diuretics** to treat fluid retention must be used with caution because many patients with AMS have been exerting themselves in a dry environment and thus may be dehydrated.

6. **Disposition.** Most AMS victims can be managed as outpatients. Patients with severe AMS require close observation and hospitalization.

7. **Prevention** of AMS is accomplished by educating the traveler and pretreating with acetazolamide.
   a. The likelihood of developing AMS can be diminished by **ascending gradually** and by initiating **acetazolamide therapy** 12–24 hours before ascent. Acetazolamide speeds acclimatization and aborts illness. It acts by inhibiting the enzyme carbonic anhydrase, resulting in bicarbonate diuresis and metabolic acidosis, which stimulates ventilation. Ventilation and oxygenation are increased, and sleep apnea resolves. The diuretic action of acetazolamide counteracts the fluid retention of AMS.
   b. High-altitude travelers should be advised of the following measures that they can take should they develop symptoms of AMS:
      (1) They should not ascend to higher sleeping altitudes.
      (2) They should descend if symptoms do not resolve, or if they become worse despite treatment.
      (3) They should descend and seek immediate treatment if they develop an altered level of consciousness, ataxia, or pulmonary edema (20% of cases).

C HAPE is the **most frequently lethal of all altitude illnesses.**

1. **Discussion**
   a. **Definition.** HAPE is a noncardiogenic pulmonary edema (NCPE) in which pulmonary artery pressure is markedly elevated owing to increased pulmonary vascular resistance. The exact cause of the pulmonary edema is not known.
   b. **Incidence.** The incidence varies from 0.01%–15%.
   c. **Risk factors** include rapid ascent, cold, excessive salt ingestion, use of sleeping medication, prior history of HAPE, and heavy exertion. Women are less susceptible, but children are more susceptible.

2. **Clinical features**
   a. **History.** HAPE usually occurs 2–4 days after ascent above 14,500 feet. Most cases occur during the second night at altitude. HAPE may occur at altitudes as low as 8000–10,000 feet, but these cases usually are associated with heavy exercise.
   b. **Symptoms**
      (1) **Early symptoms** include dyspnea on exertion, fatigue with minimal to moderate effort, and a dry hacking cough.
      (2) **Symptoms of AMS usually occur concurrently** with the development of HAPE. As the HAPE patient deteriorates (usually on the second night), the dyspnea worsens and is unrelieved by rest. This dyspnea at rest is a serious sign, and descent is urgently needed.
      (3) **Later symptoms** include fever, cough productive of clear, watery sputum, and hemoptysis. Cerebral edema and hypoxia with mental status changes may occur.
   c. **Physical examination findings** include a few localized **rales** in early HAPE, which progress to patchy unilateral or bilateral rales, then diffuse rales and rhonchi, and gurgles that can be heard without the stethoscope. **Cyanosis** of the nail beds may progress to central cyanosis as hypoxia worsens. **Tachypnea** and **tachycardia** also worsen, and a concomitant respiratory tract infection may occur.

3. **Differential diagnoses** include pneumonia, high-altitude bronchitis and pharyngitis, pulmonary embolism, pneumothorax, and exacerbation of cardiac and pulmonary disease.

4. **Evaluation**
   a. **Laboratory studies. ABG determinations** reveal a respiratory alkalosis with hypoxemia.
   b. **Diagnostic tests.** The **ECG** demonstrates right-sided heart strain due to pulmonary hypertension.
   c. **Imaging studies.** A **chest radiograph** reveals fluffy alveolar infiltrates, with areas of clearing between the patches.

5. **Therapy.** If HAPE is recognized early and treated properly, death can be avoided in most cases.
   a. The highest treatment priority is **immediate descent.** Descent of 1500–3000 feet is adequate in most cases.
   b. Other treatment should include **oxygen** and, ideally, **bed rest.** Oxygen lowers the pulmonary artery pressure, decreases vasoconstriction, increases arterial oxygen saturation, and relieves symptoms.
      (1) AMS and HAPE victims have been treated in **hyperbaric chambers,** but hyperbaric chamber therapy has not been demonstrated to be more effective than oxygen therapy.
      (2) A **Gamow bag,** a portable pressurized bag inflated using a foot pump, has been used; inflation to 2 pounds per square inch (psi) above ambient pressure simulates a descent of 5000 feet.
   c. Several authors have suggested that **furosemide,** 80 mg twice daily, is beneficial in treating HAPE, and may be helpful in treating patients with AMS when antidiuresis is present.

6. **Disposition.** Rapid recovery often occurs after descent to lower altitudes, but supplemental oxygenation should be continued until the victim is completely recovered. Patients with more severe cases should be hospitalized and closely monitored. Once oxygen saturation is greater than 90% on room air and clinical improvement is apparent, the patient may be discharged from the hospital. After 2–3 days of rest, reascent may be undertaken if the patient is fully recovered.

D HACE is the **least common** form of high-altitude illness (the incidence is less than 1% in climbers), but it is the **most severe.**

1. **Discussion.** HACE is characterized by progressive neurologic deterioration in a person with AMS or HAPE. Mild AMS may progress rapidly to HACE, with coma occurring within 12 hours. Most cases develop over 1–3 days and occur above 12,000 feet, but death has occurred as low as 8400 feet.

2. **Clinical features. Evidence of global cerebral dysfunction in people with AMS is the chief indication of HACE.** Signs and symptoms include severe headache, nausea and vomiting, and altered mental status. Confusion, hallucinations, ataxia, slurred speech, seizures, and focal neurologic deficits may precede coma.
   a. **Once coma develops, death occurs in over 60% of victims.**
   b. The most telltale sign of early HACE is **cerebellar ataxia,** which is by itself an indication for immediate descent.
   c. Because of elevated intracranial pressure (ICP) resulting in dislocation of brain structures, **focal neurologic signs** such as third and sixth cranial nerve palsies may be identified.

3. **Differential diagnoses** include cerebrovascular accident, unidentified trauma, intracranial hemorrhage, hypoglycemia, and exacerbation of underlying illness.

4. **Evaluation.** Laboratory and advanced testing usually is not available in remote regions. Upon arrival at the hospital, the patient with suspected HACE should be carefully assessed and other causes for altered mental status considered.

5. **Therapy.** The treatment for HACE is the same as for AMS and HAPE: descent, rest, and oxygen.
   a. **Evacuation** to hospital facilities at lower altitude is of prime importance. If descent is not possible, **hyperbaric therapy** (using a Gamow bag) should be initiated if possible.

   b. **Oxygen** should be given at a rate of 2–4 L/min as early in the rescue as possible.

   c. **Steroids** have been shown to be of benefit by several studies. Dexamethasone (8 mg orally, intramuscularly, or intravenously) should be given initially, followed by 4 mg four times daily.

   d. **Airway management** and **advanced care** are necessary for comatose victims. Cautious use of hyperventilation is needed because of the pre-existing alkalosis. Administration of mannitol and diuretics should be considered.

6. **Disposition.** Minor psychological changes may persist after a severe episode of HACE; any severe sequelae mandate exclusion of other possible causes. After stabilization and resolution of altered mental status, the victim should be cautioned about future high-altitude travel and the risk of HACE recurrence.

E **Other high-altitude illnesses**

1. **Ultraviolet keratitis (snow blindness).** Ultraviolet light penetrates the atmosphere to a greater degree at high altitudes where the air is "thinner" with less particulate matter and fewer clouds. The amount of ultraviolet radiation increases by 5% for every 300 meters (1000 feet) of elevation, and ultraviolet light is reflected by snow and rocks found at high elevations.

   a. **Pathophysiology.** Ultraviolet B radiation is absorbed by the cornea and can produce burns in less than 2 hours.

   b. **Clinical features.** Symptoms appear 6–12 hours after exposure and include severe eye pain, a gritty sensation, tearing, chemosis, photophobia, and eyelid swelling.

   c. **Therapy.** Ultraviolet keratitis usually heals within 24 hours and is self-limited, but it is extremely painful and often requires systemic analgesics. Prevention is possible by wearing proper sunglasses with side shields.

2. **Exacerbation of pre-existing illnesses.** Several diseases may be exacerbated by ascent to high altitudes:

   a. Patients with **chronic obstructive pulmonary disease (COPD)** may experience increased dyspnea and reduced exercise ability owing to worsened alveolar hypoxia.

   b. Patients with **arteriosclerotic heart disease** do not have good adaptive capabilities for high altitudes and are at risk to suffer from earlier onset of angina.

   c. Patients prone to **CHF** may experience a worsening of their condition owing to fluid retention. These patients should continue or increase their diuretic medications, and should consider low-flow oxygen during sleep.

   d. Patients with **sickle cell disease** are at higher risk for a vaso-occlusive crisis owing to the hypoxemia and dehydration encountered at high altitude.

V   SCUBA DIVING INJURIES

A **Discussion**   Scuba diving is often associated with accidents and illness, especially in the untrained. Many adverse physical conditions are encountered while diving, including cold, wetness, absence of air to breathe, changes in light and sound, and increased ambient pressure. The diving injuries discussed here are those caused by changes in pressure and air volume (dysbarism), and most often include barotrauma, dysbaric air embolism (DAE), and decompression sickness (DCS).

1. **Physiology**

   a. **Pressure.** The direct or indirect effects of pressure account for most diving injuries. Pressure (force per unit area) is greater underwater because of the weight of water. The density of water increases with depth, and large changes in pressure accompany small fluctuations in depth. At the surface (i.e., at sea level), pressure is 14.7 psi, or one atmospheric pressure absolute (ATA). For every 33 feet of depth in sea water, the pressure increases by 1 ATA. For example, at a depth of 33 feet, the pressure doubles to 2 ATA; at 165 feet it is 6 ATA. Scuba diving generally is done at a maximum depth of 120 to 130 feet (4 ATA).

b. Gas laws. Three gas laws of diving physiology help explain the nature of diving injuries:

(1) **Boyle's law** states that the volume of a gas is inversely proportional to its pressure at a given temperature. Thus, when the pressure is doubled, the volume of a unit of gas is halved. An easy way to remember this is the mnemonic **BOYLE**: "**B**reathe (as you ascend) **O**r **Y**our **L**ungs **E**xplode."

(2) **Dalton's law** states that the total pressure of a mixture of gases is equal to the sum of the partial pressures of the component gases.

(3) **Henry's law** states that the amount of gas dissolved in a given volume of fluid is proportional to the pressure of the gas with which it is in equilibrium. This explains why more nitrogen dissolves in the diver's body as ambient pressure increases with descent.

2. Types of scuba diving injuries

a. Barotrauma, the most common affliction of divers, is the tissue damage resulting from expansion or contraction of gas within an enclosed space, occurring during either ascent or descent.

(1) **Barotrauma of descent ("squeeze").** If the air-filled space (e.g., ears, sinuses) is not collapsible, the resulting pressure imbalance results in mucosal edema, vascular engorgement and hemorrhage, and tissue distortion with accompanying pain.

   (a) **Aural barotrauma** is the most common type.

   (b) **Paranasal sinus barotrauma** can also occur. The maxillary and frontal sinuses are most often affected.

(2) **Barotrauma of ascent** occurs when obstruction of air passages prevents the venting of expanding gases to the atmosphere. It is the reverse process of squeeze. **Ears and sinuses are unlikely to be affected** unless a nasal decongestant has worn off and the eustachian tubes are blocked.

   (a) **Odontalgia (tooth pain)** occurs because of a change of enclosed air spaces in the teeth, which exert pressure on sensitive tissues.

   (b) **Gastrointestinal barotrauma** may occur because of expansion of intraluminal bowel gas during ascent.

b. DAE is the presence of gas bubbles in the systemic vasculature as the result of the rupture of pulmonary tissue and veins. One of the most serious injuries, it is a major cause of death and disability among scuba divers.

(1) **Etiology.** Most cases result from the diver ascending too rapidly or while holding his or her breath, often because of panic in the event of running out of air or other emergency circumstances.

(2) **Pathophysiology.** If a diver holds his or her breath while ascending, the expanding gas is not able to escape from the lungs.

   (a) As a result, the alveoli may rupture, leading to **pulmonary overpressurization syndrome (POPS),** or "burst lung." Injuries include pneumomediastinum, pneumothorax, and subcutaneous and interstitial emphysema.

   (b) In **systemic air embolism,** the most feared complication of POPS, air bubbles are pumped by the left ventricle into systemic arteries where they occlude the more distal circulation.

c. DCS ("the bends")

(1) **Pathophysiology.** DCS results from the formation of gas bubbles in blood and body tissues when the ambient pressure is decreased. The decreased pressure effect is similar to opening a champagne bottle, when the rapid liberation of inert gas from solution causes bubble formation. Many factors determine the rate at which the gases reach a new equilibrium, but the primary mechanism is ascending too rapidly.

   (a) Although the bubbles may form anywhere in the body, the major mechanical effect is **vascular occlusion.**

   (b) If a right-to-left cardiac shunt exists, **neurologic embolism** may occur.

(c) The blood–bubble interface is viewed by the immune system as foreign matter and may incite an inflammatory response, Hageman factor activation, and clot formation. The net effect of this response is decreased tissue perfusion and ischemic injury.

(2) **Types**

(a) **Type I DCS** is the mild form involving the skin and the musculoskeletal system.

(b) **Type II DCS** includes neurologic, cardiac, and other serious organ system involvement.

B Clinical features

1. **Barotrauma**

   a. **Aural barotrauma**

      (1) **Middle ear aural barotrauma** is characterized by **pain,** which occurs when eustachian tube dysfunction prevents equalization of the middle ear pressure, leading to a pressure differential of more than 100–150 mm Hg. If descent is continued despite pain, **tympanic membrane rupture** can occur and is characterized by **vertigo, disorientation,** and **vomiting,** which may then cause panic and drowning.

      (2) **Inner ear aural barotrauma,** which is rare, is characterized by **severe vertigo, tinnitus,** and **deafness.**

   b. **Paranasal sinus barotrauma.** Clinical signs include fullness, pain, or hemorrhage of the affected sinus.

2. **DAE.** The symptoms produced by DAE are related to the site of the air embolus, and vary from pain to severe complications, including death from stroke or cardiac ischemia.

   a. The **onset of symptoms immediately upon reaching the surface** is the hallmark of DAE. Sudden loss of consciousness upon reaching the surface should be considered DAE until proven otherwise.

   b. **Neurologic signs** usually predominate because the brain is the organ most frequently affected. Even a small embolus can produce significant neurologic dysfunction. The symptoms are typical of an acute stroke and are varied. **Asymmetric multiplegias** are the most common presentation.

3. **DCS.** The clinical findings of DCS depend on the site of vascular occlusion.

   a. **Cutaneous effects** include mottled rashes, pruritus, subcutaneous emphysema, and swelling.

   b. **Periarticular joint pain** is typically described as a deep, dull ache, often exacerbated by movement, with the shoulders and elbows most often affected.

   c. **Neurologic findings** are varied; the symptoms seen in a given case depend on the vasculature affected. A "hit" within the spinal cord that causes focal neurologic deficits is a common presentation. The brain may also be affected.

   d. **Pulmonary findings** are not usually apparent unless more than 10% of the lung vasculature is obstructed.

C Differential diagnoses

The symptoms of decompression sickness and DAE do not always resolve following recompression. In these cases, other diagnoses need to be considered, such as **trauma** and **intracranial hemorrhage.**

D Evaluation

Because diving illness may present with a wide variety of symptoms, careful evaluation is needed to make a definitive diagnosis.

1. **History.** Information related to the diving trip or accident often is important in making the diagnosis.

   a. Any symptom that occurs in the immediate postdive phase (within 10 minutes of surfacing) should be considered **DAE** until proven otherwise.

   b. Symptoms that begin more than 10 minutes after exiting the water should be viewed as **DCS** until explained otherwise. Over half of all DCS patients experience symptoms within the first hour after surfacing.

2. **Imaging studies. Magnetic resonance imaging (MRI) scanning** permits assessment of brain and spinal cord damage from air emboli.

E **Therapy** Overall, the rate of success with recompression is 80%–90%. Greater success is associated with early institution of hyperbaric oxygen therapy. (Hyperbaric treatment according to well-established protocols provides oxygen and pressure, which are needed to treat DCS and DAE.)

1. **Prehospital management**
   a. **Stabilization**
      (1) **Life support measures** should be instituted as soon as possible.
      (2) Exposure and hypothermia should be considered in all cases.
      (3) The patient should be placed supine, and **100% oxygen** should be administered by mask, which facilitates "offgassing" of the nitrogen bubbles and improves oxygenation.
   b. **Transport.** Once stabilized, the patient should be transported without delay to a medical facility with a hyperbaric/recompression chamber. If air transportation is used, the aircraft should be pressurized to 1 ATA or should fly low at 1000 feet. If the location of the nearest facility is uncertain, assistance is available 24 hours a day from the National Diving Alert Network (DAN) at Duke University [(919) 684-8111].

2. **ED management**
   a. **Stabilization.** Advanced life support drugs and measures should be administered if needed. Victims with altered level of consciousness may require intubation and ventilatory support. The use of continuous positive airway pressure (CPAP) and positive end-expiratory pressure (PEEP) should be avoided whenever possible because of the increased risk of overpressurizing the noncompliant lung and causing air embolism.
   b. **Fluid resuscitation.** Intravascular volume depletion and hemoconcentration are common in serious DCS, and fluids should be replaced as needed.
   c. **Glucocorticoids are no longer indicated.**

F **Disposition** All seriously ill victims require **hospitalization and close observation.**

G **Prevention** Education is important for prevention of future accidents.

VI DROWNING AND NEAR-DROWNING

A **Discussion**

1. **Definitions**
   a. **Drowning** is death by suffocation from submersion in a liquid medium, usually water.
   b. **Near-drowning** is survival following submersion.
   c. **Secondary drowning** is eventual death from drowning after an initial brief period of recovery (minutes to days).
   d. **Immersion syndrome** is sudden death occurring as a result of contact with very cold water. The mechanism is unclear, but it is likely due to vagally induced bradycardia or cardiac arrest with resultant loss of consciousness. Alcohol ingestion is considered an important predisposing factor.
   e. **Postimmersion syndrome** may be seen in near-drowning victims within 72 hours. It is a type of adult respiratory distress syndrome (ARDS) caused by inactivation or washout of surfactant, alveolar capillary membrane damage with leakage, and an inflammatory response in the lung.

2. **Incidence.** Drowning is a significant cause of morbidity and mortality, accounting for more than 4000 deaths annually in the United States and 140,000 annually throughout the world.

3. **Predisposing factors.** In drowning and near-drowning, there is often a precipitating condition or event, such as an inability to swim, muscle cramps, exhaustion, cervical spinal cord injury, alcohol or drug intoxication, hypothermia, seizures, hypoglycemia, or a diving accident.

4. **Pathophysiology**
   a. The **sequence of events** may include initial panic and struggle, breath-holding, swallowing of water, and vomiting. When unable to suppress respiratory drive, most victims gasp for air, aspirating water in the process. The resulting hypoxia leads to unconsciousness, loss of reflexes, and eventual asphyxiation. Approximately 10%–20% of drownings occur without aspiration; in these cases intense laryngospasm prevents water from entering the lungs.
   b. **Fresh water versus salt water aspiration.** Although there are differences in the body's physiologic response to fresh water versus salt water aspiration, the complications and treatments of each are similar. The end result of both types of water aspiration is pulmonary edema with shunting and hypoxemia.
      (1) **Fresh water** is hypotonic relative to plasma, and is rapidly absorbed into the circulation. RBC lysis may occur as a result of fresh water aspiration, causing hyperkalemia and hemoglobinuria in severe cases; however, these changes are transitory and rarely of sufficient magnitude to warrant treatment. Of greater concern is the pulmonary injury resulting from loss of surfactant and disruption of membranes.
      (2) **Salt water** is three times more concentrated than plasma, and thus is not absorbed into the circulation. Instead, fluid from the circulation is drawn into the alveoli, producing pulmonary edema, shunting, decreased gas exchange, and hypoxemia. The potential exists for hypovolemia and hemoconcentration, but only rarely are these significant.

B Clinical features   Near-drowning victims can present with a wide range of signs and symptoms, depending on the seriousness of the initial insult and the extent of organ system involvement. The submersion victim often has **severe hypoxia** with diffuse systemic effects. **Altered mental status** may result from cerebral hypoxia and edema. **Cardiac arrhythmias** may be seen, and **renal failure** sometimes occurs.

C Differential diagnoses   If the patient presents in full arrest, consider as possible causes anoxia, immersion syndrome, hypothermia, and trauma.

D Evaluation   The diagnosis of near-drowning is obvious to rescue personnel involved in the initial resuscitation.

1. **History and physical examination.** An **accurate history** and **core body temperature** measurement should be obtained. Associated conditions and injuries (e.g., cervical spine fracture) should be sought.

2. **Laboratory studies.** A CBC, a serum electrolyte panel, and an ABG determination should be obtained to evaluate for hemolysis and hypoxia.

3. **Diagnostic tests.** An ECG and cardiac monitoring should be used to assess for arrhythmias.

4. **Imaging studies.** A chest radiograph should be obtained to evaluate the lungs, and a spinal radiograph should be obtained to rule out fractures. CT scanning may be appropriate for patients with head injuries or an altered level of consciousness.

E Therapy

1. **Prehospital management**
   a. **Removal from water.** Treatment of near-drowning begins at the scene with rapid, cautious removal of the victim from the water. **Spinal precautions** should be observed.
   b. **Stabilization.** A **patent airway** and **ventilation** must be established. **CPR** should be initiated and continued on any arrested patient if there is even a remote possibility of success.
   c. **Removal of water from the lungs.** No drainage procedure is necessary to empty the lungs of aspirated water unless a large amount of salt water is present in the lungs. Drainage may be accomplished by briefly lowering the patient's head and upper torso to allow dependent drainage.

2. **ED management.** Hospital management includes standard advanced life support measures, and the following:
   a. **Oxygenation** should be monitored by pulse oximetry. If a PaO$_2$ greater than 60 mm Hg cannot be maintained even following the administration of high-flow oxygen, or if the patient cannot adequately protect the airway, the patient should be intubated and mechanically ventilated. PEEP or CPAP is often required, and hyperventilation may be used to decrease cerebral edema.
   b. **Rewarming measures** should be undertaken if the patient is hypothermic. External or internal methods may be used, depending on the patient's core body temperature.
   c. **Monitoring.** Cardiac monitoring and ICP monitoring (in pediatric patients) should be instituted. Reassessment should be performed at frequent intervals.
   d. **Treatment of complications.** Standard treatment of bronchospasm, electrolyte imbalance, seizures, hypothermia, arrhythmias, and hypotension should be undertaken as needed. Neither steroids nor antibiotics should be given prophylactically.

F **Disposition**   The near-drowning victim should be closely monitored. The patient who demonstrates no evidence of significant exposure and who remains asymptomatic may be discharged after several hours of observation if the situation allows adequate follow-up. Victims with mild to moderate hypoxemia require hospitalization, as do critically ill patients.

VII   SMOKE INHALATION INJURIES

A **Discussion**   Fire-related inhalation injuries and fatalities are caused by heat, flames, altered gas levels (low oxygen, high carbon dioxide and carbon monoxide), direct irritation and damage to the respiratory tract, indirect injuries, and smoke.

1. **Heat-related inhalation injuries.** Breathing heated air may cause damage to the respiratory tract. Air temperatures of 93°C (200°F) may be tolerated for 30 minutes, but temperatures of 250°C (480°F) will be tolerated for only 3 minutes, with death more likely with longer exposures.

2. **Smoke-related inhalation injuries.** Fire is the most common cause of exposure to toxic inhalants. Smoke contains a large variety of substances that may cause injury or death when inhaled. The contents of smoke from a fire are related to the substances burning. Many products of combustion may be inhaled:
   a. **Simple asphyxiants** include dust, ash, and nontoxic carbon particles.
   b. **Pulmonary irritants** include hydrogen chloride, phosgene, and other toxins. Inhalation may result in laryngospasm, bronchospasm, and pulmonary epithelium damage, and may possibly lead to NCPE.
   c. **Chemical asphyxiants** result in tissue anoxia despite a normal PaO$_2$.

3. **Altered gas level–related inhalation injuries.** Hydrogen cyanide, hydrogen sulfide, carbon monoxide, and agents that produce methemoglobinemia interfere with oxygen delivery and utilization.
   a. **Carbon monoxide poisoning** is the most common toxicologic cause of death and fire-related mortality (see Chapter 20 VI).
   b. **Open space versus closed space fires.** In open wilderness fires, hypoxia is rare due to the constant fresh air available. However, in a closed burning space (e.g., house, factory), the oxygen level may be quite low and toxic gases may accumulate.

B **Clinical features**   Most victims have coughing and upper airway irritation. Patients with more severe exposures have stridor, worsening dyspnea and hypoxia, headache, confusion, and seizures.

1. **Smoke inhalation.** Simple irritants found in smoke often cause a cough and upper airway irritation. Symptoms often resolve spontaneously without specific treatment.

2. **Airway burns.** Signs of potential airway burns include facial and upper chest burns, singed facial or nasal hair, black carbonaceous particles in the airway, and local erythema and swelling of the upper airway.

3. **Pulmonary signs.** Pulmonary irritants such as hydrogen chloride may cause significant burning and stinging to the eyes, mucous membranes, nasal passage, and lower respiratory tract. Bronchospasm may result and, if severe chemical burning occurs, stridor and pulmonary edema may be seen.

4. **Chemical asphyxiation.** Chemical asphyxiants cause varying degrees of symptoms depending on the amount and duration of exposure. Carbon monoxide, hydrogen cyanide, and hydrogen sulfide poisoning symptoms range from a mild headache and nausea to severe headache, psychiatric disturbance, seizures, coma, and death.

C Evaluation

1. **History.** Knowledge of the circumstances, products burned, location, odors at the fire, and symptoms of other victims can provide important clues. It is important to focus on the mechanism of injury and, if possible, to identify the inhalation agents, because specific toxins may require specific antidotes and treatment.

2. **Laboratory and diagnostic studies**
   a. If the history and physical examination suggest toxic exposure, specific tests such as an ABG determination, carboxyhemoglobin and cyanide levels, chest radiographs, a CT scan, and toxicology screens should be considered.
   b. If the patient is at risk for delayed pulmonary complications (e.g., in the case of phosgene thermal burn), observation and further testing are indicated.
   c. In patients with subacute complications such as NCPE or thermal injury, which may present with delayed respiratory distress, serial ABGs, chest radiographs, and endotracheal intubation may be indicated.

D Therapy

1. **Prehospital management**
   a. **Removal from the scene.** The victim should be removed from the fire and smoke while paying attention to scene safety. An adequate airway must be ensured, and supplemental 100% oxygen should be provided. Precautions must be taken to avoid exposure to possibly toxic chemicals on the patient's clothes and body.
   b. **Stabilization** of the patient is with standard prehospital protocols. Spine protection must be ensured. Initial treatment for burns, cuts, and other coexisting trauma can be provided.

2. **ED management.** Airway, breathing, and circulatory support should be continued, and intravenous access obtained.
   a. **Minor bronchospasm and airway irritation.** Patients may require supportive care only.
   b. **Simple asphyxiant exposure.** Patients may require only administration of oxygen and observation for complete resolution of symptoms.
   c. **Thermal burns to the airway.** Patients likely require intubation, which should be performed before stridor or compromise occurs.
   d. **Bronchospasm.** Patients should be treated with nebulized bronchodilators and close observation.
   e. **Stridor** indicates that thermal injury to the vocal cords has occurred. Intubation should be performed to prevent obstruction as a result of swelling.
   f. **NCPE.** Patients may require CPAP or PEEP.
   g. **Altered level of consciousness.** Patients require standard treatment and evaluation. Administration of naloxone, thiamine, and glucose should be considered.
   h. **Chemical asphyxiation**

    (1) Carbon monoxide poisoning is discussed in Chapter 20 VI E.

    (2) Hydrogen cyanide poisoning. A specific treatment kit, the Lilly Cyanide Antidote Kit, is available in the United States. Cyanide binds tightly to the ferric (Fe^{3+}) cytochrome complex and blocks the cytochrome oxidase system. The goal of treatment is to provide alternative ferric ions, which can be accomplished by generating methemoglobin with nitrites. The antidote kit contains amyl nitrite (inhalation), sodium nitrite, and sodium thiosulfate (which provides sulfur to help eliminate the cyanide molecules).

    (3) Hydrogen sulfide poisoning. Hydrogen sulfide inhalation may result in poisoning similar to hydrogen cyanide poisoning, except that the cytochrome oxidase system is reversibly blocked. Standard resuscitation techniques are usually sufficient to reverse hydrogen sulfide toxicity; in severe cases, nitrites may be used as with hydrogen cyanide poisoning. Sodium thiosulfate is not used in the treatment of hydrogen sulfide poisoning.

    (4) Mixed inhalations. In patients with mixed inhalations, treatment with nitrites should be avoided because they may form 25% or more methemoglobin if a coexistent carbon monoxide poisoning occurs, causing more severe tissue hypoxia. Instead, a sodium thiosulfate infusion should be started and a carboxyhemoglobin level obtained.

      (a) If the carboxyhemoglobin level is low and the patient has persistent acidosis or unstable vital signs, the entire cyanide antidote kit can be used.

      (b) If the carboxyhemoglobin level is high, the patient should be transferred to a hyperbaric oxygen facility; once inside, the sodium nitrite portion of the kit is infused.

E Disposition

1. **Discharge.** Patients with resolution of major symptoms and who are not at risk for toxic inhalation may be discharged.

2. **Admission**

    a. Any patient who is persistently symptomatic (cough, dyspnea, bronchospasm) requires admission to the hospital, close observation, and treatment of complications.

    b. If the inhaled chemicals may result in delayed pulmonary or systemic complications, prolonged observation (over 6 hours) or admission is required to detect any development of NCPE or ARDS.

    c. Most smoke inhalations involve uncertain combustion products. Therefore, any patient with significant respiratory distress will need to be fully evaluated and observed for at least 24 hours.

VIII   LIGHTNING INJURIES

A Discussion

1. **Incidence and mortality rates.** Lightning kills 30% of its victims, over 200 people annually in the United States. More than 60% of lightning strike victims have injuries and long-term sequelae.

2. **Severity.** The voltage from a lightning strike averages about 10 to 30 million direct-current (DC) volts, with a duration of 0.1 to 1 millisecond. Duration of exposure is the primary determinant of degree of injury.

3. **Pathophysiology.** The skin is a good insulator; most lightning strikes pass over the outside of the body (the "flashover phenomenon"). If the victim is wet from rainwater or sweat, the moisture turns to steam and superficial burns may result. Clothes may be suddenly ripped away by the energy involved.

4. **Types of lightning injuries**

    a. Direct strike: lightning strikes victim

    b. Side flash: near-miss, but some voltage strikes

    c. Contact voltage: injury results from touching an object that is struck by lighting

    d. Ground voltage: walking near ground strike

    e. Thermal burning: clothing or object burns victim

    f. Blunt injury: victim is thrown, concussion

B **Clinical features** Injuries vary depending on the mechanism, the duration of exposure, and the area of the body involved in the lightning strike.

1. **Cardiopulmonary arrest.** Death from a lightning strike is usually due to immediate cardiopulmonary arrest. Lightning's DC energy often causes cardiac asystole [as opposed to household electricity's alternating current (AC), which more often causes ventricular fibrillation]. The asystole produced by lighting is frequently temporary in a healthy adult; however, the accompanying respiratory arrest may last significantly longer, causing hypoxia, which induces a second cardiac arrest from arrhythmias.

2. **Burns** are usually superficial unless the clothing has ignited. Superficial burns often have a pathognomonic arborescent (branch or feather-like) pattern and do not require treatment. Patients should be evaluated for deep muscle damage, although it occurs rarely. Fasciotomy is rarely, if ever, indicated. Entry and exit wounds, like those that occur with high-voltage AC electrical burns, are unusual.

3. **Injuries to the eyes** may cause cataracts and ocular trauma. Often the pupils are initially unreactive or unequal.

4. **Tympanic membrane rupture** occurs in more than 50% of victims.

5. **Fractures** and **dislocations** may occur, but are uncommon.

6. **Neurologic signs** and **symptoms** occur frequently following lightning injury.

    a. A majority of victims with severe injury (60%) have **transient lower extremity paralysis,** usually due to vascular spasm and nerve instability, which resolves in several hours. The **upper extremities** are **paralyzed 30% of the time.**

    b. Permanent paresis can result from direct injury to the spinal cord.

    c. Confusion and **amnesia** for several days may occur, and **personality changes** have been reported.

    d. Coma. Comatose patients have a poor outcome; a full evaluation is required to rule out a surgically correctable cause.

C **Differential diagnoses** include seizure, trauma, cerebrovascular accident, subarachnoid hemorrhage, cardiac arrhythmias, spinal cord and head injury, heavy metal poisoning, and drug exposure.

D **Evaluation**

1. **History and physical examination.** A history of being outdoors in a thunderstorm should suggest lightning, especially if there are multiple victims. The physical examination should focus on clues such as tympanic membrane rupture, superficial burns with pathognomonic arborescent patterns, and clothing burns or disintegration.

2. **Laboratory studies.** A urinalysis should be obtained to check for myoglobinuria. A serum electrolyte panel, CBC, and cardiac isoenzymes (even in asymptomatic patients) should also be obtained.

3. **Diagnostic tests.** The patient should be placed on cardiac and pulse oximetry monitors, and an ECG should be obtained.

4. **Imaging studies.** Radiographs and CT scans may be appropriate.

E **Therapy**

1. **Prehospital management**

    a. Rescuers should be cautious when treating victims outdoors in a thunderstorm, because lightning can strike the same place twice.

b. Basic and advanced life support measures may be needed; advanced cardiac life support (ACLS) protocols do not need to be modified for victims of lightning injury.

c. In triage of multiple victims, priority should be given to persons without signs of life; this differs from normal triage principles, which advise not spending time or resources on the patient in cardiopulmonary arrest. Lightning strike victims in arrest may only require ventilatory support for several minutes until the respiratory arrest resolves.

2. ED management includes establishing intravenous access, fluid restriction if possible, treatment of burns and trauma, and supportive care, including psychosocial support for the likely neurologic changes.

F Disposition   Seriously injured or symptomatic patients require admission. Asymptomatic patients must be observed for several hours to ensure that CHF does not develop and to monitor for delayed signs of injury and neurologic damage.

IX   VENOMOUS SNAKEBITES

A Discussion   Venomous snakes inhabit all states with the exceptions of Maine, Alaska, and Hawaii. In addition, exotic venomous snakes are kept in zoos and private collections throughout the United States. Therefore, the potential for bites by venomous snakes exists everywhere.

1. Incidence

a. Each year in the United States, over 8000 victims of venomous snakebites are treated; of these, 50 victims die. An additional 38,000 bites by harmless snakes are recorded.

b. July and August are the peak months for snakebites. Snakes are poikilothermic and therefore are most active in the summer. Most snakes prefer to retreat when disturbed, but will bite when provoked or suddenly surprised.

2. Identification of snakes. If possible, the type of snake responsible for the snakebite should be identified to determine whether the snake is venomous and the type of venom injected.

a. Venomous snakes may be classified as crotalids (pit vipers), elapids, or colubrids. Most venomous snakes in the United States are pit vipers.

(1) Crotalids are snakes with **movable front fangs.** Three types of crotalid pit vipers are native to the United States: the **rattlesnake,** the **water moccasin ("cottonmouth"),** and the **copperhead** (the most prevalent but least venomous of the pit vipers). Characteristics of pit vipers include:

(a) Small "pit" indentation between the snake's eye and nostril

(b) Vertical slit pupils

(c) Arrowhead-shaped head

(d) A single caudal row of plates from the anal plate to one third of the way from the tail (nonpoisonous snakes have two rows of plates)

(e) May have "rattles" on the tail (in rattlesnakes)

(2) Elapids are snakes with **fixed front fangs** (e.g., **coral snakes**). Coral snakes are small and shy, and have red and black bands that are wider than the interspaced yellow rings. ["Red on yellow, kills a fellow (coral snake); red on black, venom lack (harmless snake)."]

(3) Colubrids have **hind fangs.** None are native to the United States, although they are found in exotic collections.

b. Harmless snakes have round eyes, oval heads, two rows of plates near the anal plate, and no pit.

3. Pathogenesis. Many venomous snakes have long, sharp hollow fangs that easily penetrate clothing. Venom is injected through these fangs in 70%–80% of bites.

a. Crotalid venom is composed of a mixture of enzymes, polypeptides, and glycoproteins that, when injected, causes tissue destruction, hemolysis, nerve damage, capillary damage, and breakdown of the host cells and coagulation factors.

b. Coral snake venom, composed of a strong neurotoxin and several enzymes, causes systemic neurologic symptoms but very little local tissue damage.

B Clinical features

1. **Severity of symptoms** is related to:
   a. Amount of venom released
   b. Type of snake (strength of venom varies)
   c. Age and size of snake
   d. Age and size of victim
   e. Prior health of victim
   f. Location of the bite (bites to the head and trunk are three times as dangerous as bites to the extremity)
   g. Treatment received

2. **Local effects**
   a. **Fang marks that continue to ooze nonclotting blood** indicate envenomization. Marks without bleeding or with clotted blood probably represent a lack of envenomation or an insect bite, or are factitious.
   b. **Immediate severe pain** that is out of proportion to the appearance of the wound suggests pit viper envenomation.
   c. **Numbness** may occur following envenomation by coral snakes.
   d. **Local swelling** occurs within several hours. Edema, cyanosis, hemorrhagic blebs, and lymphangitis may occur, and may spread progressively.

3. **Systemic effects**
   a. Shock and hypotension
   b. Compartment syndrome (see Chapter 18 VII)
   c. Fluid shift
   d. Hemolysis
   e. Coagulopathies
   f. Petechiae and bleeding
   g. Pulmonary edema
   h. Neurotoxicity (especially with coral snake and Mojave rattlesnake)

C Differential diagnoses Most snakebites are memorable experiences, but some victims are unable to recall the event. Unless obvious signs and symptoms of venomous snakebite are present, consideration should be given to a "dry bite" without venom, chigger bites, insect stings, animal bites, local trauma with cellulitis or other infection, other trauma producing two-puncture irritated skin lesions, and systemic illness.

D Evaluation Many snakebite victims are intoxicated with alcohol, which makes evaluation more difficult.

1. **Snake identification.** Efforts should be made to safely retrieve and identify the snake. Dead snakes should be handled carefully because some snakes may "bite" as a result of reflexes even after death.

2. **Laboratory studies.** For severely symptomatic victims, the tests ordered should include a CBC with platelet count; BUN, creatinine, and electrolyte levels; coagulation profile; urinalysis; and blood type and cross match.

3. **Diagnostic tests and imaging studies.** An ECG and appropriate radiographs, including chest radiographs, are indicated.

E Therapy

1. **Prehospital management**

    a. Transport. The victim should be transported rapidly to a hospital. Attempts should be made to calm the patient, to prevent the spread of venom. If possible, the patient should be carried, with the site of the bite immobilized and placed in a dependent position. If possible, the snake should be brought to the ED for identification, using safety precautions.

    b. The use of ice, incision and suction, tourniquets, electrical shock, and administration of antivenin should be avoided by prehospital providers. Most victims are bitten within short travel distance to a hospital, hence the saying, "A set of car keys is the best first aid for snakebite."

  2. ED management

    a. Stabilization. Management of the patient's ABCs, with fluid resuscitation for shock and hypotension, should be initiated. Tourniquets or constrictive bands should be removed slowly, and only after an intravenous line has been established.

    b. Examination. The patient should be examined carefully to determine the extent of injury. Mark the skin to identify the rate of spread of erythema and swelling, observing closely for the development of compartment syndrome. Monitor for systemic signs such as hypotension, pulmonary edema, coagulopathy, and neurologic abnormalities.

    c. Prophylaxis. Tetanus toxoid should be administered as dictated by the patient's immunization status. The use of prophylactic broad-spectrum antibiotics is recommended by many authorities, but studies supporting the administration of antibiotics are rare.

    d. Debridement. The site of injury should be cleansed and débrided.

    e. Antivenin is the definitive treatment for snake envenomation. Antivenin is an equine antibody solution that binds and neutralizes the harmful components of snake venom. There are two types produced in the United States used for crotalid and elapid bites.

      (1) Indications. Antivenin administration is indicated for significant envenomations. There is a **four-grade classification system** used to evaluate severity of envenomation: from grade I (minimal symptoms, no antivenin required) to grade IV (very severe, with rapid swelling, ecchymosis, CNS symptoms, convulsions, and shock).

      (2) Administration. Antivenin should be administered within 4 hours if possible. After 12 hours, the risk–benefit ratio is questionable. **Guidelines for antivenin administration** are included with the antivenin. Examples of usual dose ranges are 2–4 vials for grade II envenomation, and 10–15 vials for grade IV envenomation.

      (3) Adverse reactions. The **risks of antivenin** include serum sickness and anaphylaxis, which can be life-threatening.

        (a) Horse serum sensitivity. The patient should be asked about a history of sensitivity to horses or horse serum, or a past infusion of antivenin (which would indicate a higher risk for reaction). All patients without a history of horse serum sensitivity should be tested for sensitivity with a dilute intradermal injection of horse serum.

        (b) Contraindications. Antivenin should not be administered if the patient is definitely sensitive to horse serum and the pit viper bite is within grade I or II. However, if it is a severe grade III or IV bite, then lack of antivenin therapy could be fatal, especially to an infant or older adult. Diphenhydramine, steroids, and epinephrine should be available to treat possible anaphylaxis during antivenin infusion.

F **Disposition**   All patients with serious snakebite envenomations should be hospitalized for continued care and observation. If the snakebite is minor, and no systemic effects or significant local findings are found, the patient can be discharged home with a responsible relative or friend.

X   INSECT AND ARACHNID BITES AND STINGS

A **Introduction**   Problems caused by the bites and stings of insects and arachnids include primary toxicity from envenomation, local infection, immediate hypersensitivity to the venom, delayed hypersensitivity, and transmission of infectious diseases.

B **Black widow spider bites**

1. **Discussion**
   a. The black widow spider (*Latrodectus mactans*) is found throughout the United States (except Alaska). It lives in protected locations such as woodpiles, basements, and garages. The term "black widow" comes from the occasional observation that the larger female kills and eats the smaller male soon after copulation.
   b. **Description.** Both male and female are venomous, but only the female can envenomate a human. The female is twice as large as the male, with a body about 1 cm long, and a total length, including legs, of 3 cm. The body is glossy black with two red spots—the classic "hourglass"—located on the central abdomen. The female is not aggressive except when guarding her nest.
   c. **Pathogenesis.** Envenomation occurs through modified digestive glands attached to appendages (chelicera) of the spider's head. The most toxic component of the venom is a neurotoxin that causes depletion of acetylcholine from nerve terminals, leading to diffuse muscle spasm.
   d. **Risk for severe reaction.** Small children and infants are at increased risk for severe reaction because of their small body size. Adults with pre-existing illness also are at greater risk.

2. **Clinical features**
   a. **Symptoms**
      (1) **Local.** A sharp pinprick may be felt from the spider's bite, but often the bite is not remembered by the victim. A dull, crampy pain or numbness develops around the bite and slowly spreads.
      (2) **Systemic** symptoms include dizziness, nausea, headache, itching, increased salivation, weakness, and warmth over the affected area. Intense pain from abdominal muscle cramps may simulate an acute abdomen. Upper extremity bites may cause chest wall cramps that simulate an acute infarction or other serious disorder. Symptoms begin to resolve after several hours.
   b. **Physical examination findings** may include muscle spasm, ptosis, facial edema, hypertension, and moderate fever. A rigid abdomen may be found without true deep tenderness. Close examination of the skin may reveal two small fang marks.

3. **Differential diagnoses** include bites of other insects or animals, and puncture wounds. Systemic symptoms can mimic an acute abdomen or serious chest pain etiology, dystonic reactions, tetanus, strychnine poisoning, or hypocalcemia.

4. **Evaluation.** The history may not reveal the circumstances of the bite because the patient may not remember being bitten. If in doubt, serious causes of chest and abdominal pain should be ruled out.
   a. **Laboratory studies.** All patients with serious symptoms require a CBC, serum electrolyte panel, BUN and creatinine levels, clotting studies, and urinalysis.
   b. **Diagnostic tests.** An ECG may reveal changes similar to those produced by digitalis toxicity.

5. **Therapy**
   a. **Prehospital management** may include placing ice on the bite wound to reduce swelling and symptoms. If possible, the spider should be brought to the hospital carefully for identification, to aid in diagnosis and treatment.
   b. **ED management**
      (1) **Stabilization.** The patient's vital signs should be monitored, and life support measures should be instituted as indicated. Hypertension may be treated with nitroprusside or diazoxide if the diastolic blood pressure is greater than 130 mm Hg.
      (2) **Local cleansing of the bite** and **tetanus prophylaxis** are required.
      (3) **Muscle relaxants** and **analgesics** are used to treat muscle spasm. Slow intravenous infusion of **calcium chloride** has long been a standard treatment and may be used also; the dosage is 10 mL of a 10% solution given intravenously over 20 minutes, which may be repeated every 2–4 hours. Cardiac rhythm and serum calcium levels should be monitored.

(4) **Antivenin** should be administered to very old and very young victims, pregnant women, patients with pre-existing illness, and seriously symptomatic victims. The dosage of antivenin is 1 vial diluted in 50 mL of normal saline administered over 15 minutes. All patients should be tested for horse serum sensitivity [see IX E 2 e (3) (a)].

6. **Disposition.** All patients with serious signs and symptoms require admission to the hospital and close observation. If asymptomatic after 2 hours, the patient may be sent home with instructions to return to the ED if any symptoms develop.

C Brown recluse spider bites

1. **Discussion.** The brown recluse spider (*Loxosceles reclusa*) is located predominantly in the south-central United States. It prefers secluded spots such as in woodpiles or under dry bark, and it can be found indoors in attics or storage areas. The brown recluse tends not to bite unless disturbed. It is brown, as its name indicates; is smaller than the black widow (about 2 cm in overall length); and usually has a violin-shaped mark on the back of the cephalothorax.

2. **Clinical features**
   a. **Local effects.** The initial bite may feel sharp, or it may cause little or no pain. Pain gradually develops after 1–2 hours. An erythematous area surrounded by a white area of vasoconstriction may appear. A central dark-red blister or bleb with a "bull's-eye" appearance may form. The lesion slowly grows in size, with rupture of the bleb and formation of an ulcer after several days. Underlying tissue, including muscle, may be affected. A black eschar then forms over a large tissue defect. Pain can be severe.
   b. **Systemic effects.** Although local destruction of skin and subcutaneous tissue is the hallmark of the brown recluse bite, the victim may also develop chills, fever, malaise, nausea, and vomiting. Children and, rarely, adults may develop intravascular hemolysis, hemorrhage, DIC, thrombocytopenia, renal failure, and death.

3. **Differential diagnoses** include other insect bites (far more common), puncture wounds, local infection, foreign body, and cutaneous manifestation of infectious or systemic disease.

4. **Evaluation**
   a. **History and physical examination** lead to suspicion or confirmation. Observation and repeated examination over several days may be needed to confirm the diagnosis. Early diagnosis is not easy to make without a positive identification of the spider or insect.
   b. **Laboratory tests.** CBC, electrolytes, urinalysis, coagulation studies, and cardiac monitoring are indicated if the patient has signs of systemic involvement or a confirmed bite with symptoms. Type and cross match and transfusion of blood may be required for patients with severe hemolysis.

5. **Therapy.** Treatment of the brown recluse bite is controversial, but **local supportive care** and careful **cleansing** with soap and water are important. **Tetanus prophylaxis** is required. Vital signs and urinary output should be closely monitored.
   a. **Steroids.** Many authors recommend systemic steroids for bites if the patient is seen within 24 hours. Methylprednisolone, 100 mg intravenously, followed by oral prednisone for 5 days may be used.
   b. **Dapsone** has not been found to be effective and is no longer recommended by most practitioners.
   c. **Antibiotics** and **analgesics** should be used as indicated during the course of the disease.
   d. **Wound management.** A surgical consultation should be obtained for optimum wound management. Excision of the wound, recommended in the past, has not been shown to improve the outcome.

6. **Disposition**
   a. **Discharge.** If no symptoms are present and suspicion of a brown recluse bite is low, outpatient management is acceptable.

b. Admission. All patients with signs of envenomation should be admitted to the hospital and monitored closely for hemolysis and other complications. Dialysis may be necessary. If the victim is significantly ill or develops systemic hemolysis, an ICU bed may be required.

D Scorpion stings

1. **Discussion.** The scorpion is a nocturnal arachnid found in the southwestern United States. It has a stinger in its tail with two venom glands. Most species are relatively harmless, and their sting usually causes a localized reaction such as occurs with a bee sting. However, the bark scorpion (*Centruroides sculpturatus*) has a neurotoxin in its venom that can cause a severe reaction. This dangerous scorpion is found on or near trees in Arizona and New Mexico. **Children are at greatest risk for complications;** they may develop respiratory compromise within 30 minutes.

2. **Clinical features**
   a. **Local effects.** The symptoms from the *C. sculpturatus* scorpion sting include immediate severe pain at the sting site, swelling, and later numbness. The injured area is hypersensitive, and the involved extremity may be paralyzed.
   b. **Systemic effects.** The neurotoxin is strongly cholinergic and can cause excessive salivation, blurred vision, muscular spasms, hypertension, and respiratory difficulties.

3. **Differential diagnoses** include snakebite, puncture wound or other trauma, insect sting, drug intoxication, and spider bite.

4. **Evaluation.** For local symptoms only, supportive treatment and observation are sufficient. For severely ill patients with respiratory distress, ICU monitoring and screening laboratory tests are required. ABGs help to assess the patient's respiratory status.

5. **Therapy**
   a. **Prehospital management** includes rapid transportation of the patient, application of an ice pack to the sting site, and safe transport of the scorpion for identification. If severe symptoms occur, life support measures should be initiated.
   b. **ED management**
      (1) **Antivenin** should be administered in all cases of severe envenomation.
      (2) **Ventilatory support** may be required, with intubation and oxygen for patients with severe systemic response or anaphylaxis.
      (3) **Atropine** may be required to counteract the cholinergic effects; the dose is titrated to relieve the cholinergic signs.
      (4) **Diazepam** may be used for seizures and muscle spasms.
      (5) **Opiates** (morphine and meperidine hydrochloride) and **barbiturates are contraindicated** because they seem to increase the toxic effects of the venom.

6. **Disposition.** All victims should be observed for 24 hours. Children should be admitted to the hospital and monitored closely. Symptomatic patients should be admitted also and transferred to the ICU if symptoms are severe.

E Hymenoptera stings

1. **Discussion**
   a. Hymenoptera include **honeybees, wasps, hornets, yellow jackets, fire ants,** and **harvester ants.**
   b. **Identification of the offending insect** can be difficult, except for the honeybee, which leaves its stinger (with venom sac attached) at the sting site. Other Hymenoptera have a retractable stinger and thus may sting many times.
   c. **Pathogenesis.** The venom injected may contain histamine, serotonin, amines, phospholipase, hyaluronidase, and other substances; the components vary with the insect type. Some components may induce an allergic reaction. Toxic reactions to Hymenoptera insect stings are quite common in the United States. There are five types of reaction to Hymenoptera stings:

(1) **Local reaction** consists of significant edema, pain, and erythema at the sting site. If the sting site is around the mouth or throat, airway obstruction may occur. The fire ant and harvester ant can sting repeatedly and cause local tissue damage, blisters, and severe pain.

(2) **Toxic reaction.** If there are 10 or more stings, a systemic reaction may develop because of the large toxin load. Vomiting, dizziness, syncope, edema, and diarrhea may develop. Multiple stings may result in convulsions and death, although this is quite rare in the United States. The Africanized bees ("killer bees") that are now in the southern United States actually have weaker, smaller sting envenomations than other bees, but they may cause more illness and death because the victim is usually stung by more bees.

(3) **Anaphylactic reaction** is the major cause of death associated with bee or wasp stings. The allergen component of single or multiple stings may cause an antigen–antibody, IgE-mediated systemic anaphylactic reaction. Histamine, slow-reacting substance of anaphylaxis (SRS-A), and other factors are released that within minutes produce generalized urticaria, pruritus, dry cough, and wheezing. Severe symptoms include dyspnea, bronchospasm with bloody and frothy sputum, cyanosis, cramps, nausea and vomiting, laryngeal stridor, hypotension, shock, loss of consciousness, and death.

(4) **Delayed reaction** consists of serum sickness–like symptoms of headache, malaise, generalized pruritus, fever, and polyarthritis. These symptoms appear 10–15 days after a sting.

(5) **Unusual reaction.** Rare reactions include encephalopathy, vasculitis, neuritis, and autonomic dysfunction.

2. **Differential diagnoses** include infection, local trauma, foreign body, and skin disorder. Few patients forget a painful sting, but identification of the exact insect may be difficult. If anaphylaxis is present, the history may be impossible to obtain; in such cases the skin should be carefully searched for sting sites.

3. **Evaluation.** If moderate or severe symptoms are present, a CBC, ABG determination, chest radiograph, and ECG should be obtained. Cardiac monitoring and close observation are indicated.

4. **Therapy**
   a. **Local reactions.** If a stinger is present in the wound, it should be scraped out (not squeezed out). The wound should be thoroughly washed and ice packs administered. Oral antihistamines and analgesics should be administered to relieve discomfort. For moderate swelling, elevation and use of oral steroids for several days are indicated.
   b. **Anaphylactic reactions** are treated with **local care, intravenous fluids, antihistamines** (diphenhydramine, 50–100 mg intravenously), and **steroids** (methylprednisolone, 125 mg intravenously, or hydrocortisone, 2 mg/kg intravenously).
      (1) If life-threatening symptoms occur, **epinephrine** should be administered, 1:1000, 0.3–0.5 mL subcutaneously, and repeated in 10 or 15 minutes.
      (2) **Albuterol nebulizer treatments** are indicated if bronchospasm is present. If severe airway compromise exists, **endotracheal intubation** may be indicated.
      (3) Hypotensive patients require large volumes of intravenous fluids; if the hypotension is persistent, **dopamine** infusion is indicated.

5. **Disposition**
   a. **Discharge.** Patients with minor local reactions may be treated symptomatically and discharged.
   b. **Admission.** Any patient with a systemic reaction should be treated, observed closely, and admitted for continued symptoms. Patients with anaphylactic reactions require intensive care monitoring in the hospital.
   c. **Long-term management** is indicated for patients with serious reactions to Hymenoptera stings. The patient should be referred to an immunologist for desensitization. All patients with systemic reactions should be prescribed three insect sting kits containing premeasured epinephrine (one kit for the car, one for home, and one to carry). A medical alert tag is advised.

XI VENOMOUS MARINE ANIMAL INJURIES

A Discussion

1. More than 2000 species of animals found in the ocean can deliver venom to humans. The number of victims continues to rise as increasing numbers of people take to the water for sport and recreation. In addition, growing interest in home salt water aquariums has put people at risk hundreds of miles from the ocean!

2. Most marine injuries occur when a victim comes into contact with an animal that is stationary in the water. Venomous marine animals usually are not aggressive, and many are immobile.

3. Injuries may be divided into three classes according to the mechanism of venom delivery: bite, nematocyst, and stinger.

   a. **Envenomation by bite.** Sea snakes and octopuses have been known to kill humans by biting with their beaks and secreting venom into the wound through their salivary glands. There is no known antivenin; treatment is supportive.

   b. **Envenomation by nematocysts.** The coelenterates (Portuguese man-of-war, fire corals, sea wasps, anemones, jellyfish, and corals) use stinging organelles called nematocysts for obtaining food and for self-defense. Most coelenterates are sessile (*attached at the base*), but some are free floating and may rub against a swimmer or diver. The most common nematocyst is a small "spring-loaded" venom gland that can penetrate human skin in most cases; it ejects venom through a connecting tube. The nematocyst may function even after the animal has been dead for some time. The severity of the envenomation depends on the species, the number of nematocysts discharged, and the victim's response to the venom. Although nematocyst envenomation may result in fatal anaphylaxis, most envenomations are minimal; the greatest danger is that of drowning after a sting or an allergic reaction to the venom.

   c. **Envenomation by stinger.** Animals possessing a stinging mechanism include sea urchins, bloodworms, stingrays, starfish, scorpion fish, catfish, lionfish, and cone shells.

B Clinical features

1. **Bites.** Pain at the site is common. Variable neurologic symptoms may be present, depending on the species, toxin, and site of the bite wound. Bleeding is not usually a problem unless a major blood vessel is involved.

2. **Nematocysts** cause a severe burning sensation with raised erythematous lesions wherever they have discharged venom into the skin. Symptoms may persist for several days. Systemic signs may include nausea, vomiting, muscle cramps, angioedema, and respiratory arrest. Patients are at risk for wound infection and foreign body reaction with delayed healing.

3. **Stings**

   a. **Bony fish stings.** The bony fishes inflict wounds through spines located on their fins when they are stepped on or handled by fishermen or aquarium keepers. Symptoms and toxicity vary depending on the species.

   b. **Catfish stings** are associated with pain and local inflammation.

   c. **Scorpion fish stings** are said to produce the most severe pain in the animal kingdom. The sting produces edema, local inflammation, and erythema, as well as systemic effects including dyspnea, hypotension, sweating, and syncope.

   d. **Stonefish stings** may kill the victim within 1 hour through cardiopulmonary arrest.

   e. **Stingray stings.** The stingray has a stinger located midway down its long, whip-like tail. When aggravated or stepped on, the stingray will thrust the tail upward, piercing its victim's skin. A sheath containing venom glands surrounds the stinger; if the stinger breaks off into the wound, severe pain and inflammation result, with systemic symptoms of salivation, diarrhea, syncope, nausea, vomiting, cramps, fasciculations, convulsions, and cardiac arrhythmias.

    f. Sea urchin stings. The sea urchin secretes a toxin on the surface of its long spines. The spines pierce the skin of the sea urchin's victim and may break off into the wound, causing a foreign body reaction with severe burning pain. Systemic symptoms are uncommon.

    g. Cone shell stings. Cone shells have a tubular gland with several teeth that may puncture skin and inject venom when a victim handles the shell. The toxin acts on skeletal muscle, causing paralysis. Weakness, diplopia, slurred speech, respiratory arrest, and death may result.

C **Differential diagnoses** The causative animal is usually difficult to determine because of the enormous variety of venomous organisms in the ocean. However, an informed swimmer or diver may be able to identify or describe the organism.

D **Evaluation** History and physical examination assist in the diagnosis, and in most cases symptomatic treatment suffices. If there is suspicion of a foreign body in the wound, soft tissue radiographs or xerograms should be obtained.

E **Therapy**

1. **Rescue.** The first priority is to rescue the victim from the water to prevent drowning. Anaphylactic reactions should be treated before addressing the wound.

2. **Neutralization of venom.** Most of the venom can be neutralized during prehospital treatment.

    a. Nematocyst injuries are treated by washing the affected area with sea water (fresh water may cause the nematocysts to discharge). Vinegar should then be poured over the wound to inactivate the nematocysts. Talcum powder or shaving cream should be applied, and the skin should be scraped with a knife to remove the nematocysts. Finally, steroid cream should be applied. Antihistamines, analgesics, antibiotics, and tetanus immunization may be required. Patients with severe envenomations and anaphylactic reactions should be admitted and treated as indicated.

    b. Puncture injuries are treated by screening for and removing foreign bodies if possible. Thorough irrigation of the wound and prophylactic antibiotics decrease infection. If venomous gland tissue remains in the wound (such as from a stingray), submersion in water as hot as the victim can tolerate for 1 hour will neutralize the heat-labile venom. Severely symptomatic patients, such as those stung by a stonefish, should be admitted and given antivenin if available.

F **Disposition** Most patients have minor injuries and skin involvement only, and can be managed as outpatients. If the type of spiny fish or degree of envenomation is questionable, cautious monitoring in the hospital may be indicated. Seriously ill patients should be admitted.

Study Questions

Directions: Each of the numbered items or incomplete statements in this section is followed by answers or by completions of the statement. Select the ONE lettered answer or completion that is BEST in each case.

1. Hypothermia is defined as a core temperature below

   A 32°C
   B 37°C
   C 35°C
   D 30°C
   E 28°C

2. The last reflex to disappear in hypothermic patients is the same reflex that first appears with rewarming. This reflex is the

   A patellar (knee-jerk) reflex
   B Achilles (ankle) reflex
   C diving reflex
   D biceps reflex
   E plantar reflex

3. Which of the following accounts for the greatest percentage of body heat loss from a person who is dry, has a normal basal metabolic rate, and is exposed to windless, cool air?

   A Radiation
   B Conduction
   C Respiration
   D Convection
   E Evaporation

4. A confused, 78-year-old woman is found outside her home in January during subzero temperatures. Large blisters have developed on the plantar and dorsal surfaces of her feet, and she has cold, mottled, dusky-colored, sensationless toes. The diagnosis for this patient is frostbite. After rewarming her, the correct treatment should include

   A rupturing all clear and hemorrhagic blisters and admitting her to the hospital
   B immediately amputating the toes that are without blood flow or sensation
   C discharging her home with instructions to keep the feet elevated and wrapped with a heating pad, and to return in 6 days
   D admitting her to the hospital for close observation and isolation from infectious agents, with possible eventual amputation
   E débriding the blisters, prescribing an analgesic, and discharging the patient to a nursing home immediately

5. The most efficient mechanism for the human body to dissipate heat in environmental temperatures at or above body temperature is

   A convection
   B conduction
   C respiration
   D radiation
   E evaporation

6. A 58-year-old man travels to Panama to perform research. While exposed to the hot, humid climate, he develops minor swelling of the feet and ankles. What is the best treatment for resolving heat edema?

- **A** Elevating legs and rest
- **B** Drinking more water and increasing salt intake
- **C** Administering furosemide or other diuretics
- **D** Donning tight stockings and increasing salt intake
- **E** Applying ice packs to feet

7. What is the primary factor differentiating heat stroke from heat exhaustion?

- **A** Heat stroke patients will always have a core body temperature higher than 40°C (105°F).
- **B** Heat exhaustion patients are able to sweat, but heat stroke patients stop sweating.
- **C** Heat stroke patients have an altered mental status.
- **D** Heat exhaustion patients usually do not have volume depletion, but heat stroke patients most often are hypovolemic.
- **E** An altered mental status is usually found in both heat stroke and heat exhaustion victims, but sweating is absent in heat stroke victims.

8. Which one of the following statements regarding classic versus exertional heat stroke is true?

- **A** Exertional heat stroke victims are not at risk for rhabdomyolysis and acute renal failure.
- **B** Classic heat stroke victims are usually sweating when found.
- **C** Risk factors for exertional heat stroke include being elderly, being without an air conditioner or fan, and polypharmacy.
- **D** Exertional heat stroke often occurs in previously healthy young people who have exercised or exerted themselves strenuously.
- **E** People with psychiatric or chronic disease are rarely at risk for classic heat stroke.

9. Which one of the following medications is useful for treating neuroleptic malignant syndrome (NMS) and malignant hyperthermia?

- **A** Intravenous calcium gluconate
- **B** Furosemide
- **C** Dantrolene
- **D** Diphenhydramine
- **E** Calcium channel blocking agents

10. A mountain climber is ascending a very high mountain. He develops a bifrontal headache, anorexia, weakness, and fatigue. That night he finds it difficult to sleep, and he develops a worsening fatigue and malaise. The likely diagnosis and potential treatment options include

- **A** acute mountain sickness (AMS); treat with acetazolamide, hydration, rest, possibly oxygen, and, if symptoms worsen, descent
- **B** acute cerebral edema; treat with steroids, and sleep at higher altitudes each night until acclimated
- **C** AMS; treat with rest, increased fluids, breathing into a bag to increase the carbon dioxide levels and stimulate respiration, and ascent to acclimate quickly
- **D** acute cerebral edema; no specific treatment is necessary because the climber will get better as he climbs higher
- **E** acute high-altitude pulmonary edema (HAPE); treat with oxygen and descent to a lower altitude

11. What is the most lethal of all high-altitude illnesses?

- **A** Acute mountain sickness (AMS)
- **B** High-altitude cerebral edema (HACE)
- **C** High-altitude pulmonary edema (HAPE)
- **D** Ultraviolet keratitis

12. Most serious scuba diving injuries are a result of

    A barotrauma
    B decompression sickness (DCS)
    C "the bends"
    D dysbaric air embolism (DAE)
    E "squeeze"

13. A 4-year-old girl is found underwater in a swimming pool, unresponsive, after being "missing" for several minutes. She has vital signs at the scene, but then dies en route to the hospital and is not resuscitated. The correct term for this girl's death is

    A drowning
    B secondary drowning
    C immersion syndrome
    D near-drowning
    E postimmersion syndrome

14. Most venomous snakes in the United States may be recognized by which one of the following features?

    A Round eyes
    B Absence of hollow fangs
    C Small "pit" indentation between each eye and nostril
    D Double row of caudal plates from the anal plate to one third of the way from the tail
    E Round, oval head

15. Lightning strikes to humans are associated with a mortality rate of

    A 10%
    B 30%
    C 75%
    D 90%
    E 100%

Answers and Explanations

1. **The answer is C** Hypothermia is defined as a core temperature below 35°C or 95°F.

2. **The answer is A** The ankle, diving, biceps, and plantar reflexes disappear and reappear later than the patellar (knee-jerk) reflex in hypothermic patients. The reflexes become hypoactive at core body temperatures below 32°C (90°F), and disappear at core body temperatures below 26°C (79°F).

3. **The answer is A** Radiation accounts for 55%–65% of heat loss in a cold climate for a person who is dry, has a normal basal metabolic rate, and is exposed to windless, cool air. The amount of heat lost through radiation depends on the temperature gradient between the body and the environment. When the environmental temperature exceeds body temperature, evaporative heat loss accounts for the greatest percentage of body heat lost (it normally accounts for 10% of heat loss). The other mechanisms account for lower percentages of heat loss (conduction = 3%, convection = about 10%, respiration = 2%–9%).

4. **The answer is D** All patients with significant frostbite should be admitted to the hospital for close observation and wound management, and isolated as much as possible from risk of infections. Elevation of the extremity, aloe vera treatments, daily whirlpool therapy, treatment for infections, and allowing time for margination of viable and nonviable tissue to occur are indicated. Blister treatment is controversial, with most experts recommending débriding clear blisters to optimize wound healing; hemorrhagic (third-degree) blisters should be left intact. Amputation may be delayed for several weeks to months.

5. **The answer is E** Evaporation is the most efficient method to remove heat because of the vaporization energy lost. In the emergency department (ED), a simple way to maximize evaporation of body heat in an overheated patient is to undress the patient, spray or pour warm water on the patient's exposed skin, and blow air over the skin with a fan. Cold water causes vasoconstriction and thus decreases the potential heat loss.

6. **The answer is A** Heat edema is seen mostly in unacclimatized older people who are exposed to tropical stresses and who sit or stand for long periods of time. There is no evidence that diuretic therapy is effective. The edema will resolve with simple leg elevation, acclimatization, or return to the home climate. Salt and water intake do not play a role in relieving heat edema, and tight stockings are excessive treatment for this benign, self-limited disorder.

7. **The answer is C** Heat stroke is a true medical emergency. It is defined as hyperpyrexia and neurologic symptoms or altered mental status. The mental status is always normal in heat exhaustion victims. Sweating may be absent or present in either heat exhaustion or heat stroke, and thus is an unreliable finding. Many heat stroke victims will have a normal or mildly elevated temperature upon arrival at a medical facility owing to cooling during transport.

8. **The answer is D** Exertional heat stroke is often seen in young people who have exerted themselves too strenuously in hot weather (e.g., athletes, military personnel). Exertional heat stroke victims are at risk for rhabdomyolysis and renal failure. Classic, rather than exertional, heat stroke is found in the elderly and in people with poor socioeconomic status. People with psychiatric and chronic disease, as well as the very young and the very old, are at risk for classic heat stroke. In most cases, classic heat stroke victims have ceased sweating when found.

9. **The answer is C** Dantrolene lowers myoplasmic calcium levels and decreases muscular contraction in both these syndromes, thus decreasing the muscular rigidity and hyperthermia that occurs in these rare conditions.

10. The answer is A AMS is treated with rest, oxygen, ensuring adequate hydration and nutrition, acclimatization, and acetazolamide. For moderate and severe cases, dexamethasone may be used. If symptoms do not resolve or worsen, descent is necessary. AMS victims are at risk for developing high-altitude cerebral edema (HACE) and HAPE.

11. The answer is C HAPE is the most lethal of all high-altitude illnesses. Most cases develop on days 2–4 after ascent above 14,500 feet.

12. The answer is D DAE is a major cause of death and disability among scuba divers. It often results from gas bubbles entering the systemic vasculature when pulmonary tissues rupture, causing strokes and other serious problems. Any symptom that occurs in the immediate postdive phase (within 10 minutes of surfacing) is likely to be DAE until proven otherwise.

13. The answer is B Secondary drowning describes death that follows a brief period of recovery after the initial submersion event. Drowning is death by submersion in a liquid medium. Near-drowning is submersion followed by survival. Immersion syndrome is sudden death after immersion in cold fluid, thought to be caused by dysrhythmias or bradycardia. Postimmersion syndrome is similar to adult respiratory distress syndrome (ARDS)—that is, due to washout of pulmonary surfactant—and may develop within 72 hours of immersion.

14. The answer is C Most venomous snakes in the United States are pit vipers, and are recognized by a small "pit" indentation (a heat-detecting organ) near each slit-shaped eye. Pit vipers also have an arrow-shaped head, a single row of caudal plates, fangs (hinged and near the front of the mouth), and (on rattlesnakes) rattles.

15. The answer is B Lightning strikes to humans are associated with a mortality rate of 30%.

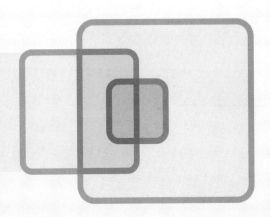

PART **V**

Special Considerations

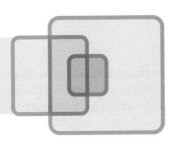

chapter **22**

Emergency Medical Services

DAVID C. CONE

I   **HISTORY OF EMERGENCY MEDICAL SERVICES (EMS)**

A   **The premodern era**

1. **Military EMS**
   a. **Napoleonic and Crimean Wars.** The first attempt at organized medical care on the battlefield reportedly occurred under the direction of Dr. Jean Dominique Larrey, Napoleon's field physician, during the Napoleonic and Crimean Wars.
   b. The **Civil War** brought the first semblance of battlefield care to the United States. Nonphysician "corpsmen" were trained to provide crude treatment for wounded soldiers where they lay.
   c. During **World War I, World War II,** and the **Korean War,** gradual improvements in field care, evacuation, and medical knowledge in general helped increase survival rates.

2. **Civilian EMS**
   a. Several large cities in the United States, notably New York and Cincinnati, established horse-drawn ambulance services during the late nineteenth century. These services were frequently staffed by physicians.
   b. Most rural areas had no ambulance services available until the second half of the twentieth century, instead relying on hearses from funeral homes to transport patients.

B   **The early 1960s**   The 1960s saw the early development of EMS along two lines:

1. **Civilian/cardiac models** were designed to take the hospital to the patient.
   a. **Myocardial infarction (MI) treatment models.** The early model of Dr. Frank Pantridge in Belfast, Ireland, and later the "Heartmobile" in Columbus, Ohio, were specifically aiming to treat MI.
   b. **Advanced life support (ALS) models.** Paramedics in Los Angeles, Miami, and Seattle took ALS care into the field to treat victims of all types of emergencies, including sudden cardiac death.

2. **Military/trauma model.** The techniques of trauma treatment and rapid evacuation learned in the military, particularly during the Korean and Vietnam wars, were eventually taken into the civilian setting, primarily for the treatment of victims of motor vehicle accidents.

C   **The modern era: 1966 to the present**   In 1966, the National Academy of Sciences published "Accidental Death and Disability: The Neglected Disease of Modern Society." This paper demonstrated the inadequate state of EMS and hospital emergency departments (EDs) in the United States, and was strongly critical of the care that citizens received when faced with a medical emergency. A list of 24 recommendations was presented, which became the guide for the development of EMS for the next few years. This was the first systematic look at organizing and developing EMS systems.

1. **Highway Safety Act (1966).** Congress responded to the National Academy of Sciences' report by passing the Highway Safety Act of 1966.

a. The act created the **Department of Transportation,** and charged it with improving EMS, giving the agency both legislative authority and financial support.

b. The act required the development of **highway traffic safety programs** in all states.

c. The act also provided **federal funds for EMS projects** and improvements throughout the country. This funding supported much of the development of modern EMS.

d. As a result of the act, a 70-hour **emergency medical technician (EMT)—ambulance curriculum** was developed, representing the first standardized training for prehospital providers in the United States. A similar **paramedic curriculum** was later developed and implemented.

2. **Emergency Medical Services System Act (1973)**

a. **Funding of EMS.** The act provided hundreds of millions of dollars for EMS research, training, and services. The "golden age of EMS" saw the development of EMS systems throughout the country, using federal dollars to purchase ambulances and equipment and to train prehospital personnel. The development of basic and ALS techniques, the transferring of technology from the hospital to the field, and the development of regional systems all resulted in the rapid advancement of emergency care in the United States.

b. **Establishment of essential components of EMS.** The act also outlined 15 essential components of EMS (Table 22–1). While this list is not considered complete by today's standards—for example, there is a notable lack of physician-level medical direction—it helped organize efforts to develop modern EMS systems.

3. **The Omnibus Budget Reconciliation Act (OBRA) (1981).** OBRA brought an end to the golden age of EMS. All federal funding for EMS was converted into block grants to the states, which could be used as each state saw fit. The former EMS funds were placed into the block of money designated for preventive health, and many EMS programs saw their funding terminated when states chose to fund other projects. While several federal agencies remain active in various aspects of EMS (such as the National Highway Traffic and Safety Administration, and the Federal Emergency Management Agency), OBRA effectively ended federal involvement in the development of EMS.

4. **Current trends.** Today, financing concerns continue to plague EMS. The overall changes in the healthcare climate, the development of managed care organizations, and the trend toward fiscal accountability have all resulted in the stagnation of EMS growth. A tighter regulatory environment and changes in the legal atmosphere of medical care have also checked the previously unencumbered development of EMS.

TABLE 22–1   Fifteen Essential Emergency Medical System (EMS) Components, As Outlined by the Emergency Medical Services System Act of 1973

1. Manpower
2. Training
3. Communications
4. Transportation
5. Emergency facilities
6. Critical care units
7. Public safety agencies
8. Consumer participation
9. Access to care
10. Patient transfer
11. Standardized record keeping
12. Public information and education
13. System review and evaluation
14. Disaster planning
15. Mutual aid

II **MODELS OF EMS DELIVERY**

A **Basic life support (BLS) versus ALS**

1. **BLS** is the provision of noninvasive care to a patient, including delivery of oxygen by masks and cannulas, first aid (e.g., splinting, bandaging), and assessment of vital signs.

2. **ALS** is the provision of invasive care to a patient, including insertion of invasive airways, administration of intravenous fluids and medications, cardiac monitoring, defibrillation, cardioversion, and transcutaneous pacing.

3. The **distinctions between BLS and ALS** are not always clear. For example, the use of automated external defibrillators is now considered a BLS skill, and some BLS systems use semi-invasive airway adjuncts (e.g., the esophageal obturator airway or double-lumen pharyngeal–tracheal airway).

B **Paid personnel versus volunteer personnel**

1. **Volunteer EMS systems** tend to dominate in suburban and rural areas, where call volumes are low. Frequently, there is difficulty maintaining an ALS level of response in these systems, because skill maintenance may be difficult when few patients are encountered, and continuing education may be less accessible.

2. **Paid EMS systems** prevail in urban areas, where EMS providers are generally full-time career staff.

C **Single-tier model versus multi-tier model**

1. In a **single-tier system,** all ambulances are ALS-capable. This is a common, but by no means dominant, model in urban areas.

2. In a **multi-tier system,** some ambulances provide ALS while others provide BLS. The type of ambulance dispatched depends on the apparent nature of the call and the resources available at the time. A nonambulance first-responder tier may be available, consisting of police or fire personnel who respond to provide immediate care but not transport.

D **Traditional models**

1. **Fire department–based model**
   a. Many EMS systems are part of the fire department serving a given area. This is currently the dominant model in urban areas of the United States. In some systems, the EMS crews also serve in fire suppression roles ("cross-trained, dual role"), whereas in others, EMS crews provide only EMS services.
   b. Even in systems where EMS is not fire department–based, fire department personnel may act as first responders, with an engine or ladder truck carrying certified first responders, EMTs, or even paramedics to a scene to provide care until the ambulance arrives.

2. **Hospital-based model**
   a. In many suburban areas, EMS is hospital-based. The EMS crews are employed by the hospital, and ambulances are stationed at the hospital or in the community, depending on the geography and demographics of the response area.
   b. Another common model is for the ALS portion of EMS to be hospital-based with paid personnel, while the BLS portion is community-based and frequently volunteer. In such a model, an ALS crew is dispatched along with the community BLS crew when there is an anticipated need for ALS.

3. **Third-service model.** In the third-service model, the EMS is separate from the fire and police departments, acting as an independent government service or as part of another department. Notable examples include the EMS systems in Boston (part of the Health Department) and in Pittsburgh (part of the Public Safety Department).

4. **Private model.** Almost all areas of the country are served by private, for-profit ambulance companies. These companies generally focus on nonemergency, prearranged transportation of

patients for a fee. Examples include transportation to and from dialysis, transfers between hospitals, and transport to physicians' offices.

    a. Types of service. Many private ambulance companies offer only **BLS service,** but some also offer **ALS service** (e.g., for interfacility transfer of a patient who needs cardiac monitoring, or who has intravenous fluids infusing). **Critical care transport** is also provided by some services (e.g., for the transfer of a patient with complicated ventilator needs, or multiple intravenous drips of cardioactive medications). Many of these critical care services use nurses as part or all of the crew.

    b. Transport contracts. Some private services contract with hospitals or other agencies to provide transport. For example, some hospital transport teams will rely on a private ambulance company to provide the ambulance and crew, and will supplement the crew with nurses or physicians from the hospital as needed, based on the anticipated needs of a given patient.

E Newer models

1. The **public utility model** emerged in 1978 in Kansas City, Missouri, and recently has been adopted by several small cities in the United States. Under the supervision of a governmental oversight body, a private ambulance company contracts with the city to provide EMS. The private service is accountable to the oversight body and must meet certain performance standards as outlined in their contract.

2. With the rapid penetration of **managed care organizations (MCOs)** and capitated service in many areas of the country, some private ambulance companies are contracting with MCOs to provide all ambulance service. In areas where a certain MCO has a large enough portion of the market share, there may be efforts for that company's contracted ambulance service to provide all ambulance service, both emergency and nonemergency, for the entire region.

III EMS PERSONNEL

A Introduction

1. **Levels of training**

    a. Basic training. There are four basic levels of EMS provider training in the United States:

       (1) First responder

       (2) EMT—basic (EMT-B)

       (3) EMT—intermediate (EMT-I)

       (4) EMT—paramedic (EMT-P)

    b. Special training. There are a number of areas in which EMS providers can seek additional training and expertise. They may then serve on special response teams, designed to provide specialized skills and equipment for certain types of emergencies.

       (1) Tactical EMS requires special training to support high-risk law enforcement operations.

       (2) Hazardous materials. Completion of an introductory awareness course is required by Occupational Safety and Health Administration (OSHA) regulations for hazardous materials rescues. Four other levels of hazardous materials training are available.

       (3) High-angle and technical rescue. Special training is required for cliff rescues and for elevator shaft and other skyscraper rope work.

       (4) Water rescue. Special training for water rescue includes swift water and scuba certification.

       (5) Other areas requiring special training include:

         (a) Wilderness EMS

         (b) Urban search and rescue

         (c) Confined space medicine

2. **Training standards and testing.** Each state is responsible for establishing criteria for levels of training. As a result, there are many different definitions and training standards for these levels. Several organizations have attempted to standardize the levels of training:

    a. The **United States Department of Transportation (DOT)** has established standardized curricula for the four levels of training. There is no requirement, however, that a given state adopt these standards.

    b. The **National Registry of EMTs** will provide testing for EMT-Bs, EMT-Is, and EMT-Ps who have completed a DOT-approved training program. While some states require National Registry certification, others conduct their own testing.

3. Personal safety

    a. Infection control is of major importance to EMS providers, who are in frequent contact with blood, respiratory secretions, and other body fluids.

      (1) Immunization against hepatitis B is recommended for field personnel, and some systems also recommend annual flu vaccinations.

      (2) Universal precautions. Knowledge and routine application of OSHA guidelines for blood-borne pathogens are essential.

    b. Physical safety

      (1) Low back injuries caused by improper lifting techniques are a common problem among EMS providers.

      (2) Violent patients. EMS providers must know when and how to safely and properly restrain patients, as well as when to remove themselves from a hazardous situation and request law enforcement assistance in handling a potentially dangerous patient.

      (3) Contaminated patients. Although EMS is rarely the principal agency in hazardous materials response, all EMS personnel must be able to safely and effectively handle and treat contaminated patients. Cooperation with the principal agency (generally the fire department) to ensure that patients are adequately decontaminated prior to EMS contact is essential.

    c. Critical incident stress management helps EMS providers cope with particularly emotional or stressful situations. Many areas offer critical stress debriefing teams that provide counseling after or even during disturbing events.

B First responder   The first responder is taught basic lifesaving techniques using minimal equipment (e.g., manual opening of an airway, assessment of breathing and circulation). The role of the first responder is to provide initial stabilizing care at the scene. In many areas of the country, non-EMS public safety personnel, such as police officers and firefighters, are trained to the first-responder level. As the most likely personnel to arrive first at the scene of a medical emergency, their training allows them to render immediate aid while awaiting more advanced providers.

1. The first responder course is approximately 40 hours in length and teaches cardiopulmonary resuscitation (CPR) and advanced first aid, as well as emergency uncomplicated obstetric delivery and spinal immobilization.

2. The first-responder national standard curriculum is currently under revision. The use of fully- or semi-automated defibrillators will likely be added to the curriculum.

C EMT-B

1. The EMT-B course is approximately 110 hours in length. In addition to covering the first-responder scope of practice, this course teaches a number of skills necessary for a BLS level of response, including the use of oxygen and oxygen delivery equipment (nasal cannulas and various types of masks), vehicle rescue and extrication, splinting, patient movement and transfer, and on-scene triage.

2. In many areas of the country, particularly rural areas, the EMT-B is the most advanced EMS provider available. The majority of ambulances in this country are staffed with EMT-Bs.

3. A recent revision of the EMT-B national standard curriculum is expected to help standardize EMT-B teaching, which historically has varied from state to state. A controversial 10-hour optional module was added to the course to teach endotracheal intubation to EMT-Bs. The course now also teaches the use of fully- or semi-automated defibrillators.

D **EMT-I**

1. There are numerous types of EMT-I certifications throughout the country. Some states offer several different levels of EMT-I certification, whereas other states have none. Training is typically 150 hours, in addition to EMT-B training.

2. The EMT-I is generally trained to perform some, but not all, of the ALS skills used by paramedics. The use of intravenous fluids and the use of the esophageal obturator airway are among the skills most frequently used by EMT-Is, and some EMT-Is can administer a limited number of medications.

E **EMT-P** A full range of ALS skills is taught at the EMT-P level, including intravenous access techniques, fluid and medication administration, advanced airway techniques (e.g., endotracheal intubation, needle thoracostomy), cardiac monitoring, and defibrillation, pacing, and cardioversion. States vary widely regarding which medications paramedics may administer, and what pieces of adjunct equipment may be used such as pulse oximeters, capnometers, and airway devices (e.g., the double-lumen pharyngeal–tracheal airway).

1. **EMT-P training** takes approximately 1000 hours. As with the other levels of training, the national standard EMT-P curriculum is currently undergoing revision.
   a. **EMT-B certification** is a **prerequisite** for EMT-P education. Many states require a certain number of years of field experience as an EMT-B prior to starting the EMT-P class.
   b. **Didactic (classroom) training** is typically 200–250 hours.
   c. **Clinical training** is generally 200–250 hours. It is usually hospital-based, with exposure to a number of hospital areas (ED, labor and delivery, operating room, pediatrics) for controlled exposure to different patient types and development of assessment and procedural skills. The areas chosen and skills emphasized are designed to mimic those the EMT-P will encounter in the field.
   d. **Internship** is usually 250–500 hours as a preceptorship. The student is paired with an experienced EMT-P in the field.

2. While all urban areas of the country have paramedics as an integral part of the EMS system, many rural areas do not have the resources to support ALS-level providers.

F **Nurses** In many areas of the country, nurses are used for **critical care interfacility transport.** For example, pediatric emergency nurses often staff ambulances used by tertiary pediatric hospitals for **interfacility transfers.** Nurses frequently make up part or all of the crew complement for **air medical services.** The use of nurses for **emergency response** is less common, though some states offer a certification process by which nurses may qualify to practice as field ALS providers.

G **Physicians** may:

1. **Care for patients on their arrival in the ED.** This is the primary role for many emergency physicians.

2. **Provide online medical control for EMS providers in the field.** Some states offer a certification process by which physicians may qualify to practice as ALS field providers, while in some areas this is done ad hoc. In general, the use of physicians for emergency response is rare. Several areas of the country, most notably Pittsburgh, use emergency medicine residents for field supervision as part of the local EMS system.

3. **Assist in critical care transport** and **air medical services.** The use of physicians in critical care transport and air medical services is more common at institutions offering residency training. For example, a number of emergency medicine residencies offer flight experience to residents, while a number of pediatric hospitals use pediatric residents for ground transport services.

4. **Serve as medical directors for local EMS agencies or companies**

H **Firefighters** Many EMS providers begin their careers as firefighters. In cities that use a dual-purpose model, personnel may serve as both firefighters and EMS providers.

IV EMS DISPATCH

A **Roles of dispatchers** Dispatchers perform two primary roles:

1. **Answering calls from the public** involves both gathering information, such as the location and nature of the problem, and providing prearrival instructions to help the caller or bystanders assist the patient until help arrives.

2. **Communicating by radio with field units.** In large systems, a dispatcher may perform only one role, and may only handle EMS calls. In smaller systems, a dispatcher may perform both functions, and may handle police, fire, and EMS for a given area.

B **"911"** Although "911" has been promoted as a common, single phone number for public access to emergency assistance of any type (police, fire, medical), it is far from universal. In many areas of the country, different seven-digit numbers must be used to access the different types of emergency assistance. "Enhanced 911" technology allows the location of the caller to be displayed on the dispatcher's computer screen, based on information from the telephone service provider. In some cases, very precise information (e.g., an office suite number) can be displayed, helping field units locate a caller who may become unable to communicate.

C **Medical priority dispatching** is designed to provide the right resources for a given call. Particularly in systems that offer both ALS and BLS ambulances, efficiency can be increased by correctly determining the severity of a call and assigning the proper unit.

D **Training and certification** While formal EMT dispatcher training and certification is available and recommended, it is by no means universal. Some jurisdictions require their dispatchers to have EMT-B training or field experience.

V MEDICAL DIRECTION OF EMS

A **History**

1. **Physicians in the field.** In the early days of "modern" EMS, physicians frequently went into the field, both to directly treat patients (as was the case with the Columbus "Heartmobile") and to teach and mentor the newly developing paramedics.

2. **Decline of physician presence in the field.** As paramedics' skills developed, EMS physicians gradually allowed them to perform unsupervised in the field. Relationships between the early paramedics and their physician mentors were generally very close, and the concept of paramedics performing ALS "under the license" of a physician medical director developed out of the confidence and trust the physicians had in these paramedics. As a result, physician participation in the field gradually died out.

3. **Rebirth of physician medical direction.** Physician medical direction (also called medical oversight and medical control) has experienced a rebirth in the past decade or so, due to several factors:

   a. **More complicated treatment protocols.** Paramedics today must have a much wider range of knowledge and skills as more drugs and equipment are taken into the field and as the expectations of the paramedic advance. More complicated treatment protocols and options for intervention have necessitated more comprehensive physician input.

   b. **Medical accountability.** The era of medical accountability has resulted in a general expectation of thorough oversight of paramedics by physicians, both by the rest of the medical community and the public.

c. **Research.** The need for research in all aspects of EMS, to satisfy such demands as documentation of high-quality patient care, financial responsibility, and the implementation of advanced technology, has attracted emergency physicians with research interest. Although EMS research is still a young field, such research provides an opportunity for the emergency physician to interact with and influence EMS personnel and systems.

B **Types of medical direction** Emergency physicians can participate in two types of medical direction: (1) direct (on-line) medical control, in which the physician gives advice, and perhaps orders, to a provider who is with a patient in the field; and (2) indirect (off-line) medical control, in which the physician helps manage the EMS system.

1. **Direct medical control**
   a. **On-line physician direction** is the provision of direct, one-on-one discussion between the paramedic in the field and the medical command physician. This discussion generally takes the form of a structured report to the physician regarding the patient (much as a medical student will "present" a patient to a supervising physician), followed by advice or orders from the physician (e.g., treatment options, medications and other interventions, destination selection). Many emergency physicians provide on-line command as part of their daily ED activities. Direct medical control is thus more commonly practiced by general emergency physicians than is indirect medical control. Although direct medical command may serve a quality assurance role, and may occasionally result in significant alteration of the care delivered to a patient, there is little evidence to date that the routine use of direct medical command, particularly for uncomplicated patient situations, is of significant benefit in terms of patient outcome.
   b. **On-line nurse direction.** In some areas, including Chicago and the state of California, nurses with EMS training provide on-line medical direction. These nurses, often known as mobile intensive care nurses (MICNs), generally have physician back-up immediately available.
   c. **On-scene medical direction.** On-scene medical command occurs in a few systems that use emergency physicians as scene supervisors.
   d. **Physician bystander intervention.** A physician bystander may offer to intervene and assist EMS personnel at a scene. This often is more of a hindrance than a help, because the majority of physicians do not have a working understanding of the field environment, the paramedics' need for adherence to protocols and standing orders, and legal issues involved in assuming responsibility for the care of a patient in the field.

2. **Indirect medical control**
   a. **Prospective**
      (1) **Initial training and certification of EMS personnel** at all levels should be supervised by emergency physicians. Although attendance at every lecture is clearly not required, physician involvement in the development and delivery of EMS education is essential. The recent and ongoing revisions of national standardized EMS curricula may help facilitate this.
      (2) **Continuing education for all levels of field providers.** Technology and knowledge bases are evolving rapidly in EMS, as throughout medicine; physician input is necessary to help determine how these advances are incorporated into the daily practice of EMS, and how providers will be educated regarding these changes.
      (3) The **development and periodic revision of treatment protocols and standing orders** should be carried out by the EMS-specialized physician. Examples of recent revisions to the protocols of many systems include the 1992 update of the American Heart Association (AHA) advanced cardiac life support (ACLS) guidelines, and the addition of adenosine to the pharmacopeia of emergency medicine and EMS.

(4) The EMS physician should play a role in **overall management of the EMS system.** While this role will vary significantly, the system medical director must be active in ensuring that resources are managed effectively.

b. Retrospective

(1) A variety of **quality assurance** models and mechanisms exist to provide for after-the-fact review of system and provider performance. A recent trend in EMS, as throughout medicine, is to move away from a quality assurance system that looks for "bad apples" toward a system of continuous quality improvement.

(2) Trauma registries, cardiac arrest registries, and other **data-collecting and statistical analysis methods** may be of value in determining quality issues for a given system.

C **Physician experience and training**

1. **Urban model versus suburban and rural models.** Most urban systems employ or involve emergency physicians with particular interest and expertise in EMS, primarily for the indirect medical direction activities. Many smaller suburban and rural systems do not have such physicians available and rely on physicians from other specialties who volunteer their time but who may bring less expertise and interest to the endeavor.

2. **EMS fellowship training programs** have been developed to provide a 1- or 2-year experience for emergency physicians who intend to specialize in EMS, after completion of an emergency medicine residency. Fellowship programs are generally affiliated with residency training sites, and offer a combination of research, administrative duties, provider education, field experience, and other academic activities. Several of these programs offer the completion of a master's degree as part of the program. Formal epidemiology, public health, and health administration training all provide skills that can be of value to the EMS provider. Fellowship programs will likely be of value in the development of academic recognition and possible subspecialty recognition for the EMS-specialized emergency physician.

VI **EMS EQUIPMENT**

A **Ambulances**

1. **Types.** There are several styles of ambulances, including modified vans, and larger box-body vehicles.

2. **Federal standards** have been developed for ambulance design and construction, both to enhance safety and to ensure that a certain minimum equipment complement is carried.

B **Medical equipment** It is important for the emergency physician to be knowledgeable in the use of medical equipment used by EMS units, because patients will be transported to the ED with this equipment in place. Certain pieces of equipment, such as the Hare traction splint for femur fractures and military antishock garments, can cause significant harm to the patient if used or removed incorrectly.

1. **BLS equipment**
   a. Oxygen delivery devices (masks, cannulas) and oxygen tanks (small portable tanks and large on-board tanks)
   b. Bandages, splints, slings, and other trauma equipment
   c. Spinal immobilization devices
      (1) Cervical collars
      (2) Long spine boards
      (3) Short extrication devices
   d. Childbirth kits

    e. Military antishock trousers (MAST), also known as pneumatic antishock garments (PASG) and pressure pants

    f. Automated and semi-automated external defibrillators

2. ALS equipment

    a. Invasive airway equipment and airway monitoring equipment (e.g., pulse oximeters)

    b. Intravenous access equipment and fluids (normal saline, dextrose in water, Ringer's lactate)

    c. Cardiac monitors, defibrillators, external pacemakers, and 12-lead electrocardiogram (ECG) equipment

3. ALS drugs. There are state, regional, and local variations in the drugs carried by ALS units. The more common agents include:

    a. Cardiac agents: lidocaine, epinephrine, atropine, bicarbonate, adenosine, nitroglycerin, furosemide, aspirin

    b. Diabetic agents: dextrose, glucagon

    c. Neurologic agents: morphine, diazepam, naloxone

    d. Other agents: albuterol, diphenhydramine, magnesium

C Communications equipment

1. Radio hardware for communication with dispatchers and other public safety agencies

2. Radio hardware for communication with hospitals (may be capable of transmitting single-lead ECG telemetry)

3. Hand-held radios for use away from the ambulance

4. Cellular telephones

5. Radio- or satellite-based positioning equipment

D Rescue equipment In some systems, EMS is the primary rescue and extrication service, while in other systems, fire or occasionally police units provide rescue, with EMS providing medical care and transport.

1. Hand-powered equipment

    a. Standard hand tools

    b. Hand-powered hydraulic cutting and spreading equipment

2. Gas- and electric-powered equipment

    a. Hydraulic cutting and spreading equipment

    b. Power saws

    c. Lifting air bags

3. Specialized patient-movement equipment

    a. Wire "Stokes" baskets

    b. Plastic sled-style stretchers for confined-space and upright lifts

    c. Longitudinally split "scoop" stretchers

4. Hazardous materials equipment (inclusion depends on the role of EMS in the local hazardous materials response plan)

    a. Personal protective equipment

        (1) Level A: complete encapsulation, with self-contained breathing apparatus (SCBA) or supplied-air masks

        (2) Level B: splash-resistant suits with SCBA or supplied-air masks

        (3) Level C: splash-resistant suits with full-face filtered-air respirator masks

    b. Decontamination equipment (for patients and responders)

    c. Other equipment and supplies for protecting the ambulance, bystanders, and the environment from secondary contamination

VII   AIR EMS

Some air medical services, particularly in remote areas, will have both helicopters and airplanes available. The helicopters may be used for local operations, whereas the airplanes may transport patients to distant specialty centers.

A **Rotor-wing aircraft (helicopters)** are used primarily for short- and medium-distance transports. Their ability to use helipads at hospitals and land at scenes for evacuation of patients makes them extremely versatile; however, they are very expensive to operate.

1. **History.** Helicopters were first used for battlefield evacuations in the Korean War, then more extensively in Vietnam. Early civilian air medical services often used helicopters that were not specifically designed for EMS operations, and in many cases were shared with other services, such as police departments. Most programs today use helicopters that are configured for medical missions.

2. **Staffing.** Various combinations of physicians, nurses, and paramedics generally staff a medical helicopter. There has been no clear advantage demonstrated to including a physician on the flight crew.

3. **Safety** has been a concern in air medical services, with statistics showing that medical helicopters crash at roughly twice the rate of other civilian helicopter services. Safety records have improved in recent years, perhaps owing to an increased use of twin-engine helicopters and limitations on pilots' work hours. Additionally, pilots are generally not informed of the nature of the flight until a determination has been made regarding the safety of weather conditions, to avoid psychological pressure to complete a flight in unsafe conditions.

4. **Use.** Most air medical programs perform a mix of interfacility transfers and scene flights, with the specific mixture dictated by local geography and demographics and tertiary referral patterns.
   a. **Interfacility flights** generally transport patients to specialty centers from outlying community facilities. Examples include transport of high-risk neonates needing neonatal intensive care unit (NICU) care, cardiac patients for emergent catheterization, and burn victims for burn center care. Specialized equipment, such as intra-aortic balloon pumps and infant isolettes, may be carried for certain interfacility missions.
   b. **Scene flights** provide rapid transport of trauma patients directly to trauma centers. Ground EMS crews that call on helicopters for evacuation of trauma patients must know how to establish a safe landing zone and how to work safely around the helicopter. In some rural areas that do not have ALS ground units, a helicopter from a distant city may be the only source of ALS care.

B **Fixed-wing aircraft (airplanes)**   Airplanes are used for longer distance transports, where their greater speed and range compensate for the need to use airport runways. Ground transport is needed to and from the aircraft.

VIII   EMS AT MASS GATHERINGS

Medical services are essential at mass gatherings. Medical needs will typically resemble those in the ED, mixing a few emergency cases with a larger number of urgent and less urgent cases. Emergency physicians are thus well suited to provide care in this setting.

A **Planning**   Emergency physicians (EMS physicians in particular) frequently play a role in planning medical services for mass gatherings and often cover such events.

1. The **size of the event** will help determine the resources needed. Events spread over large areas (such as golf tournaments, regattas, and festivals) generally require more resources than confined events (such as stadium sports).

2. **Nature of attendees.** The medical needs of events with many participants (such as marathons) will be very different from events with many spectators (such as concerts).

3. **Length of the event.** Multiple-day events (e.g., the Olympics) will require significantly more planning and resource expenditure than single-day events (e.g., the Super Bowl).

4. **Transport and evacuation needs.** Receiving hospitals and potential evacuation routes must be identified in advance.

5. **Anticipated incidents.** Plans should account for both routine medical care for participants and spectators who become ill or injured, and for the possibility of a mass casualty incident. Formulas exist for approximating the number of medical incidents to be expected at certain types of events.

6. **Other factors** to consider include whether the event is indoors or outdoors, the weather or climate, and the age range of the anticipated crowds.

B **Personnel and equipment requirements**

1. Some states and jurisdictions have **regulatory requirements** for medical staffing, based on the anticipated size of the crowd.

2. Most mass gatherings are covered by **EMS personnel, occasionally supplemented by physicians.** Various combinations of mobile BLS and ALS teams (e.g., in ambulances, on golf carts, on foot) and fixed-site treatment teams (in aid rooms, tents, trailers) are generally used.

3. Private ambulance companies often hold **contracts** with stadiums, concert halls, and other fixed venues to provide medical coverage.

IX EMS RESEARCH

A **Background** EMS techniques, technology, and ideas have often been taken from the relatively controlled hospital setting to the poorly controlled field environment, with no evidence that they are beneficial or even safe in the prehospital arena. EMS research has typically been lacking, and what research has been done has not always followed accepted scientific methods. The majority of EMS research has been focused on the provision of a given therapy to a given patient (e.g., drug A versus drug B for treatment of condition X, mortality of patients treated with method 1 versus method 2). While such research is important, examining the overall structure and function of the system and all of the patients it serves will likely be more productive.

B **Potential benefits of EMS research**

1. Improvement in patient care

2. Academic recognition for EMS and for EMS physicians

3. Improved cost-effectiveness and system efficiency

4. Development of new questions to explore

C **Problems encountered conducting EMS research**

1. It is difficult to secure funding for projects.

2. The uncontrolled field environment is not conducive to data collection.

3. EMS personnel are not well trained in research techniques. (Research training is one major goal of EMS fellowships.)

4. Field providers (EMTs, paramedics) are not trained in data collection and research methodologies.

5. There is difficulty in securing institutional review board (IRB) approval, often due to a lack of familiarity and comfort with EMS concepts.

6. There is difficulty in obtaining informed consent in emergency situations.

7. There is difficulty in adapting classic study techniques, such as the randomized double-blind placebo-controlled trial, to the field environment.

8. The large number of system models, lack of standardized training, and equipment/drug variations make multicenter trials and intersystem comparisons difficult.

D **Recent trends**   Several recent trends in EMS have helped move research efforts forward:

1. Development of academic EMS organizations (National Association of EMS Physicians, National Association of EMS Educators)
2. Development of EMS fellowships for emergency physicians
3. Pursuit of master's level training (e.g., in public health, epidemiology) by EMS physicians
4. Development of publication and presentation venues for EMS research
5. Efforts toward subspecialty recognition for EMS physicians

Study Questions

Directions: Each of the numbered items or incomplete statements in this section is followed by answers or by completions of the statement. Select the ONE lettered answer or completion that is BEST in each case.

1. Which of the following therapies falls within the emergency medical technician—basic (EMT-B) scope of practice?

   A Initiation of intravenous fluids
   B Administration of high-flow oxygen via a nonrebreather mask
   C Cardioversion of ventricular tachycardia with a manual defibrillator
   D Administration of intravenous dextrose for hypoglycemic coma
   E Administration of sublingual nitroglycerin for chest pain

2. Which one of the following is an example of retrospective medical direction?

   A Initial training of a paramedic
   B Developing a new protocol for the use of adenosine in supraventricular tachycardia
   C Ensuring proper training of the paramedic in the use of this new drug
   D Discussing the use of adenosine with the paramedic when he or she calls for on-line medical command
   E Reviewing ambulance call reports to determine the trends of adenosine use and to be sure it is being used correctly

3. Which one of the following is the most likely emergency medical system (EMS) activity for the general emergency physician?

   A Performing an audit of a trauma registry for a large urban EMS
   B Providing direct (on-line) medical direction for an acute life support (ALS) unit in the field
   C Revising protocols to incorporate recent changes in the practice of prehospital medicine
   D Supervising an EMS fellowship program
   E Performing EMS research

4. Which one of the following was included in the list of 15 essential emergency medical system (EMS) components that was developed in 1973?

   A Air medical services
   B Physician medical direction
   C Disaster planning
   D International EMS development
   E Recommended immunizations for EMS personnel

5. A first responder can perform which one of the following medical interventions?

   A Emergency obstetric delivery
   B Delivery of oxygen via a nonrebreather mask
   C Cardiac monitoring
   D Extrication of the entrapped patient from a motor vehicle
   E Administration of intravenous fluids

6. Which one of the following missions would most likely be performed by an emergency medical system (EMS) helicopter?

[A] Transport of a patient with a dissecting thoracic aneurysm from a rural community hospital to a tertiary center 35 miles away

[B] Transport of a patient requiring a liver transplant to a specialty center 750 miles away

[C] Medical coverage of a major-league baseball game

[D] Transport of a patient with chest pain from home to a local community hospital 10 miles away

[E] Substitute for ground units during a snowstorm

7. Which one of the following is closest to universal in emergency medical systems (EMS) in the United States?

[A] "911"

[B] Basic life support (BLS) ambulance service

[C] Advanced life support (ALS) ambulance service

[D] Public utility model EMS systems

[E] Emergency physicians specializing in EMS

Answers and Explanations

1. The answer is B The emergency medical technician—basic (EMT-B) training covers noninvasive skills, including advanced first aid, cardiopulmonary resuscitation (CPR), and oxygen administration by non-invasive methods such as nasal cannulas and masks. The EMT-B is not trained in the use of intravenous therapies. Although the EMT-B is trained in the use of fully or semi-automatic external defibrillators, cardioversion with a manual defibrillator is not an EMT-B skill. The recently revised EMT-B curriculum will allow the EMT-B to assist the patient in taking his or her own medications (e.g., nitroglycerin), but in general the EMT-B does not administer medications independently.

2. The answer is E Reviewing ambulance call reports to determine the trends of adenosine use and to be sure it is being used correctly represents retrospective medical direction; it is a review or quality improvement activity. Initial training of a paramedic, development of a new drug protocol, and ensuring the proper training of the paramedic in the use of a new drug protocol represent prospective medical direction, because these activities help prepare the provider and the system for a certain type of patient. Discussing the use of a drug with a paramedic when he or she calls for on-line medical command represents direct medical control (i.e., assisting the provider with a specific patient encountered in the field).

3. The answer is B Many general emergency physicians provide on-line, or direct, medical direction for paramedics in the field, because many emergency departments (EDs) serve as base stations for ALS units. Performing an audit of a trauma registry for a large urban EMS, revising protocols to incorporate recent changes in the practice of prehospital medicine, supervising an EMS fellowship program, and performing EMS research are activities that are generally performed by physicians with specific interest in EMS, although in many areas with no such EMS specialists, general emergency physicians may be asked to perform these tasks.

4. The answer is C Disaster planning was among the 15 essential EMS components, and has been fairly well developed. The lack of physician medical direction has been of major concern to emergency physicians, and is being overcome gradually. Air medical services, international EMS efforts, and provider safety and well-being were all later developments.

5. The answer is A A first responder is taught basic, lifesaving first aid, cardiopulmonary resuscitation (CPR), and emergency delivery. Oxygen administration and the extrication of a motor vehicle accident victim are emergency medical technician—basic (EMT-B) skills, whereas cardiac monitoring and the administration of intravenous fluids are emergency medical technician—paramedic (EMT-P) skills. In some states, these latter skills are emergency medical technician—intermediate (EMT-I) skills.

6. The answer is A A helicopter would be most appropriate for the transport of a patient with a dissecting thoracic aneurysm from a rural community hospital to a tertiary center 35 miles away. The speed and versatility of helicopters make them very useful for transportation where time is of the essence and moderate distances are involved. The cost of EMS helicopters, though, makes them impractical for routine use in cases where ground units would perform well. Airplanes are more practical for distances beyond about 150 miles.

7. The answer is B Many areas of the United States are not yet covered by "enhanced 911" or even by "basic 911" systems for access to emergency aid. While almost all areas of the country have BLS emergency service, many areas do not have ALS services available, or emergency physicians with a subspecialty interest in EMS. The public utility model, while almost 20 years old, is still found in only a few cities in the United States.

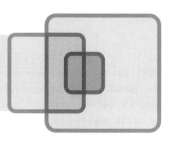

chapter 23

Disaster Medicine

DAVID C. CONE

I **DEFINING DISASTERS**

There is no clear agreement on terminology for disasters, which may cause significant confusion in the areas of disaster research and reporting. Disasters can be considered along a spectrum of severity from small, local events to catastrophic, international events.

A **Multicasualty incidents (MCIs)**   An MCI is any incident that generates more than one significant victim. Most local disaster plans are designed to handle MCIs, not true disasters.

B **Disasters**

1. Traditionally, disasters have been classified as **natural** (e.g., earthquakes, tornadoes, hurricanes) or **manmade** (e.g., building collapses, terrorist attacks). This distinction actually has little value in terms of responses, research, and data collection.

2. A disaster is generally considered to be **an event that overwhelms** the ability of local resources to respond effectively. For example, a multivehicle accident with a dozen victims may be managed routinely by an urban emergency medical services (EMS) system; however, this same event may be a disaster in a rural area if outside resources need to be called in to supplement the limited local resources.

3. There are numerous **recent examples** of disasters in the United States.
   a. The February 1993 bombing of the **World Trade Center** was handled primarily by New York City resources, with some outside assistance in the initial response. This event, which would have been a true disaster in almost any other city, was treated essentially as a large MCI.
   b. Many **airliner crashes** are disasters, requiring multijurisdictional responses.
      (1) The July 1989 crash in **Sioux City, Iowa,** with a significant number of survivors, required a coordinated response from agencies in three states.
      (2) Some crashes, such as the September 1994 crash outside **Pittsburgh, Pennsylvania,** are not disasters or even MCIs because there are no survivors.
   c. In April 1995, the **Oklahoma City Federal Building** was bombed. Although several buildings in the immediate area also were damaged or destroyed, the EMS, fire, and medical infrastructures were minimally affected.
      (1) The **immediate response** (i.e., first 12 hours) was handled by the Oklahoma City Fire Department, with assistance from a number of nearby cities and private ambulance companies with whom pre-existing mutual aid agreements existed.
      (2) A number of federal Urban Search and Rescue task forces responded during the next few days to assist in the **search and removal process.**
   d. Major acts of international terrorism such as the Twin Towers on Sept. 11, 2001, and bombings in Spain and London often require regional as well as a national response.

C **Catastrophic disasters**   A catastrophic disaster is one that not only generates many casualties, but also may destroy hospitals, EMS stations, and other infrastructure needed to provide care. Examples include a major hurricane or earthquake.

1. **Recent examples** of catastrophic disasters in the United States include:
   a. **Mississippi Valley floods (summer 1993).** Some catastrophic events destroy or paralyze much of an area's infrastructure, but they may not generate many casualties. This is often the case with floods, blizzards, and droughts. Most of the medical concerns in the Midwest floods involved primary care and public health, particularly sanitation, provision of potable water, and access to routine care.
   b. **Hurricane Andrew, Florida (August 1992).** Much of the infrastructure was destroyed in the most heavily affected areas. Total damage exceeded $25 billion. Several federal Disaster Medical Assistance teams responded to the area in the days following the hurricane. Although these teams did provide some emergency care, mostly for injuries sustained during the cleanup process, it was found that the greatest need was for primary care. The teams essentially replaced the local primary care system while it was rebuilt.
   c. **Northridge, California earthquake (1994).** In the most heavily affected area, the medical infrastructure was destroyed. Several hospitals were rendered unsafe and were evacuated, and several fire and EMS stations were damaged. Several federal Disaster Medical Assistance teams responded to the area in the first few days after the earthquake. One team operated in the parking lot outside the emergency department (ED) of one of the affected hospitals, while others operated in a local park. As with Hurricane Andrew, the teams did provide some emergency care, mostly for injuries sustained during the cleanup, but again, the greatest need was for routine primary care.
2. There is frequently an **international response** to a catastrophic disaster, as occurred following earthquakes in **Armenia** in 1988, and **Kobe, Japan,** in 1995. The United States, however, has tended to be self-reliant in disaster responses.

D **Complex emergencies** are often **societal events** [e.g., **famines** (Ethiopia), **refugee crises** (Rwanda), **civil wars** (Afghanistan and Bosnia)].

1. Complex emergencies are defined by the Centers for Disease Control (CDC) as being characterized by at least two of the following:
   a. **Civil strife**
   b. **Armed conflict**
   c. **Population migration**
   d. **Economic collapse**
   e. **Food scarcity**
   f. **Famine**
2. Generally, complex emergencies are the focus of international disaster agencies, which concentrate on the long-term, public health aspect of these disasters.

II PHASES OF DISASTER RESPONSE

A Planning

1. **Simplicity** and **familiarity** are key elements to a successful plan. The best MCI and disaster plans do not invoke new organizational structures, complex management plans, and elaborate communications schemes, but instead are **simply expansions of the day-to-day operations** of the responders. This allows for the expansion of the plan to fit the size of the incident.
2. **Common approach.** Disaster plans, whether for communities, hospitals, or even entire states, should be designed to work for any type of incident.
   a. A **generic, "all-hazards" approach** is much simpler than having a separate plan for each type of disaster that might occur.
   b. **Hospital disaster plans** must account for the possibility that internal and external resources may be disrupted. By having a generic, all-hazards plan, the hospital will be able to deal with

an internal problem, such as a power failure or fire, or an external problem, such as an MCI that brings large numbers of patients to the hospital. **Realistic drills** of the hospital disaster plan not only serve to familiarize staff with the plan and their assigned roles, but also help find problems and deficiencies that need attention.

3. **Coordination.** EMS agencies and EMS physicians must ensure that **all agencies** that might be involved in a disaster response participate in the development and practice of the plan. Police, fire, hospitals, utilities, military, and various local, state, and federal government agencies all have roles in disaster responses and must be integral parts of the planning process to ensure smooth integration of needed resources.

4. **Designation.** It is crucial that disaster plans designate who will fill various roles. The **incident command system (ICS),** which has become a fairly standardized approach to multiagency emergency responses, has several specific command roles that must be filled, and these personnel must be designated and agreed on in advance to avoid confusion at that scene.

B **Notification** Some disasters occur with significant warning (e.g., hurricanes), while others do not (e.g., terrorist attacks, earthquakes). Improvements in weather tracking and warning systems over the past few decades have allowed for notification of pending hurricanes hours or even days before they strike, allowing for a coordinated evacuation and preparation process. At present, computer and Doppler radar technology is being developed to provide better warning for tornadoes; the information provided by this technology may allow people in the potential path of a tornado to take shelter by giving them several minutes' warning.

C **Immediate search and rescue** is performed generally by untrained civilians initially. An organized, professional search and rescue response may follow, but the most significant numbers of victims are typically rescued by bystanders.

D **Response** The **incident commander (IC)** has overall charge of managing the aftermath of an MCI or disaster. The IC has at his or her disposal several subcommanders, each in charge of one particular aspect of the response (e.g., police, fire, EMS, finance, public information). Depending on the size and type of incident, some commands may or may not be needed.

1. **Initial activities.** The **first emergency response personnel** who arrive on the scene have the following responsibilities:
   a. **Perform a rough assessment of the event,** and notify the dispatcher of the nature and scope of the event and what resources will likely be needed. There is a tendency to call for many more resources than needed, and this can actually complicate scene management and hinder an effective response.
   b. **Establish a command post in a safe location.** The senior member of the first unit on the scene serves as the IC until relieved by more senior personnel who have been designated in the plan.
   c. **Initiate triage.** In most cases, first-in personnel should avoid providing detailed treatment for patients they encounter; instead, they should begin sorting patients by severity.

2. **Scene** and **crowd control** are essential. The convergence phenomenon guarantees that unrequested emergency responders, the media, and the curious public will converge on a disaster or MCI scene.

3. **Establishment of EMS sectors.** The EMS commander should establish a number of EMS sectors, each with a sector commander. Certain sectors may be needed in some events but not in others. **Typical sectors** include:
   a. Communications
   b. Triage
   c. Treatment
   d. Transportation
   e. Resources

4. **Triage**
   a. A **formal triage process,** with organized transportation, helps distribute victims more evenly to the receiving facilities and can help match patient needs with available hospital resources. Many victims are transported to hospitals by bystanders or may transport themselves. This can cause significant problems if one hospital receives most of the patients, as tends to happen in MCIs, or if the hospitals are not functional.
   b. Triage should be initiated by the **first responding unit,** then be continued by the **most experienced personnel.** In a widespread disaster (e.g., a hurricane), patients may be spread out over many miles, making coordination of triage difficult.
   c. A number of different **triage systems** and types of **triage tags** exist. There is no firm agreement on the relative value of the different systems or even the value of triage tags, but patients generally are divided into three or four categories.
      (1) **First priority.** Patients who have the most serious injuries yet are salvageable receive the first attention.
      (2) **Second priority.** Patients with significant injuries but who are at least temporarily stable are second priority.
      (3) **Third priority.** Patients who are ambulatory with minimal injuries are third priority.
      (4) **No treatment.** Patients who are deceased or who are expected to die receive no attention. Patients with major injuries that are not clearly salvageable do not receive treatment because large numbers of personnel and treatment resources cannot be dedicated to one patient.

5. **Treatment in the field**
   a. **Equipment depots** are established at the casualty collection point or other designated area to avoid the necessity of taking large quantities of equipment and supplies into the site. The **resource sector commander** is responsible for collection, placement, and distribution of equipment and supplies.
   b. **Minimal stabilizing care** should be delivered at the site, particularly if the site itself is still hazardous. In most MCI settings, patients are quickly removed to a casualty collection point some distance from the site, where further stabilizing treatment is administered, and secondary triage is performed.

6. **Transportation.** The **transportation sector commander** is responsible for matching patient needs with available hospital resources. Depending on the circumstances, the transportation commander may want to use both ground and air transport. In a catastrophic disaster, damage to transportation resources and to receiving facilities may hinder evacuation efforts.

7. **Hospital activities**
   a. **Handling of incoming patients.** Roles and responsibilities should be clearly delineated in each hospital's disaster plan to ensure the smooth handling of arriving patients. Certain areas of the hospital should be assigned to certain tasks, such as waiting areas for families, temporary morgue space, areas for incoming staff to report for assignments, and minor treatment areas.
   b. **Communications.** During a disaster, each hospital should keep the **EMS dispatcher** or **transportation sector commander** apprised of its ability to handle further casualties. The assessment of the ED's functional capacity is usually made by the ED attending physician. Communications is always one of the largest problems in a disaster or MCI response. It may not be possible to get an accurate assessment of the expected patient load, and communication between the hospitals and the scene may be difficult.
   c. **Triage.** Each patient who arrives at the hospital should be triaged again, and then resources should be assigned based on need. Some **tracking system,** such as tags, should be used to expedite patient flow and ensure accurate data collection.

E **Recovery.** The recovery effort may take days, weeks, or months, depending on the type and extent of damage. In catastrophic disasters, primary care may need to be supplemented until the infrastructure is rebuilt. Public health issues are often of major concern during the recovery period.

III ROLE OF THE EMERGENCY PHYSICIAN

Experience has demonstrated that physicians, including emergency physicians, are generally of little help at a disaster or MCI scene. Physicians typically lack the knowledge and skills to operate safely and effectively in the field environment, and they are likely to be a significant liability to the overall response. In general, the most useful place for an emergency physician to be during a disaster or MCI is in the ED.

A In some systems, emergency physicians have been integrated into disaster or MCI plans to function as triage or treatment personnel or to assist the EMS commander. This may be effective if the physician has the training and experience to operate in the field, works within the system to develop the plan, and drills with the EMS personnel frequently.

B Emergency physicians have been able to effectively provide primary care following disasters. Physicians whose facilities are rendered unusable by a disaster may wish to direct their efforts at primary care in field hospitals or temporary facilities.

IV FEDERAL DISASTER RESOURCES

The federal government spends approximately $1 billion per week on disaster response, relief, and recovery in the United States.

A The **federal response plan** is a coordinated organizational structure under which numerous federal agencies work to provide resources to 12 emergency support functions (ESFs), which represent the functional areas that are involved in disaster response, relief, and recovery. Examples of ESFs include health and medical care, fire, mass care, urban search and rescue, food, and energy. Each ESF is under the direction of a lead agency, with other agencies in support roles.

B **National disaster medical system (NDMS)**
1. NDMS was created in 1984 to **develop a nationwide network** of hospitals that could provide beds for casualties in a catastrophic disaster. Participating hospitals agree to make available a certain number of beds should the system be activated.
2. NDMS is a **cooperative effort** of the Department of Defense, Department of Health and Human Services, Federal Emergency Management Agency (FEMA), Veterans Administration, civilian hospitals, and governments at the federal, state, and local levels.
3. NDMS can only be activated by **presidential disaster declaration** (for a civilian event) or by the Secretary of Defense (for a military event).

C **Federally sponsored response teams**
1. **Disaster medical assistance team (DMAT)**
   a. **Definition.** A DMAT, which is a component of NDMS, generally consists of 100–250 people representing a wide range of medical and logistic talents, including physicians, EMTs and paramedics, nurses, pharmacists, public health specialists, and communications personnel. Positions generally are double- or triple-filled to ensure a full complement when deployed.
   b. **Purpose.** Teams can provide triage, medical and surgical intervention, and public health services to supplement or replace local resources.

    c. Jurisdiction. Teams are available for local response or for nationwide response when deployed by federal order. For large events, typically more than one DMAT is deployed, and other DMATs may be called in a week or so later to relieve the first-in teams.

2. **Urban Search and Rescue Task Forces.** The primary mission of these task forces is the search and recovery of patients from collapsed structures.

    a. The task force is composed of 50–70 members, including two physicians and four medical technicians. Other team members are heavy rescue specialists, search dogs and handlers, communications technicians, and structural engineers.

    b. There are currently approximately 25 Urban Search and Rescue Task Forces in the United States, under the sponsorship of the Department of Defense, FEMA, and several other supporting agencies.

V   DISASTER RESEARCH

A Obstacles   Efforts to conduct research in disaster medicine are hampered by a number of factors:

1. The unpredictable nature of these events makes them difficult to study.

2. During an actual disaster, resources are directed to response and mitigation. Data collection is generally a low priority.

3. A lack of standardized definitions, data sets, and research methodologies makes comparisons between events difficult.

4. By the time disaster researchers can reach a scene, the primary response is generally over, and most potential data have been lost.

5. Funding for disaster research is sparse. The "it-will-never-happen-to-us" mentality tends to limit the number of grants and other funding sources available for disaster medicine.

B Recent efforts

1. **Funding.** A number of coordinated disaster research efforts have begun recently. Most of these are sponsored by government agencies (e.g., CDC, FEMA) or academic institutions.

2. **Training.** Emergency physicians have assumed a leadership role in the new fields of disaster medicine and disaster research. Formal training in public health and epidemiology has proven to be of significant value to disaster specialists.

Study Questions

Directions: *Each of the numbered items or incomplete statements in this section is followed by answers or by completions of the statement. Select the ONE lettered answer or completion that is BEST in each case.*

1. Which one of the following incidents qualifies as a catastrophic disaster?

   (A) A subway derailment with 125 major injuries
   (B) A nerve-gas attack at a professional baseball game with 35,000 injuries
   (C) An earthquake with significant damage to hospitals and numerous casualties
   (D) A fire aboard a cruise ship
   (E) A nursing strike at a community hospital

2. Which one of the following plans is the best hospital disaster plan?

   (A) One plan for internal disasters, one plan for external disasters
   (B) A physician plan, an administrative plan, and a nursing plan
   (C) A plan that can expand as needed to fit the size of the event
   (D) A plan that emphasizes the steps needed to evacuate the hospital
   (E) A complex plan that accounts for every possible contingency on paper, leaving nothing to chance

QUESTIONS 3–6

The patients in questions 3–6 all arrive at the same emergency department (ED) simultaneously, brought in by basic life support (BLS) ambulances from a motor vehicle accident. It is 3 A.M., and the ED physician has two nurses and a clerk to assist him. There is no physician backup in the hospital. The physician should triage these patients, matching each patient with the correct priority, as listed below:

   (A) First priority
   (B) Second priority
   (C) Third priority
   (D) No treatment

3. A 30-year-old man with an open femur fracture and facial contusions, a heart rate of 100 beats/min, a blood pressure of 100/60 mm Hg, and evidence of moderate alcohol intoxication

4. A 45-year-old woman with difficulty breathing, decreased breath sounds over the left chest, tracheal deviation to the right, and a heart rate of 120 beats/min

5. A 25-year-old woman with no vital signs and evidence of closed head and abdominal injuries

6. A 4-year-old boy, found by emergency workers in a child safety seat, crying loudly, with contusions to both arms but no other apparent injuries and normal vital signs for his age

Answers and Explanations

1. **The answer is C** Catastrophic disasters generally are considered to be those with destruction of infrastructure, making the provision of care difficult. Therefore, an earthquake causing significant damage to hospitals and numerous casualties would qualify as a catastrophic disaster. A small nursing strike, while causing significant internal problems for the affected hospital, is not considered a catastrophic disaster; however, a large regional nursing strike could be considered catastrophic if it paralyzes the ability of the region to provide medical care.

2. **The answer is C** A hospital disaster plan must be simple, flexible, and expandable to handle all types of emergencies. Separate plans for each department should be discouraged, in favor of an integrated plan.

3–6. **The answers are 3-B, 4-A, 5-D, 6-C** The patients with the most serious yet salvageable injuries receive first priority. The 45-year-old woman with the tension pneumothorax can be treated quickly with needle thoracostomy followed by tube thoracostomy and/or intubation, depending on the extent of her other injuries. Patients with serious but stable injuries (e.g., the man with the femur fracture) are treated next, but careful attention must be given to this patient's mental status to be sure he has simple intoxication and not a head injury or other occult injury. Patients who appear to have minimal injuries, such as the child, are treated last, and patients who are deceased or have minimal chance of salvage are not treated. An attempt to resuscitate the 25-year-old woman would use all the resources currently available, with little chance of success.

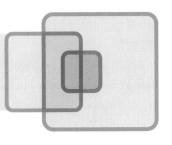

chapter **24**

Legal Issues

B. ZANE HOROWITZ • R. KONANE MOOKINI

I   INTRODUCTION

The American legal system allows those who feel they have been wronged to argue their cases in court.

A Criminal versus civil law

1. **Criminal law.** A **criminal action** is a wrong committed against the public or the public good. For an action to be a crime, there must be both an intent to commit the illegal act as well as the commission of the act itself. Seldom is criminality an issue in treating patients. As long as the patient consents to medical care, charges such as assault (i.e., confrontation causing reasonable apprehension of unpermitted personal contact) or battery (i.e., unpermitted personal contact) rarely occur. Although both assault and battery may be crimes, they may also be used as the basis of a claim of intentional tort.

2. **Civil law.** Civil cases **(torts)** involve wrongs committed against private parties. When a patient or family member is angered by an interaction with a healthcare provider, he or she may, as a legal recourse to achieve satisfaction, bring a lawsuit against the physician and hospital. Although many claims can be made in a lawsuit, the most frequent tort is that of **negligence.**

B Medical negligence is the failure to follow acceptable standards of care in a way that results in injury to the patient. Medical negligence is the most common claim in a malpractice lawsuit.

1. **Elements of negligence.** In order to bring a successful lawsuit on the tort of negligence, four elements must be proven:
    a. **Duty to treat.** A physician has a duty to treat the patient if a doctor–patient relationship is established. For the purposes of emergency medicine, all patients, regardless of their ability to pay, establish a physician–patient relationship by presenting themselves to the emergency department (ED); therefore, the physician must render care.
    b. **Breach of duty.** To prove this element of negligence, the law requires that a physician's actions must be demonstrated to be below the acceptable standard of care.
        (1) The standard of care is established by an expert's testimony. It is not necessarily defined by information in reference books, nor is it established by common local practice, cost-cutting guidelines, hospital protocols, or policies.
        (2) If a plaintiff's attorney can produce an expert that is willing to testify that the defendant's practice is below the standard of care in his or her opinion, the case will move forward. Defense hinges on producing appropriate experts to testify that documentation of the case reflects the level of care someone in the same field of medicine would provide under similar circumstances. Some states have limited experts to those board-certified in the field of emergency medicine with a minimum number of years of direct clinical practice.
    c. **Injury.** The patient must have suffered an injury as a result of the physician's breach of duty. Injuries are defined differently by lawyers than by physicians. Although the patient may appear healthy, injuries such as pain and suffering, loss of consortium (inability to have sexual intercourse), loss of wages, and mental anguish have been claimed.

d. **Proximate cause.** The injury must be a direct result of either the physician's action or his or her failure to act or diagnose a condition that led to the injuries.

2. **Avoiding malpractice.** Excessive diagnostic testing will not reduce the likelihood of being sued. Physicians can do much to reduce lawsuits by:
   a. **Practicing good medicine.** This is the primary way of preventing malpractice suits.
   b. **Communicating well.** The physician should attempt to allay anger and minimize unreasonable expectations on the part of patients and family. Patients will be less likely to sue if they believe that the physician genuinely cares about them.
   c. **Documenting thoroughly.** Accurate documentation of all assessments, care rendered, and discussions with patients regarding treatment options is essential. If a patient is refusing recommendations or is being noncompliant, these facts should be noted as well.

II   INFORMED CONSENT

The concept of informed consent was laid down in 1914 by Justice Cardozo in *Schloendorff v. New York Hospital:* "Every human being of adult years and sound mind has a right to determine what shall be done to his body; a surgeon who performs an operation without his patient's consent commits an assault for which he is liable in damages."

A **Implied consent** applies in all true emergencies. A true emergency exists when there is an immediate threat to life or limb. In this situation, the physician should perform what a "reasonably prudent person" would want done under the same circumstances and document the rationale for the procedure in the patient's chart.

B **Express written consent** is required for all nonemergency procedures. Even in the busiest of EDs, fewer than 5% of all patients represent true life or limb emergencies.

1. **Adults.** The patient must:
   a. **Give consent voluntarily** (not under duress or financial inducement)
   b. **Be informed.** The patient must:
      (1) Understand the nature of the procedure
      (2) Understand the risks and benefits of the procedure
      (3) Understand the alternatives to the procedure
      (4) Have the opportunity to ask questions and receive answers to them
   c. **Be competent.** The patient must:
      (1) Display normal mental capacity
      (2) Not be under the influence of drugs or alcohol
      (3) Not be cognitively impaired as a result of injury or illness

2. **Minors.** The child's legal guardian (if not the mother or father) must be identified. The adult consenting must meet all of the criteria outlined in II B 1. In the following situations, it may not be necessary to obtain the express written consent of the minor's guardian, although rules vary from state to state:
   a. **Emancipated minors** live on their own and are responsible for their own expenses. Military personnel are usually considered emancipated minors.
   b. **Minors who request treatment of pregnancy or sexually transmitted diseases (STDs).** Because these situations may be embarrassing, some states allow a minor to consent for examination and treatment of suspected venereal disease or pregnancy.
   c. **Minors in police custody.** For example, a 16-year-old suspected of driving under the influence of alcohol may be required to undergo a blood alcohol determination and treatment of injuries by police who have placed the minor under arrest or into protective custody.

C **Refusal** is the right of a competent adult to not give consent, and thereby forego recommended treatment or evaluation.

1. **Adults.** In order to refuse, the adult must meet all of the requirements outlined for consent in II B 1. The patient's medical record should document that the patient:
   a. Is alert and oriented
   b. Has normal mental capacity
   c. Is not under the influence of alcohol or drugs
   d. Has received an explanation of the proposed procedure, its alternatives, and the risks and benefits of both the procedure and the alternatives
   e. Understands that refusing may lead to death or permanent loss of health
   f. Was invited to return at any time to have the procedure done
   g. Was offered all other reasonable treatments (e.g., oral antibiotics given in a situation where intravenous antibiotics are indicated)

2. **Minors.** Exceptions to the rules of consent include the following when a parent or guardian refuses treatment on behalf of a child:
   a. If the physician believes that the refusal of treatment by the parent or guardian would seriously jeopardize the child's health, then a court order can be sought to compel treatment. For example, if the parents of a child with suspected meningitis refuse a lumbar puncture and antibiotics, the child should be held in the ED and Risk Management called to initiate a request to a judge for court-ordered treatment.
   b. If the physician believes the child is a victim of abuse or neglect, then evaluation and treatment should occur and the appropriate investigating agency notified.

III PATIENT CONFIDENTIALITY AND REPORTABLE CONDITIONS

A **Patient confidentiality**   The physician has a legal and moral duty to hold what a patient discloses to him or her, or what is discovered through examination or medical testing, to be confidential. This information should not be disclosed to anyone, even well-meaning family members, the patient's insurance company, or other caregivers, without the patient's consent. The following are examples of situations where it is inappropriate to provide information regarding the patient's condition without consent from the patient:

1. A family member requests information regarding the patient's diagnosis.

2. An insurance company requests information regarding the presenting complaint of the patient.

3. An employer inquires about an employee's injuries or ability to return to work.

4. The media requests information on hospitalized "newsworthy" patients.

5. An outside hospital requests release of the patient's medical records.

6. An attorney "just wants to talk about a case."

B **Reportable conditions**   Although the physician–patient relationship is held in highest scrutiny of confidentiality, society has recognized that sometimes a greater duty is owed to the public than to the patient. Many states have specific statutes regarding when to report certain conditions that would provide for the greater good to society, despite violating a patient's confidentiality. Although statutes vary among states, most require that a physician violate patient confidentiality in the following situations:

1. **Threats.** If a patient makes a threat of violence against a specific person, then the physician must ensure that the person is contacted and warned. The person notified, the specific warning, and the date and time must be recorded in the medical record of the patient who made the threat.

2. **Domestic violence.** Reporting of domestic violence is mandatory in most states. This mandate requires the physician to prepare a written report of injuries sustained as a result of the action of any member of the patient's household, even if the patient does not want to file a police report or seek help.

3. **Sexual assault.** In most states, clear written documentation, usually on a standardized reporting form, is required for victims of alleged sexual assault. Samples obtained from the patient must be labeled and handled as a "chain of evidence" (i.e., each person handling the evidence sample must sign for its receipt until the sample is received at a crime laboratory). Occasionally, the physician may also be asked to obtain hair or blood samples from the alleged perpetrator, and similar chain of evidence procedures apply.

4. **Child abuse.** A physician who suspects that a child has been the victim of physical abuse, sexual assault, or neglect is required to notify the appropriate investigating agency (e.g., the police or Social Welfare Services). The child must be protected from further harm, which may require separating the child from his or her parents and preventing the parents from removing the child from the ED. In this situation, the parent's or guardian's right to consent for the child is negated, and a police or court order is required to treat the child for non–life-threatening problems.

5. **Elder abuse.** Like child abuse and domestic violence, the mistreatment or abandonment of an incapacitated elder may require reporting to police, Adult Protective Services, or an elder ombudsman. If a physician believes that a patient has been mistreated in a skilled nursing facility, state law may also require that the incident be reported to the state licensing agency that oversees nursing homes.

6. **Wounds**
   a. **Weapon-inflicted.** Some states require that a physician notify the police immediately of patients with wounds believed to be inflicted by a weapon. The intent of this law is to aid in the investigation of crimes. However, in the absence of a specific reporting statute, the physician must not disclose a confidential statement by a patient stating that he or she committed a crime.
   b. **Animal bite wounds.** In some states, bite wounds may have to be reported to local health authorities or animal control agencies. The physician may also be obligated to report the harboring of illegal animals, such as exotic snakes. The intent of these laws is to prevent other citizens from being bitten and to control the spread of rabies and other diseases spread by animal vectors.

7. **Public health issues.** Most states require certain types of illnesses to be reported to public health authorities for investigation and follow-up. Laws vary from state to state, and local health departments should be consulted for requirements. Examples of some of the more common situations that require reporting include:
   a. **Communicable diseases**
      (1) STDs
      (2) HIV and AIDS
      (3) Hepatitis, especially in food handlers
      (4) Childhood diseases (e.g., measles, meningitis)
      (5) Unusual infections (e.g., rabies, Hantavirus infection)
   b. **Food poisoning outbreaks**
      (1) Staphylococcal food poisoning
      (2) Shellfish-related food poisoning
      (3) Botulism
   c. **Pesticide exposure.** California has extensive regulations requiring physicians to report all cases, no matter how minor, of pesticide-related illness. Surveillance of farm workers is required for many products used in agriculture.
   d. **Disorders that lead to lapse of consciousness** (e.g., epilepsy). Often, it is necessary to notify the Health Department, which may secondarily release the information to the Department of Motor Vehicles (DMV) or other mandated licensing authorities. Some states may allow the physician to report directly to the DMV.

8. **Impaired physicians.** Some states require a physician to protect the public good if he or she believes a physician is too impaired to treat patients but continues to do so. It is advisable to con-

tact local hospital counsel to determine the exact reporting requirements. Knowledge of physician incompetence and failure to report it may make a fellow physician liable for tort action by an injured party.

| **IV** | **INVOLUNTARY HOLDS** |

A patient may have his or her right to leave the hospital suspended under certain conditions. However, the patient's right to refuse treatment remains his or her own unless superseded by a life-threatening emergency or a court order to treat.

A **Mental illness**   A patient who, as a result of mental illness, is unable to care for him- or herself, or poses a danger to him- or herself or others, may be placed on a psychiatric hold. In some jurisdictions the ability to place this type of hold is granted to medical personnel, police agencies, social workers, and mental health agencies. Laws may differ from county to county, as well as from state to state. The intent of this law is to provide psychiatric treatment to the patient; it usually does not give the physician consent to treat medical problems. In a true emergency, the concept of implied consent still applies.

B **Inebriation**   A patient who, as a result of alcohol intoxication, is unable to understand the elements of consent or refusal may be placed on an inebriation hold. Even if local statutes do not specifically address this issue, an emergency physician may document in the medical record that the patient is a danger to him- or herself or others as a result of inebriation and that it is necessary to restrain the patient until such time that sobriety is obtained. When the patient is sober, medical care should again be offered. If the patient refuses once sober, notation of all the elements of refusal and an invitation to return should be documented in the medical record.

C **Inability to care for self**   Some patients may be unable to care for themselves as a result of their medical illness. Statutes may call for the reporting of abandonment in such cases. The patient should be treated under the concept of implied consent.

1. An application for conservatorship of the patient may need to be presented before a judge to best serve the patient's needs. Social service agencies within the hospital can assist the physician in such an application. Admission or nursing home placement may be necessary in the interim.

2. Once conservatorship is granted, the patient's conservator has the right to consent or refuse for the patient.

D **Police holds**   A police officer may place in his or her custody any person suspected of a crime. That person might be brought to an ED for medical clearance prior to incarceration.

1. The person under arrest has the same rights of consent and refusal as anyone else.

2. Frequently, in an attempt to be manipulative, an individual under arrest will refuse treatment. If the patient refuses to be seen, the treating physician should note that the patient refused examination and treatment, and instruct the police to return the patient to the ED if the patient changes his or her mind regarding treatment. All of the elements of consent and refusal, the patient's mental state, the advice to the patient and law enforcement officer, and the officer's department and badge number should be documented.

E **Requests for blood samples**   In most states, as a condition of accepting a license to operate a motor vehicle, the operator waives his or her right to refuse blood or breath testing for alcohol. Police may bring a person to the ED and request an alcohol or drug test. The patient need not be under arrest for a request to be made.

1. The physician's first priority should be stabilization and treatment of the patient's medical condition. Once the patient is stabilized, police requests should be honored.

2. In some states, the law even allows noninjurious restraint of the patient to obtain the sample. However, a physician cannot be compelled to perform an act that he or she believes would result in injury to him- or herself, the staff, or the patient. Good judgment in these cases will balance the issue of patient safety against the need of society to prosecute drunken drivers.

V PATIENT TRANSFER LAWS

In response to an epidemic of hospitals refusing to treat or stabilize uninsured emergency patients, Congress passed the first "antidumping" law in 1986. This law was strengthened further, in a second congressional act, in 1989. Violation of these laws carries a fine of $50,000 per occurrence, which is not covered under a physician's malpractice insurance. The Health Care Finance Administration (HCFA) may also suspend or revoke an involved hospital's Medicare reimbursement privileges. A single alleged violation allows HCFA to inspect all transfers to search for other violations. Emergency physicians are often in the middle of these potential transfer law violations, so a thorough understanding of these laws is crucial to the practice of emergency medicine.

A **Consolidated Omnibus Budget Reconciliation Act (COBRA)/Emergency Medical Treatment and Active Labor Act (EMTALA)** These acts provide every person with a medical emergency or active labor (defined by the presence of contractions) the right to be examined and stabilized prior to transfer. The requirements of these laws are as follows:

1. Any person who enters the hospital property (including hospital-owned clinics and ambulances, as well as the ED) is entitled to medical evaluation and stabilization.

2. A screening medical examination must be performed to determine if an emergency medical condition exists. An emergency medical condition is defined as a condition that "without immediate treatment could place the health of the patient in serious danger or cause significant impairment of a bodily function or organ; or in the case of a pregnant woman, could cause harm to the woman or unborn child."

3. Stabilization of the emergency medical condition must occur prior to transfer. Stabilization is not clearly defined, but the court will find the physician at fault if any deterioration in the patient's medical condition occurs during transfer.

4. Transfer of unstable patients may occur only if all six of the following conditions are met:
   a. The physician signs a certificate stating that the medical benefits of transfer outweigh the risks of remaining at the treating hospital.
   b. The patient or guardian gives consent to transfer.
   c. The transferring hospital and physician have provided all medical treatment to minimize the risks of transfer.
   d. The receiving physician and facility agree to accept the patient in transfer.
   e. All medical records, laboratory results, and radiographs are sent with the patient.
   f. The transfer is carried out with appropriate and qualified personnel and equipment (e.g., ambulance, aeromedical, or other specialized units). The emergency physician transferring the patient is responsible for the medical care of the patient while in transit, unless care is transferred to a transporting physician.

B **Omnibus Budget Reconciliation Act (OBRA)** Additional refinements to COBRA include the following:

1. It is inappropriate to inquire regarding the patient's ability to pay or the patient's insurance status until after the screening medical examination occurs.

2. When requested to do so by an emergency physician who identifies an unstable condition, on-call specialists have a duty to respond to the ED and treat the patient.

a. The on-call physician must attend the patient physically.

b. The emergency physician who is forced to transfer a patient because the on-call physician failed to respond may be protected from liability. Excellent documentation by the emergency physician of attempts to contact the on-call physician and the nature of phone conversations with the on-call physician is vital.

3. Hospitals with specialized facilities (e.g., burn units, trauma centers, tertiary pediatric centers, high-risk obstetric units) may not refuse a transfer if bed space is available.

4. A special "whistle-blower" regulation calls for hospitals to report other hospitals that have transferred a patient to them in violation of these laws. Anyone who reports a transfer violation is protected from sanctioning by the hospital or medical staff.

Study Questions

Directions: Each of the numbered items or incomplete statements in this section is followed by answers or by completions of the statement. Select the ONE lettered answer or completion that is BEST in each case.

1. A 16-year-old army private who sprained his ankle in a basketball game wants to leave the emergency department (ED) to seek treatment at the base clinic tomorrow. What should the emergency physician do?

- A Seek the patient's parents' consent.
- B Allow the patient to refuse treatment.
- C Have the patient sign out against medical advice.
- D Insist on completing all Consolidated Omnibus Budget Reconciliation Act (COBRA) transfer paperwork.
- E Seek the patient's commanding officer's consent.

2. A 15-year-old runaway thinks she got "the clap" while working as a prostitute to support herself. She refuses blood tests. What should the emergency physician do?

- A Hold her in the emergency department (ED) until she reveals the names and whereabouts of her parents.
- B Initiate treatment with oral antibiotics because she is a minor requesting treatment for a sexually transmitted disease (STD).
- C Notify the police that a "missing person" has been found.
- D Consult Child Protective Services regarding a protective custody arrangement.
- E Admit the patient to the pediatrics ward and consult the hospital attorney.

3. A 20-year-old house painter fell 20 feet to the ground and was unconscious when the paramedics arrived. He is now conscious, but unsteady on his feet. When questioned, he is unable to relay what has happened to him or correctly identify the day of the week. Nevertheless, the patient insists that he wants to go home and "just rest" for his headache. The emergency physician should

- A call the painter's employer to inform him that a work-related injury has occurred
- B call the painter's wife and ask her to consent for his treatment
- C hold the patient against his will, continue to reason with him regarding the need for treatment, and try to obtain a head computed tomography (CT) scan
- D call the police to place the patient on an inebriation hold
- E let the patient sign out against medical advice if he is oriented and can walk unassisted

4. A 48-year-old attorney is having crushing chest pains and is brought to the emergency department (ED) at Suburban Hospital. He tells the emergency physician that he thinks the pains are stress-related and that he wants to go home because, ironically, he has to be in court tomorrow to represent a plaintiff in a malpractice case against Suburban. Which of the following would be the most prudent course of action on the part of the emergency physician?

- A Offer to call the patient's wife, his personal physician, his clergy member, or anyone else who might help persuade him to accept treatment.
- B Allow the patient to sign out against medical advice because he is competent and an attorney.
- C Allow the patient's wife to drive him to another hospital.
- D Notify the judge who will be hearing the malpractice case and tell him one of the attorneys in the case is ill.
- E Admit the patient against his will as a threat to himself.

5. A 34-year-old science teacher has four bite marks on her hand. During questioning, she admits that the injury occurred while feeding her pet javelina. She tells the physician that she brought the javelina across the border from Mexico on her last vacation, and asks him not to tell anyone about it because they are illegal in this country. What should the physician do?

    (A) Call the police to report a crime.

    (B) Treat the wounds like a cat bite and avoid documenting the type of pet in the chart.

    (C) Respect the patient's confidentiality but document that the patient was told she should call the local animal control agency to ascertain the legality of the pet.

    (D) Call the local animal control agency to report a bite by an exotic animal and inquire as to the need for rabies vaccination.

6. A 26-year-old exterminator presents with several injuries, including a possible hand fracture. The physician notices blood on the back of the patient's shirt. The patient is hesitant to allow the physician to examine his back, but eventually agrees. Upon examination, the physician discovers what appears to be a bullet wound. A chest radiograph shows a small-caliber bullet lodged above the patient's right shoulder. The patient asks the physician not to report the injury, saying that "he can take care of the problem himself." What should the physician do?

    (A) Treat the patient and honor his statements as confidential between physician and patient.

    (B) Call the police to report a patient with a bullet wound.

    (C) Call the other hospital emergency departments (EDs) in the area to see if a similarly injured person was brought in.

    (D) Refuse treatment until the patient reveals details of the assault.

QUESTIONS 7–8

7. A 57-year-old pilot has a syncopal episode while urinating. Extensive work-up reveals no cardiac or neurologic cause, and the patient is discharged from the emergency department (ED). Prior to discharge, the patient asks the physician to bill him directly so that he can pay cash for his treatment. What should the physician do?

    (A) Tell the patient that according to hospital policy, the patient's insurance company must be billed.

    (B) Direct the patient to the billing department to make whatever arrangements for payment he desires.

    (C) Allow the patient to pay cash, but notify the patient's employer.

    (D) Allow the patient to pay cash, but notify the patient's insurance company anyway.

8. Two days later, a man identifying himself as the company physician at TransWest Airlines calls the physician who treated the pilot. He tells the physician that he has been notified of the patient's lapse of consciousness and that he wants to verify it before suspending him temporarily. The pilot is scheduled to pilot flight 747 to Dallas tonight. The physician should

    (A) tell the caller that no patient information is available over the phone, but he might want to question the employee directly

    (B) direct the caller to the Medical Records department

    (C) tell the caller that no patient information is available over the phone and then contact the Federal Aviation Administration (FAA) after consulting with the hospital attorney

    (D) tell the caller that no patient information is available over the phone, but advise him to cancel the flight

    (E) tell the caller that with the patient's written consent, he can obtain a faxed copy of the patient's chart

9. A 22-year-old chronic schizophrenic is brought in to the emergency department (ED) by police for disturbing the peace. The police ask the physician on duty to sedate the patient and hold her until morning. Can the physician treat this patient without her consent?

- (A) No—this patient has the right to refuse treatment.
- (B) No—although this patient may not be able to consent or refuse, no life- or limb-threatening emergency exists.
- (C) Yes—this patient is too impaired to consent.
- (D) Yes—this patient has an acute psychiatric emergency.
- (E) Yes—because the police have requested treatment, it is legal to treat the patient.

QUESTIONS 10–11

10. A 17-year-old is brought in by police for weaving down the street while driving. No accident occurred, and the patient pulled over when directed. According to the officer, the patient failed a field sobriety test, which involved walking a straight line. The officer plans to cite the teenager for driving under the influence of alcohol but not arrest him. The police officer requests that the physician obtain a blood sample from the patient. Can the physician carry out this request?

- (A) No—the patient can refuse or consent as long as he is not under arrest.
- (B) No—the patient's parents should be called for consent because he is a minor.
- (C) No—the patient may refuse even if he is under arrest.
- (D) Yes—the patient may not refuse a reasonable police request.
- (E) Yes—otherwise, the physician could be charged with obstructing justice.

11. The father of the teenager arrives in the emergency department (ED). He tells the physician that his son has diabetes, and that he had been due home from a date with his girlfriend. The girlfriend is contacted, and she relates that they could not get seated at a restaurant in time, so they went to a movie instead. She said that her boyfriend had seemed fine all night, and that he dropped her off just minutes before he was stopped by the police. The father demands that the blood sample be relinquished to him because he never consented to treatment for his son, and threatens a lawsuit. How should the physician proceed?

- (A) He should relinquish the blood sample.
- (B) He should tell the father that he needs the blood sample to determine whether the patient is hypoglycemic.
- (C) He should evaluate the patient for a medical emergency, but retain the blood sample.
- (D) He should refer the father to the police.

12. A 73-year-old woman with advanced Alzheimer's disease is found in a cold apartment by her landlord. The landlord says he thinks the patient's grand-niece, who was her conservator, was caring for her and buying her food with the patient's Social Security check. He does not know how to contact the niece. Can the patient be treated without her conservator's permission?

- (A) No—the conservator must consent to treatment on her great-aunt's behalf.
- (B) No—only the patient can consent if the conservator is not available.
- (C) Yes—the landlord may consent for the patient if he agrees to pay her bills.
- (D) Yes—because the patient is mentally impaired and suffering from hypothermia, implied consent applies.
- (E) No—police consent must be obtained to treat the neglected elderly woman.

13. The chief of surgery, the hospital administrator, and a nurse who witnessed an anesthesia resident injecting fentanyl in a back room arrive in the emergency department (ED). They confront the resident and demand a comprehensive blood and urine drug screen as part of their investigation and disciplinary action. The resident seems dazed and has pinpoint pupils but refuses to cooperate. Can a spontaneously voided urine specimen be submitted for drug testing?

- (A) Yes—the resident has committed a crime and time is of the essence to preserve evidence.
- (B) Yes—physicians are obligated to report colleagues who may represent a hazard to patients and the specimen will provide necessary evidence.
- (C) No—the anesthesiologist may refuse to have any body fluid analyzed unless he consents.

14. The urgent care clinic owned by the hospital is located across the street from the emergency department (ED). A nurse at the urgent care clinic calls the ED, requesting that the ED provide a monitored bed for a 67-year-old patient awaiting transfer to his health maintenance organization (HMO)-approved hospital. The patient presented to the clinic with jaw pain, but his electrocardiogram (ECG) revealed abnormalities. Why is transferring this patient to another hospital a bad course of action?

- (A) It is a Consolidated Omnibus Budget Reconciliation Act (COBRA) violation to transfer the patient from the clinic to the ED.
- (B) It is a COBRA violation to transfer the patient to another hospital without stabilizing him.
- (C) It is a COBRA violation to ascertain that the patient belongs to an HMO before stabilizing treatment is initiated.
- (D) It is a COBRA violation to not accept the patient at a facility with a higher level of care.

15. Just as a pregnant 22-year-old woman with contractions 12 minutes apart is registering at the emergency department (ED) of Hospital A, her insurance company calls after being notified by her husband. The insurance company representative insists that the woman's husband should drive the patient 2 miles to Hospital A's sister hospital, which has inpatient obstetric services. Hospital A does not offer inpatient obstetric services, but shares an on-call list with the sister institution. How should this situation be handled?

- (A) The husband should be advised to drive his wife to the sister hospital.
- (B) The husband and wife should be escorted to the sister hospital by a midwife with a delivery kit.
- (C) An obstetric and neonatal transfer team should be requested to escort the patient to the sister hospital, unless delivery is imminent.
- (D) The on-call obstetrician should be consulted to see if he will accept the patient in transfer, and then the patient should be sent in an ambulance, even if delivery is imminent.

Answers and Explanations

1. The answer is B Military personnel, even those younger than 18 years, are generally considered emancipated minors. In this case, the physician should allow the 16-year-old army private to refuse treatment because he is considered an emancipated minor and a sprained ankle is not a true emergency.

2. The answer is D Although superficially it might appear that this runaway is an emancipated minor who is requesting treatment for a condition exempt from parental notification, and who handles her own expenses by prostituting, there may be overriding considerations that would make this child a possible victim of abuse or neglect. Child protective services should be consulted for their input.

3. The answer is C This patient is not of normal mental capacity, and easily may have a life-threatening emergency. The physician should document his unsteady gait and retrograde amnesia in the medical record and attempt to proceed with the needed evaluation (e.g., a CT scan).

4. The answer is A This patient is not making a decision that reflects what a "reasonably prudent person would want done under similar circumstances." The physician should try to reason with the patient and involve his family in the decision. If all else fails, the hospital attorney may be contacted for advice. As always, everything that happens should be fully documented in the patient's medical record. The patient may very well sign out against advice, but the physician should attempt to offer every option for treatment, including transferring the patient to his own physician at another facility.

5. The answer is D Javelinas, small mammals indigenous to northern Mexico, can become infected with the rabies virus, and, therefore, it is necessary to report this bite wound to local public health authorities. Furthermore, because javelinas are illegal, there may be a second reporting requirement to a police agency.

6. The answer is B In many states, injuries inflicted by weapons must be reported to police. It is uncertain whether this patient committed a crime or was a victim of a crime, but either way, it is something for the police to investigate.

7. The answer is B Although the safety issue involved here may seem significant, the patient has a right to confidentiality and the physician may not disclose his diagnosis to his insurance company. The patient should be directed to the billing department to make whatever payment arrangements he desires; however, the lapse of consciousness may be reported to the Health Department in accordance with state laws. Health Insurance Portability and Accountability Act of 1996 (HIPAA) legislation is designed to prevent unauthorized sharing of confidential information, but state health laws require some diagnoses to be reported.

8. The answer is C No information should be given to the employer or company physician over the phone; however, the physician is obligated to warn the passengers on TransWest flight 747, because their lives may be threatened if the pilot loses consciousness. The physician should contact the hospital attorney immediately regarding Federal Aviation Administration (FAA) procedures. Because time is of the essence, simply reporting the incident to the Health Department may not be timely enough to prevent a mishap.

9. The answer is B Although the patient may be suffering from a mental illness, her outburst does not pose a threat to herself or others, nor is she obviously incapable of taking care of herself based on the facts presented. Therefore, because no emergency exists, the physician cannot treat the patient if she refuses treatment.

10. The answer is D A blood sample for alcohol should be obtained and turned over to the police. Some states may have statutes that vary, but in general, a reasonable police request for evidence of a crime committed should be honored as long as obtaining the evidence does not endanger the patient or delay his care. Because the patient may be too intoxicated to be released, and because he is a minor and cannot legally sign out on his own accord, the patient's parents must be contacted, but their consent is not necessary to obtain the blood sample.

11. The answer is C The blood sample is in the custody of the police and the physician has no control over what it will be used for; therefore, it cannot be returned to the father. The physician's first priority is to check the patient's blood sugar by a fingerstick method and administer glucose if the patient is found to be hypoglycemic. Once the emergency has been resolved, the physician should, in a caring and professional manner, explain to the father what has happened, request permission to treat the teenager, and offer to make the medical records available to the father if needed to exonerate his son in this incident. By exhibiting a caring, professional manner, the physician may diffuse the father's anger.

12. The answer is D The physician should treat the patient on the basis of implied consent, because a potential medical emergency exists. The conservator, for whatever reason, has abandoned this patient. The incident should be reported to Adult Protective Services, and the assistance of a hospital social worker should be obtained in seeking a petition for a new conservator by court order. Because the patient's medical record may be evidence in a court hearing or criminal trial against the original conservator, good documentation of the patient's health status and injuries is essential.

13. The answer is C The anesthesiology resident has a right to refuse to submit a urine sample. Although the patient may require treatment for drug intoxication, no obvious emergency exists, and no treatment or diagnostic testing can be performed against his consent at this point. The medical record should be appropriately documented. The hospital attorney should be notified. If the hospital attorney or administrator decides to pursue this as a crime of theft of controlled substances, the police may be notified. Once the police arrive, if they place the resident under arrest, then blood and urine samples may be legally requested as part of a criminal investigation.

14. The answer is B Because the patient is on hospital property, there is an obligation to examine and stabilize him. A full examination, including an ECG, laboratory studies, and radiographs, should be performed, and the patient transferred by advanced life support ambulance only when he is pain free and completely stable.

15. The answer is C The patient must be examined because she presented in labor (defined by the presence of contractions). If the patient is found to be in labor, all elements of the emergency transfer law must be met, including a written assertion by the emergency physician that states that transfer to another hospital outweighs the benefits of staying at a facility with no obstetric services. If the emergency physician feels the patient will deliver imminently, the on-call obstetrician must be called and must come to the hospital to stabilize, deliver, or accompany the patient in transfer.

Index

Page numbers in *italics* denote figures; those followed by t denote tables. Q and A indicate questions and answers.